FIRST RESPONDER

8th Edition

J. David Bergeron

Chris Le Baudour

Medical Reviewer

Keith Wesley, M.D.

Legacy Author

Gloria Bizjak

PEARSON

Prentice Hall

Upper Saddle River, New Jersey 07458

Library of Congress Cataloging-in-Publication Data

First responder / J. David Bergeron ... [et al.]; medical reviewer,
Keith Wesley. — 8th ed.
    p.; cm.
Includes bibliographical references and index.
ISBN-13: 978-0-13-614059-7
ISBN-10: 0-13-614059-9
    1. Medical emergencies. 2. Emergency medical technicians.
I. Bergeron, J. David, 1944-
[DNLM: 1. Emergency Medical Services. 2. Emergencies.
3. Emergency Medical Technicians. 4. Emergency Treatment. WX 215
F527 2008]
RC86.7.B47 2008
616.02'5—dc22
                                                    2008015701

Publisher: Julie Levin Alexander
Publisher's Assistant: Regina Bruno
Executive Editor: Marlene McHugh Pratt
Acquisitions Editor: Sladjana Repic
Senior Managing Editor for Development: Lois Berlowitz
Development Editor: Josephine Cepeda
Associate Editor: Monica Moosang
Director of Marketing: Karen Allman
Executive Marketing Manager: Katrin Beacom
Marketing Specialist: Michael Sirinides
Marketing Assistant: Lauren Castellano
Managing Production Editor: Patrick Walsh
Production Liaison: Julie Li
Production Editor: Peggy Hood
Media Product Manager: John Jordan
Media Project Manager: Stephen J. Hartner
Manufacturing Manager: Ilene Sanford
Manufacturing Buyer: Pat Brown
Managing Photography Editor: Michal Heron
Senior Design Coordinator: Christopher Weigand
Interior Design: Wanda España
Cover Photo: Ray Kemp/911 Imaging
Director, Image Resource Center: Melinda Reo
Manager, Rights and Permissions: Zina Arabia
Manager, Visual Research: Beth Brenzel
Manager, Cover Visual Research and Permissions: Karen Sanatar
Image Permission Coordinator: Joanne Dippel
Composition: Aptara
Printing and Binding: Courier Kendallville
Cover Printer: Phoenix Color Corporation

Notice on Care Procedures

It is the intent of the authors and publisher that this textbook be used as part of a formal First Responder education program taught by qualified instructors and supervised by a licensed physician. The procedures described in this textbook are based upon consultation with First Responder and medical authorities. The authors and publisher have taken care to make certain that these procedures reflect currently accepted clinical practice; however, they cannot be considered absolute recommendations.

The material in this textbook contains the most current information available at the time of publication. However, federal, state, and local guidelines concerning clinical practices, including, without limitation, those governing infection control and universal precautions, change rapidly. The reader should note, therefore, that new regulations may require changes in some procedures.

It is the responsibility of the reader to familiarize himself or herself with the policies and procedures set by federal, state, and local agencies as well as the institution or agency where the reader is employed. The authors and the publisher of this textbook and the supplements written to accompany it disclaim any liability, loss, or risk resulting directly or indirectly from the suggested procedures and theory, from any undetected errors, or from the reader's responsibility to stay informed of any new changes or recommendations made by any federal, state, and local agency as well as by his or her employing institution or agency.

Notice on Gender Usage

The English language has historically given preference to the male gender. Among many words, the pronouns "he" and "his" are commonly used to describe both genders. Society evolves faster than language, and the male pronouns still predominate our speech. The authors have made great effort to treat the two genders equally, recognizing that a significant percentage of First Responders are female. However, in some instances, male pronouns may be used to describe both males and females solely for the purpose of brevity. This is not intended to offend any readers.

Pearson Prentice Hall™ is a trademark of Pearson Education, Inc.
Pearson® is a registered trademark of Pearson plc
Prentice Hall® is a registered trademark of Pearson Education, Inc.

Pearson Education, Ltd., *London*
Pearson Education Australia Pty. Limited, *Sydney*
Pearson Education Singapore Pte. Ltd.
Pearson Education North Asia Ltd., *Hong Kong*
Pearson Education Canada, Ltd., *Toronto*

Pearson Educación de Mexico, S.A. de C.V.
Pearson Education—Japan, *Tokyo*
Pearson Education Malaysia, Pte. Ltd.
Pearson Education, Upper Saddle River, New Jersey

10 9 8 7 6 5 4 3 2 1

ISBN-10:   0-13-614059-9
ISBN-13:   978-0-13-614059-7

Brief Contents

Contents

MODULE 1   **Preparatory**   1

MODULE 5 **Illness and Injury** 245

Photo Scans

Algorithms

Algorithms

Letter to Students

As the authors of this textbook, we want to personally congratulate you on your decision to become an Emergency Medical Responder. Your decision is one of service, and to serve others, especially in a great time of need, is one of the most rewarding opportunities anyone can experience. One of the first things you may notice is the name change from First Responder to Emergency Medical Responder. This change serves to more accurately reflect the roles and responsibilities inherent in this training program. Emergency Medical Responder programs were originally developed to provide individuals with the skills necessary to assess and begin caring for patients at the scene of an emergency. In many areas of the nation, Emergency Medical Responders are able to provide life-saving care long before more advanced providers arrive. Their quick response and quality of care save thousands of lives each year.

The availability of Emergency Medical Responder programs is growing each year and we are very proud to continue to play an important role in that training. In fact, as this book goes to print, a new training curriculum is being developed in an effort to increase the quality of care being provided by Emergency Medical Responders all across the nation. This commitment has allowed the Emergency Medical Responder to become an important part of the EMS system in the United States.

This textbook has been an important component of thousands of training programs over the past 25 years and has contributed to the success of hundreds of thousands of students just like you. This new 8th Edition retains all of the features found to be successful in previous editions and includes some new topics and concepts that have recently become a part of most Emergency Medical Responder courses. The basis of this text is the U.S. Department of Transportation's First Responder National Standard Curriculum. The brand new 8th Edition also includes the most current American Heart Association (AHA) guidelines for CPR and the use of AEDs.

Your decision to become an Emergency Medical Responder is a significant one. We believe strongly that being able to assess and care for patients requires much more than just technical skills. It requires you to be a good leader, and good leaders demonstrate characteristics such as integrity, compassion, accountability, respect and empathy. We have introduced components in the 8th Edition that we feel will help you become the best EMR you can be. One of these components is the "First on Scene" scenarios at the beginning of each chapter. In these scenarios we throw you right in the middle of a real life emergency and attempt to offer you a perspective you will not get with any other training resource. You will see first hand how individuals just like yourself make decisions when faced with an emergency. You will feel the fear and anxiety that is such a normal part of being a new Emergency Medical Responder. Not everyone you meet will make the best decisions and we want you to consider each scenario carefully and discuss them with your classmates and instructor.

Becoming an Emergency Medical Responder is just the first step in what is likely to be a lifetime of service. Just a warning to you, the feeling you get when you are able to help those in need is contagious. We encounter students all across the country who have discovered that their passion is helping others. We hope that we can be a part of discovering your passion! We welcome you to EMS and a life of service!

J. David Bergeron & Chris Le Baudour

Emergency Medical Responder Training Programs

Throughout this textbook, you will notice that we have replaced the name First Responder with the new title, Emergency Medical Responder. This change comes as the curricula for all levels of EMS providers are undergoing an important update and revision. The designation Emergency Medical Responder was identified in the *National EMS Scope of Practice Model,* a recently published document that defines the level of EMS personnel and specifies practices and minimum competencies at each level. Although all Emergency Medical Responder courses follow the same national standard education objectives, some jurisdictions may require specific prerequisites. For instance, some training programs may require completion of American Heart Association (AHA) CPR course, or an equivalent course, before entering an Emergency Medical Responder training program. This textbook includes the most recent AHA Basic Life Support and automated external defibrillator (AED) guidelines for the Health Care Provider at the time of printing.

The content of the 8th Edition is summarized here, with emphasis on "what's new" in each unit of this edition. Note, please, that in addition to the items listed below, the 8th Edition includes new features: "First on Scene" scenarios, "Is It Safe?" and "Geriatric Focus" sections in the body of text, text/objectives correlations in the margins, and at the end of each chapter the "Quick Quiz."

Module 1, Preparatory: Chapters 1–5

The first module sets a framework for all of the modules that follow by introducing essential concepts, information, and skills. The EMS system and the role of the Emergency Medical Responder within the system are introduced. Issues of Emergency Medical Responder safety, well-being, and legal and ethical issues are covered, as are basic anatomy and physiology and techniques of safe lifting and moving.

What's New in the Preparatory Module?

- In Chapter 1, *Introduction to EMS Systems:*
  - Updated terms for EMS personnel: Emergency Medical Responder, Emergency Medical Technician, Advanced Emergency Technician, and Paramedic.
  - Information on the history of EMS.
  - Expanded definitions and examples of *protocols, standing orders, scope of practice,* and *patient advocate.*
  - New information on the use of global positioning system (GPS) technology.
  - Photo scan of different types of Emergency Medical Responders.

- In Chapter 2, *Legal and Ethical Issues:*
  - Definitions of *scope of practice* and *standard of care* have been revised.
  - The section on ethics has been expanded.
  - Information on HIPAA has been added.
  - New and expanded terms and definitions of *duty, breach of duty, damages,* and *causation* have been added.

- In Chapter 3, *Well-Being of the Emergency Medical Responder:*
  - Definitions and examples of stress and accumulative stress have been added.
  - Information on SARS, West Nile Virus, MRSA, and avian flu have been added.
  - A new photo scan on the proper technique for removing gloves has also been added.

- In Chapter 4, *The Human Body:*
  - Detailed illustrations of the circulatory, respiratory, musculoskeletal, nervous, and digestive systems, plus illustrations of the skin, have been added with enhanced descriptions of each.

- In Chapter 5, *Lifting, Moving, and Positioning Patients:*
  - Additional cautions have been added about the appropriate use of cervical collars.
  - Updated definitions and new photos of single-operator, dual-operator, and the new pneumatic/electric lift stretchers have been added.
  - New photos have been added, including ones for the slider board and slider bag.

Module 2, Airway: Chapter 6

There is only one chapter in Module 2, but it may be considered the most important one in the text because no patient will survive without an open airway. Basic airway management techniques are covered in detail.

What's New in the Airway Module?

- In Chapter 6, *Airway Management:*
  - The 2005 AHA Guidelines on basic life support techniques are included in the chapter.
  - Information on "tidal volume" has been added.
  - Bag-valve mask ventilation has been incorporated into the chapter.

Module 3, Patient Assessment: Chapter 7

This module explains and illustrates some of the most important skills of a Emergency Medical Responder. All steps of the assessment and their application to different types of trauma and medical patients, as well as the skills of measuring vital signs, taking a patient history, communication, and hand-off to EMTs are discussed.

What's New in the Patient Assessment Module?

- In Chapter 7, *Assessment of the Patient:*
  - The mnemonic BP-DOC has been added as an alternative to DCAP-BTLS.

Module 4, Circulation: Chapter 8

This module discusses one- and two-rescuer CPR, the chain of survival, the responsibilities of the Emergency Medical Responder, and using automated defibrillators.

- In Chapter 8, *Resuscitation and Use of the AED:*
  - The chapter has a new, more up-to-date title.
  - The 2005 AHA Guidelines on basic life support techniques are included in the chapter.
  - Information on hypothermia and resuscitation has been added.

Module 5, Illness and Injury: Chapters 9–12

The Illness and Injury module covers medical emergencies such as chest pain and respiratory emergencies; environmental emergencies such as heat and cold emergencies; behavioral emergencies; emergencies related to alcohol and other drugs; and poisoning, bites, and stings. Also contained in this module are a chapter on bleeding and soft-tissue injuries, which covers types of bleeding, shock, and burns, and a chapter on muscle and bone injuries, which discusses the musculoskeletal system; injuries to the extremities; injuries to the head, spine, and chest; and helmet removal.

What's New in the Illness and Injury Module?

- In Chapter 9, *Caring for Medical Emergencies:*
  - Terms and definitions have been added or expanded, including *cardiac compromise, myocardial infarction, nitroglycerin, hypertension, tidal volume, accessory muscles, wheezing, inhaler, cerebrovascular accident, syncope, generalized seizure, complex seizure, grand and petite mal seizures, incontinence, aortic aneurysm, pancreatitis, referred pain, guarding, poison,* and *core temperature.*
  - Discussions on the topics of heart attack, MI, angina pectoris, and snake bite have been expanded.
  - Topics added include OPQRST assessment tool and the Cincinnati stroke scale.

- In Chapter 10, *Caring for Bleeding, Shock, and Soft-Tissue Injuries:*
  - The definition of the term *perfusion* has been updated, and the term *tracheal deviation* has been added.

- In Chapter 11, *Caring for Muscle and Bone Injuries:*
  - The definitions of the terms *extremity, ligament, tendon, appendicular skeleton,* and *axial skeleton* have been added.

- In Chapter 12, *Caring for the Geriatric Patient:*
  - ALL NEW!

Module 6, Childbirth and Children: Chapters 13–14

This module offers an understanding of childbirth and the complications and emergencies that may arise from delivery. Also discussed are the characteristics of infants and children and providing emergency care to pediatric patients.

Module 7, EMS Operations: Chapters 15–16

This module deals with nonmedical operations and special situations, including gaining access in motor-vehicle collisions and buildings; hazards such as fire, hazardous materials, and radiation emergencies; multiple-casualty incidents; triage; and the incident management system.

What's New in the EMS Operations Module?

- Chapter 16, *Multiple-Casualty Incidents, Triage, and the Incident Management System*:
  - The information on the role of the Emergency Medical Responder at the scene of a multiple-casualty incident has been expanded.
  - Information on the National Incident Management System has been added.

Appendices

Seven appendices cover determining blood pressure, breathing aids and oxygen therapy, pharmacology, air medical transport operations, EMS response to terrorism and weapons of mass destruction, swimming and diving accidents, and student learning skill sheets.

What's New in the Appendices?

- Appendix 4, *Air Medical Operations:*
  - ALL NEW!
- *Appendix 7, Student Learning Skill Sheets:*
  - ALL NEW!

Our Goal: Improving Future Training and Education

Some of the best ideas for better training and education methods come from instructors who can tell us what areas of study caused their students the most trouble. Other sound ideas come from practicing Emergency Medical Responders and from students who are new to the field. We welcome any of your suggestions. Please write to us at:

Brady/Prentice Hall Health
c/o EMS Editor
Pearson Education
One Lake Street
Upper Saddle River, NJ 07458
Visit Brady's web site at www.bradybooks.com

If you experience a problem with the companion CD, please write to technical support at media.support@pearsoned.com or call 800-677-6337.

Acknowledgments

Medical Advisor

Keith Wesley, MD FACEP

Our special thanks to Dr. Keith Wesley. His reviews were carefully prepared, and we appreciate the thoughtful advice and keen insight offered.

Dr. Wesley is the Wisconsin State EMS Medical Director and is a board certified emergency medicine physician living in Eau Claire, Wisconsin. He is the Chair of the National Council of State EMS Medical Directors. Dr. Wesley is the author of many articles and EMS textbooks and a frequent speaker at EMS conferences across the nation. He is an active EMS medical director currently providing medical oversight to the Chippewa Fire District in Chippewa Falls, Wisconsin, and to the EMT-Basic Services of Ashland and Bayfield counties, as well as the Apostle Islands Lake Shore National Park.

Contributors

Our appreciation to the contributors below for their ideas and advice.

Bob Elling, MPA, REMT-P

Clinical Instructor, Albany (NY) Medical Center; Instructor, EMT-Basic and Paramedic courses, Hudson Valley Community College's Institute of Prehospital Emergency Medicine, NY; Professor of Management, American College of Prehospital Medicine; Regional Faculty, NYS Department of Health, EMS Bureau; Regional Faculty, American Heart Association; Paramedic, Colonie, NY

Donny Boyd

Firefighter, Montgomery County, MD; Montgomery County Urban Search and Rescue Team; Engineering Technician and Fire Instructor, Maryland Fire and Rescue Institute, College Park, MD

James L. Jenkins, Jr., BA, NREMT-P

Tuckahoe Volunteer Rescue Squad, LifeNet, Richmond, VA

Craig Edward Smith

Fire Service Instructor, Prince George's County Fire/EMS Department, Fire/EMS Training Academy, MD

Brian D. Bricker, NREMT

REACH Air Medical Services, Santa Rosa, CA

Reviewers

We wish to thank the following EMS professionals who reviewed material for the 8th Edition of First Responder. The quality of their reviews has been outstanding, and their assistance is deeply appreciated.

John L. Beckman, AA, FF/EMT-P, Instructor, Affiliated with Addison Fire Protection District; Fire Science Instructor, Technology Center of DuPage, IL

Cheryl Blazek, EMT-P; Southwestern Community College, Creston, IA

Brian D. Bricker, NREMT
REACH Air Medical, Santa Rosa, CA

Leo M. Brown, Lafe Bush, EMT-P; NJ Administrative Deputy Chief, Long-
boat Key Fire Rescue, FL

David J. Casella, M.Ed, EMT-B; Osseo OEC Program, Osseo, MN

Henry Cortez, LP, AAS; Texas Emergency Response Training and Consulting, McAllen, TX

Christopher Ebright, BEd, NREMT-P; University of Toledo Division of EMS
Education, Toledo, OH

James W. Fox, EMT-PS, EMS-I; EMS Assistant Coordinator, Des Moines
Fire Department, Des Moines, IA

Les Hawthorne, BA, NREMT-P; EMS Coordinator, Southwestern Illinois
College, Belleville, IL

Bernard Kay, BSME, EMT-D, North Seattle (WA) Community College

James S. Lion, Jr., AEMT-I; EMS Intructor, Erie County, EMT Lt;
Williamsville Fire Department, NY

T. J. MacKay, Glendale Community College, Glendale, AZ

Michael O'Brien, M.A., EMT-P; Illinois Medical Emergency Response Team;
Chicago, IL

Jeff Och, Carver Fire & Rescue, Carver, MN

Robert D. Parker, B.S., NREMT-P; Associate Professor of EMS, Johnson
County Community College, Overland Park, KS

Wade Skinner, Advisor, Safety and Health, Kennecott Utah Copper Corp.,
Bingham Canyon, UT

We also wish to express appreciation to the following EMS professionals who
reviewed earlier editions of Emergency Medical Responder. Their suggestions and
insights helped to make this program a successful teaching tool.

Chad D. Andrews, BA, EMT-P, EMS-I; Program Director of Emergency
Medical Services, Kirkwood Community College, Cedar Rapids, IA

Sgt. Charles Angello, Essex County Police Academy, Cedar Grove, NJ

Vicki Bacidore, RN, MS; EMS Instructor, Loyola University Medical Center,
Maywood, IL

John L. Beckman, FF/EMT-P; Affiliated with Addison Fire Protection
District, Highland Park Hospital, IL

Kenneth O. Bradford, EMT-P; Santa Rosa Junior College, Emergency Medical Care Programs, Windsor, CA

Steven M. Carlo, BS, FNAEMD, EMT-I, EMD; Erie Community College-
North, Emergency Medical Technology Department, Williamsville, NY

Patricia A. Ciara, B.S., EMT-P; Assistant Deputy Chief Paramedic;
EMS/CME Supervisor, Chicago Fire Department, Chicago, IL

William H. Clark, Paramedic, ACLS Instructor; Chief and EMS Coordinator,
Escatawpa Volunteer Fire Department, MS

Jo Ann Cobble, M.A., NREMT-P, RN; Chair, Department EMS, University
of Arkansas for Medical Sciences, Little Rock, AR

Tony Crystal, Director, EMS, Lake Land College, Mattoon, IL

Captain Dale A. Crutchley, NREMT-P; EMS Administrator/Training Coordinator; Annapolis Fire Department, Annapolis, MD

Jeff Daleske, NREMT-P; Program Coordinator, Mercy School of EMS, Des
Moines, IA

Gary Dean, Education Coordinator, East Texas Medical Center EMS,
Tyler, TX

Garry L. DeJong, NREMT-P; EMS Training Coordinator; Captain, Albuquerque Fire Department, Albuquerque, NM

Jerry Domaschk, NREMT-P; Instructor, Louisiana Technical Colleges, Schriever, LA

T.J. Feldman, MA, EMT-B, West Hartford, CT

Alejandro Garcia, EMT-P; EMS Coordinator, Wichita Falls Fire Department, Wichita Falls, TX

Stephen Garrison, RN, NREMT-P; EMS Manager, Memorial Hospital, South Bend, IN

Donald Graesser, Bergen County EMS Training Center, Paramus, NJ

Jaime S. Greene, BA, EMT-B; EMT Education Program Director, Palm Beach County Schools, West Palm Beach, FL

Robert Hancock, B.S., L.P., MS-IV; University of North Texas Health Science Center, Fort Worth, TX

Steve Harrell, EMT-P; Associate Professor, Daytona Beach Community College, Daytona Beach, FL

Glenn R. Henry, NREMT-P; Transport Coordinator-Rainbow Response, Egleston Children's Hospital, Atlanta, GA

Attila Hertelendy BHSc, CCEMT-P, NREMT-P, ACP; University of Mississippi Medical Center, Jackson, MS

Sgt. David M. Johnson, NREMT-P; Emergency Services Unit, Montville Township Police, Montville, NJ

Jerry W. Jones, MPA, BA, EMT-IV; Paramedic Program, Columbia State Community College, Shelbyville, TN

Kathleen M. King, BA, MS, EMT-B; Instructor, Northampton County EMS Training Institute,Northampton Community College, Bethlehem, PA

Barbara L. Klingensmith, MS, NREMT-P; Director, Public Services Programs, Edison Community College, Fort Myers, FL

Doug Lawson, Devil Lake, ND

Tom LeGros, NREMT, Fire District 12, St. Tammany, LA

Jon F. Levine, Medical Director, Boston Emergency Medical Services, Boston, MA

John A, Lewin, EMT-P; EMS Coordinator, Illinois State Police Academy, Springfield, IL

Glenn H. Luedtke, NREMT-P; Director, Cape & Islands Emergency Medical Services System, Cape Cod, MA

Sergeant David M. Magnino, EMT-P; Paramedic, California Highway Patrol Academy, Emergency Medical Services, West Sacramento, CA

William D. McElhiney, Massachusetts State Police, Medical Unit, New Braintree, MA

Geoffrey T. Miller, Assistant Professor, Institute of Public Safety, Santa Fe Community College, Gainesville, FL

Ronold Morton, EMS Coordinator, Marshall Fire/EMS, Marshall, TX

Billy Murray, NREMT-P, Nags Head Fire and Rescue, NC

Nikhil Natarajan, NREMT-P, CCEMT-P, I/C; Adjunct Instructor, Ulster Community College, NY

Ronald A. Olson, Milwaukee Police Department Training Bureau, Milwaukee, WI

Ham Robbins, Rent-A-Medic, Eastport, ME

Bryan Scyphers, Chairperson, Public Safety Services, Davidson County Community College, Winston-Salem, NC

Mark Slettum, North EMS Education, Division of North Memorial Health Care, Robbinsdale, MN

E.A. Sowinski, BSN, RN, NREMT-B; Delaware State Fire School, Dover, DE

Michael Strong, FF/EMT-P, Public Safety Training Associates, Paw Paw, MI

Jack L. Taylor, BA, EMT-P; I/C, EMS Program Director, Kalamazoo Valley Community College, Kalamazoo, MI

Tim Taylor, NREMT-P; Captain, Department of Fire and Rescue, Prince William County, Woodbridge, VA

Ronald C. Thomas, Jr., Training and Research Manager, Florida State Fire College, Ocala, FL

Larry Thompson, FAE/Paramedic; EMT Program Coordinator, College of Marin; Marin County Fire Department, Kentfield, CA

Pat D. Trevathan, MS; EMT-Instructor/Coordinator, Kentucky Tech Fire/Rescue Training, West Kentucky State Technical Institute, Paducah, KY

James E. Walker, Special Projects Coordinator, Northeastern University, Burlington, MA

Holly Weber, REACH Air Medical Services, Santa Rosa, CA

Willard Wright, EMT-B, eic SIEMT; Staten Island EMT, NY

Jeff Zuckernick, EMS Department, Kapiolani Community College, Honolulu, HI

Photo Acknowledgments

All photographs not credited adjacent to the photograph or in the photo credit section below were photographed on assignment for Brady/Prentice Hall Health/Pearson Education.

Organizations

We wish to thank the following organizations for their valuable assistance in creating the photo program for the 8th Edition:

Ken Bradford, Public Safety Training Center, Windsor, CA

Dan & Pat McDonald, REACH Air Medical Services, Santa Rosa, CA

Bill, Cindy, Kasey, and Ryder Schalich, Schalich Construction, Santa Rosa, CA

Gary Tennyson and Sean Sullivan, veriHealth Ambulance Service, Petaluma, CA

Lt. Scott Dunn, Sonoma County Sheriffs Department, Santa Rosa, CA

Chief Bob Uboldi, Kenwood Fire Protection District, Kenwood, CA

Chief Bruce Varner, Santa Rosa Fire Department, Santa Rosa, CA

Technical Advisors

Thanks to the following people for providing valuable technical support during the photo shoots for the 8th Edition:

Brian Bricker, NREMT

Chris Le Baudour, NREMT

John Martin, EMT

Scott Snyder, EMT-P

Ted Williams, EMT-P

Photograph Models

A very special thanks to the following friends, family, and colleagues who gave of their time and talent and opened their homes during the photo shoots for the 8th Edition.

Sam Adams
Allyson Bricker
Alexis Bricker
Cheryle Belli
Dylan Bricker
Donald Calhoun
Paul Carter
Loren Davis
Scott Dunn
Tashia Fitzgerald
Billy Gomez
Michael Hani
Shaun Hani
Hope Hunt
Derrick Johnson
Audrey Le Baudour
Joanne Le Baudour
Sheila McQueeny
Nicole Medeiros
Casey Meints
Kayla Meints
Kevin Morrow
Wendy Morrow
Roya Nikzad
Katie Nolan
John Owen
Sean Padgett
Randy Palma
Teresa Reiss
Greg Sarpy
Barbara Seubert
Scott Snyder
Joan Sorenson
Sarah Stimach
Hannah Taylor
Leah Taylor
Brianne Webster
James West
Sam Willard
Ted Williams
Dick Youngs
Faye Youngs

Chris Le Baudour

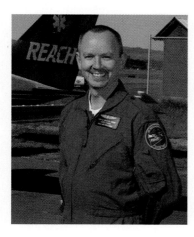

Chris Le Baudour has been working in EMS since 1978 as an EMT-I and an EMT-II in both the field and clinical settings. In 1984 Chris began his teaching career in the Department of Public Safety–EMS Division at Santa Rosa Junior College in Santa Rosa, California.

Chris holds a Master's Degree in Education with an emphasis in online teaching and learning as well as numerous certifications. Chris has spent the past 24 years mastering the art of experiential learning in EMS and is well known for his innovative classroom techniques and his passion for teaching and learning in both the traditional and online classrooms.

Chris is very involved in EMS education at the national level as a Board Member of the National Association of EMS Educators. He is a frequent presenter at both state and national conferences and a prolific EMS writer. Chris also serves as the Director of Communications for REACH Air Medical Services in Santa Rosa, California.

David Bergeron

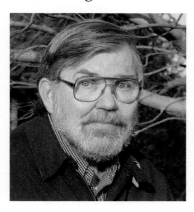

David Bergeron has been active in the development of instructional and training programs for the emergency medical services (EMS) for over 35 years. His early work included "a front row seat" to the development of modern patient assessment and care inspired by the studies of Dr. R Adams Cowley, Maryland Shock Trauma Center, Maryland Institute of EMS Systems, and Maryland Fire and Rescue Institute (MFRI).

David's work in instructional development for emergency medicine has included EMT-Basic, Emergency Medical Responder (First Responder), EMT-Intermediate, and EMT-Paramedic student and instructor programs. He is credited for writing the first comprehensive textbook for the First Responder, for establishing the first behavioral objectives for EMTs, and for being the first to develop a full-course glossary for EMT instruction.

As well as serving as an instructional technologist on leading textbooks in emergency medicine, David has been on the teaching faculty of the University of Maryland, Longwood University, numerous community colleges, and schools of nursing. His publications include textbooks that have been translated into Spanish, Portugese, French, German, Italian, Lithuanian, and Japanese.

His development of this current edition of FIRST RESPONDER has benefited from the work being done by many EMS systems and the creative co-authorships of Gloria Bizjak and Chris Le Baudour.

Welcome to First Responder

ONE LAKE STREET
UPPER SADDLE RIVER, NJ 07458

Dear Instructor:

Brady, your partner in education, is pleased to bring you the Eighth Edition of the classic text *First Responder*. We continue to offer the high-quality content and innovation that you have come to know and trust from Brady, but you will immediately notice one important change in this exciting new edition. While retaining thorough coverage of the U.S. DOT First Responder National Standard Curriculum, the authors—having incorporated the new designations for EMS personnel licensure levels from the National EMS Scope of Practice model—have replaced the term "First Responder" with "Emergency Medical Responder." This revision also contains a wealth of valuable tools to make your job easier as you help your students prepare for success.

More instructors use *First Responder* than any other First Responder text on the market. Our authors, editors, marketers, and salespeople regularly receive comments from customers who tell us what they like, what they don't like, what works, what doesn't, what's new, what's obsolete, and what they would change. One message comes through clearly: you lead a busy life, juggling multiple roles, and you need all the help and support you can get. You need a solid book you can rely on and a supplements package that helps you to easily and quickly prepare for an engaging class.

The following walkthrough outlines the features found throughout the text as well as provides information for the extensively revised and updated student and instructor supplements that make this the most complete learning system for Emergency Medical Responders. We also highlight several related resources that can be used to make your program the best it can be.

First Responder is proud to continue the tradition of bringing to Emergency Medical Responder education the highest standards of writing, development, production, and service that our customers expect and deserve.

Sincerely,

Julie Levin Alexander
VP/Publisher

Marlene McHugh Pratt
Executive Editor

Lois Berlowitz
Senior Managing Editor

Katrin Beacom
Executive Marketing Manager

Sladjana Repic
Acquisitions Editor

Thomas Kennally
National Sales Manager

Guide to Key Features

■ **First on Scene**—*New!* Scenarios challenge the Emergency Medical Responder to consider roles and responsibilities and patient care priorities. Appear at the start of each chapter and continue to be referenced throughout the chapter as specific content applies.

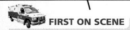

FIRST ON SCENE

"Micah!" There was a shout from somewhere. "Micah, will you wake up!" Micah Garibaldi shot up in his bed and quickly looked around the dorm room. Nothing seemed out of place. His vacationing roommate's movie posters still hung at odd angles from multicolored pushpins, clothing and books were still scattered around in piles, and the filter on the little octagon-shaped goldfish tank was still humming away, even though the fish were long gone. Just as he was starting to lie back down, someone pounded on the door, rattling it with each booming impact.

"Micah! Are you in there?" Micah slid out of bed and stomped across the room to the door.

"What?" he shouted as he pulled the door open. The look on that new freshman Frank Kline's face told him immediately that something really was wrong.

"There's this girl down in our room," Frank was wide-eyed and whispering hoarsely. "And she's like, like having some sort of, I think she's dying or something!" Micah, the dorm "doctor" ever since completing an Emergency Medical Responder course, quickly threw on a robe as he ran down the hall.

"Airway, breathing, circulation," he repeated in a running whisper, his nerves tightening his stomach and making his hands shake. "Remember the ABCs. Remember the ABCs."

■ **Geriatric Focus**—*New!* Highlights unique experiences and considerations when dealing with this special population.

Geriatric Focus

Due to the drying out of the bones in the elderly, the ribs can become much less flexible and therefore allow far less chest wall movement during breathing. As you check for breathing or provide ventilations, you might not see as much chest rise and fall as on a younger patient. Observe the abdomen for signs of movement, when you assess breathing or provide ventilations. You should see a steady rise and fall of the abdomen much like you normally would of the chest. Of course, a lack of movement is never good, and you must consider the possibility of a total airway obstruction and provide care accordingly.

■ **Quick Quiz**—*New!* At the end of every chapter, presents multiple-choice questions that directly tie to DOT objectives and Additional Learning Tasks.

■ **Is It Safe?**—New! Emphasizes specific safety considerations for the EMR.

Is It Safe ?

It is important to carefully consider the potential for spine injury before opening the patient's airway. For example, the absence of an obvious mechanism of injury does not automatically rule out spine injury. A patient found unresponsive in an alley could have been assaulted and therefore may have a neck or back injury. When in doubt, always take appropriate spinal precautions. ■

■ **Text/Objective Correlations**—*New!* Marginal references appear as close as possible to specific content being addressed.

Bleeding

Having an idea of how blood and blood vessels work within the body will assist you in assessing patients with bleeding problems. Keep the following general considerations in mind while you learn how to care for patients:

- *Body substance isolation (BSI) precautions.* The risk of infectious disease should always be assessed and minimized when caring for bleeding patients. BSI precautions must be taken routinely to avoid skin contact with mucous membranes and body fluids. Gloves should be worn during every patient encounter. Additional equipment (goggles, gown, mask) should also be used when there is an increased risk of contact with blood or other body fluids (for example, in cases of childbirth or when a patient is spitting or vomiting blood).
- *Severity of blood loss.* The severity of blood loss should be based on the patient's signs and symptoms and an estimation of blood loss. If signs and symptoms of shock are present, bleeding should be considered serious.
- *Body's normal response to bleeding.* The body's automatic response to bleeding is blood vessel constriction and clotting. In cases of major bleeding, however, clotting might not occur because the flow of blood washes the clot away before it can form. The factors affecting the body's response are discussed throughout this chapter.

Uncontrolled bleeding should be taken seriously. If not stopped, it will lead to shock and death.

> 5–2.3 Establish the relationship between body substance isolation (BSI) and bleeding.
>
> 5–2.6 Establish the relationship between body substance isolation (BSI) and soft-tissue injuries.

Quick Quiz

1. Which one of the following is NOT a typical characteristic of arterial bleeding?
   a. Blood spurts from the wound.
   b. Blood flows steadily from the wound.
   c. The color of the blood is bright red.
   d. Blood loss is often profuse in a short period of time.

2. For each bruise the size of a patient's fist, assume a blood loss of:
   a. 2%.
   b. 4%.
   c. 10%.
   d. 20%.

3. Which one of the following procedures is usually the last resort used to control bleeding?
   a. direct pressure
   b. tourniquet
   c. elevation combined with direct pressure
   d. pressure points

4. Most cases of external bleeding may be controlled by:
   a. applying direct pressure.
   b. using a tourniquet.
   c. securing a pressure dressing.
   d. applying the closest pressure point.

7. The tearing loose or the tearing off of a large flap of skin is which one of the following types of wound?
   a. abrasion
   b. amputation
   c. laceration
   d. avulsion

8. The first step in caring for an open wound is to expose the wound surface. The next step is to:
   a. control bleeding.
   b. clear the wound surface.
   c. care for shock.
   d. prevent further contamination.

9. When providing care for an open injury to the cheek in which the object has entered through the skin into the mouth, ensure an open airway and:
   a. remove the impaled object.
   b. turn the patient's head to one side.
   c. dress and bandage the outside of the wound.
   d. place dressings into the mouth.

10. When providing care for an open injury to the external ear:
   a. pack the ear canal.
   b. use a cotton swab to clear the ear canal.
   c. wash out the ear canal.
   d. apply dressings and bandage in place.

■ **Enhanced Illustrations**—Updated art and photos provide students with visual schematics to help them learn and apply patient assessment and other skills critical to Emergency Medical Responders.

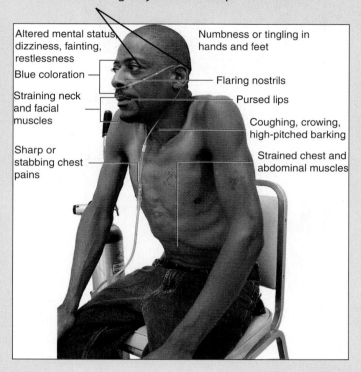

Altered mental status, dizziness, fainting, restlessness

Blue coloration

Straining neck and facial muscles

Sharp or stabbing chest pains

Numbness or tingling in hands and feet

Flaring nostrils

Pursed lips

Coughing, crowing, high-pitched barking

Strained chest and abdominal muscles

■ **New Appendix on Air Medical Transport Operations**—Presents information on the role of Emergency Medical Responders in patient care during air medical transport.

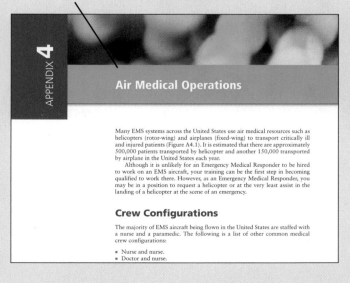

APPENDIX 4

Air Medical Operations

Many EMS systems across the United States use air medical resources such as helicopters (rotor-wing) and airplanes (fixed-wing) to transport critically ill and injured patients (Figure A4.1). It is estimated that there are approximately 500,000 patients transported by helicopter and another 150,000 transported by airplane in the United States each year.

Although it is unlikely for an Emergency Medical Responder to be hired to work on an EMS aircraft, your training can be the first step in becoming qualified to work there. However, as an Emergency Medical Responder, you may be in a position to request a helicopter or at the very least assist in the landing of a helicopter at the scene of an emergency.

Crew Configurations

The majority of EMS aircraft being flown in the United States are staffed with a nurse and a paramedic. The following is a list of other common medical crew configurations:

■ Nurse and nurse.
■ Doctor and nurse.

■ **New and Updated Content**—Includes new designations for EMS Personnel: Emergency Medical Responder, Emergency Medical Technician, Advanced Emergency Technician, and Paramedic; an all-new chapter on Caring for the Geriatric Patient; information on HIPAA and the National Information Management System; and new and expanded definitions throughout.

TABLE 1–2	Levels of EMS Training

■ *Emergency Medical Responder*—This level of EMS training is designed specifically for the person who is often first to arrive at the scene. Many police officers, firefighters, industrial workers, and other public service providers are trained as Emergency Medical Responders. This training emphasizes scene safety and how to provide immediate care for life-threatening injuries and illnesses as well as how to assist ambulance personnel when they arrive.

■ *Emergency Medical Technician (EMT)*—In most areas, an EMT is considered the minimum level of certification for ambulance personnel. The training emphasizes assessment and the care and transportation of the ill or injured patient. The EMT may also assist with the administration of certain common medications. (This was formerly called the *EMT-Basic* level of training.)

■ *Advanced Emergency Medical Technician (AEMT)*—An AEMT, or advanced EMT, is a basic-level EMT who has received specific additional training in specific subjects, allowing some level of advanced life support. Some of the additional skills an AEMT may be able to perform are starting IV (intravenous) lines, inserting advanced airways, and administering medications. (This was formerly called the *EMT-Intermediate* level of training.)

■ *Paramedic*—Paramedics are trained to perform what is commonly referred to as advanced life support care, such as inserting endotracheal (ET) tubes and starting IV lines. They also administer medications, interpret electrocardiograms, monitor cardiac rhythms, and perform cardiac defibrillation. (This was formerly called the *EMT-Paramedic* level of training.)

■ **New Appendix on Student Learning Skill Sheets**—Aid in organizing steps needed to perform skills and in identifying criteria used for performance evaluation

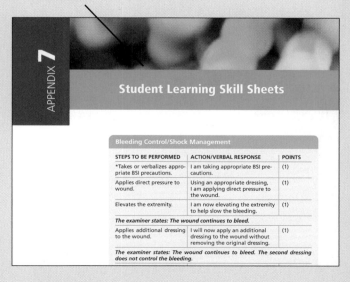

APPENDIX 7

Student Learning Skill Sheets

Bleeding Control/Shock Management

STEPS TO BE PERFORMED	ACTION/VERBAL RESPONSE	POINTS
*Takes or verbalizes appropriate BSI precautions.	I am taking appropriate BSI precautions.	(1)
Applies direct pressure to wound.	Using an appropriate dressing, I am applying direct pressure to the wound.	(1)
Elevates the extremity.	I am now elevating the extremity to help slow the bleeding.	(1)
The examiner states: The wound continues to bleed.		
Applies additional dressing to the wound.	I will now apply an additional dressing to the wound without removing the original dressing.	(1)
The examiner states: The wound continues to bleed. The second dressing does not control the bleeding.		

Guide to Key Features

Student CD-ROM

An exciting multimedia tool, the Student CD-ROM helps reinforce key concept and is ideal for the way today's students learn. The CD ROM includes:

- **Chapter Review** All new multiple-choice quizzes for each chapter to test and reinforce knowledge.

- **Making It Real** Scenarios with questions and rationales throughout to walk students through the critical thinking process.

- **Skill Videos** Video clips are accompanied by essay-style questions to encourage critical thinking.

- **Triage Simulations** Test student knowledge of proper triage in MCI scenarios.

- **Games** Basketball and hangman games make terminology easy and fun.

- **Virtual Airway Tour** A tour through the entire airway with an audio walkthrough. Helps students visualize this complex and critical component of care.

- **Animations** Highly visual exercises that enhance and reinforce anatomy, physiology, biology, and specific processes.

- **Anatomy and Physiology Illustrations** Highlight basic anatomy and physiology.

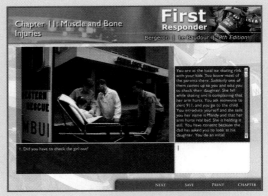
Making It Real

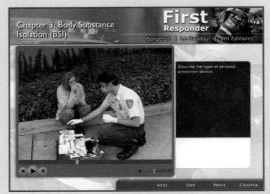
Skill Videos

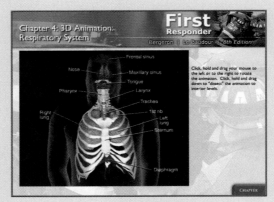
Animations

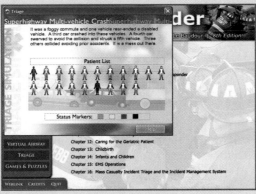
Triage Simulations

Teaching and Learning Package

In today's fast-paced learning environment, training takes place beyond the printed page. **FIRST RESPONDER'S** rich supplemental resources expand upon the book content to provide additional enrichment opportunities.

For the Student

- **Companion Website**
(www.prenhall.com/bergeron)
Contains chapter-by-chapter interactive review quizzes with immediate scoring and feedback, A&P matching exercises, a Trauma Gallery, and annotated links to appropriate EMS resources. Additionally, a link to Brady's EMT-Achieve Test Prep—a valuable tool to help prepare you for your national and state exams—can be found here.

- **Student Workbook** (0-13-244747-9)
Features activities—including key term definitions, labeling, listing, matching and short essays—and personal development and application exercises are designed to reinforce key concepts.

- **Review and Reference Tools**
Achieve: First Responder Test Preparation
(www.prenhall.com/emtachieve)
by Bob Elling is a dynamic online test preparation product for both students and instructors that includes test and quiz questions, DOT objectives, rationales, video, animation, and photos as well as score reports by content that show area progress and areas for improvement. Instructors will be able to monitor each student's progress in order to quickly identify problem areas so that corrective action can be taken.

Review Manual for the First Responder
(0-13-118439-3) by Joseph J. Mistovich is the text to help students pass their National Registry and other certification exams. All items are written and tested by educators and offer proven authoritative information with rationales. Blending a comprehensive collection of practice exam questions with helpful test-taking tips and student hints, all items reference the Department of Transportation's objectives. As you build confidence by digging into this rich content review, you'll find that the Brady/Pearson test preparation system is a blueprint for success across the boards.

Pocket Reference for BLS Providers, 3rd ed
(0-13-173730-9) by Bob Elling is written specifically for EMT-Bs and First Responders. A must-have for every EMT-B and First Responder, this handy, easy-to-carry pocketsize field reference complements all Brady First Responder and EMT-Basic textbooks and includes patient assessment flow charts and skills sequences.

For the Instructor

- **First Responder PowerPoint Slides** (0-13-513333-5)
An updated PowerPoint Slide set provides you with everything you need for a dynamic presentation.

- **Instructor's Resource Manual** (0-13-513301-7)
A brand new Instructor Manual includes objectives, presentation outlines, handouts with answer keys, and unique classroom activities designed to engage students and enhance the "First on Scene" feature in the text.

- **TestGen** (0-13-513331-9)
Thoroughly reviewed and updated. Contains hundreds of exam-style questions, as well as references to DOT objectives and text pages where answers can be found or supported.

- **Distance Learning Options**
Based on Course Compass, Black Board, and WebCT platforms, all instructor resources, student CD, and companion website content is provided to enable instructors to set up and run online courses or portions thereof.

First Responder Certificate Program

The American Safety & Health Institute

The American Safety & Health Institute (ASHI) is an association of safety and health educators providing nationally recognized training programs. ASHI's mission is to make learning to save lives easy. ASHI authorizes qualified individuals to offer First Responder training and certification programs for corporate America, government agencies, and emergency responders. To learn more about ASHI, visit www.ashinstitute.org.

About the ASHI First Responder Certification Program

In the early 1970s, officials at the U.S. Department of Transportation National Highway Traffic Safety Administration (NHTSA) recognized a gap between basic first aid training and the training of Emergency Medical Technicians (EMTs). Their solution was to create "Crash Injury Management: Emergency Medical Services for Traffic Law Enforcement Officers," an emergency medical care course for "patrolling law enforcement officers." As it evolved, the course expanded to include other "First Responders" – public and private safety and service personnel who, in the course of performing other duties, are likely to respond to emergencies (firefighters, highway department personnel, etc.). The Crash Injury Management course provided the basic knowledge and skills necessary to perform lifesaving interventions while waiting for EMTs to arrive. The original program was never intended for training EMS personnel. Because the Crash Injury Management course was designed to fill the gap between basic first aid training and EMT, it was considered "advanced first aid training." In 1978, the Crash Injury Management course was renamed *Emergency Medical Services: First Responder Training Course* and was specifically targeted at "public service law enforcement, fire, and EMS rescue agencies that did not necessarily have the ability to transport patients or carry sophisticated medical equipment." Then in 1995, the course went through a major revision and its name was changed to *First Responder: National Standard Curriculum*. At that time, the First Responder was described as "an integral part of the Emergency Medical Services System."

The ASHI First Responder program is not intended for those individuals seeking state licensure or credentialing as an EMS professional. Rather, the ASHI program is designed to fill the original need for an "advanced first aid course" for non-EMS providers who, in the course of performing other duties, are likely (or expected) to respond to emergencies; law enforcement officers, firefighters, and other public and private safety and service personnel. The original First Responder program was intended to provide these "pre-EMS" responders with the basic knowledge and skills necessary for lifesaving interventions while waiting for the EMS professionals to arrive. That original intent – filling the knowledge and skill gap between basic first aid training and EMS – is the intent of ASHI's First Responder program.

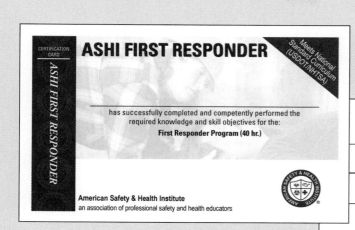

CERTIFICATION CARD

ASHI FIRST RESPONDER

ASHI FIRST RESPONDER

Meets National Standard Curriculum (USDOT/NHTSA)

has successfully completed and competently performed the
required knowledge and skill objectives for the:

First Responder Program (40 hr.)

American Safety & Health Institute
an association of professional safety and health educators

ASHI APPROVED CERTIFICATION CARD

_____
Authorized Instructor (Print Name)

_____
Holder's Signature

_____   _____
Date Completed   Renewal Date

_____   _____
Training Center Phone No.   Training Center Note

Successful completion indicates card holder has met the required knowledge and skill objectives of the curriculum
to the satisfaction of an ASHI authorized Instructor. Successful completion does not guarantee future performance,
nor imply state licensure or credentialing. The ASHI FR curriculum is based on the objectives of the First
Responder: National Standard Curriculum (USDOT/NHTSA). Rate this program online at www.ashinstitute.org or
call (800) 246-5101.

Evaluation of knowledge and skill competence is required for ASHI certification as a First Responder. The student must successfully complete the 50-question ASHI First Responder Exam and demonstrate the ability to work as a lead first responder in a scenario–based team setting, adequately directing the initial assessment and care of a responsive and unresponsive medical and trauma patient.

STATE LICENSURE AND CREDENTIALING

ASHI's First Responder program is designed to train and certify—not to license or credential—First Responders. EMS Provider licensing and credentialing are legal activities performed by the state, not ASHI. Individuals who require or desire licensure and credentialing within the state EMS system as a First Responder or Emergency Medical Responder must complete specific requirements established by the regulating authority. It is not the intent of ASHI's First Responder program to cross the EMS scope of practice threshold.

INTERNATIONAL USE OF ASHI FIRST RESPONDER

Given the current state of globalization and the increasing international reach of ASHI-authorized Instructors, the *ASHI First Responder* program has expanded outside of the United States. As appropriate actions by First Responders alleviate suffering, prevent disability and save lives, ASHI encourages this international expansion, particularly in areas with emerging but undeveloped EMS systems. However, as in the United States, the scope of practice for medically trained persons is often subject to federal, state, provincial or regional laws and regulations. It is not the intent of *ASHI's First Responder* program to cross the EMS (or medical) scope of practice threshold in any country.

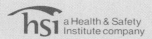
a Health & Safety Institute company

American Safety & Health Institute
1450 Westec Drive, Eugene, OR 97402.
Phone 800-800-7099 Fax 541-344-7429

MODULE 1 Preparatory

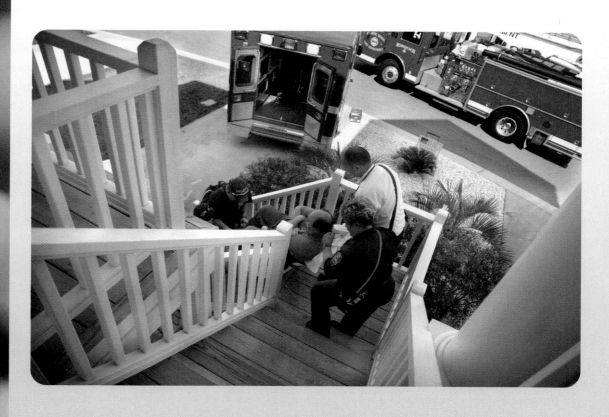

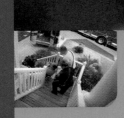

CHAPTER 1

Introduction to EMS Systems

Thousands of people become ill or are injured every day, and physicians are seldom close by when these emergencies occur. In fact, some time usually passes between the onset of an injury or illness and the delivery of medical care. Emergency medical services (EMS) systems have been developed for this very reason. The purpose is to get trained medical personnel to the patient as quickly as possible and to provide emergency care at the scene of the emergency and en route to the hospital. Emergency Medical Responders are an essential part of that EMS team.

You have made a great choice in deciding to become part of the EMS team by being trained as an Emergency Medical Responder. However, the realization that people will depend on you to provide assistance during an emergency can be overwhelming. To gain confidence in your knowledge and skills, it is important that you learn and understand what is expected of you in this new role. When you do, you can act more quickly to provide efficient and effective emergency care.

To begin, this chapter introduces you to EMS systems and to the roles and responsibilities of the Emergency Medical Responder.

OBJECTIVES

This chapter is based on the objectives of the U.S. DOT's First Responder National Standard Curriculum. Note that cognitive objectives are listed below and beside corresponding text throughout the chapter. You will also notice as you read each objective that the term Emergency Medical Responder is used. This is simply a name change and reflects the new name for the First Responder.

By the end of this chapter, you should be able to (from cognitive or knowledge information):

1–1.1 Define the components of Emergency Medical Services (EMS) systems. (p. 4)

1–1.2 Differentiate the roles and responsibilities of the Emergency Medical Responder from other out-of-hospital care providers. (p. 7)

1–1.3 Define medical oversight and discuss the Emergency Medical Responder's role in the process. (p. 8)

1–1.4 Discuss the types of medical oversight that may affect the medical care of an Emergency Medical Responder. (p. 8)

1–1.5 State the specific statutes and regulations in your state regarding the EMS system. (p. 9)

By the end of this chapter, you should be able to feel comfortable enough to (by changing attitudes, values, and beliefs):

1–1.6 Accept and uphold the responsibilities of an Emergency Medical Responder in accordance with the standards of an EMS professional. (pp. 10, 12, 14–16)

1–1.7 Explain the rationale for maintaining a professional appearance when on duty or when responding to calls. (p. 14)

1–1.8 Describe why it is inappropriate to judge a patient based on a cultural, gender, age, or socio-economic model, and to vary the standard of care rendered as a result of that judgment. (p. 14)

ADDITIONAL LEARNING TASKS

As you participate in this program and practice your skills, you should also be able to:

➤ Identify the six major duties of an Emergency Medical Responder and discuss how those duties apply directly to patient care.

➤ Demonstrate knowledge of and be able to perform the tasks that fall within the Emergency Medical Responder scope of practice.

➤ State the major milestones in the development of the modern EMS system.

➤ Discuss how recent advances in technology such as global positioning systems (GPS) have enhanced the efficiency of the Emergency Medical Responder.

 FIRST ON SCENE

It's a bright sunny spring day and Colin just left what he felt was one of his best interviews yet. All that time playing on the computer and messing around with video games was starting to pay off. If all went well, he would soon be working for a major video game development company right in his own hometown.

Things were looking up, and there was a noticeable bounce in his step as he descended the stairs to the visitor parking lot. Just as he reached the sidewalk, he heard a yell for help from across the lot. He hesitated for a moment and looked around to see if anyone else heard what he did. Again, he heard a female voice yelling for help, but he could not see anyone. He decided to investigate and go in the direction of the call.

Two rows over, he saw a middle-age woman leaning over a young boy on the ground. He appeared to be shaking, and there was a white foamy substance coming from his mouth. The woman saw Colin and yelled in a panicked voice for him to call an ambulance.

"Yes. Okay," Colin said. "I'll go back to the lobby and call for help. I'll be right back!"

He made it back to the lobby in record time and, in short bursts of words, advised the receptionist that someone was down in the parking lot and that she needs to call 9-1-1. She made the call and also alerted the building's Medical Emergency Response Team. With some hesitation, Colin returned to the scene in the parking lot.

The EMS System

People have likely been providing emergency care for one another since humans first walked on the Earth. Although many of those early treatments may seem primitive by today's standards, what has not changed is the awareness that treatment of some kind was needed. A formal system for responding to emergencies has only existed for a relatively short time (Table 1–1). It was during the American Civil War that the Union army first began training soldiers to provide first aid to the wounded on the battlefield. These "corpsmen," as they were known, were trained to provide care for the most immediate life threats such as bleeding. After their initial care, the injured were transported by horse-drawn carriage to waiting physicians. Thus, the first formal ambulance system in the United States had begun.

The first civilian ambulance services began in the late 1800s, with the sole purpose of transporting injured and ill patients to the hospital for care. It was not until 1928 that the concept of civilian "on-scene" care was first implemented with the organization of the Roanoke Life Saving and First Aid Crew in Roanoke, Virginia.

In 1966, the National Academy of Sciences released its report entitled, "Accidental Death and Disability: The Neglected Disease of Modern Society." This report revealed for the first time the inadequacies of prehospital care and provided suggestions for the development of formal EMS systems.

COMPONENTS OF THE EMS SYSTEM

1–1.1 Define the components of Emergency Medical Services (EMS) systems.

emergency medical services (EMS) system ■ the chain of human resources and services linked together to provide continuous emergency care from the onset of care at the prehospital scene, during transport, and on arrival at the medical facility.

If hospital personnel waited for patients to come to them, many people would die before getting medical care. Fortunately, it has become possible to extend life-saving care to the patient through a chain of resources known as the **emergency medical services (EMS) system** (Scan 1-1). Once the system is activated, care begins at the emergency scene and continues during transport to a medical facility. At the hospital, a formal transfer of care to the emergency department (ED) staff at the medical facility ensures a smooth continuation of care. Note that the ED may still be commonly referred to as the emergency room, or ER, in some areas.

The following is a list of common resources found in a typical EMS system:

■ Specially trained personnel.
■ Ambulances.
■ Fire departments.
■ Rescue squads.
■ Communication centers.
■ Air medical transport services.
■ Hospitals.
■ Law enforcement agencies.

The events that occurred on September 11, 2001, increased public awareness of the EMS system and rescue personnel who are called "first responders." Unfortunately, the media coverage helped confuse the distinction between a rescuer who appears first on scene and an EMS First Responder, who is a trained medical-care provider. Thus, the U.S. Department of Transportation (DOT) has embarked on renaming this level of EMS from "First Responder" to "Emergency Medical Responder." To encourage this logical and necessary change, this textbook uses the new title only.

Refer to Table 1–2 to compare the roles and responsibilities of the four types of EMS responders. They are based on the U.S. DOT's national standard curricula but vary slightly from state to state. Your instructor will explain variations in your area.

TABLE 1–1 | EMS Time Line

1790s	Napoleon's chief physician develops a system designed to triage and transport the injured soldiers from the battlefield to established aid stations.
1805–1815	Jean Larrey formed the *Ambulance Volante* (flying ambulance). It consisted of a covered horse-drawn cart designed to bring medical care closer to the injured on the battlefields of Europe.
1861–1865	Clara Barton coordinates the care of sick and injured soldiers during the American Civil War.
1865	First civilian ambulance company is formed in Cincinnati, Ohio.
1869	New York City Health Department Ambulance Service begins operation out of what was then known as the Free Hospital of New York, now Bellevue Hospital.
1915	First recorded air medical transport occurs during the retreat of the Serbian army from Albania.
1928	The concept of "on-scene care" was first initiated in 1928, when Julian Stanley Wise started the Roanoke Life Saving and First Aid Crew in Roanoke, Virginia.
1941–1945	Highly trained medical corpsmen are used to treat and transport injured soldiers from the battlefield.
1950–1973	In the Korean and Vietnam Wars, helicopters are used to evacuate injured soldiers and deliver them to waiting field hospitals.
1960	Cardiopulmonary resuscitation (CPR) makes its first public debut.
1966	Publication of the report entitled, "Accidental Death and Disability: The Neglected Disease of Modern Society," commonly referred to as the "White Paper." The study concluded that many of the deaths occurring every day were unnecessary and could be prevented through better prehospital treatments. Resulted in Congress passing the National Highway Safety Act.
1969	Emergency Medical Technician–Ambulance program is made public.
1973	Congress passes the Emergency Medical Services Act, which provided funding for a series of projects related to trauma care.
1988	National Highway Transportation & Safety Administration (NHTSA) defines elements necessary for all EMS systems.
1990	The Trauma Care Systems and Development Act encourages the development of improved trauma systems.
1995	Release of the most recent update to the EMT Basic and First Responder National Standard Curricula.
1996	Publication of the EMS Agenda for the Future, outlining the most important directions for the future of EMS development.
1998	Release of the most recent update to the EMT Paramedic National Standard Curricula.
1999	Release of the most recent update to the EMT Intermediate National Standard Curricula.

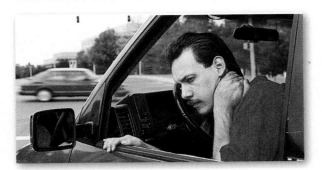

1 ■ Emergency scene.

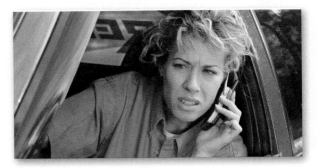

2 ■ Recognition of the crash scene and activation of EMS.

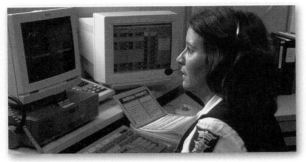

3 ■ Emergency Medical Dispatcher (EMD).

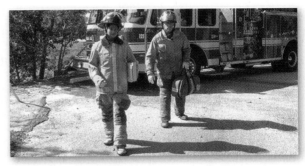

4 ■ Arrival of Emergency Medical Responders.

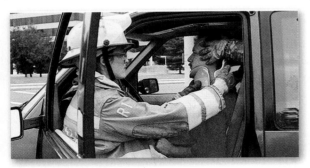

5 ■ Care given at the scene.

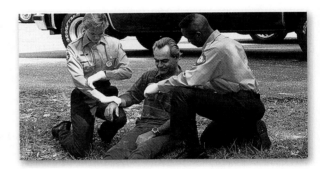

6 ■ Arrival of additional EMS personnel.

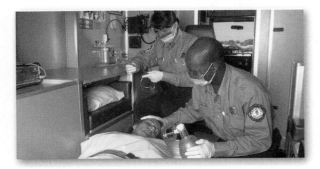

7 ■ Care during transport.

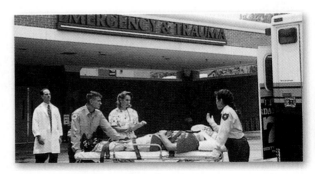

8 ■ Transfer to hospital emergency department (ED).

TABLE 1–2	Levels of EMS Training

- *Emergency Medical Responder*—This level of EMS training is designed specifically for the person who is often first to arrive at the scene. Many police officers, firefighters, industrial workers, and other public service providers are trained as Emergency Medical Responders. This training emphasizes scene safety and how to provide immediate care for life-threatening injuries and illnesses as well as how to assist ambulance personnel when they arrive.

- *Emergency Medical Technician (EMT)*—In most areas, an EMT is considered the minimum level of certification for ambulance personnel. The training emphasizes assessment and the care and transportation of the ill or injured patient. The EMT may also assist with the administration of certain common medications. (This was formerly called the *EMT-Basic* level of training.)

- *Advanced Emergency Medical Technician (AEMT)*—An AEMT, or advanced EMT, is a basic-level EMT who has received specific additional training in specific subjects, allowing some level of advanced life support. Some of the additional skills an AEMT may be able to perform are starting IV (intravenous) lines, inserting advanced airways, and administering medications. (This was formerly called the *EMT-Intermediate* level of training.)

- *Paramedic*—Paramedics are trained to perform what is commonly referred to as advanced life support care, such as inserting endotracheal (ET) tubes and starting IV lines. They also administer medications, interpret electrocardiograms, monitor cardiac rhythms, and perform cardiac defibrillation. (This was formerly called the *EMT-Paramedic* level of training.)

1–1.2 Differentiate the roles and responsibilities of the Emergency Medical Responder from other out-of-hospital care providers.

NOTE

As of this writing, a specialized task force led by the National Association of State EMS Directors and the National Council of State EMS Training Coordinators has been asked to redefine The National Scope of Practice Model. The purpose of the task force is to look closely at our current national EMS model and make suggestions for change that will reflect the future of EMS in the United States and how EMS systems can best meet the needs of the populations we serve.

ACTIVATING THE EMS SYSTEM

Once an emergency occurs and is recognized, the EMS system must be activated. Most citizens activate it by way of a 9-1-1 phone call to an emergency dispatcher, who then sends available responders—**Emergency Medical Responders, Emergency Medical Technicians (EMTs),** and **Paramedics**—to the scene. Some areas of the country may not have a 9-1-1 system in place. In those areas, the caller may need to dial a seven-digit number for the ambulance, fire, police, or rescue personnel. The most desirable 9-1-1 service is referred to as *enhanced* 9-1-1, which enables the communications center to automatically receive caller information, such as phone number and address, making it easier to confirm location and reconnect should the call be lost.

Is It Safe ?

One of the most important concepts to remember as you become a part of the EMS team is that of safety. Many people are injured and even killed each year when they

Emergency Medical Responder ■ a member of the EMS system who has been trained to render first aid care for a patient and help EMTs at the emergency scene.

Emergency Medical Technician (EMT) ■ a member of the EMS system whose training emphasizes assessment, care, and transportation of the ill or injured patient. Depending on the level of training, emergency care may include starting IV (intravenous) lines, inserting advanced airways, and administering some medications.

Paramedic ■ a member of the EMS system whose training includes advanced life support care, such as inserting endotracheal (ET) tubes and starting IV lines. Paramedics also administer medications, interpret electrocardiograms, monitor cardiac rhythms, and perform cardiac defibrillation.

rush into an unsafe scene to help an injured victim. Take the time to stop and observe the scene before rushing in. Do your best to identify any obvious hazards that could endanger you or others arriving at the scene. ■

For some 9-1-1 services, personnel are trained as **Emergency Medical Dispatchers (EMDs)**. EMDs receive specialized training to provide pre-arrival instructions to callers, thereby helping to initiate life-saving care before EMS personnel arrive. Once the EMS system is activated, resources such as personnel and vehicles are dispatched. EMS personnel will then provide care at the scene and during transport. They also will deliver the patient to the most appropriate medical facility.

IN-HOSPITAL CARE SYSTEM

For most patients, the care destination will be a hospital emergency department. There the patient is further evaluated using advanced technology such as laboratory tests and diagnostic exams. The emergency department is the gateway to the rest of the services that hospitals offer. If a patient has a serious injury or illness, the role of emergency department personnel is to stabilize all immediate life threats and transfer care to the most appropriate in-hospital resources, such as the medical/surgical or intensive care units, or to have the patient transferred to a more specialized hospital.

FIRST ON SCENE

By the time he returned to the scene, Colin could see that the young boy had stopped shaking. Within seconds, a pair of women arrived at the scene and introduced themselves as Elizabeth and Nora, members of the company's Medical Emergency Response Team. They had equipment with them and seemed to know what they were doing. Elizabeth knelt beside the patient and appeared to be listening for something. Nora took the woman aside and asked questions about the boy.

Some hospitals handle all routine and emergency cases but have a specialty that sets them apart from other hospitals. One specialty designation is a trauma center, in which specific services and surgery teams are available 24 hours a day. Some hospitals specialize in the care of certain conditions such as burns and cardiac problems. Other hospitals may specialize in a particular type of patient such as pediatric and neonatal patients.

MEDICAL OVERSIGHT

1–1.3 Define medical oversight and discuss the Emergency Medical Responder's role in the process.

Medical Director ■ a physician who assumes the ultimate responsibility for medical oversight of the patient care aspects of the EMS system.

protocols ■ written guidelines that direct the care that EMS personnel provide for patients.

1–1.4 Discuss the types of medical oversight that may affect the medical care of an Emergency Medical Responder.

FIRST ➤ Each EMS system has a **Medical Director**. The Medical Director is a physician who assumes the ultimate responsibility for direction and oversight of all patient care aspects of the EMS system. The Medical Director also oversees training and develops treatment **protocols** (written guidelines that direct the care that EMS personnel provide for patients). Most EMS systems have prescribed protocols for how to manage the most common types of patients, such as patients with chest pain, cardiac arrest, difficulty breathing, and severe allergic reaction. Emergency Medical Responders act as designated agents of the Medical Director. ■

The physician cannot physically be present at every emergency, so the EMS system provides **standing orders**. These orders are in the form of protocols, which authorize rescuers to perform specific skills in specific situations without actually speaking to the Medical Director. For instance, the protocol for how to care for a patient with chest pain may include a standing order for oxygen. Thus, the Emergency Medical Responder may provide oxygen to any patient with chest pain based on this standing order. That kind of "behind the scenes" medical direction is called **off-line medical direction** (or *indirect medical direction*). Procedures

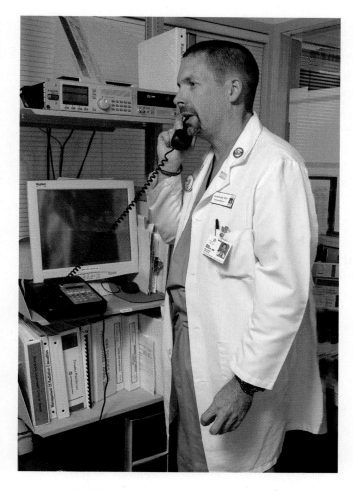

FIGURE 1.1 On-line medical direction being provided by an EMS physician.

not covered by standing orders or protocols require the Emergency Medical Responder to contact medical direction by radio or telephone prior to performing a particular skill or administering care (Figure 1.1). Orders from medical direction given in this manner—by radio or phone—are called **on-line medical direction** (or *direct medical direction*).

As an Emergency Medical Responder at the scene of an emergency, you may have limited access to the Medical Director. It will be necessary for you to adhere to the training you receive or to follow the orders of on-scene EMS providers who have a higher level of training or certification. Like all EMS personnel, you must only provide care that is within your scope of practice. The **scope of practice** is defined as the care that an Emergency Medical Responder is allowed and supposed to provide according to local, state, or regional regulations or statutes. The scope of practice includes protocols and guidelines set in place by the local jurisdiction.

The scope of practice is based on the DOT National Standard Curriculum for the Emergency Medical Responder but may vary from state to state and region to region. Your instructor will inform you of any local protocols and policies that may define your scope of practice. Always follow your local protocols.

The Emergency Medical Responder

The lack of people with enough training to provide care before more highly skilled EMS providers arrive at a scene is the weakest link in the chain of the EMS system. Training Emergency Medical Responders will help correct this problem.

standing orders ■ specific instructions developed by the medical director, which authorize the Emergency Medical Responder, EMT, or Paramedic to provide care for specific medical conditions or injuries.

off-line (indirect) medical direction ■ standing orders and protocols developed by an EMS system that authorize rescuers to perform particular skills in certain situations without actually speaking to the Medical Director.

on-line (direct) medical direction ■ orders to perform a skill or administer care from the on-duty physician, given to the rescuer in person, by radio, or by phone.

1–1.5 State the specific statutes and regulations in your state regarding the EMS system.

scope of practice ■ the care that an Emergency Medical Responder, an EMT, or Paramedic is allowed and supposed to provide according to local, state, or regional regulations or statutes. Also called *scope of care*.

emergency care ■ the prehospital assessment and basic care for the sick or injured patient. The physical and emotional needs of the patient are considered and attended to during care.

FIRST ➤ Emergency Medical Responders are trained to reach patients, find out what is wrong, provide **emergency care** and, only when necessary and without causing further injury, move patients. These individuals are usually the first trained personnel to reach the patient. An Emergency Medical Responder may be a law enforcement officer, a member of the fire service, an office coworker, or a private citizen (Scan 1-2). In all cases, an Emergency Medical Responder is trained and has successfully completed an Emergency Medical Responder course. Many police officers and firefighters are trained to this level. Industrial companies are beginning to train employees as Emergency Medical Responders as well. The more private citizens who become trained as Emergency Medical Responders, the stronger the EMS system becomes. ■

Since the beginning of Emergency Medical Responder training programs, hundreds of thousands of people have completed formal courses, with many going on to provide essential care. In most areas of the United States, the care Emergency Medical Responders provide reduces suffering, prevents additional injuries, and saves many lives.

FIRST ON SCENE

Within minutes, the sirens of responding emergency vehicles could be heard. By then, there were five members of the Medical Emergency Response Team caring for the young boy, who was beginning to wake up. The team of responders placed the boy on his side, cleared out his mouth with some kind of suction device, and gave him some oxygen. That must have been what he needed, because after they cleared his mouth, he woke up.

ROLES AND RESPONSIBILITIES

Personal Safety

FIRST ➤ Your primary concern as an Emergency Medical Responder at an emergency scene is your own *personal safety*. The desire to help those who are in need of care may tempt you to ignore the hazards at the scene. You must make certain that you can safely reach the patient and that you will remain safe while providing care. ■

Part of an Emergency Medical Responder's concern for personal safety must include the proper protection from infectious diseases. All Emergency Medical Responders who assess or provide care for patients *must* avoid direct contact with patient blood or other body fluids. Personal protective equipment (PPE) that minimizes contact with infectious material includes:

- Disposable protective gloves.
- Barrier devices, such as pocket face masks with one-way valves and special filters for rescue-breathing procedures.
- Protective eye wear, such as goggles or face shields, to avoid contact with droplets expelled during certain care procedures such as ventilating and suctioning.
- Special face masks with filters that minimize contact with airborne microorganisms.
- Gowns or aprons that minimize contact of splashed blood or other body fluids.

Typically, you will only need protective gloves and possibly face masks for most patient care situations. However, the items in the preceding list should be on hand so that you can protect yourself and provide care safely. (More is said about infectious diseases and personal protection in Chapter 3.)

Emergency Medical Responders who are in law enforcement, the fire service, or industry may be required to carry out their specific job tasks before they provide

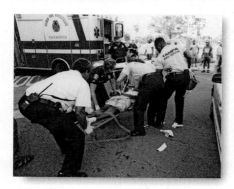

1 ■ Emergency Medical Responders work in many different fields and environments. They may be full-time fire service personnel. (© Craig Jackson/In the Dark Photography)

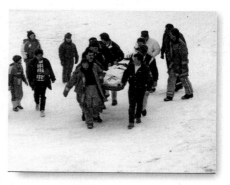

2 ■ They may be firefighter volunteers. (© Craig Jackson/In the Dark Photography)

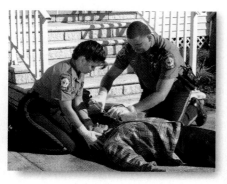

3 ■ Emergency Medical Responders may be law enforcement personnel, including state troopers, ATF, DEA, and FBI agents.

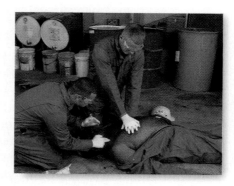

4 ■ They are homeland security personnel, campus security police, shopping mall and factory security personnel, and industrial Medical Emergency Response Teams (MERTs).

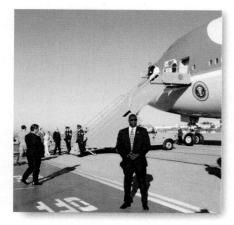

5 ■ Emergency Medical Responders are park rangers, lifeguards, athletic trainers, military combat life savers (CLSs), and executive protection personnel such as Secret Service agents.

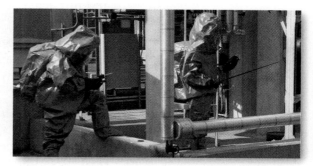

6 ■ Emergency Medical Responders are also rescue team specialists for specific disciplines, such as hazardous materials, confined space, swift water, ice, trench, high angle, cave, and urban rescues.

patient care (controlling traffic, stabilizing vehicles, shutting down machinery). If this applies to you, always follow department or company standard operating procedures.

FIRST ➤ As an Emergency Medical Responder, you are part of the EMS system. Your activities at the scene and the care you provide will help save lives, prevent additional injury, and give comfort to patients. ▪

Patient-Related Duties

Prior to receiving care, the injured or ill person is referred to as a *victim*. Once you start to carry out your duties as an Emergency Medical Responder, the victim becomes a *patient*. Your presence at the scene means that the EMS system has begun its first phase of care. True, the patient may need a physician at the hospital to survive, but the patient's chances of reaching the hospital alive are greatly improved because an Emergency Medical Responder has initiated emergency care.

FIRST ➤ As an Emergency Medical Responder, you have six main patient-related duties to carry out at the emergency scene. These duties are (Scan 1-3):

1. *Size up the scene.* Scene safety is your first concern, even before patient care. Evaluate how to protect yourself and the patient, try to determine what caused the injury or illness, how many patients you have, and what kind of assistance you will need. You must control the scene to protect yourself and the patients and to minimize additional injuries. At the same time, make sure that the dispatcher is alerted so more highly trained personnel can be sent. Should you need the police, fire service, rescue squad, power company, or others at the scene, you must make sure that the dispatcher is aware of this need.

2. *Determine the patient's chief complaint or primary injury.* To do so, gather information from the patient and by assessing the patient, as well as from the scene and bystanders. Using the supplies you have, provide emergency care to the level of your training. Remember, emergency care deals with both illness and injury. It can be as simple as providing emotional support to someone who is frightened because of a crash or mishap. Or it can be more complex, requiring you to deal with life-threatening emergencies, such as starting basic life support (BLS) measures for a heart attack victim. In later chapters, you will learn how to provide a combination of emotional support and physical care skills to help the patient until more highly trained personnel arrive.

3. *Lift, move, or reposition the patient only when necessary.* You need to judge when safety or care requires you to move or reposition a patient. When you must move a patient, use techniques that minimize the chance of injuring yourself.

4. *Transfer the patient and patient information.* Provide for an orderly transfer of the patient and all patient-related information to more highly trained personnel. You may also be asked to assist such personnel and work under their direction.

5. *Protect the patient's privacy and maintain confidentiality.* This responsibility is not only a matter of good patient care, but also a matter of legality.

6. *Be the patient's advocate.* You must be willing to be an advocate for the patient and do what is best for him as long as it is safe to do so. ▪

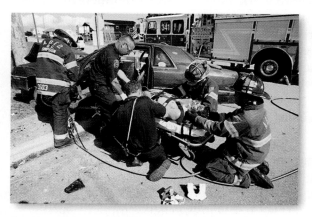

1 ■ Emergency Medical Responder is to safely gain access to the patient. *(Photo by Nathan Eldridge)*

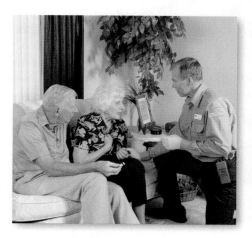

2 ■ Emergency Medical Responders must find out what is wrong with the patient.

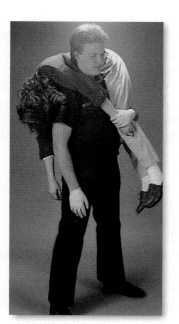

3 ■ Emergency Medical Responders lift or move patients when necessary without causing further injury.

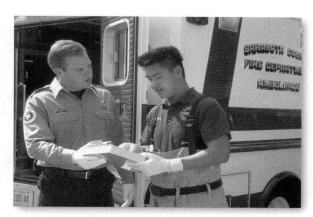

4 ■ The Emergency Medical Responder transfers the patient and patient information to appropriate medical personnel, protects the patient's privacy and maintains confidentiality, and acts as the patient's advocate.

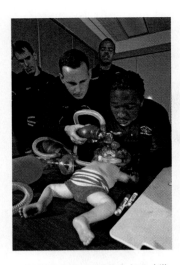

FIGURE 1.2 Maintaining skill proficiency is an important part of being an Emergency Medical Responder. (© Richard T. Nowitz/Corbis)

TRAITS

To be an Emergency Medical Responder, you must be willing to take on certain duties and responsibilities. It takes hard work and study to be an Emergency Medical Responder. Because you must keep your emergency care skills sharp and current (Figure 1.2), you may be required to recertify or relicense periodically.

You also have to be willing to deal with people. Individuals who are sick or injured are not at their best. You must be able to overlook rude behavior and unreasonable demands, realizing that patients may act this way because of fear, uncertainty, or pain. Dealing with patient reactions is often the hardest part of the job. To do so in a professional manner is sometimes very difficult.

FIRST ➤ All patients have the same right to the very best of care. Your respect for others and acceptance of their rights are essential parts of the total patient care that you provide as an Emergency Medical Responder. You cannot modify the care you provide according to your view of religious beliefs, cultural expression, age, gender, social behavior, socioeconomic background, or geographic origin. Every patient is unique and deserves to have his or her needs met by a consistent standard of care. ▪

To be an Emergency Medical Responder, you must be honest and realistic. When helping patients, you cannot tell them that they are okay if they are truly sick or hurt. You cannot tell them that everything is all right, when they know that something is wrong. Telling someone not to worry is not realistic. When an emergency occurs, there is truly something to worry about. Your conversations with patients can help relax them, if you are honest. By telling patients that you are trained in emergency care and that you will help them, you ease their fears and gain their confidence. Letting patients know that additional aid is on the way also will help them relax.

As an Emergency Medical Responder, there may be limits to what you can say to a patient or a patient's loved ones. Telling a patient that a loved one is dead may not be appropriate if you are still providing care for the patient. In such circumstances, it is often necessary for you to be tactful. Remember, people under the stress of illness or injury often do not tolerate additional stress well.

Being an Emergency Medical Responder requires that you control your own feelings at the emergency scene. You must learn how to care for patients, while controlling your emotional reactions to their injury or illness. Patients do not need sympathy and tears. They need your professional care.

As an Emergency Medical Responder, you have to be a highly disciplined professional at the emergency scene. You must not make inappropriate comments about patients or the horror of the incident. You must maintain your focus on the patient and avoid unnecessary distractions.

Providing the appropriate care requires you to admit that the stress of responding to emergency scenes will affect you. You may have to speak with other EMS care providers or a specialist within the EMS system to resolve the stress and emotional challenges caused by responding to emergencies.

No one can demand that you change your lifestyle to be an Emergency Medical Responder. However, first impressions are important. Your appearance alone can earn a patient's confidence. So, keep your uniform neat and clean at all times. Also, how you approach the patient and the respect you show is important. Refer to the patient in a manner that is appropriate for his or her age. All elders should be referred to as Mr., Mrs., or Ms., while children respond well to their first names. The significance of these actions can greatly affect the willingness of the patient to share information and feel comfortable in your care.

In addition, to be an Emergency Medical Responder, you must keep yourself in reasonably good physical condition. You may be of little help to the patient if you are unable to bend over or catch your breath. So watch your diet, exercise regularly, and be sure to get a yearly checkup with your doctor. You do not want to become another patient on the scene.

When you complete your training and become an Emergency Medical Responder, you are filling a vital need in your community.

SKILLS

In addition to learning facts and information, you will be required to perform certain skills as part of your Emergency Medical Responder training. These skills vary from course to course. The following list is an example of the skills learned by the typical Emergency Medical Responder. You are not expected to memorize this list. Read the list and check off each skill as you learn it in your course.

As an Emergency Medical Responder, you should be able to:

- Assess for and manage potential hazards at the scene.
- Gain access to patients in vehicles.
- Gain access to patients in buildings.
- Evaluate the possible cause of an illness or injury.
- Gather pertinent information from patients and bystanders.
- Properly use all items of personal safety.
- Conduct an appropriate patient assessment.
- Gather accurate vital signs (pulse, respiration, skin signs, pupils).
- Properly document assessment findings.
- Relate signs and symptoms to illnesses and injuries.
- Evaluate and manage a patient's airway and breathing status.
- Perform cardiopulmonary resuscitation (CPR) for adults, infants, and children.
- Set up and use the automated external defibrillator (AED) on patients in cardiac arrest.
- Control bleeding by using direct pressure, elevation, pressure dressings, and pressure points.
- Assess and manage the patient who is showing signs of shock.
- Assess and provide care for patients with closed and open injuries, including face and scalp wounds, nosebleeds, eye injuries, neck wounds, chest injuries, and abdominal injuries.
- Perform basic dressing and bandaging techniques.
- Assess and care for injuries to bones and joints.
- Assess and care for possible head and face injuries.
- Assess and care for possible injuries to the neck and spine.
- Assess and care for possible heart attacks, strokes, seizures, and diabetic emergencies.
- Identify and care for poisoning cases.
- Assess and care for burns.
- Assess and care for heat- and cold-related emergencies.
- Assist a mother in delivering her baby.
- Provide initial care for the newborn.
- Identify and care for drug- and alcohol-abuse patients.
- Perform nonemergency and emergency patient moves when required.

- Perform triage at a multiple-patient emergency scene.
- Work under the direction of an Incident Commander in an incident command system (ICS) or incident management system (IMS) operation.
- Work under the direction of EMTs or more highly trained personnel to help them provide patient care, doing what you have been trained to do at your level of care as an Emergency Medical Responder.

In some systems, Emergency Medical Responders may be required to perform all or any of the following:

- Deliver oxygen.
- Apply or assist in applying a traction splint.
- Apply or assist in applying a cervical collar.
- Assist in securing a patient to a long spine board (backboard) or other device used to immobilize the patient's spine.

EQUIPMENT, TOOLS, AND SUPPLIES

Most Emergency Medical Responders carry very few pieces of equipment, tools, and supplies. Some may carry special or separate kits for trauma emergencies, medical emergencies, and childbirth. It is easier to grab a small kit containing the items needed for the incident than to pick up and carry a large kit with everything in it. If you are assigned to a special event, such as a football game or a carnival, you may want to include items that will meet the needs of that event in addition to the standard dressings and bandages.

The DOT has recommended that Emergency Medical Responders know how to use, and have available whenever possible, the following items (Figure 1.3):

- Appropriate personal protective equipment (masks and gloves).
- Triangular bandages.
- Roller-type bandages.

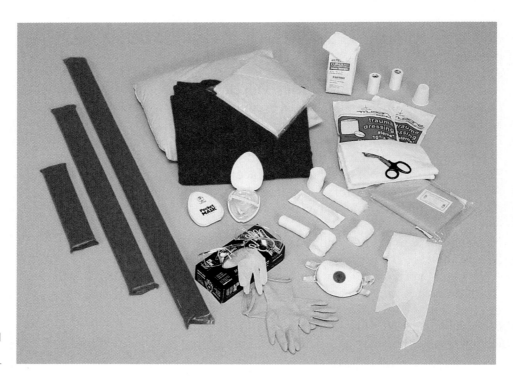

FIGURE 1.3 Emergency medical care equipment and supplies.

- Gauze pads and trauma dressings.
- Occlusive dressings.
- Adhesive tape.
- Bandage shears.
- Eye protector (paper cup or cone).
- Stick (for tourniquet).
- Blanket and pillow.
- Upper and lower extremity splint sets.

In some localities, Emergency Medical Responders are expected to take a patient's blood pressure. In those areas, the kit would include a blood pressure cuff and a stethoscope. Some jurisdictions may have Emergency Medical Responders administer oxygen, and also suction the patient's mouth and nose when needed. In those jurisdictions, Emergency Medical Responders carry oxygen delivery systems and suctioning equipment.

The DOT has suggested that all Emergency Medical Responders should be able to use the following tools and equipment for gaining access to patients (your course may include other items):

- Jack and jack handle.
- Pliers, screwdriver, hammer, and knife.
- Rope.

ADVANCES IN TECHNOLOGY

In recent years, there have been several advances in technology that have made the job of the EMS team more effective and efficient. One of the most important of those advances is the introduction of the GPS to the civilian marketplace (Figure 1.4). GPSs are becoming more common as they are being installed in all types of public safety vehicles, including police cars, fire engines, and ambulances. The use of GPS technology allows emergency personnel to more easily navigate to the location of the emergency, thus reducing response time. It also allows dispatch personnel to track the location of emergency vehicles within the system and use resources more efficiently.

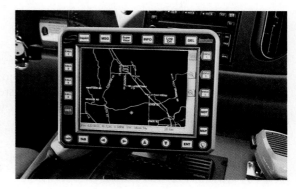

FIGURE 1.4 A typical GPS device installed in an emergency vehicle.

FIRST ON SCENE WRAP-UP

It looked like the cavalry was arriving. There were so many vehicles with lights and sirens. First, there were the fire trucks, two of them! Then an ambulance showed up, and behind that was another SUV-type vehicle painted just like the ambulance. Before Colin knew it, there was what seemed like a dozen people all hovering over the young boy.

He stuck around to observe the excitement and even forgot for a minute why he was actually there. He heard Elizabeth give a report to the ambulance team about the boy and how she thought he might have had a seizure.

Wow, what an exciting day. He couldn't stop thinking about the poor boy and how he must have felt when he woke up and saw so many people hovering over him. The woman with the boy turned out to be his mother, and she took the time to thank Colin for making sure the call to 9-1-1 was made quickly.

Summary

The EMS system is a chain of resources established to provide care to the patient at the scene of an emergency and during transport to the hospital emergency department (ED). There are four levels of EMS training: Emergency Medical Responder, EMT, and Paramedic. EMS personnel are dispatched to the scene of an emergency when a dispatcher receives a 9-1-1 call. Dispatchers may be specially trained as Emergency Medical Dispatchers (EMDs) who offer pre-arrival care instructions to bystanders at the scene.

Every EMS system is required to designate a Medical Director, a physician who assumes the ultimate responsibility for medical oversight of the patient care aspects of the EMS system. Medical direction can be off-line (indirect), which includes established protocols that authorize rescuers to perform particular skills in certain situations without actually speaking to the Medical Director. Medical direction can also be on-line (direct) via radio or phone contact with the on-duty physician prior to performing a skill or administering care.

Emergency Medical Responders are an important part of the EMS system and are usually the first trained personnel to arrive at the emergency scene. The EMS system's primary goal is personal safety, which must begin with the Emergency Medical Responders themselves. No one should enter or approach an emergency scene until it is safe to do so. No one should begin patient assessment and care without first donning personal protective equipment (PPE).

An Emergency Medical Responder's main duties are sizing up the scene to ensure the scene is safe to enter, gaining access to the patient, finding out what is wrong with the patient and providing emergency care, moving patients (when necessary), transferring the patient and any patient information to more highly trained personnel when they arrive at the scene, protecting the patient's privacy and maintaining confidentiality, and being the patient's advocate.

Included in those duties are responsibilities such as controlling the scene, calling the Emergency Dispatcher, obtaining help from bystanders, and assisting more highly trained personnel when they arrive.

The Emergency Medical Responder will be expected to care for patients of both injury and illness. Care can range from emotional support to basic life support (BLS) measures. Emergency Medical Responders have to maintain skills, keep up to date, and deal with people. They also must know what they should and should not say to patients and their families. Performing as professionals is an important Emergency Medical Responder responsibility.

Remember and Consider

The decision to become an Emergency Medical Responder is an important one. You should give full consideration to all aspects of emergency care and the training program before taking the steps to become an Emergency Medical Responder. Once you have decided, however, you will find it to be very rewarding.

➤ Become familiar with the Emergency Medical Responder scope of practice in your area or region.

➤ Know your roles and responsibilities as an Emergency Medical Responder.

➤ Think about the qualities you would like to see in an Emergency Medical Responder who renders care to you or your loved ones. Do you have those qualities? If not, think about how you can come closer to being that kind of Emergency Medical Responder. If possible, talk to someone who is an Emergency Medical Responder or EMT to gain additional insight.

Investigate

➤ Determine the locations of medical facilities in your area and the level of care or special services they provide. Also find out where specialty centers are located and how patients are transported to them if they are not in the immediate area.

➤ Learn what you must do to refresh your knowledge and maintain your certification. Find and attend continuing education classes whenever possible.

➤ Investigate the specific statutes and regulations in your state or province regarding the EMS system.

Quick Quiz

1. Which of the following is NOT a common component of an EMS system?
   a. ambulances
   b. hospitals
   c. homeless shelters
   d. fire service

2. All care provided by EMS personnel within an EMS system is overseen by a(n):
   a. Medical Director.
   b. Fire Chief.
   c. Ambulance Supervisor.
   d. Nursing Supervisor.

3. Which one of the following best describes the role of the Emergency Medical Responder in an EMS system?
   a. identifies hazards and transport patients
   b. cares for immediate life threats and assists EMTs
   c. secures the scene and serves as Incident Commander
   d. assists Paramedics with advanced skills

4. Emergency Medical Dispatchers receive training that allows them to:
   a. control the scene via the radio.
   b. triage patients via the radio.
   c. declare a mass-casualty incident.
   d. provide pre-arrival care instructions.

5. Which one of the following receives the highest level of training in an EMS system?
   a. Emergency Medical Responder
   b. Emergency Medical Technician
   c. Advanced EMT
   d. Paramedic

6. Guidelines written by the Medical Director describe the care that EMS personnel provide for patients. Those guidelines are called:
   a. dispatching.
   b. protocols.
   c. on-line direction.
   d. prescriptions.

7. Which one of the following would MOST likely be considered a standing order?
   a. Stay clear of an unsafe scene.
   b. Run with lights and sirens.
   c. Begin CPR on a victim of cardiac arrest.
   d. Dispatch an ambulance to an emergency scene.

8. Protocols and standing orders are forms of:
   a. off-line medical direction.
   b. on-line medical direction.
   c. pre-arrival instructions.
   d. standby guidelines.

9. The care that an Emergency Medical Responder is allowed and supposed to provide according to local, state, or regional regulations or statutes is known as:
   a. scope of practice.
   b. standard of care.
   c. national standard curricula.
   d. Emergency Medical Responder care.

10. As a member of the EMS team, your primary role is one of:
    a. patient care.
    b. safety.
    c. transport.
    d. documentation.

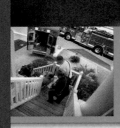

CHAPTER 2

Legal and Ethical Issues

As an Emergency Medical Responder, you must make many decisions when responding to an emergency and while caring for patients. Understanding the related legal and ethical issues will help you make the best decisions possible.

You may already have concerns about some legal and ethical issues. For example, should an off-duty Emergency Medical Responder stop to aid victims of an automobile crash? Should you release information about your patient to an attorney over the telephone? May a child with a suspected broken arm be treated, even if a parent is not present? What should happen when a patient who needs emergency medical care refuses it?

This chapter provides you with an overview of the legal and ethical aspects of being an Emergency Medical Responder who provides care to ill and injured patients of all ages.

OBJECTIVES

This chapter is based on the objectives of the U.S. DOT's First Responder National Standard Curriculum. Note that cognitive objectives are listed below and beside corresponding text throughout the chapter. You will also notice as you read each objective that the term Emergency Medical Responder is used. This is simply a name change and reflects the new name for the First Responder.

By the end of this chapter, you should be able to (from cognitive or knowledge information):

1–3.1 Define the Emergency Medical Responder scope of care. (p. 22)

1–3.2 Discuss the importance of Do Not Resuscitate (DNR) orders (advance directives) and local or state provisions regarding EMS application. (pp. 27–28)

1–3.3 Define consent and discuss the methods of obtaining consent. (pp. 24–26)

1–3.4 Differentiate between expressed and implied consent. (pp. 25–27)

1–3.5 Explain the role of consent of minors in providing care. (pp. 26)

1–3.6 Discuss the implications for the Emergency Medical Responder in patient refusal of transport. (pp. 24–25)

1–3.7 Discuss the issues of abandonment, negligence, and battery, and their implications to the Emergency Medical Responder. (pp. 28–30)

1–3.8 State the conditions necessary for the Emergency Medical Responder to have a duty to act. (pp. 28–29)

1–3.9 Explain the importance, necessity, and legality of patient confidentiality. (pp. 30–32)

1–3.10 List the actions that an Emergency Medical

Responder should take to assist in the preservation of a crime scene. (pp. 33–34)

1–3.11 State the conditions that require an Emergency Medical Responder to notify local law enforcement officials. (p. 32)

1–3.12 Discuss issues concerning the fundamental components of documentation. (p. 34)

By the end of this chapter, you should be able to feel comfortable enough to (by changing attitudes, values, and beliefs):

1–3.13 Explain the rationale for the needs, benefits, and usage of advance directives. (pp. 27–28)

1–3.14 Explain the rationale for the concept of varying degrees of DNR. (pp. 27–28)

ADDITIONAL LEARNING TASKS

As you participate in this program and practice your skills, you should also be able to:

➤ Find out if your state has Good Samaritan laws, as well as who they protect and to what extent.
➤ Become familiar with the forms and policies pertaining to DNR orders in your state or jurisdiction.

 FIRST ON SCENE

"Hold on!" Mike yells. She feels his body tense under the smooth leather jacket. The motorcycle leans far to the right and then quickly back to the left, causing the tires to squeal and wobble as the bike comes to a clumsy stop. Heather looks over Mike's shoulder and feels her stomach go cold. Two deep gouges scar the asphalt all the way to the far side of the road, where a small sports car is overturned and partially wrapped around a tree. Behind her, amazingly close to the black skid marks left by the motorcycle, a man is lying in a heap on the road.

"Wait," Mike says as Heather climbs from the bike and pulls her helmet off. "Let's keep going. There's got to be a pay phone up ahead somewhere!" In a matter of seconds, the entire Emergency Medical Responder class that Heather took two months ago flashes through her head.

"No," she says, quickly pulling her wind-whipped hair back into a ponytail. "That guy in the road needs help right now!"

Legal Duties

FIRST ➤ Most of us have heard stories about people being sued because of something they did or did not do when they stopped to help someone at the scene of an emergency. However, successful suits of this type are not common. Most states have established laws that minimize exposure to liability and encourage passersby to provide emergency care to those in need. These laws require the individual who is providing care to be doing so without promise of or actual compensation and to remain within a specified *scope of practice* (sometimes called *scope of care*). ■

SCOPE OF PRACTICE

1–3.1 Define the Emergency Medical Responder scope of care.

Recall from Chapter 1 that the term *scope of practice* refers to what is legally permitted to be done by some or all individuals trained or licensed at a particular level, such as an Emergency Medical Responder, EMT, or Paramedic. The scope of practice, however, *does not* define what must be done for a given patient or in a particular situation.

The scope of practice for a layperson might be based on nothing more than common sense or an eight-hour first-aid class taken many years ago. However, the scope of practice for Emergency Medical Responders and other EMS personnel is based in part on the U.S. Department of Transportation's (DOT's) national standard curricula and, in most cases, is more clearly defined by local and state statutes and regulations. Questions relating to scope of practice typically ask, "Were you allowed to perform the care that you did?"

STANDARD OF CARE

standard of care ■ the care that should be provided for any level of training based on local laws, administrative orders, and guidelines and protocols established by the local EMS system.

The term **standard of care** is more subjective and deals with questions such as "Did you do the right thing, at the right time, and for the right reasons?" It is defined by several factors, such as scope of practice, common practice, current research, and sometimes juries. Just like the scope of practice, standard of care can and does vary from county to county, state to state, and region to region (Figure 2.1).

A standard of care allows you to be judged based on what is expected of someone with your training and experience working under similar conditions. Your Emergency Medical Responder course follows guidelines developed by the U.S. DOT as well as other authorities that have studied what is needed to provide the most appropriate standard of care required at your level in your region. You will be trained so that you can provide this standard of care. If the care you provide is not up to the expected standard, you may be held liable for your actions.

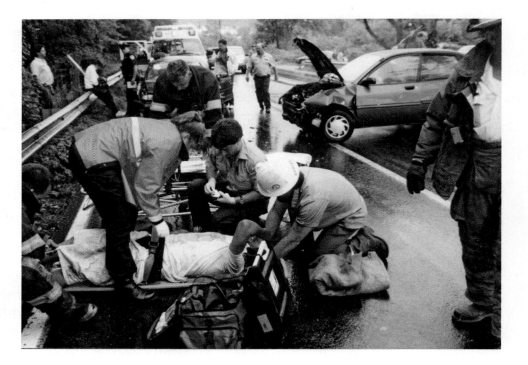

FIGURE 2.1 Different emergency personnel may be assisting during an emergency, including police, firefighters, and EMTs. Each must adhere to a specific standard of care. *(© Mark C. Ide)*

You may be required to communicate with your Medical Director by telephone or radio, and you will be expected to follow approved standing orders or protocols for your EMS system.

Keep written notes of what you do at the emergency scene, especially if a crime has occurred. You may be called on to provide this information at a later date. If your EMS system requires you to complete forms, submit reports, or sign patient transfer papers, complete these forms thoroughly and in a timely manner. Your documentation must be able to show that you provided an appropriate standard of care.

ETHICAL RESPONSIBILITIES

Ethics can be simply defined as "behavior." However it is not any behavior, but behavior that is right, good, and proper. As an Emergency Medical Responder, you have an ethical obligation to behave in a way that puts your patient's needs before your own, as long as it is safe to do so (Figure 2.2). You have a responsibility to see that the patient receives the most appropriate medical care possible, even when he does not think any care is needed. Another ethical responsibility as a member of the EMS team is to constantly maintain your skills and knowledge. This includes keeping abreast of recent research by reading professional publications and attending conferences when practical. It also means practicing your skills in order to maintain confidence and an appropriate level of mastery. You also must attend continuing education and refresher programs because it is necessary to keep yourself ready to perform at all times. Remember, every patient deserves the best care possible.

It is also important for you to be honest in reporting the care you provided to a patient, even if a mistake was made. Although EMS providers should always attempt to provide the appropriate care, mistakes do occur. Errors should be reported immediately so corrective steps, if needed, may be taken as soon as possible.

Behavior (ethics) is determined by beliefs (values). Doing the right thing is not always easy and can cause you internal struggles. Many groups and professions have a common set of shared values. These values serve as a "moral compass" and help guide an individual's decision-making process. Because EMS personnel are frequently faced with making difficult decisions, several EMS groups, agencies, and institutions have adopted the following set of values:

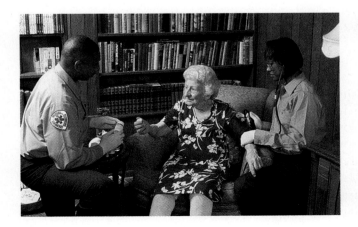

FIGURE 2.2 Ethical conduct means that Emergency Medical Responders give all patients respectful and considerate care.

- Integrity.
- Compassion.
- Accountability.
- Respect.
- Empathy.

1–3.3 Define consent and discuss the methods of obtaining consent.

competence ■ the state of being competent, or properly or sufficiently qualified or capable of making appropriate decisions about one's own health or condition.

Consent

COMPETENCE

A discussion about consent would not be complete without a clear definition of the word *competence*. **Competence** is the patient's ability to understand an Emergency Medical Responder's questions and the implications of decisions made. For an Emergency Medical Responder to get consent or accept a refusal of care, he should establish whether or not the patient is competent to make such decisions. A patient may not be competent to make medical decisions in certain cases, such as when intoxicated, under the influence of drugs, or has a serious injury or mental illness. To determine competency, the Emergency Medical Responder may begin by asking questions that a competent adult should be able to answer, such as where the patient is at the time, what day or month it is, and what has happened to him. Answering these questions, however, does not always establish competence, as in the case of suicidal patients.

Geriatric Focus

Approximately 15% of all people in the United States older than the age of 65 demonstrate some degree of dementia. *Dementia* is the deterioration of specific mental capacities such as memory, concentration, and judgment. One of the most common causes of dementia is Alzheimer's disease.

An elderly patient with dementia may not fully comprehend the seriousness of his situation and may not want you to provide care. In other words, the elderly patient with dementia may not be competent to make decisions regarding his own medical care.

When presented with an elderly patient who is showing signs of disorientation, a short attention span, confusion, or hallucinations, obtain a detailed history from family members or caregivers. It will be important to determine if the patient's mental status is normal for him or if it has gotten worse.

Do not allow patients who are showing signs of dementia to refuse care without further investigation into their normal state of mind. In most cases, you will want to wait for the EMTs to arrive and take over care before you leave the scene.

REFUSAL OF CARE

1–3.6 Discuss the implications for the Emergency Medical Responder in patient refusal of transport.

FIRST ➤ Alert and competent adults have the right to refuse care. Their refusal may be based on a variety of reasons, including their economic situation or religious views. They may even base it on a lack of trust. Or, they may have reasons that you find senseless. For whatever reason, competent adults may refuse care. You may not force care on them, nor may you restrain them. Restraining any patient against his or her wishes could result in a charge of battery for the Emergency Medical Responder. Your only course of action is to try to gain a patient's confidence through conversation. If this fails and you feel the patient is at risk, you may have to call in law enforcement.

A patient does not have to speak to refuse your care. If the patient shakes his head to signal "no" or if he holds up a hand to signal you to stop, the patient has refused your help. If the patient pulls away from you, this may also be viewed as refusal of care.

It is important for you to understand the laws that govern patient refusal in your area. In many jurisdictions, an Emergency Medical Responder cannot leave a patient who is refusing care until an EMT has arrived and taken over patient care. ■

When your services are refused:

■ Do not argue with a patient.
■ Do not question a patient's reasons if they are based on religious beliefs.
■ Do not touch a patient. If you do, this could be considered battery.
■ Stay calm and professional.
■ Make certain that dispatch is alerted, even if a patient has stated that he does not want help.
■ Talk with the patient. Let him know that you are concerned. Tell him that you respect his right to refuse care, but that you think he should reconsider your offer to help.
■ Explain in plain and simple terms what the consequences are of refusing care. In other words, a patient with chest pain who refuses care may be at risk of cardiac arrest. This must be explained to the patient.
■ Carefully document the refusal of care. Document your offer of help, an explanation of your level of training, why you think care is needed, the consequences of not accepting care, and the patient's refusal to accept your care. Also document the names of anyone who witnessed your efforts to assist the patient. If your EMS system provides you with release forms, ask the patient to please read and sign the form. Make certain that you ask him if he understands what he has read before he signs the form.

A parent or legal guardian can refuse to let you care for a child. If the reason is fear or lack of confidence, simple conversation may change the individual's mind. In cases involving children, if the adult takes the child from the scene before EMTs arrive, you must report the incident to the EMTs or to the police. All states have special laws protecting the welfare of children. Such information may have to be passed on to the courts in order to find out if the child eventually received needed care. Know the laws in your state and jurisdiction regarding reporting such events. In all cases, know and follow local protocols.

EXPRESSED CONSENT

FIRST ➤ An adult patient of legal age, when alert and competent, can give consent to provide care. In Emergency Medical Responder care, a patient's consent is usually oral and commonly referred to as **expressed consent** (also referred to as informed consent). To qualify as expressed consent, the patient must be making an informed decision (Figure 2.3).

For a patient to make an informed decision, you need to advise the patient of the following:

■ Your level of training.
■ Why you think care may be necessary.
■ What care you plan to provide.
■ Any consequences related to refusing care. ■

1–3.4 Differentiate between expressed and implied consent.

expressed consent ■ consent to emergency care that is given to an Emergency Medical Responder by a competent adult who has made an informed decision. Also referred to as *informed consent*.

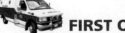

FIRST ON SCENE

Heather approaches the man lying in the road and finds him unresponsive. With each raspy breath, blood pours from his mouth and collects on the pavement in a shining pool. Unsure exactly what to do, she walks over to the overturned car where she finds a woman, clad in a bright bikini top and cut-off jean shorts, pinned between the passenger door and the tree.

"Hello?" Heather says. "Are you okay?" The woman moans softly, but her eyes remain closed.

Mike is now off the motorcycle and staring at the man in the road. "Come on!" he shouts to Heather. "My cell phone has no signal. Let's go find a pay phone!"

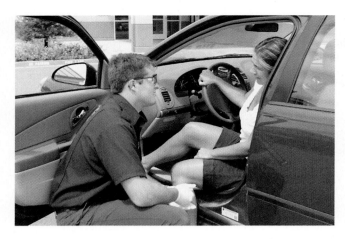

You must receive consent before caring for any patient. A simple way to gain this consent can be by stating something like, "Hi, my name is Chris. I am an Emergency Medical Responder. May I help you?" A patient who is responsive may answer verbally or simply allow you to continue your care. Expressed consent does not need to be verbal. By *not* pulling away or stopping you, the patient is giving consent.

There are occasions when a child refuses care. By law, only a parent or guardian of the child may give consent or refuse care. Of course, gaining the child's confidence and easing any fears should be part of your care.

FIGURE 2.3 Obtaining consent from an adult patient prior to providing care.

1–3.5 Explain the role of consent of minors in providing care.

unresponsive ■ no reaction to verbal or painful stimuli; previously referred to as *unconscious*.

implied consent ■ a legal position that assumes an unresponsive or incompetent adult patient would consent to receiving emergency care if he could. This form of consent may apply to other types of patients (for example, the mentally ill).

IMPLIED CONSENT

In emergency situations in which a patient is **unresponsive**, confused, or so severely ill or injured that expressed consent cannot be given, you may legally provide care based on **implied consent**. It is implied that the patient would want to receive care and treatment if he or she was aware of the situation and able to respond. Because children are not legally allowed to provide consent or to refuse medical care, a form of implied consent is used in most states when parents or guardians are not on the scene and cannot be reached quickly. The law assumes that the parents would want care to be provided for their child (Figure 2.4). The same holds true in cases involving the developmentally disabled, the mentally ill, or patients experiencing a behavioral emergency. It is assumed that their parents or legal guardians would give consent for treatment.

FIGURE 2.4 You may provide care to a minor based on implied consent when a parent or guardian is not available.

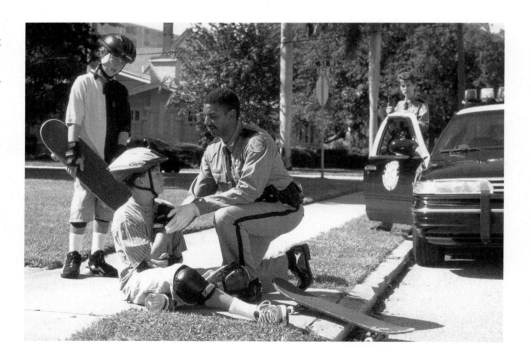

Do Not Resuscitate Orders

FIRST ➤ At some time, you will come upon a patient who has a Do Not Resuscitate (DNR) order. This is typically in the form of a written document, usually signed by the patient and his or her physician, which states that the patient has a terminal illness and does not want to prolong life through resuscitative efforts. A DNR order is one type of *advance directive* because it is written and signed in advance of any event where resuscitation may be undertaken (Figure 2.5). A DNR order is more than the expressed wishes of the patient or family. It is an actual legal document. In some cases, the patient will be wearing a DNR bracelet. This should

1–3.2 Discuss the importance of Do Not Resuscitate (DNR) orders (advance directives) and local or state provisions regarding EMS application.

PREHOSPITAL DO NOT RESUSCITATE ORDERS

<u>ATTENDING PHYSICIAN</u>

In completing this prehospital DNR form, please check part A if no intervention by prehospital personnel is indicated. Please check Part A and options from Part B if specific interventions by prehospital personnel are indicated. To give a valid prehospital DNR order, this form must be completed by the patient's attending physician and must be provided to prehospital personnel.

A) _____ **Do Not Resuscitate (DNR):**
No Cardiopulmonary Resuscitation or Advanced Cardiac Life Support be performed by prehospital personnel

B) _____ **Modified Support:**
Prehospital personnel administer the following checked options:
_____ Oxygen administration
_____ Full airway support: intubation, airways, bag/valve/mask
_____ Venipuncture: IV crystalloids and/or blood draw
_____ External cardiac pacing
_____ Cardiopulmonary resuscitation
_____ Cardiac defibrillator
_____ Pneumatic anti-shock garment
_____ Ventilator
_____ ACLS meds
_____ Other interventions/medications (physician specify)
_____

Prehospital personnel are informed that (print patient name)_____ should receive no resuscitation (DNR) or should receive Modified Support as indicated. This directive is medically appropriate and is further documented by a physician's order and a progress note on the patient's permanent medical record. Informed consent from the capacitated patient or the incapacitated patient's legitimate surrogate is documented on the patient's permanent medical record. The DNR order is in full force and effect as of the date indicated below.

_____

Attending Physician's Signature

_____

_____

Print Attending Physician's Name

Print Patient's Name and Location
(Home Address or Health Care Facility)

_____

Attending Physician's Telephone

_____

Date

Expiration Date (6 Mos from Signature)

FIGURE 2.5 A DNR order is one example of an advance directive. Other examples include health-care proxies and living wills.

not be mistaken for a medical identification bracelet, which gives information about medical conditions and/or allergies. ∎

There are varying degrees of DNR orders, expressed through a variety of detailed instructions. For example, one DNR order might stipulate that resuscitation be attempted only if cardiac or respiratory arrest is observed, but *not* attempted if the patient is found already in cardiac arrest. Another DNR order might specify that only assisted ventilations may be administered should the patient stop breathing, but if the heart stops, chest compressions are not to be provided.

The presence of a DNR order does not mean "do not care." As an Emergency Medical Responder, you have a duty to provide appropriate comfort and care within the bounds of the DNR. It is also within the patient's rights to withdraw the DNR order at any time.

Many states also have laws governing living wills. These are statements signed by the patient, commonly about the use of long-term life support and comfort measures such as respirators, IV feedings, and pain medications.

Negligence *Refusals also have lots lawsuits*

FIRST ➤ The basis for most medical lawsuits involving prehospital emergency care is **negligence**. This is a term often used to indicate that a care provider either did not do what was expected or did something carelessly. However, from a legal standpoint, negligence is much more complicated.

For a lawsuit alleging negligence to be successful, the following four elements must be established:

- *Duty to act.* The Emergency Medical Responder had a legal duty to provide care.
- *Breach of duty.* Care for the patient was not provided to an acceptable standard of care.
- *Damages.* The patient was injured (damaged) in some way as a result of improper care or the lack thereof.
- *Causation.* A direct link can be established between the damages and the breach of duty on the part of the Emergency Medical Responder. ∎

In many cases, Emergency Medical Responders have a legal **duty to act**. Those functioning as part of a fire service, rescue squad, police agency, or formal response team may be legally obliged to respond and render care. This means that they are required, at least while on duty, to provide care according to their agency's standard operating procedures. In some localities, this duty to act may also apply to paid Emergency Medical Responders when they are off duty.

The concept of a "duty to act" can be less clear in the case of Emergency Medical Responders working in a business office or industrial environment. When in doubt, it is best to provide care and call for help.

Because the laws governing the duty to act vary from state to state, your instructor can inform you of the specifics in your state or region. In most cases, an Emergency Medical Responder is considered to have a duty to act once help is offered to a patient. If care is offered and then accepted by the patient, a legal

negligence ∎ a failure to provide the expected standard of care.

duty to act ∎ a legal requirement that Emergency Medical Responders while on duty must provide care according to their department's standard operating procedures.

1–3.8 State the conditions necessary for the Emergency Medical Responder to have a duty to act.

duty to act has been established, and the Emergency Medical Responder must remain at the scene until someone of equal or higher training takes over for them.

After a duty to act has been established, the second condition for negligence would be applicable if care was substandard for the Emergency Medical Responder's level of training and experience under the conditions of the emergency scene. The same would apply if the care rendered was beyond the scope of practice.

Finally, if there was a duty to act and the standard of care was not met, a suit for negligence may be successful if the patient was injured (damaged) in some way due directly to the inappropriate actions of the Emergency Medical Responder. This is a complex legal concept, made more difficult by the fact that the damage may be physical, emotional, or psychological.

Physical damage is the easiest to understand. For example, if an Emergency Medical Responder moved a patient's injured leg before applying a splint and the standard of care states that the Emergency Medical Responder should have suspected a fracture and placed a splint on the limb, then the Emergency Medical Responder may be negligent if this action worsened the existing injury.

The same case becomes much more involved when the patient claims that the Emergency Medical Responder's inappropriate action caused emotional or psychological problems. The court could decide that the patient has been damaged and establish the third requirement for negligence.

Inappropriate care does not always involve splinting, bandaging, or some other physical skill. As a general rule, you should always advise a patient to seek treatment by EMTs and to go to the hospital. If you tell an ill or injured patient that he does not need to be seen by more highly trained personnel, you could be negligent if you had a duty to act and the patient accepted your care, but:

- The standard of care stated that you should have alerted or had someone activate the EMS system to request an EMT response, and you failed to do so.
- Delay in more advanced care caused complications that led to additional injury.

FIRST ➤ As stated previously, a requirement for proof of negligence is the failure of the Emergency Medical Responder to provide care to a recognized and acceptable standard of care. There is no guarantee that you will not be sued, but a successful suit is unlikely if you provide care to an acceptable standard. ■

If your state has **Good Samaritan laws**, you may be protected from civil liability if you act in good faith to provide care to the level of your training and to the best of your ability. You will be trained to deliver the standard of care expected of Emergency Medical Responders in your area. Your instructor will explain the laws specific to your locality.

Good Samaritan laws ■ laws designed to protect care providers who deliver care in good faith, to the level of their training, and without compensation.

Abandonment

FIRST ➤ Once you begin to help someone who is sick or injured, you have established a legal duty and must continue to provide care until you transfer patient care to someone of equal or higher training (such as an EMT or physician). If you leave

1–3.7 Discuss the issues of abandonment, negligence, and battery, and their implications to the Emergency Medical Responder.

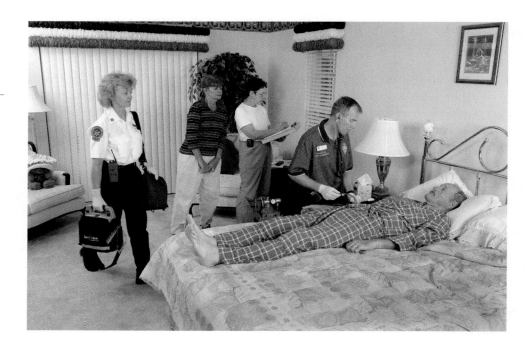

FIGURE 2.6 Once care is initiated, the Emergency Medical Responder assumes responsibility for the patient until relieved by more highly trained personnel.

abandonment ■ to leave a sick or injured patient before equal or more highly trained personnel can assume responsibility for care.

REMEMBER

Patient confidentiality does not apply if you are required by law to report certain incidents (such as rape, abuse, or neglect), if you are asked to provide information to the police, or if you receive a subpoena to testify in court. Maintain notes about each incident to which you respond, and keep a copy of any official documents filled out by you or responding EMTs.

1–3.9 Explain the importance, necessity, and legality of patient confidentiality.

the scene before more highly trained personnel arrive, you may be guilty of abandoning the patient and may be subject to legal action under specific laws of **abandonment** (Figure 2.6).

Because you are not trained in medical diagnosis or in how to predict the stability of a patient, you should not leave a patient even if someone with training equal to your own arrives at the scene. The patient may develop more serious problems that would be better handled by two Emergency Medical Responders.

Some legal authorities consider abandonment to include the failure to turn over patient information during the transfer of the patient to more highly trained personnel. You must inform those providers of the facts that you gathered, the assessment made, and the care rendered. ■

Is It Safe ?

One of the most common places abandonment is likely to occur is in the emergency department of the hospital. This occurs when an Emergency Medical Responder or EMT arrives at the emergency department with a patient and then leaves without a proper hand off to an appropriate ED staff member. If the patient suddenly becomes worse and a proper hand off was not performed, it can be said that the Emergency Medical Responder or EMT abandoned the patient and therefore may be liable for any damages the patient may suffer. Never leave a patient anywhere without properly handing them over to the next level of care, which includes a full verbal report. ■

CONFIDENTIALITY

Confidentiality is an important concept for those who deal with and care for patients. As an Emergency Medical Responder, you should not speak to your friends, family, and other members of the public (including the press and media)

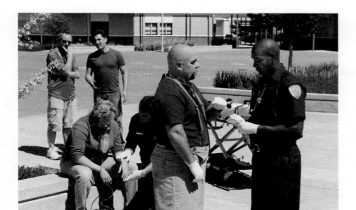

FIGURE 2.7 To maintain patient confidentiality, discuss your patient only with those who will be continuing patient care.

about the details of care you have provided to a patient. You should not name the individuals who received your care. If you speak of the emergency, you should not relate specifics about what a patient may have said, any unusual aspects of behavior, or any descriptions of personal appearance. To do so invades the privacy of the patient. Your state may not have specific laws stating these limitations, but most individuals in emergency care feel strongly about protecting the patient's right to privacy.

confidentiality ■ refers to the treatment of information that an individual has disclosed in a relationship of trust and with the expectation that it will not be divulged to others.

Information about an emergency and patient care should only be released if the patient has authorized you to do so in writing or you receive an appropriate request from a court or law enforcement agency. In all other cases, refer requests for patient information to your supervisor or other appropriate person.

Authorization is not required for you to pass on patient information to other health-care providers who are part of the continued care of the patient (Figure 2.7). This sharing of information with those involved in the care of the patient is a necessary and important part of good patient care (Figure 2.8).

One law that governs confidentiality, the *Health Insurance Portability and Accountability Act (HIPAA)*, went into effect in 2003 and dictates the extent to which patient information can be shared. HIPAA gives patients more control over their own health care information and limits the way that information is stored and shared with others. It also establishes strong accountability for the use and sharing of patient information.

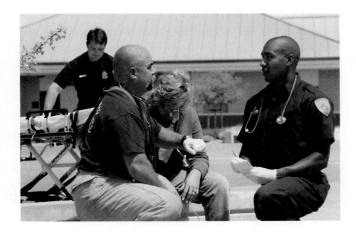

FIGURE 2.8 During transfer of patient care, sharing of information with those involved in the care of the patient is a necessary and important part of good patient care.

Is It Safe ?

It is only natural to want to discuss the calls you respond to and the patients you care for with your colleagues, friends, and family. However, be cautious. One of your legal and ethical obligations is patient confidentiality. Discuss with your instructor with whom and what you can talk about before you accidently share something that you should not. It is better to be safe than sorry. If in doubt, don't share! ▪

A good rule of thumb regarding the sharing of patient information is: when in doubt, do not share. Your instructor will explain in detail what types of information may be shared and in what situations.

1–3.11 State the conditions that require an Emergency Medical Responder to notify local law enforcement officials.

Reportable Events

All 50 states have laws that define "mandatory reporters" and what types of events they must report. What differs from state to state is who is considered a mandatory reporter. For example, all Emergency Medical Responders must report certain events or conditions that they know or suspect have occurred. These events may include such things as exposures to certain infectious diseases, suspicious burns, vehicle crashes, drug-related injuries, crimes that result in knife or gunshot wounds, child and elder abuse, domestic violence, and rape. Check with your chief officer, EMS division chief, or with state and federal agencies to learn which incidents are reportable in your area and to whom or to which agency you should report them.

Most states have included Emergency Medical Responders in the list of mandatory reporters for cases of known or suspected child or elder abuse and neglect. You must ask your instructor to share with you the list of defined mandatory reporters in your state. You may also find this information by performing a simple search on the Internet for "mandatory reporter" plus your state's name.

FIRST ON SCENE

Heather realizes that she can't safely reach the woman pinned by the car and decides to try to help the man in the road. She shakes off her backpack, rummages through it, and pulls out two large beach towels.

"Help me roll him onto his side," she says to Mike. "Slow and careful!"

They are able to get the man onto his side and clear much of the blood from his mouth and nose.

"Hey, here comes a car," Mike says as he holds the man's head still. "Let's have them stay here with these people while we go get help."

"I've already started helping them," Heather says and grabs one of her oversized beach towels to flag down the oncoming car. "I can't leave now."

The approaching car slows to a stop, and the windows are suddenly filled with round, curious faces.

"Listen," Heather runs to the driver's side. "These people are really hurt. I need you to find a phone and call 9-1-1!"

Special Situations

ORGAN DONORS

You may respond to a call where a critically injured patient is near death and has been identified as an *organ donor*. An organ donor is a patient who has completed a legal document that allows for donation of organs and tissues in the event of his or her death. A family member may give you this information, or you may find an organ donor card in a patient's personal effects. Sometimes this information is indicated on the patient's driver license.

Emergency care of a patient who is an organ donor must not differ in any way from the care of a patient who is not a donor. All emergency care measures must be taken regardless of donor status.

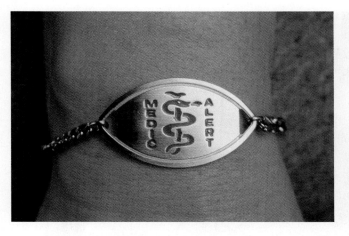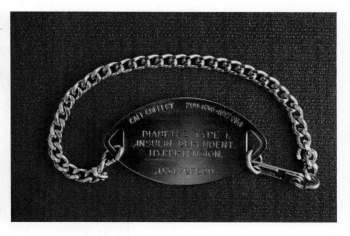

FIGURE 2.9 The MedicAlert bracelet is one example of a medical identification device (front and back shown).

MEDICAL IDENTIFICATION DEVICES

Another special situation involves the patient who wears a medical identification device (Figure 2.9). This device—a necklace, arm or ankle bracelet, or card—is meant to alert EMS personnel to the patient's particular medical condition, such as a heart problem, allergies, diabetes, or epilepsy. If the patient is unresponsive or unable to answer questions, this device may provide important medical information.

In some areas of the country, the "Vial of Life" program is currently in use. This program includes a special vial where important medical information is stored and a window sticker that alerts EMS personnel to the presence of the vial. The vial is kept in the patient's refrigerator, where it can be found easily by rescuers.

CRIME SCENES

A *crime scene* is defined as the location where a crime has been committed or any place where evidence relating to a crime may be found. Many crime scenes involve injuries to people and therefore require the assistance of EMS personnel. If you suspect a crime has been committed, do not enter the scene until instructed to do so by law enforcement personnel.

When an Emergency Medical Responder is providing care at a crime scene, certain actions should be taken to preserve evidence. Make as little impact on the scene as possible, only moving items necessary for patient care. Take special care to note the position of the patient and preserve any clothing you may remove or damage. Try not to cut through holes in clothing from gunshot wounds or stabbings. Remember to report any items you move or touch.

1–3.10 List the actions that an Emergency Medical Responder should take to assist in the preservation of a crime scene.

Documentation

Documentation is an important part of the patient care process and may last long after the call is over. Some states do not require Emergency Medical Responders to complete specific types of documentation, but you would be wise to keep records of all calls to which you respond (Figure 2.10). They may be needed in the event of subpoena or lawsuit. Your instructor will inform you of legal requirements in your area.

1–3.12 Discuss issues concerning the fundamental components of documentation.

FIGURE 2.10 Even if you are not required to do so, keep records of all calls to which you respond in case they are needed as evidence in court.

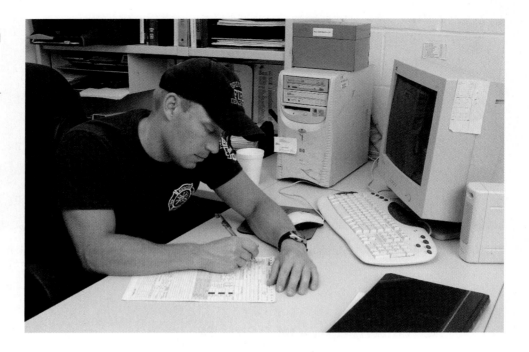

In special situations, you may be required by law to make written or verbal reports. Special situations include child, elder, or spouse abuse; wounds sustained or potentially sustained by violent crime; sexual assault; or infectious disease exposure. Again, your instructor will inform you of requirements in your area.

FIRST ON SCENE WRAP-UP

About 30 minutes later, just when Heather was beginning to think that the people in the car might have just kept on driving, she hears sirens approaching. "What a sweet sound!" she thinks to herself. Within moments, the scene is filled with firefighters in bulky yellow coats and pants, carrying multicolored bags and shouting information to each other.

The man on the road is quickly loaded into an ambulance, which rushes away with sirens blaring. Heather turns and walks over to see what they are doing to help the trapped woman. The firefighters have peeled most of the car away using large, noisy power tools. Once the woman is finally freed, Heather sees that the woman's left leg is nearly severed at about midthigh.

With a sigh, Heather makes her way past the blood and bent pieces of the small car and finds Mike over by the motorcycle. She hugs him, and they both watch silently as the second ambulance pulls away and disappears around the same bend as the first.

Summary

Emergency Medical Responders have to learn and maintain their skills and knowledge to a level where they can perform patient care to the expected standard of care. In many states, specific laws known as Good Samaritan laws have been written to allow you to provide emergency care to patients without fear of civil legal action being taken against you. That is, you may be protected if you act in good faith, not for compensation, to a standard of care at your level of training and to the best of your abilities.

You must have expressed (informed) consent from a responsive, competent adult patient before you may provide care. This consent is usually verbal but may be nonverbal as well. In cases in which the patient is unable to give consent, such as when he is unresponsive, you may care for the patient under the law of implied consent. Implied consent also applies to children and emotionally or mentally disturbed patients when their parents or legal guardians are not present.

A patient may refuse your care.

An Emergency Medical Responder may be guilty of negligence if the following elements can be established:

duty to act, breach of duty, damages, and causation. That is, negligence is proved when it can be established that EMS personnel had a legal duty to provide care, did not provide care to an acceptable standard of care, and the inappropriate care caused damage (injury) to the patient. When you stop to provide care, you are responsible for the patient until someone more highly trained takes over.

If you begin to care for a patient and then leave the scene, you can be charged with abandonment.

Keep in mind that patients have a right to privacy, so you must respect patient confidentiality. Also remember that care for organ donors should not differ from care given to any other patient, that medical identification devices worn or carried by a patient can provide important medical information, and that you should try to preserve evidence when caring for a patient at a crime scene.

Documentation is part of the patient care process. Always keep detailed and accurate records of the care you provide.

Remember and Consider

Every time you respond to a call, you will be faced with some aspect of a legal or ethical issue. It may be as simple as making sure the patient is willing to accept your help or as complex as a terminally ill patient who refuses your care. You may have to decide whether or not to stop and help even though you are off duty. You may worry about being sued.

Investigate

Knowledge is your best protection. Each state enacts laws that protect citizens, but state laws vary. Be sure you are familiar with the laws of your state that guide the actions of Emergency Medical Responders. Check with your agency's legal office or with your supervising officers on the legal details of patient consent and care.

➤ Find out what types of consent forms and run sheets for documentation are used in your jurisdiction.

➤ Obtain and review a sample DNR order from the library or an attorney. Find out if DNR bracelets are used and accepted in your jurisdiction.

➤ Learn about different types of evidence and the ways you may help preserve a crime scene.

Quick Quiz

1. Which one of the following terms is best defined as what an Emergency Medical Responder is allowed to do based on DOT National Standard Curricula as well as state and local statutes and regulations?

    a. standard of care
    b. scope of practice
    c. duty
    d. negligence

2. Which one of the following is an example of an advanced directive?

   a. protocols
   b. standing orders
   c. Do Not Resuscitate (DNR) order
   d. medical direction

3. What type of consent is necessary from responsive, competent adult patients?

   a. implied
   b. applied
   c. absentee
   d. expressed

4. Which one of the following is NOT true about expressed consent?

   a. It is also known as informed consent.
   b. It must always be given verbally by the patient.
   c. It can be given by parents of minors on their behalf.
   d. The patient must be informed of your intentions.

5. What type of consent is used when a patient is unresponsive?

   a. informed
   b. expressed
   c. assumed
   d. implied

6. Which one of the following patients may legally refuse care at the scene of an emergency?

   a. 11-year-old boy who was hit by a car while riding his bicycle
   b. 26-year-old unresponsive overdose patient
   c. 46-year-old intoxicated driver of a vehicle involved in a collision
   d. 68-year-old alert woman having chest pain

7. Which one of the following is NOT an element required for a claim of negligence?

   a. duty
   b. absence of duty
   c. damages
   d. causation

8. Most states require Emergency Medical Responders and other EMS personnel to report incidents involving known or suspected:

   a. gun use.
   b. addiction.
   c. child abuse or neglect.
   d. sexual activity.

9. Which one of the following should take place BEFORE you enter a known crime scene?

   a. The scene must be made safe by law enforcement personnel.
   b. The scene must be made safe by fire personnel.
   c. You must have the permission of your supervisor.
   d. You must wait for the EMTs to arrive.

10. Which one of the following is MOST likely a breach of patient confidentiality by an Emergency Medical Responder?

   a. provides detailed information about the patient to the nurse in the emergency department
   b. returns to the station and shares details of the call with colleagues
   c. shares details of the patient's condition with the EMTs who are taking over care
   d. provides details about the emergency after being subpoenaed to the court

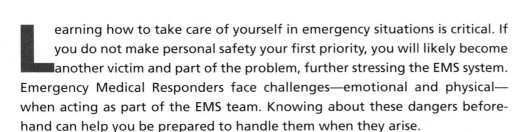

Well-Being of the Emergency Medical Responder

Learning how to take care of yourself in emergency situations is critical. If you do not make personal safety your first priority, you will likely become another victim and part of the problem, further stressing the EMS system. Emergency Medical Responders face challenges—emotional and physical— when acting as part of the EMS team. Knowing about these dangers before- hand can help you be prepared to handle them when they arise.

This chapter helps you learn what to expect and describes how you can assist yourself, the patient, the patient's family, your own family, and other Emergency Medical Responders in dealing with stress. Aspects of personal safety, including how you can protect yourself from infectious diseases, are also presented.

OBJECTIVES

This chapter is based on the objectives of the U.S. DOT's First Responder National Standard Curriculum. Note that cognitive objectives are listed below and beside corresponding text throughout the chapter. You will also notice as you read each objective that the term Emergency Medical Responder is used. This is simply a name change and reflects the new name for the First Responder.

By the end of this chapter, you should be able to (from cognitive or knowledge information):

1–2.1   List possible emotional reactions that the Emergency Medical Responder may experience when faced with trauma, illness, death, and dying. (pp. 40–43)

1–2.2   Discuss the possible reactions that a patient's family member may exhibit when confronted with the patient's death or dying. (pp. 39–40)

1–2.3   State the steps in the Emergency Medical Responder's approach to the family confronted with death and dying. (p. 40)

1–2.4   State the possible reactions that the family of the Emergency Medical Responder may exhibit. (p. 43)

1–2.5   Recognize the signs and symptoms of critical incident stress. (p. 43)

1–2.6   State possible steps that the Emergency Medical Responder may take to help reduce/alleviate stress. (pp. 43–45)

1–2.7   Explain the need to determine scene safety. (pp. 53–55)

1–2.8   Discuss the importance of body substance isolation (BSI). (pp. 47–53)

1–2.9   Describe the steps the Emergency Medical Responder should take for personal protection from airborne and bloodborne pathogens. (pp. 49–53)

1–2.10   List the personal protective equipment neces- sary for each of the following situations: hazardous materials, rescue operations, exposure to bloodborne and airborne pathogens, violent scenes, crime scenes, and electricity. (pp. 47–53, 53–55)

By the end of this chapter, you should be able to feel comfortable enough to (by changing attitudes, values, and beliefs):

1–2.11 Explain the importance of serving as an advocate for the use of appropriate protective equipment. (p. 47)

1–2.12 Explain the importance of understanding the response to death and dying and communicating effectively with the patient's family. (pp. 39–40)

1–2.13 Demonstrate a caring attitude toward any patient with illness or injury who requests emergency medical services. (pp. 40, 52)

1–2.14 Show compassion when caring for the physical and mental needs of patients. (pp. 39–40)

1–2.15 Participate willingly in the care of all patients. (p. 52)

1–2.16 Communicate with empathy to patients being cared for, as well as with family members and friends of the patient. (pp. 39–40)

By the end of this chapter, you should be able to show how to (through psychomotor skills):

1–2.17 Use appropriate personal protective equipment, given a scenario with potential infectious exposure. At the completion of the scenario, the Emergency Medical Responder will properly remove and discard the protective garments. (pp. 48–49)

1–2.18 Complete disinfection/cleaning and all reporting documentation, given the above scenario. (pp. 47–50)

ADDITIONAL LEARNING TASKS

Many states and regions have a crisis intervention or a critical incident stress management (CISM) team in place to help responders deal with the stress of a difficult emergency. Talk with your agency and find out about crisis intervention resources. Be able to:

➤ Identify the crisis intervention or CISM team in your region and determine how to access its services.

Protecting yourself—and your patients—from infectious diseases is important. You must wear protective equipment when responding to emergencies, and you should use special disinfectants to clean equipment. As an Emergency Medical Responder, you must be able to:

➤ Put on and use all personal protective equipment in appropriate situations.
➤ Take off and appropriately discard or dispose of all personal protective equipment.
➤ Disinfect or clean all nondisposable equipment used in patient care.
➤ Properly dispose of all disposable equipment used in patient care.

One of your most important jobs is to stay safe, both physically and emotionally. If you become a victim, you will be of little or no use to a patient, and you may actually put other rescuers in danger. Safeguard yourself by doing the following:

➤ Learn about stressors and understand how to deal with them, especially those that accompany critical incidents.
➤ Constantly evaluate scene safety.
➤ Before providing emergency care to a patient, always use appropriate body substance isolation (BSI) precautions. That includes wearing gloves at a minimum, and eye protection or face mask and gown as necessary.

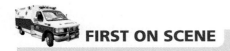

FIRST ON SCENE

Jake swallows the last of his hot chocolate, steps carefully across the rubber flooring, and glides back onto the smooth ice of the skating rink. He can't help but smile. Everything is perfect, from the crispness of the air to the sweet aftertaste of the chocolate and the warmth radiating from his exercising muscles. He glides toward a woman who is helping a small boy with wobbly ankles to skate—like a scene from a Norman Rockwell painting. Just as he passes them, the woman pinwheels her arms and grabs for the railing that runs around the edges of the rink.

Jake digs his blades in for a quick stop, sending a spray of ice shavings into the air, and grabs for the woman's flailing arms. He just misses her fingers and watches as she crashes onto her back, her head bouncing off the ice with a thud. She immediately sits up, laces both hands together on the back of her head, and begins to rock back and forth. Her cry of pain echoes across the rink.

"Are you okay?" Jake asks. He kneels next to her and places a hand on her shaking shoulders. "I'm an Emergency Medical Responder," Jake says. "May I help you?"

She doesn't respond but continues weeping and rocking. The boy is now sobbing, too, and trying to hold on to her jacket as he watches Jake fearfully.

It's then that Jake notices blood falling in large round splatters onto the ice. "Oh hey, you're bleeding," he says.

The woman suddenly looks wide eyed at Jake and then at the boy and scoots frantically backward away from both of them. "Stay away!" She hisses between sobs. "Just stay away."

Emotional Aspects of Emergency Medical Care

DEATH AND DYING

As an Emergency Medical Responder, you will at some time have to deal with a patient who has a terminal illness. Such patients and their families will have many different reactions to the illness. A basic understanding of what they are going through will help you deal with their stress and your own.

When a patient finds out that he is dying, he will go through several stages, each varying in duration and magnitude. Sometimes those stages are not experienced in the same order given below, and sometimes they overlap one another. Whatever the length or order of these stages, they all affect both the patient and his family. The stages include:

- *Denial, or "not me."* The patient denies that he is dying and puts off having to deal with the situation. Often, the patient displays strong disbelief.
- *Anger, or "why me?"* The patient is angry about the situation. This anger is often vented on family members or even EMS personnel.
- *Bargaining, or "OK, but first let me . . ."* The patient feels that making bargains will postpone the inevitable.
- *Depression, or "OK, but I haven't . . ."* The patient becomes sad, depressed, and often mourns things that he has not accomplished. He then may become unwilling to communicate with others.
- *Acceptance, or "OK, I'm not afraid."* The patient works through all the stages and finally is able to accept death, even though he may not welcome it. Frequently, the patient will reach this stage before family members do, in which case he may find himself comforting them.

1–2.2 Discuss the possible reactions that a patient's family member may exhibit when confronted with the patient's death or dying.

1–2.3 State the steps in the Emergency Medical Responder's approach to the family confronted with death and dying.

Many times a patient's family member or loved one will respond by going through these same stages. Be mindful. Do not neglect their need for information and compassion. Several approaches are appropriate when dealing with situations such as these. Emergency Medical Responders may offer patients and their families the following courtesies:

- Recognize patient needs. Treat your patient with respect and do whatever is possible to preserve his dignity and sense of control. Speak directly to the patient and avoid talking about him to family members or friends in his presence. Try to respond to his choices about how to handle the situation. Allow the patient to talk about feelings, even though it may make you uncomfortable. Respect the patient's privacy if he does not want to express personal feelings.
- Be tolerant of angry reactions from the patient or family members. Sometimes they will direct their anger at you, but do not take it personally. The patient and family need a chance to vent, and they will often choose whoever is nearby as a target.
- Listen empathetically. That is, try to understand the feelings of the patient or family member. There is seldom anything you can do to fix the situation, but sometimes just listening is helpful.
- Do not give false hope or reassurance. Avoid saying things like "everything will be all right." The family knows things will not be all right, and they do not want to try to justify what is happening. A simple "I'm sorry" is sufficient.
- Offer comfort. Let both the patient and the family know that you will do everything you can to help or that you will help them find assistance from other sources if needed. Remember, a gentle tone of voice and possibly a reassuring touch, if appropriate, can be helpful.

EMERGENCY MEDICAL RESPONDERS AND STRESS

stress ■ an emotionally disruptive or upsetting condition that occurs in response to adverse external influences. Stress is capable of affecting physical health.

Stress is an emotionally disruptive or upsetting condition that occurs in response to adverse external influences. It is capable of affecting physical health with increased heart rate, a rise in blood pressure, muscular tension, irritability, and depression. Almost everyone must deal with some type of stress on a daily basis, whether driving in traffic, coping with work and family problems, meeting school and office deadlines, or waiting for an appointment. Surveys and research reports over the past two decades have revealed that 43% of all adults suffer adverse health effects from stress. In fact, stress may be a factor in up to 80% of all non-traumatic deaths. Recent research confirms that stress contributes to cardiovascular disease, stroke, diabetes, cancer, and arthritis, as well as to gastrointestinal, skin, neurological, and emotional disorders.

1–2.1 List possible emotional reactions that the Emergency Medical Responder may experience when faced with trauma, illness, death, and dying.

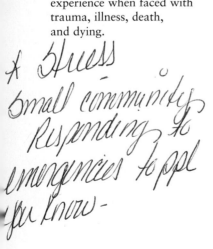

Another Side of Personal Safety

Stress is a concern for all Emergency Medical Responders. The job makes intense physical and psychological demands on your well-being. Police officers, firefighters, and disaster response personnel must respond quickly to emergencies and react appropriately to situations where lives are at risk. The need to make immediate decisions about patient care is a big responsibility. A mistake caused by their reaction to stress can cause harm to both patients and rescuers. An injury can become more serious or pain can become more intense. Care that is delayed at the scene or performed improperly may cause a chronic problem for the patient or lead to long-term disability.

Two of the best ways to minimize the stress associated with responding to emergencies and caring for patients are to work closely with other more experienced responders and to practice your skills often.

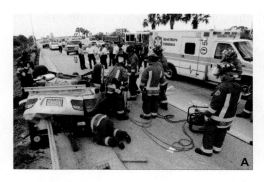

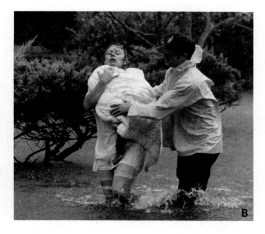

FIGURE 3.1 A range of stressful reactions can result from working at emergency scenes such as **A.** a multiple-vehicle collision (© *Craig Jackson/In the Dark Photography*) or **B.** storm-related disaster (© *Sun Herald/Corbis*).

Causes of Stress

Emergencies are stressful events, some more than others. The following are examples of very stressful situations, or **critical incidents,** encountered in EMS. The stress of any of these events can continue long after the event is over. They include:

- *Multiple-casualty incidents.* An emergency that involves multiple patients is referred to as a **multiple-casualty incident (MCI).** MCIs may range from a motor-vehicle crash that injures two drivers and a passenger to a large tropical storm that causes injury to hundreds of people (Figure 3.1).
- *Pediatric patients.* Emergencies involving infants or children are considered some of the most stressful that EMS providers—even the most experienced ones—are required to handle (Figure 3.2).
- *Death.* It can be difficult for a health-care provider to deal with the death of a patient, and even more so if the patient is young or someone the provider knows.

critical incident ▪ any situation that causes a rescuer to experience unusually strong emotions that interfere with the ability to function either during the incident or after; a highly stressful incident.

multiple-casualty incident (MCI) ▪ a single incident that involves multiple patients. Also called a *mass-casualty incident.*

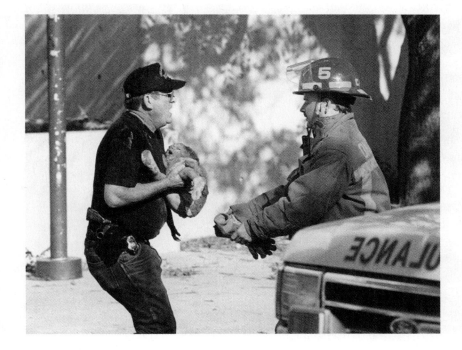

FIGURE 3.2 A stressful event can occur at any moment. (© *Charles H. Porter IV/Corbis Sygma*)

- *Violence.* Not only is it difficult to witness violence against others, but it is also dangerous. Take steps to protect yourself when responding to a violent situation or when a situation suddenly becomes violent.
- *Abuse and neglect.* As an Emergency Medical Responder, you may be called on to provide care for an infant, child, adult, or elderly patient who exhibits signs of abuse or neglect. Remember that abuse and neglect occur in all social and economic levels of society.
- *Death or injury of a coworker.* Bonds are formed among members of EMS. The death or injury of another provider, even if you do not personally know that person, can cause a stress response (Figure 3.3). It is also common in smaller communities to respond to someone you know. This can add a level of stress not seen when responding to strangers. *EMS, fire & PS*

Remember, although everyone responds to stress differently, stress and the reactions to it are common to all emergency personnel. It pays to stay aware of the stress factors you are exposed to every day as well as your immediate and long-term reactions to them. Just as important to recognizing the effects of stress in yourself is the ability to recognize the effects in your coworkers. Keep an eye out for signs of stress in others and offer assistance as appropriate.

Burnout

EMS personnel are trained to handle difficult situations, but they are not untouched by what they see and do on the job. **Stressors**—factors that cause wear and tear on the body's physical or mental resources—can take their toll. Stressors in EMS work can be as obvious as a fatal collision or the unexpected death of a child. Sometimes, however, stress can accumulate over months or even years of responding to ordinary injuries and illnesses.

Some EMS providers suffer from **burnout,** a reaction to cumulative stress or to multiple critical incidents. Emergency Medical Responders are at increased risk for burnout because of the demands and activities of the job. The signs of burnout include a loss of enthusiasm and energy replaced by feelings of frustration, hopelessness, low self-esteem, isolation, and mistrust. Many factors contribute to *alcoholism*

stressor ■ the part of a situation or the situation that causes stress.

burnout ■ an extreme emotional state characterized by emotional exhaustion, a diminished sense of personal accomplishment, and cynicism.

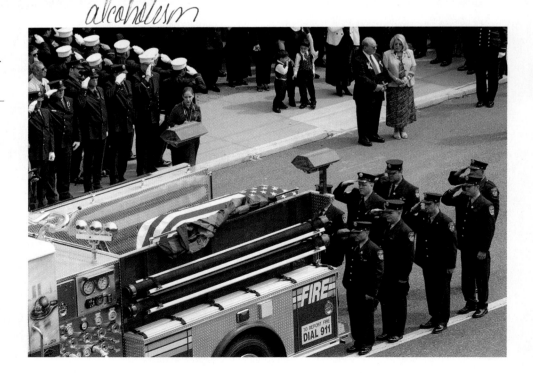

FIGURE 3.3 The death of a fellow EMS provider can be one of the most stressful events you experience. (© *Chip East/Reuters Newmedia Inc./Corbis*)

burnout, such as multiple or back-to-back emergency events involving serious medical problems, injuries, or death; facing public hostility; struggling with bureaucratic obstacles; long hours; and putting up with poor working conditions.

Shift work, 12 or 24 hours at a time, can be a significant source of stress, particularly when combined with other stress factors. This pattern of work is common in EMS. It can be found to be even more stressful now that there are so many dual-income families, who often miss time shared with their children and each other. The need for continuing education also contributes to already strained schedules. Evening meals that could be restful times, for example, even for those who dine by themselves, are too often replaced with high-caffeine beverages and high-fat fast food, all consumed on the run. A healthier diet and lifestyle can help Emergency Medical Responders combat the stressors that are an unavoidable part of the job.

Is It Safe ?

Being safe means being on top of your game at all times. Burnout can cause you to become distracted and complacent, which can cause you to miss an unsafe scene or potential hazard. You must take care of yourself both physically and emotionally in order to be at your best at all times. ▪

Both short-term and long-term stressors are occupational hazards for Emergency Medical Responders. Fortunately, research in the past 15 years has found ways to help reduce both kinds of stress. The old saying "work hard, play hard" may not be a particularly useful expression; in fact, it may actually cause more difficulties by trying to solve a complex problem with too simple a solution.

Signs and Symptoms of Stress

The way you handle stress can affect both your emotional health and the way you respond to emergencies. Emergency Medical Responders have a duty to confront the psychological effects of the work they do. Ignoring stress does not make it go away. Instead, it may crop up in unexpected forms, such as insomnia, fatigue, heart disease, alcohol use, increased incidence of illnesses, or other disruptive responses. You may find yourself suffering a loss in the level of your work performance and how you behave around others. Those who do not find ways to cope with stress can become depressed, suffer physical disorders, experience burnout, and may even have to leave the field permanently.

Recognize the signs and symptoms of stress when they appear. They include irritability with family, friends, and coworkers; inability to concentrate; changes in daily activities, such as difficulty sleeping or nightmares, loss of appetite, and loss of interest in sexual activity; anxiety; indecisiveness; guilt; isolation; and loss of interest in work or poor performance. In addition, you might experience constipation, diarrhea, headache, nausea, and hypertension.

DEALING WITH STRESS

Stress may be caused by a single event, or it may result from the combined effects of several incidents. It is important to remember that a severe incident can cause different reactions in different people. Stress may also be caused from a combination of factors, including personal problems, such as friends and family members who just do not understand the job. It is frequently necessary for health-care providers to work on holidays, weekends, and during important family events. This can be frustrating to friends and family members, which may cause stress for

1–2.4 State the possible reactions that the family of the Emergency Medical Responder may exhibit.

1–2.5 Recognize the signs and symptoms of critical incident stress.

1–2.6 State possible steps that the Emergency Medical Responder may take to help reduce/alleviate stress.

the provider. It can also be difficult when family and friends do not understand the strong emotions involved in responding to a serious incident.

Ways in which an Emergency Medical Responder can deal with stress include making lifestyle changes and counseling.

Is It Safe?

Be alert for signs of stress and burnout in those with whom you work. A large part of staying safe is having a partner who is looking out for your safety as well as his or her own. One of the best ways to deal with stress is to talk about it. If you see signs of stress in others, offer to talk to them and help them deal with the stressors that are affecting them. ■

Lifestyle Changes

It is often difficult to make changes in the habits or the lifestyle you have developed, but it is essential to consider the effects that current conditions have on your well-being. Remember that your health is of primary importance. Look carefully at your life habits and consider making adjustments.

FIRST ➤ There are several ways you can change your lifestyle when trying to deal with stress (Figure 3.4). They include the following:

- Develop more healthful and positive dietary habits. Avoid fatty foods and increase your carbohydrate intake. Also reduce your consumption of alcohol, sugar, and caffeine, which can negatively affect sleep patterns and cause irritability.
- Exercise. Properly performed exercise helps reduce stress. It also can help you deal with the physical aspects of your responsibilities, such as carrying equipment and performing other physically demanding emergency procedures.

FIGURE 3.4 Making lifestyle changes includes **A.** eating a healthy diet and **B.** exercising regularly.

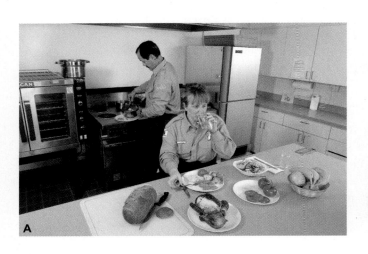

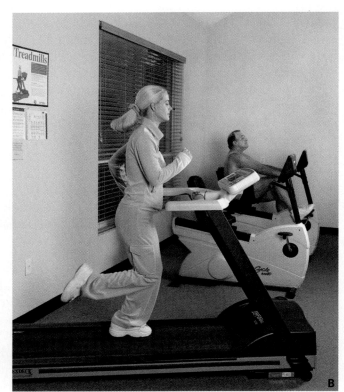

- Devote time to relaxing. Consider trying relaxation techniques, such as deep-breathing exercises and meditation.
- Change your work environment or shifts, if possible, in order to allow more time to relax with family or friends, or ask for a rotation to a less stressful assignment for a brief time.
- Seek professional help from a mental health professional, a social worker, or a member of the clergy. It is important to develop a healthy perspective about what you do. Being an Emergency Medical Responder is what you do, not who you are. ▪

Critical Incident Stress Management

FIRST ➤ **Critical incident stress management (CISM)** is an in-depth and broad plan designed to help the Emergency Medical Responder cope with job-related stress. Part of that plan includes the **critical incident stress debriefing (CISD)**. CISD is a process in which teams of trained peer counselors and mental health professionals meet with rescuers and health-care providers who have been involved in a major incident (Figure 3.5). These meetings are usually held within 24 to 72 hours after the incident, thus making the CISD part of the CISM. The goal is to assist the providers in dealing with the stress related to that incident. ▪

Participation in a CISD is strictly voluntary. No one should ever be forced or coerced to attend. Participants are encouraged to talk about their fears or their reactions to the incident. It is *not* a critique, and all participants should be made aware that whatever is said during a debriefing will be held in the strictest confidence, both by the participants themselves and the debriefing team. CISDs are usually helpful in assisting EMS personnel to better understand their reactions and feelings both during and after an incident. Attendees will also come to understand that other members of the team are likely experiencing similar reactions.

After the open discussion during which everyone is encouraged to share, but not forced to do so, the debriefing teams offer suggestions on how to deal with and prevent further stress. It is important to realize that stress after a major incident is both normal and to be expected. The CISD process can be helpful in speeding up the recovery process. Typically, CISD sessions are created to help control and then reduce the effects of the incident on emergency personnel. This includes beginning an efficient recovery process for Emergency Medical Responders and minimizing the effects of post-traumatic stress disorder.

critical incident stress management (CISM) ▪ an in-depth, broad plan designed to help rescue personnel cope with the stress resulting from a highly stressful incident.

critical incident stress debriefing (CISD) ▪ a process in which teams of professional and peer counselors provide emotional and psychological support to EMS personnel who are or have been involved in a critical (highly stressful) incident.

No critique or blame on questioning each other on action

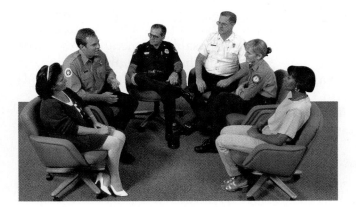

FIGURE 3.5 Emergency Medical Responders at a critical incident stress debriefing.

Your instructor will inform you of situations in which CISD should be requested and how to access the local system.

Body Substance Isolation Precautions

EMERGENCY MEDICAL RESPONDERS AT RISK

FIRST ➤ As an Emergency Medical Responder, you will deal with emergencies involving illness and injury. Therefore, you will need to protect yourself against exposure to infectious diseases. To do that, you must take **body substance isolation (BSI) precautions,** which are specific steps that help to minimize exposure to a patient's blood and body fluids. Examples of BSI precautions include wearing protective gloves, masks, gowns, and eyewear.

Consider the following situations:

■ A police officer puts handcuffs on a suspect who has a small open wound on his hand.
■ A firefighter finds his leather gloves soaked with blood after extricating a patient from a wrecked car.
■ A lifeguard touches dried blood while cleaning equipment after an emergency.
■ A sheriff's deputy is searching the front seat of a suspect's car and is stuck by a needle that the suspect dropped the night before.
■ A firefighter, who is checking his equipment, handles a tool covered with blood from an earlier call.
■ A firefighter who arrives first on the scene to care for a patient who has suddenly become ill is exposed to the patient's heavy coughing spell. ■

In each situation, the Emergency Medical Responder may be at risk of exposure to an infectious disease. What BSI precautions should be taken in each case described in the preceding list? At the start of each shift, Emergency Medical Responders should check their hands for breaks in the skin and cover the areas that are not intact. If unprotected hands come in contact with blood (wet or dry) or any other body fluids, they should be promptly washed with soap and water or a commercially produced antiseptic hand cleanser (Figure 3.6). Make sure you wear disposable synthetic gloves before touching any patient and before handling equipment that may have been exposed to blood and body fluids (Figure 3.7).

To provide care to a patient who is coughing, sneezing, spitting, or otherwise spraying body fluids into the air, wear a mask and eye protection in addition to gloves. If you must search an individual or a vehicle, use a flashlight, mirror, or probe to search in areas that are not visible, such as in pockets or between seat cushions.

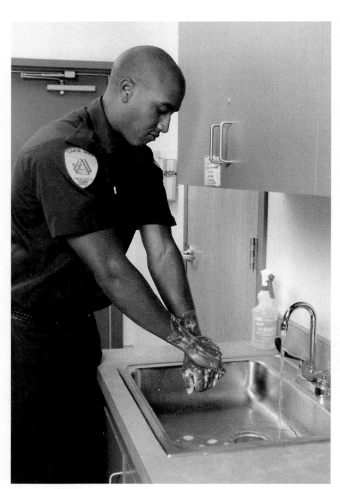

FIGURE 3.6 Hand washing is one of the most effective means of minimizing the spread of infection.

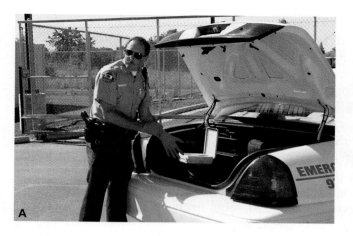
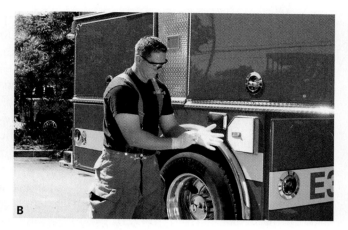

FIGURE 3.7 **A.** Even law enforcement officers need to take precautions when dealing with injured individuals in unknown situations. **B.** In nonfire emergencies, firefighters should wear synthetic gloves under their leather gloves.

Finally, to dispose of blood-soaked gloves or any other disposable equipment that has blood or body fluids on it, follow the guidelines published by the U.S. Occupational Safety and Health Administration (OSHA) or National Fire Protection Association (NFPA).

Emergency Medical Responders frequently face unpredictable, uncontrollable, dangerous, and life-threatening circumstances. Anything can happen in an emergency. Making an arrest, helping a heart attack victim, carrying a child from a burning building, stopping a brawl, helping deliver a baby—each situation has the potential to expose an Emergency Medical Responder to infectious diseases. Use good judgment. Follow OSHA guidelines.

It is not enough to simply use proper BSI precautions with each and every patient; you must also encourage others to do so. By being consistent and thorough with this practice, you become a role model for your colleagues and peers and, by your actions, encourage others to do the same.

1–2.8 Discuss the importance of body substance isolation (BSI).

DEALING WITH RISK

As an Emergency Medical Responder, you must become good at assessing risk. Yet, some emergency personnel worry more about acquired immune deficiency syndrome (AIDS) than they do about going into a burning building. The fact is that AIDS is a disease that an Emergency Medical Responder is least likely to acquire. As a member of the EMS team, your chances of being infected with the human immunodeficiency virus (HIV), the virus that causes AIDS, are very slight, even if you come in direct contact with infected blood or body fluids. You are at a much greater risk of contracting hepatitis B or C. An estimated 250 health-care workers die each year from hepatitis or its complications, more than from any other infectious disease.

Regardless of the risk of infection, all EMS personnel must follow the rules for their own safety and the safety of others. Keep in mind that an organism that can cause disease may not always do so, and it can affect different people in different ways. For example, an organism that you transfer from one patient to another may cause disease in the second patient but not the first. In other words, the way disease is spread and develops is a subject that is so complicated that its study is a specialty unto itself.

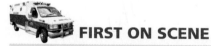

FIRST ON SCENE

"Hold on," Jake approaches the woman with his hands open and outstretched. "The worst is over. Let me help you."

She scoots back against the low carpeted wall that surrounds the rink and shakes her head. "I've got hepatitis," she whispers, tears still flowing from her red eyes. "Please just call an ambulance." Her dark hair and black jacket have been hiding the seriousness of the blood loss, but now that they are saturated, bright blood begins to pool quickly on the ice around her.

Jake hesitates and looks at his ungloved hands. There is a paper cut on the side of his left index finger. He looks from his hands to the woman's crying face. He turns and shouts to the advancing skate guard, "Call 9-1-1! Then bring me a first aid kit."

WARNING

Liquid or droplet exposure to skin, hair, gloves, clothing, and equipment requires you to find out from medical direction how to proceed. Washing with soap may not be enough. Contact with any unknown microbe or potential pathogen may require being seen by a physician.

pathogens ■ organisms such as viruses and bacteria that cause infection and disease.

personal protective equipment (PPE) ■ equipment such as gloves, mask, eyewear, gown, turnout gear, and helmet, which protect rescuers from infection and/or from exposure to hazardous materials and the dangers of rescue operations.

Do not guess at which precautions are necessary or assume that you can easily determine on your own how to prevent disease. You have entered this course prepared to help care for illness and injury. You can begin by not becoming a patient yourself and by not spreading infections.

Infections are caused by organisms such as viruses and bacteria. Viruses cause illnesses such as colds, flu, HIV, and hepatitis. Bacteria cause sore throats, food poisoning, rheumatic fever, gonorrhea, Legionnaire's disease, and tuberculosis (TB), to name a few. There are both viral and bacterial forms of pneumonia and meningitis. Viruses and bacteria are also called *pathogens*. The term **pathogen** means to generate suffering (*patho-*, suffering; *-gen*, create or form). Pathogens are spread by exposure to body fluids such as blood and semen, as well as exposure to airborne droplets, such as those that come from coughing, sneezing, spitting, or even breathing close to someone's face.

Infectious diseases are a real danger to Emergency Medical Responders. However, if you follow safety procedures and use the personal protective equipment provided by your agency, the risks can be minimized.

FIRST ➤ OSHA has issued strict guidelines on the precautions to take to reduce exposure to infectious disease. You can transmit pathogens to the patient, and the patient can transmit them to you unless you use **personal protective equipment (PPE)** (Figure 3.8):

■ *Synthetic gloves.* Inspect your hands before donning gloves and cover any broken skin. Put on your gloves before any contact with the patient. Put on a second pair of gloves if you are working around sharp objects, such as broken glass and metal edges at a collision scene. If the outer gloves are torn, the gloves underneath still provide a layer of protection. Wash hands and change gloves between patients. OSHA has stated that hand washing is one of the most important steps to take for infection control.

■ *Face shields or masks.* Wear surgical-type masks for blood or fluid splatter. For fine particles of airborne droplets (coughing), wear a high-efficiency particulate air (HEPA) or N-95 respirator. In addition, a surgical-type mask may be placed on the patient if he is alert and cooperates (monitor respirations).

■ *Eye protection.* The mucous membranes of your eyes can absorb fluids and are a route for infection. Use eyewear that protects them from both the front and the side.

■ *Gowns.* Protect your clothing and bare skin when there is spurting blood, childbirth, or multiple injuries with heavy bleeding. ■

Because you cannot tell if patients have infectious diseases just by looking at them, it is important to wear PPE for any contact with a patient. This includes wearing gloves at all times, plus face shields and eye protection whenever you may be exposed to splattering fluids or airborne droplets. This protection forms a barrier between you and the patient.

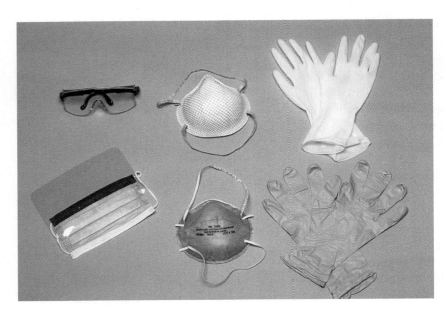

FIGURE 3.8 Personal protective equipment (PPE).

Your instructor will show you how to properly put on and use your protective equipment in a way that maintains its cleanliness (Scan 3–1). You will also learn how and where to properly dispose of all used materials (Figure 3.9). In addition, it is important that all reusable equipment is cleaned or disinfected with soap and water and/or a bleach solution (Figure 3.10). You must learn, understand the need for, and practice these infection control procedures to reduce your risk of infection. Infection control procedures are based on guidelines from OSHA and the Centers for Disease Control and Prevention (CDC), and practicing them is a part of your responsibility as an Emergency Medical Responder.

Today, governments at the local, state, and federal levels are taking steps to protect Emergency Medical Responders from exposure to infectious diseases. The CDC has created detailed guidelines for how to stay safe while caring for patients. These guidelines are referred to as *Standard Precautions*. One of the underlying concepts that form the foundation for these guidelines is the assumption that all blood and body fluids are potentially hazardous and must be treated as infectious.

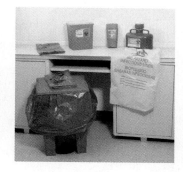

FIGURE 3.9 Examples of biohazard containers.

AIRBORNE AND BLOODBORNE PATHOGENS

FIRST ➤ Infectious diseases range from such generally mild conditions as the common cold to life-threatening diseases such as tuberculosis. The four diseases of most concern to Emergency Medical Responders are (Table 3–1):

■ Human immunodeficiency virus (HIV).

■ Hepatitis.

■ Tuberculosis (TB).

■ Meningitis. ▪

1–2.9 Describe the steps the Emergency Medical Responder should take for personal protection from airborne and bloodborne pathogens.

HIV is the pathogen that causes AIDS. As yet, there is no cure, but there are newly developed medications that help reduce the patient's symptoms. Even so, new medical developments should not prevent you from using PPE while caring for every patient. Keep in mind several facts about HIV. First, HIV does not survive well outside the body. It is not as concentrated in body fluids as is the hepatitis B virus. HIV is also much more difficult to transmit than hepatitis B. The routes of exposure to HIV are limited to direct contact with nonintact (open) skin or mucous membranes and with blood, semen, or other body fluids. Thus, it is unlikely that a rescuer taking proper BSI precautions will get the disease on the job.

In contrast to HIV, hepatitis B is a very tough virus. It can survive on clothing, newspaper, or other objects for days after infected blood has dried. HBV causes permanent liver damage in many cases and can be fatal. Several other forms of the disease, including hepatitis C, are less common than hepatitis B but still present a risk to Emergency Medical Responders.

Tuberculosis (TB), a disease most often affecting the lungs, can also be fatal. Although thought to have been nearly eradicated as recently as 1985, TB has had a resurgence. Even worse, new strains of the disease are resistant to treatment with traditional medications. Unlike HIV and hepatitis B, TB is spread by aerosolized droplets in the air, usually the result of coughing and sneezing. Thus, TB can be contracted even without direct physical contact with a carrier. Use face masks

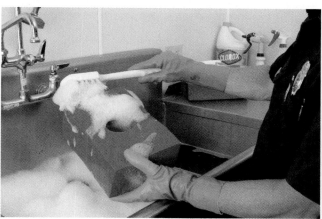

FIGURE 3.10 Safe workplace procedures include facilities for cleaning contaminated equipment and supplies.

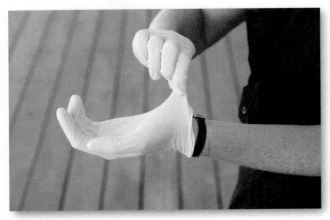

1 ■ Begin by grasping the outer cuff of the opposite glove.

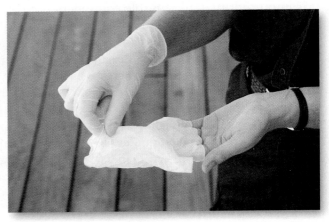

2 ■ Carefully slip the glove over the hand, pulling it inside out.

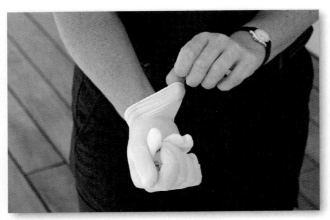

3 ■ Next, slip a finger of the ungloved hand under the cuff.

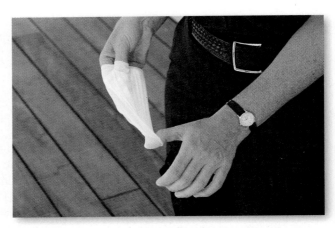

4 ■ Carefully slip it off, turning it inside out.

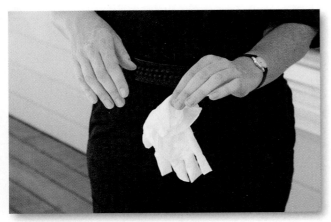

5 ■ Once removed, both gloves will end up inside out with one glove inside the other. This will contain any blood or body fluids.

TABLE 3–1 | Diseases of Concern to Emergency Medical Responders

DISEASE	HOW TRANSMITTED	VACCINE
Acquired immune deficiency syndrome/human immunodeficiency virus (AIDS/HIV)	Needle sticks, blood splash on mucous membranes (eye, mouth), or blood contact with open skin	No
Hepatitis B virus (HBV)	Needle sticks, blood splash on mucous membranes (eye, mouth), or blood contact with open skin; some risk during mouth-to-mouth CPR and exposure to contaminated equipment and dried blood	Yes
Tuberculosis (TB)	Airborne aerosolized droplets	No
Meningitis	Respiratory secretions or saliva	Yes, for one strain

with one-way valves for rescue breathing. Use a HEPA respirator or N-95 respirator when TB is suspected (Figure 3.11). These respirators greatly reduce the risk of exposure to this airborne disease.

Meningitis, an inflammation of the lining of the brain and spinal cord, is also a serious disease, especially for children. The most infectious varieties of meningitis are caused by bacteria. Meningitis is transmitted by respiratory droplets, like TB, but is far easier to contract. The disease may have a rapid onset (several hours to a few days) and needs quick treatment with antibiotics. Antibiotics taken after exposure to bacterial meningitis may prevent acquisition of the disease.

Not all pathogens are well understood. In fact, there are new pathogens emerging all the time. The following is a list of well known pathogens that

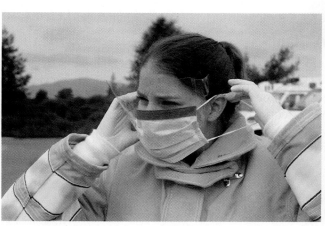

A.

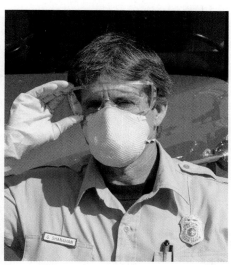

B.

FIGURE 3.11 Wear either **A.** a high-efficiency particulate air (HEPA) mask or **B.** an N-95 to minimize your chances of being exposed to an airborne pathogen.

have received significant attention from both the CDC and the media in recent years:

- *Severe acute respiratory syndrome (SARS).* First reported in Asia in 2003, the SARS virus quickly spread to more than 8,098 people in two dozen countries in North America, South America, Europe, and Asia. According to the World Health Organization (WHO), a total of 774 died before the SARS global outbreak of 2003 was contained.
- *West Nile virus (WNV).* A potentially serious illness, WNV, experts believe, has been established as a seasonal epidemic in North America that flares up in the summer and continues into the fall. The severe symptoms include high fever, headache, neck stiffness, stupor, disorientation, coma, tremors, convulsions, muscle weakness, vision loss, numbness, and paralysis. These symptoms may last several weeks, and neurological effects may be permanent.
- *Avian flu.* This is a form of influenza that is common in birds and, in rare cases, has been known to spread to humans, in which it causes a high likelihood of death.
- *Methicillin-resistant staphylococcus aureus (MRSA).* This bacteria is resistant to certain antibiotics, including methicillin and other more common antibiotics such as oxacillin, penicillin, and amoxicillin. Staph infections, including MRSA, occur most frequently among people in hospitals and health-care facilities (such as nursing homes and dialysis centers) who have weakened immune systems.

EMPLOYEE RESPONSIBILITIES

An infection control program will only work if Emergency Medical Responders learn and follow correct procedures. As an Emergency Medical Responder, you have an obligation to adhere to safe work practices in order to protect yourself, your family, and the public. Washing hands regularly, using gloves and other PPE, and making safe work practices a habit are good ways to start.

NOTE

You may not withhold emergency care from a patient who you think may have an infectious disease. With the proper precautions, you can provide emergency care to people infected with HIV or hepatitis B without putting yourself at risk. To date, there are no known cases of emergency workers contracting HIV or hepatitis B during routine patient care using gloves and appropriate PPE. Emergency Medical Responders who practice infection control should feel confident that they are not risking their lives.

FIRST ON SCENE

The woman's sobs slowly taper off and, as her bloody hands drop to the ice, Jake sees that she is losing consciousness. Her eyes are shifting groggily from him to the crowd of onlookers and to the small boy who is now being comforted by a teenage girl. Jake wants so badly to help the woman somehow, to apply pressure to stop her bleeding, to hug her and tell her that she'll be okay—anything. But hepatitis. Wow, he thinks. He doesn't want to get hepatitis.

As the small mumbling crowd watches, the woman's eyes slowly close and she slumps over onto the red ice.

IMMUNIZATIONS

One of the many ways that Emergency Medical Responders can minimize the risk of acquiring an infectious disease is by becoming immunized. Vaccines have been developed for many of the more common infectious diseases we see today. While most receive these vaccinations as part of childhood wellness checks, there are additional vaccines available to adults.

In 1992, OSHA mandated that all employees who have a reasonable risk of becoming exposed to blood or other potentially infectious material (OPIM) while performing their normal job duties must be offered hepatitis B vaccinations (Figure 3.12). Although the employer must offer the vaccine at no charge, employees do have the option to decline.

New vaccines are being developed all the time, some that could greatly decrease the likelihood that you could acquire an

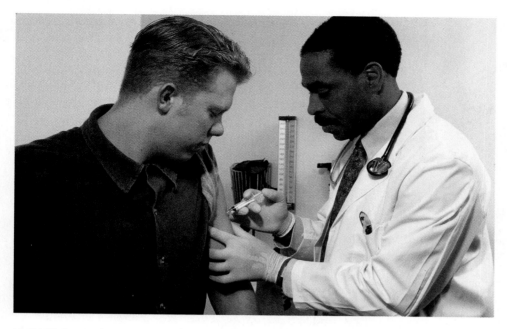

FIGURE 3.12 The OSHA-mandated infectious disease program includes immunizations against certain diseases. *(© Michal Heron)*

infectious disease. Be sure to educate yourself and consult with your own physician before receiving vaccinations.

Scene Safety

Ensuring scene safety starts before Emergency Medical Responders actually arrive at the scene. En route to the scene, it is important to get as much information as possible from dispatch about the emergency. The nature of the call will help determine what type of BSI precautions and equipment may be needed, as well as what type of approach precautions to take. Dispatchers will not always have complete or accurate details about an incident. Often, those who report an emergency are excited, nervous, confused, in pain, or in a panic. They may even hang up before they finish giving all the details. Become familiar with your response area and the types of calls typical to it, so you can be prepared for both the expected and the unexpected.

When approaching an emergency scene, look around for hazards and listen for noises in the area. Is it quiet, and is that normal for the area? Is there yelling, screaming, gunshots, dogs barking? Decide where to place the vehicle: facing the scene to provide lighting or beyond the scene to provide quick and easy supply access and patient loading, on the street to block traffic and protect the scene or off the street to protect yourself and your partner. When deciding where to position the vehicle, consider that placement must provide for access to equipment, efficient loading of the patient, and continued traffic flow where possible or at least rerouting of traffic around the scene.

Before approaching the patient, you must ensure scene safety—for yourself, the patient, and bystanders. Look for the presence of weapons, and do not attempt to provide care if you see them. There may be hazardous materials, toxic substances, downed power lines and broken poles, or unstable vehicles at the scene. Environmental conditions such as icy and slippery roads, steep grades, rocky terrain,

1–2.7 Explain the need to determine scene safety.

1–2.10 List the personal protective equipment necessary for each of the following situations: hazardous materials, rescue operations, exposure to bloodborne and airborne pathogens, violent scenes, crime scenes, and electricity.

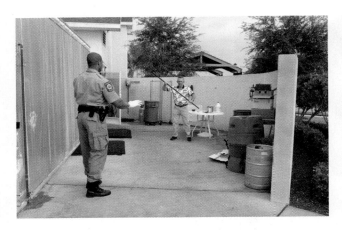

FIGURE 3.13 Safety at the scene includes looking for weapons as you approach. Do not approach anyone who is armed with any type of weapon.

or heavy traffic and a crowd of onlookers must all be considered in your approach, placement of your vehicle, and care of your patient.

Violent situations may involve weapons—not just guns but knives or bats, boards, chains, and other items (Figure 3.13). These can be used to harm you, just as they harmed the victim. You may also be responding to a crime scene where you want to be aware of the potential for violence, where you do not want to approach until it is clear, and where you do not want to disturb evidence any more than you must while caring for the patient. Crowds can also be potentially dangerous. When necessary, notify dispatch that you need assistance for crowd control and law enforcement for protection and scene security.

Keeping yourself safe is your first responsibility. Once you can ensure your own safety, approach and take care of the patient. Following are specific types of unsafe incidents where Emergency Medical Responders must take special precautions.

HAZARDOUS MATERIALS INCIDENTS

Some chemicals can cause serious illness or death, even if your exposure is brief. They may be transported by truck or rail and stored in warehouses or used in local industries. If there is a collision in which transported chemicals are spilled or if stored containers begin to leak, the spilled chemicals are likely to be considered a hazard to the community and to responding EMS personnel.

hazardous materials incident ■ the release of a harmful substance into the environment. Also called a *hazmat incident.*

Emergency Medical Responders should maintain a safe distance from the source of the hazard and treat it as a **hazardous materials incident.** Placards may help with identifying materials in motor-vehicle collisions. These placards use coded colors and identification numbers that are listed in the *Emergency Response Guidebook*, a handbook published by the U.S. DOT. This book should be placed in every emergency response vehicle. It can provide important information about a hazardous substance, as well as information on safe distances, emergency care, and suggested procedures in the event of spills or fire.

Is It Safe?

One of the most important concepts you can learn and live by is that Emergency Medical Responders are usually unprepared to deal with a hazardous materials spill. If you suspect a hazardous material is involved in a scene to which you are responding, stay clear and call in a specialized hazmat team to secure the scene before you enter. ■

It also is always wise to carry a pair of binoculars in your vehicle. Use them to identify hazardous materials placards from a safe distance, thus ensuring your own safety.

As an Emergency Medical Responder, your most important duty in a hazardous materials incident is to recognize potential problems and take action to preserve your own safety and that of others. (See Chapter 15 for a more detailed discussion of the Emergency Medical Responder's responsibilities at a hazardous materials incident.) You should also make sure an appropriately trained hazardous materials response team is notified (Figure 3.14). These teams have special training and equipment to handle such incidents, so it is important that you not take any action other than protecting yourself, your patients, and bystanders. An inappropriate action could cause a larger problem than the already existing one.

Many emergency response agencies require hazardous materials training at the awareness level. Your instructor can inform you of the requirements in your area.

RESCUE OPERATIONS

Emergency Medical Responders may be first on the scene of an emergency that involves rescue. Rescue scenes may include dangers from electricity, fire, explosion, hazardous materials, traffic, or water and ice. It is important to evaluate each situation and request assistance from the appropriately trained teams. You may need the police, fire services, the utility company, or other specialized personnel. Never perform acts that you are not properly trained to do. Secure the scene to the best of your ability, and then wait for the help you have requested to arrive. Remember that whenever you are working at a rescue operation, you must use PPE, which may include turnout gear, protective eyewear, helmet, puncture-proof gloves, and disposable synthetic gloves.

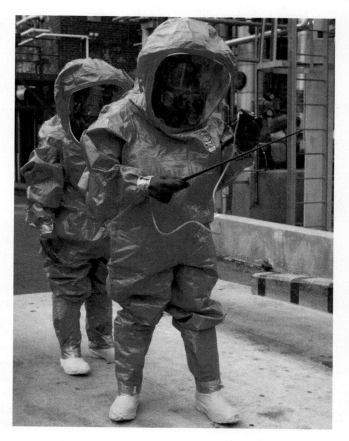

FIGURE 3.14 Emergency Medical Responders should wait for hazmat teams to arrive at the scene of any hazardous materials incident.

VIOLENCE AND CRIME SCENES

Emergency Medical Responders may also respond to scenes involving victims of violence or crime. In some areas, EMS providers are issued bulletproof vests for their protection, along with PPE. No matter what area you work in, your first priority—even before patient care—is to be certain the scene is safe before you enter it. Threatening people or pets, people with weapons, intoxicated people, and others may present problems that you are not prepared to handle. Recognize these situations and request the necessary help. Do not enter the scene until help arrives to secure it and make it safe for you to perform your duties.

FIRST ON SCENE WRAP-UP

Ten minutes after the woman fell, a group of firefighters and EMTs are walking gingerly across the ice. They are sliding a gurney piled high with equipment bags toward her. Jake explains to the first uniformed rescuer what happened and lowers his voice as he mentions the hepatitis.

The crews, already wearing gloves, quickly put an oxygen mask on the woman, control her bleeding, and secure her to a long yellow board. As they are lifting her onto the gurney, she wakes.

"I think she'll be okay," the EMT at the head of the gurney says to Jake. "It was the right thing to call us."

As Jake accompanies them to the edge of the rink and watches as the crews take her and the boy out of the arena, he again looks down at his hands. He decides never again to be caught without a pair of exam gloves.

Summary

One way an Emergency Medical Responder can help patients and their families cope with death and dying is to understand their stages of grief, which include denial, anger, bargaining, depression, and acceptance.

Stress is a daily part of an Emergency Medical Responder's job. A stressor may be a single terrible event or a series of events that, when combined, will overload the ability of a rescuer to cope. Emergencies that produce excessive stress include hazardous materials incidents or multiple-casualty incidents. Emergencies involving pediatric patients, death, violence, abuse and neglect, and the death or injury of another rescuer also are associated with excessive stress. Emergency Medical Responders may find themselves reacting unexpectedly and immediately or experiencing a delayed reaction days or weeks following an event. Typically, a rescuer will recover from an acute stress reaction in a few days or weeks. However, cumulative stress may lead to burnout, which may require professional counseling. To help reduce the stress associated with responding to emergency situations, rescuers can make lifestyle changes or adjustments. In more severe cases, professional help or counseling may be of importance in ensuring emotional well-being.

Taking the steps necessary to deal adequately with stress associated with a critical incident may be best accomplished by following your EMS system's critical incident stress management (CISM) recommendations, including peer counseling through critical incident stress debriefing (CISD).

Safeguarding your well-being is critical. Dealing with risk is often part of the rescuer's roles and responsibilities. Many situations put the Emergency Medical Responder at risk of exposure to infectious disease. It is important for the Emergency Medical Responder to be familiar with and follow OSHA guidelines for infection control. To protect yourself from pathogens, use personal protective equipment (PPE) such as gloves (always), face shields or masks, eye protection, and gowns when necessary. These protective barriers between you and the patient are called body substance isolation (BSI) precautions. Dispose of PPE properly.

Four pathogens present especially significant risks to Emergency Medical Responders. They are HIV, hepatitis (typically bloodborne), tuberculosis, and meningitis (typically airborne). Do not limit your thinking to just these four, and do not believe that an outbreak must be reported for there to be a danger.

It is the responsibility of the Emergency Medical Responder to provide emergency care to all patients, regardless of their real or potential level of infection. Ensure your personal safety by being alert to the potential for danger at every emergency call.

Remember and Consider

Remember that your safety has to come first. For you to help others, you must first take care of yourself. Keep in mind that your emotional safety is also important in order to prevent burnout, which often causes a loss of personnel to emergency response services.

➤ Identify a network of family or friends who may be able to assist you in handling stress.

➤ Make sure you have the necessary PPE available whenever you may be responding to an emergency. Use the equipment every time, on every call. If you do this, you will not have to wonder if you were protected on "that" call.

Investigate

➤ Learn how and when to access the CISM in your local area.

➤ Practice putting on PPE and determine what equipment is necessary for different types of emergency responses. Learn how to properly dispose of items after use.

➤ Learn what types of specialized assistance or specially trained personnel are available in your area and how to establish contact in case of an emergency.

Quick Quiz

1. All of the following are common emotional reactions of an Emergency Medical Responder who has faced serious trauma, illness, or death, EXCEPT:
   a. depression.
   b. burnout.
   c. low blood pressure.
   d. insomnia.

2. The best definition of the term *stressor* is anything that:
   a. produces wear and tear on the body's resources.
   b. consumes the attention of the person experiencing stress.
   c. puts pressure on the body.
   d. causes significant behavioral changes.

3. Common causes of stress for Emergency Medical Responders include all of the following EXCEPT:
   a. driving with lights and sirens.
   b. multiple-casualty incidents.
   c. severely injured pediatric patients.
   d. the scene of a violent crime.

4. All of the following are terms used for the stages a person experiencing death might experience EXCEPT:
   a. denial.
   b. anger.
   c. bargaining.
   d. refusal.

5. Which one of the following would be the best response by an Emergency Medical Responder to family members who are facing the death of a loved one?
   a. Avoid talking directly to the patient.
   b. Do not tolerate angry reactions.
   c. Try your best to understand their feelings.
   d. Tell them everything will be okay.

6. All of the following are common signs and symptoms of stress EXCEPT:
   a. irritability.
   b. difficulty sleeping.
   c. increased appetite.
   d. difficulty concentrating.

7. Which one of the following statements about critical incident stress is MOST accurate?
   a. It is rarely caused by a single incident.
   b. It can be the result of many incidents over a long period of time.
   c. It affects all people the same way.
   d. It can always be avoided with proper preparation.

8. Which one of the following is the BEST definition of critical incident stress management?
   a. It is a broad plan designed to help EMS personnel cope with job-related stress.
   b. It mainly consists of a defusing process.
   c. It is a mandatory process in which all responders must participate.
   d. It focuses on the appropriateness of patient care delivered at the scene.

9. Take body substance isolation (BSI) precautions:
   a. for TB and HBV patients only.
   b. for any ill or injured patient.
   c. only for patients who have a known infection.
   d. only for patients who are bleeding.

10. Which one of the following is the pathogen that most often affects the lungs and can be spread by a patient coughing?
    a. human immunodeficiency virus (HIV)
    b. hepatitis B
    c. meningitis
    d. tuberculosis (TB)

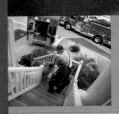

CHAPTER 4

The Human Body

As an Emergency Medical Responder, you will not be able to provide care for an ill or injured patient unless you have an idea of where the problem lies. This requires a patient assessment. To assess a patient adequately, you must be familiar with normal anatomy and the terms used to describe it. In addition, this knowledge will make it possible for you to give an accurate patient report, even over a telephone or radio.

This chapter introduces you to the anatomy of the human body, including its major systems and their basic functions. It also introduces you to terms used to describe a patient's position and condition.

OBJECTIVES

This chapter is based on the objectives of the U.S. DOT's First Responder National Standard Curriculum. Note that cognitive objectives are listed below and beside corresponding text throughout the chapter. You will also notice as you read each objective that the term Emergency Medical Responder is used. This is simply a name change and reflects the new name for the First Responder.

By the end of this chapter, you should be able to (from cognitive or knowledge information):

1–4.1 Describe the anatomy and function of the respiratory system. (p. 66; also see Chapter 6)

1–4.2 Describe the anatomy and function of the circulatory system. (p. 66; also see Chapters 8 and 10)

1–4.3 Describe the anatomy and function of the musculoskeletal system. (p. 66; also see Chapter 11)

1–4.4 Describe the components and function of the nervous system. (p. 66; also see Chapter 11)

ADDITIONAL LEARNING TASKS

A basic understanding of the normal anatomy and function of the human body will help the Emergency Medical Responder know when something is wrong with a patient. Anatomical descriptions and positional and directional terms will help you report patient problems more accurately. Practice using them and be able to:

➤ Describe the standard anatomical position.

➤ Define and properly apply the terms *anterior, posterior, midline, medial, lateral, proximal, distal, superior, inferior, patient's right and left, prone, supine,* and *right and left lateral recumbent positions.*

It is also helpful to know the five major regions of the body and the contents of the four major body cavities. Be sure you are able to:

➤ Use common terms to list the five major regions of the body and the subdivisions of each region.

➤ Name and locate the four major body cavities.

➤ Name and locate the organs contained in each body cavity.

➤ Identify the four abdominal quadrants.

➤ Name two types of structures that are found in every location in the body.

➤ List and define the major body systems.

 FIRST ON SCENE

"George 14, George 1-4," says the dispatcher, interrupting Stephanie's cell phone call.

"Go ahead for George 14," she says after snapping the phone shut.

"George 14, respond to Highway 4 between Ottoman and West Carlin for a check on the welfare of Adam 9. He was on a traffic stop about four minutes ago and we can't get a response now."

"Copy." She puts her cruiser into drive and activates the lights and siren. "George 14 responding from Okalusa Drive and Southwest 14th." She realizes her stomach is tight and growing nauseous as she covers the distance to Jason's location.

He was having radio trouble earlier in the day, so she thinks it's probably nothing. Then again, the department has been making an increasing number of drug-related arrests now that summer is here, and the lake is attracting visitors at a record pace. She forces herself to focus on the road ahead as she travels along the dusk-lit concrete surface of Highway 4.

Cresting the hill just past the West Carlin exit, she sees a patrol car on the shoulder of the highway, take-down lights still flashing, but nothing else. No other vehicles, no movement, and no police officer. As she pulls up to the empty, idling car her stomach drops. She has to force her hand to stop trembling as she grabs the radio mic. There, sprawled in the dirt on the side of the road and not moving is State Patrolman Jason Patnode.

Overview of the Human Body

Students beginning training in Emergency Medical Responder courses are often a little worried about having to learn human **anatomy**. Don't be. As an Emergency Medical Responder, you will not need to be as precise as other medical personnel are when they consider the human body. However, you will need to know the basic body structures and their locations.

anatomy ■ the study of body structure.

Do not become overly concerned with trying to learn each and every anatomical term for the human body. A head is still a head, and feet are still feet. However, you will need to learn some new terms and make them as much a part of your vocabulary as the everyday terms *heart* and *lungs*.

FIRST ➤ To be an Emergency Medical Responder, you must be able to look at a person's body and know the major internal structures and the general location of each. Your concern is not how the body looks dissected or how the body looks on an anatomical wall chart. You must be concerned with living bodies and knowing where things are located as you look from the outside.

You know about blood vessels and nerves. As you look at any region of the body, remember that for your purposes:

- Blood vessels go everywhere in the body, to every structure.
- Nerves go everywhere in the body, to every structure. ■

When you look at an arm, you must see something that is alive and part of a living organism. You know that an arm is made of muscles, bones, blood vessels, nerves, and other tissues. When you assess injuries, never forget that there could be internal bleeding and that damaged nerves may be causing pain, loss of feeling, or even loss of function.

POSITIONAL AND DIRECTIONAL TERMS

anatomical (AN-ah-TOM-i-kal) position ■ the standard reference position for the body in the study of anatomy. The body is standing erect, facing the observer. The arms are down at the sides, and the palms of the hands are forward.

FIRST ➤ The following are some basic terms that may be used to refer to the human body (Figure 4.1):

- *Anatomical position.* Consider the human body, standing up, facing you. The arms are down at the sides, and the palms of the hands are facing forward. This is referred to as the **anatomical position.** References to all body structures and locations assume the body in this position.

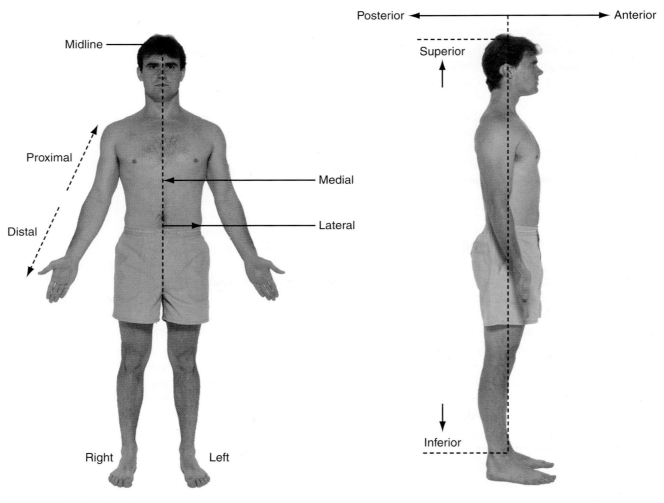

FIGURE 4.1 Directional terms.

- *Right and left.* Always refer to right and left as seen from the patient's perspective. Even though you may think this is simple, it is easy to get confused and make references to your own left and right.
- *Anterior and posterior.* The term **anterior** refers to the front of the body, and the term **posterior** refers to the back of the body.
- *Midline.* The **midline** is an imaginary vertical line that divides the body into right and left halves. Anything toward the midline is said to be **medial,** while anything away from the midline is said to be **lateral.** Remember the anatomical position, which places the thumb on the lateral side of the hand and the little finger on the medial side. ▪

There are other directional terms that can be useful. **Superior** means toward the top of the head, as in "the eyes are superior to the nose." **Inferior** means toward the feet, as in "the mouth is inferior to the nose." *Superior* and *inferior* are usually reserved for structures in the head, neck, and torso. Notice that you cannot say something is superior or inferior unless you are comparing at least two points of reference or structures. The heart is not simply superior; it is superior to the stomach. Because you are using the anatomical position for all your references to the body, any medical professional will know what you mean when you say a wound is just above the eye. For this reason, *superior* and *inferior* may be optional terms in your course.

Proximal and **distal** are also good terms to learn and use. These two terms are often used incorrectly and should be avoided unless you are certain of their correct usage. To use the terms correctly, there must be a point of reference and two structures being compared. The structure closest to the point of reference is said to be *proximal*, while the structure farthest away is *distal*. It helps to think that the close structure is in the proximity of the reference, while the far structure is some distance away. These two terms—*proximal* and *distal*—usually replace *superior* and *inferior* on the limbs. *Proximal* and *distal* also may be used for the torso when referring to vessels and tubes that have an origin and an end. An example would be the pancreatic duct, which delivers digestive enzymes into the small intestine. It starts in the pancreas (proximal) and ends in the small intestine (distal).

The most commonly used points of reference are the shoulder joint and the hip joint. Thus, the elbow is said to be proximal when compared to the wrist, which is distal. The knee is proximal when compared to the ankle. Most medical professionals only use *proximal* and *distal* in reference to the arms and legs. Thus, a structure closer to the shoulder is called *proximal*; another structure near the wrist is called *distal*. Do not refer to a structure close to the shoulder as superior or one near the elbow as inferior. Keep in mind that superior and inferior are usually used for the head, neck, and torso.

Trying to remember all this in an emergency situation could lead to some confusion. Take the opportunity to use the classroom setting to practice the proper use of these terms.

In addition to directional terms, there are specific positional terms with which you should become familiar (Figure 4.2). These terms include:

- **Supine,** which means lying face up.
- **Prone,** which means lying face down.
- **Lateral recumbent** (recovery position) is lying on one's side.

Because the term *lateral recumbent* can be used for lying on the right or left, it is proper to describe a patient as in either a right lateral recumbent position or a left lateral recumbent position. The correct recording of the patient's position may be of

anterior ▪ the front of the body or body part.

posterior ▪ the back of the body or body part.

midline ▪ an imaginary vertical line used to divide the body into right and left halves.

medial ▪ toward the midline of the body.

lateral ▪ to the side, away from the midline of the body.

superior ▪ toward the head (for example, the chest is superior to the abdomen).

inferior ▪ away from the head (for example, the lips are inferior to the nose).

proximal ▪ closer to the torso.

distal ▪ farther away from the torso.

supine ▪ the patient is lying face up.

prone ▪ the patient is lying face down.

lateral recumbent ▪ the patient is lying on his side.

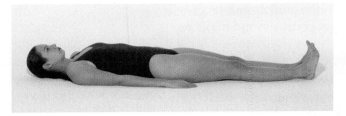
Supine

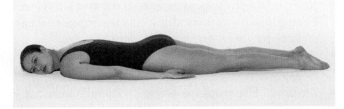
Prone

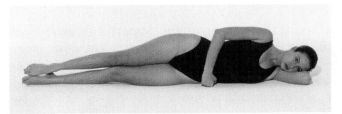
Lateral recumbent position

FIGURE 4.2 Positional terms.

medical significance and also may become part of the legal record of how a patient was first seen. As with directional terms, positional terms should be studied and practiced so that they become part of your professional vocabulary and documentation.

Most Emergency Medical Responders do not deal with emergencies on a daily basis. Unless you review and use anatomical terms often, you may forget them over time. Be aware that medical and rescue personnel are trained to take your information. They will not be confused if you say *front, back, above,* and *below.* Never let terminology stand in the way of clear communication with EMS providers, physicians, and other medical professionals.

BODY REGIONS

FIRST ➢ The human body can be divided into five regions (Figure 4.3). These regions have the common, everyday names of *head, neck, torso, upper extremities (shoulders, arms,* and *hands),* and *lower extremities (hips, legs,* and *feet).* Later in this text, you will be asked to study specific areas within each region. For now, to begin your new approach to viewing the body, start with the simplest of subdivisions:

- Head
  — Cranium, which houses the brain
  — Face
  — Mandible (MAN-di-bl), or lower jaw
- Neck
- Torso
  — Chest, or the thorax (THO-raks)
  — Abdomen, which extends from the lower ribs to the pelvic girdle
  — Pelvic cavity, which is protected by the bones of the pelvic girdle
- Upper extremities
  — Shoulder joint
  — Arm
  — Elbow
  — Forearm

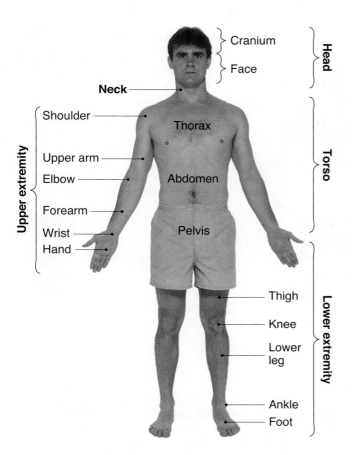

FIGURE 4.3 Body regions.

Cranium
Face
Head
Neck
Shoulder
Thorax
Upper extremity
Upper arm
Elbow
Abdomen
Forearm
Wrist
Pelvis
Hand
Torso
Thigh
Knee
Lower
leg
Lower extremity
Ankle
Foot

- — Wrist
- — Hand
- ■ Lower extremities
  - — Hip joint
  - — Thigh
  - — Knee
  - — Leg
  - — Ankle
  - — Foot ■

The terms *cranium, thorax*, and *mandible* may not be used in most daily conversations, but the other terms are already part of your vocabulary. The significant thing is to begin looking for these simple subdivisions each time you consider possible diseases and injuries. As stated previously, more specifics will be covered throughout this text.

BODY CAVITIES

FIRST ➤ There are four major body cavities—cranial, thoracic, abdominal, and pelvic (Figure 4.4). Housed in these cavities are the major vital organs, blood vessels, and nerves. ■

Cranial Cavity
The cranial cavity is the brain case of the skull, housing the brain and its specialized membranes. The spinal cord runs through the center of the backbone, protecting the cord and its specialized membranes.

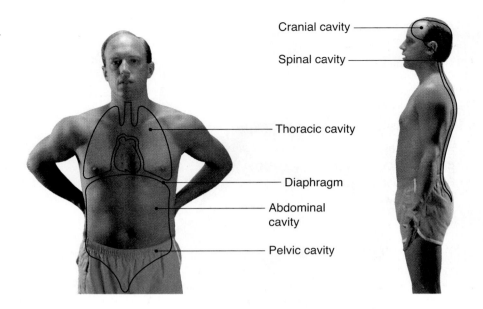

FIGURE 4.4 Body cavities.

Cranial cavity

Spinal cavity

Thoracic cavity

Diaphragm

Abdominal cavity

Pelvic cavity

thoracic (tho-RAS-ik) cavity ■ the anterior body cavity that is above (superior to) the diaphragm. Also called *chest cavity*.

diaphragm (DI-uh-fram) ■ the muscular structure that divides the chest cavity from the abdominal cavity.

Thoracic Cavity

The **thoracic cavity**, also known as the chest cavity, is enclosed by the rib cage. It protects the lungs, heart, great blood vessels, part of the windpipe (trachea), and part of the esophagus (e-SOF-ah-gus), which is the tube leading from the throat to the stomach. The lower border of the chest cavity is the **diaphragm** muscle, a dome-shaped muscle used in breathing. The diaphragm separates the chest cavity from the abdominal cavity (Figure 4.5).

FIGURE 4.5 Location of diaphragm and abdominal quadrants.

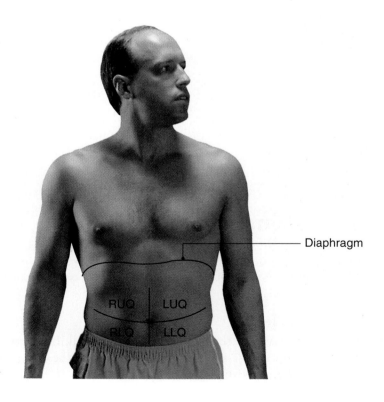

Diaphragm

RUQ | LUQ

RLQ | LLQ

Abdominal Cavity

The **abdominal cavity** lies between the chest cavity and the pelvic cavity. The stomach, liver, gallbladder, pancreas, spleen, small intestine, and most of the large intestine can be found in the abdominal cavity. Unlike the other body cavities, the abdominal cavity is not surrounded by bones. If you consider the organs in this cavity and the lack of bony protection, it is easy to see why trauma to the abdomen can result in severe injury.

abdominal cavity ■ the anterior body cavity that extends from the diaphragm to the pelvic cavity.

Pelvic Cavity

The **pelvic cavity** is protected by the bones of the pelvic girdle. This cavity houses the urinary bladder, portions of the large intestine, and the internal reproductive organs.

pelvic cavity ■ the anterior body cavity surrounded by the bones of the pelvis.

ABDOMINAL QUADRANTS

FIRST ➤ The abdomen is a large body region that contains many vital organs. The navel, or umbilicus (um-BIL-i-kus), is the main point of reference when describing the abdomen, which is divided into four quadrants (Figure 4.5). The **abdominal quadrants** are:

- Right upper quadrant (RUQ) contains most of the liver, the gallbladder, and part of the small and large intestine.
- Left upper quadrant (LUQ) contains most of the stomach, the spleen, part of the small and large intestine, and part of the liver.
- Right lower quadrant (RLQ) contains the appendix and part of the small and large intestine.
- Left lower quadrant (LLQ) contains part of the small and large intestine. ■

Some organs are located in more than one quadrant, as you can see from the preceding list. Pelvic organs also are included in these quadrants, with the urinary bladder being assigned to both lower quadrants.

FIRST ➤ When assessing a patient's abdominal area, be sure to palpate the soft areas to the rear of the abdomen on each side. These soft areas are located on the posterior, just above (superior to) the pelvic bones. They contain the kidneys and are susceptible to injury because they are not protected by bone. ■

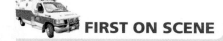

FIRST ON SCENE

"Jason!" Stephanie drops to her knees in the dirt next to her friend, pulls on a pair of gloves, and tears open his bloody uniform shirt. There is a perfectly round hole in his chest just below the right nipple, and dark blood is dripping steadily from the wound. She rolls him up onto his side to check his back, and he moans, grabbing weakly at her arms. There is a large, ragged hole just below his right shoulder blade and blood is bubbling thickly out onto the ground.

She grabs her portable radio and keys the mic. "Control, George 14, I need you to let the responding ambulance know that Adam 9 has been shot. He has an entrance wound just below the right nipple and an exit wound under the right shoulder blade. He is responsive to pain and has noisy breathing. I don't see anything else."

She then drops the radio into the dust, places one hand over each of Jason's wounds, and applies steady pressure.

The kidneys are a special case. They are not contained within the abdominal cavity because they are located behind the membrane that lines the cavity. The location of the kidneys makes them subject to injury from blows to the midback. Any pain or ache in the back may involve the kidneys. Most of the pancreas and the aorta are also located behind the abdominal cavity membrane. The pancreas is mostly in the right upper quadrant, and the aorta lies just in front of the spinal column.

REMEMBER

"Right" and "left" always refer to the patient's right and left.

Body Systems

Knowing the body systems and their functions can prove to be of value to the Emergency Medical Responder. However, most training courses do not have the time to go into great detail. Throughout this text, specific anatomy and some

abdominal quadrants ■ four divisions of the abdomen used to pinpoint the location of pain or injury: right upper quadrant (RUQ), left upper quadrant (LUQ), right lower quadrant (RLQ), and left lower quadrant (LLQ).

1–4.1 Describe the anatomy and function of the respiratory system.

1–4.2 Describe the anatomy and function of the circulatory system.

1–4.3 Describe the anatomy and function of the musculoskeletal system.

1–4.4 Describe the components and function of the nervous system.

basic functions are covered as they apply to illness, injury, and Emergency Medical Responder care.

Remembering the different body functions can be useful when trying to determine the extent of injury or the nature of an illness. The following is a list of the major body systems and their primary functions:

■ *Respiratory system.* The primary structures associated with the respiratory system include the nose, mouth, trachea, lungs, and associated muscles. The respiratory system is primarily responsible for the exchange of oxygen and carbon dioxide. Oxygen is placed into the bloodstream while carbon dioxide is removed.

■ *Circulatory system.* The primary structures of the circulatory system include the heart, blood vessels, and blood. The main job of the circulatory system is to carry well-oxygenated blood and other nutrients to the body's cells, and assist with the removal of wastes and carbon dioxide from the cells.

■ *Musculoskeletal.* (MUS-kyu-lo-SKEL-et-l) *system.* The primary structures of the musculoskeletal system include the bones, muscles, tendons, and ligaments. The main function of this system is to provide structure, support, and protection for the body and internal organs. In addition, the musculoskeletal system allows for body movement.

Geriatric Focus

One of the major effects of aging is the deterioration and weakening of the bones. Arthritis and osteoporosis are major contributors to this process. Approximately 33% of all falls involving the elderly result in at least one fractured bone. The most common fall related to fractures involves the hip and/or pelvis.

■ *Nervous system.* The primary structures of the nervous system include the brain, spinal cord, and nerves. The main function of the nervous system is to control movement, interpret sensations, regulate body activities, and generate memory and thought.

■ *Digestive system.* The primary structures of the digestive system include the esophagus, stomach, small intestines, and large intestines. Its main function is to digest and absorb food and remove certain wastes.

■ *Urinary system.* The primary structures of the urinary system include the kidneys, ureters, and bladder. The main function of this system is to remove chemical wastes from the blood and help balance water and salt levels in the blood.

■ *Reproductive system.* The primary structures of the reproductive system include the testes and penis for the male and the ovaries, fallopian tubes, uterus, and vagina for the female. This system produces hormones needed for sexual reproduction.

■ *Skin.* The largest organ in the body, the skin covers the body's many tissues, organs, and systems. It protects the body from heat and cold, as well as from toxins in the environment, such as bacteria and other foreign organisms. It regulates body temperature and senses heat, cold, touch, pain, and pressure. It also regulates body fluids and chemical balance. The skin is actually part of the integumentary (in-teg-u-MEN-tah-ree) system, which includes all the layers of the skin, nails, hair, sweat glands, oil glands, and mammary glands.

Geriatric Focus

As people age, the skin loses an important component called *collagen.* The result in the elderly is skin that is very thin and less elastic. This means that it can be easily damaged by simple falls or rough handling.

■ *Immune system.* The immune system protects the body from disease-causing organisms with white blood cells, microorganism-attacking cells, antibody-producing cells, and antibodies. It also helps to control allergies and the body's reactions to certain diseases. Some immune system reactions include the body attacking itself (autoimmune diseases).

Geriatric Focus

The following table offers an overview of systems of the body and the related changes that commonly occur with aging.

BODY SYSTEM	CHANGES WITH AGE	CLINICAL IMPORTANCE
Respiratory	Loss of strength and coordination in respiratory muscles Cough and gag reflex reduced	Increased likelihood of respiratory distress and failure
Cardiovascular	Loss of elasticity and hardening of arteries Changes in heart rate, rhythm, efficiency	High blood pressure common Greater likelihood of strokes, heart attacks Greater likelihood of bleeding from minor trauma
Neurological (brain and spinal cord)	Brain tissue shrinks Loss of memory Depression common Altered mental status common Impaired balance	Delay in appearance of symptoms with head injury Difficulty in patient assessment Increased likelihood of falls
Endocrine (glands that secrete hormones)	Lowered estrogen production (women) Decline in insulin sensitivity Increase in insulin resistance	Increased likelihood of fracture (bone loss) and heart disease Diabetes mellitus common with greater possibility of hyperglycemia
Gastrointestinal	Diminished digestive functions	Constipation common Greater likelihood of malnutrition
Thermoregulatory (heat and cold regulation)	Reduced sweating Decreased shivering	Environmental emergencies more common
Integumentary (skin)	Thins and becomes more fragile	More subject to tears and sores Bruising more common Heals more slowly
Musculoskeletal	Loss of bone strength (osteoporosis) Loss of joint flexibility and strength (osteoarthritis)	Greater likelihood of fractures Slower healing Increased likelihood of falls
Renal (kidneys)	Loss of kidney size and function	Increased problems with drug toxicity
Genitourinary (genitals and bladder)	Loss of bladder function	Increased urination and/or loss of control Increased urinary tract infection
Immune	Diminished immune response	More susceptible to infection Impaired immune response to vaccines

Relating Structures to the Body

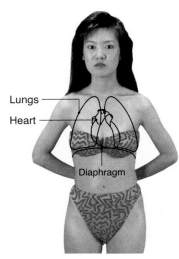

FIGURE 4.6 Position of the heart and lungs.

Look at Figure 4.6. Notice the position of the heart and lungs and their placement in the chest cavity. Then, as a quick point of reference, use your fingers to find the notch just below your own breastbone (sternum). Find a point directly over the inferior (lower) border of the heart by measuring two finger-widths up from this notch. Look at yourself in a mirror and notice this point, this is where your heart is located.

Look at Figure 4.6 again. Notice the position of the lungs in the chest cavity. The lungs are protected by the rib cage. By studying this figure, you will have a good idea of the size, shape, and position of the lungs.

Figure 4.7 shows the position of the stomach, liver, and the first portion of the small intestine, which is called the *duodenum* (du-o-DE-num). The lower ribs protect the stomach and liver. The first portion of the small intestine is important in emergency medicine because it is held in a more rigid position than the rest of the small intestine. Forceful blows to the abdomen, often received in automobile collisions, may injure the first portion of the small intestine without causing any significant damage to the rest of the intestine.

Notice that Figure 4.8 shows the gallbladder behind the liver, the pancreas behind the lower part of the stomach, and the spleen behind the left side of the stomach. Knowing these general locations will improve your chances of correctly assessing the nature of many injuries to the abdomen.

Now look at Figure 4.9. Notice the space occupied by the small intestine. As you can see, it fills most of the abdominal cavity. You also can see the space occupied by the large intestine. Notice how it passes through each of the four abdominal quadrants as it "frames" the small intestine.

It is important to know that the kidneys are behind the abdominal cavity, and the bladder is in the pelvic cavity (Figure 4.10). Although they appear well protected, injuries to these structures are common in motor-vehicle collisions. This is particularly true when occupants who are not wearing seat belts are thrown about in the passenger compartment. Internal organs may also be

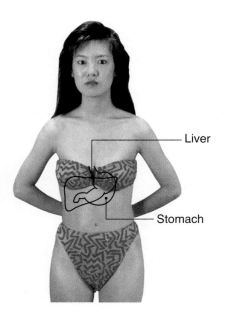

FIGURE 4.7 Position of the stomach and liver.

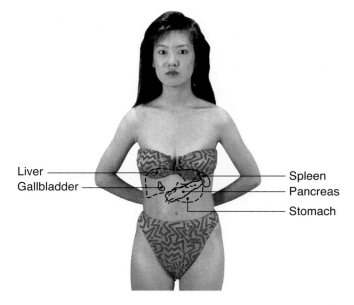

FIGURE 4.8 Position of the gallbladder, pancreas, and spleen.

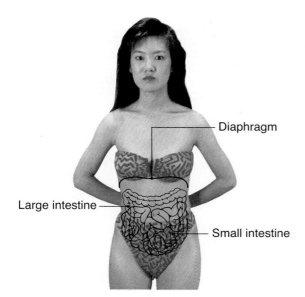

FIGURE 4.9 Position of the small and large intestine.

Diaphragm

Large intestine —

— Small intestine

injured by gunshots, stabbings, severe blows to the abdomen or back, and forces or weights that cause crushing.

Scans 4–1 through 4–10 sum up this material with an internal view of the locations of the major body organs. Study the drawings and spend the time to relate the positions of these organs to the body's exterior.

FIGURE 4.10 Position of the urinary system.

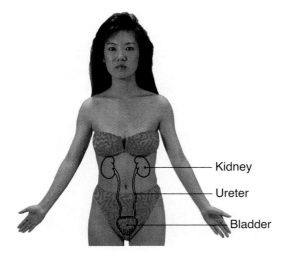

— Kidney

— Ureter

— Bladder

FIRST ON SCENE WRAP-UP

It seemed like forever before Stephanie heard sirens approaching. Jason had yet to do anything except flutter his eyelids and groan. Although the direct pressure seemed to have stopped most of the bleeding, Jason appeared to be struggling more to breathe. Thankfully, she heard vehicle after vehicle rolling to a stop nearby, and the screaming sirens are quickly replaced by a multitude of slamming doors and running feet.

"Okay, we're here now," a woman says and puts her hand on Stephanie's trembling shoulder. She lets go of Jason and stands up. He is immediately surrounded by firefighters and medics, who are tearing open packages and shouting to each other. She takes a few steps back and is caught in the tight embrace of the shift supervisor. "You did real good, kid," he says into her ear. "You did exactly what you were supposed to do."

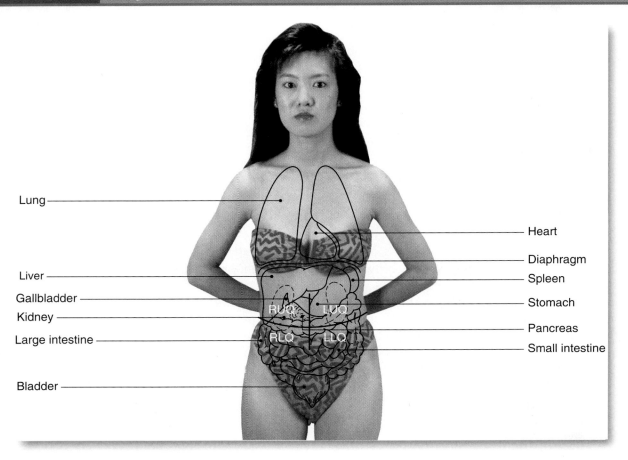

Lung

Heart

Diaphragm

Liver

Spleen

Gallbladder

Stomach

Kidney

Pancreas

Large intestine

Small intestine

RUQ   LUQ

RLQ   LLQ

Bladder

SOLID ORGANS

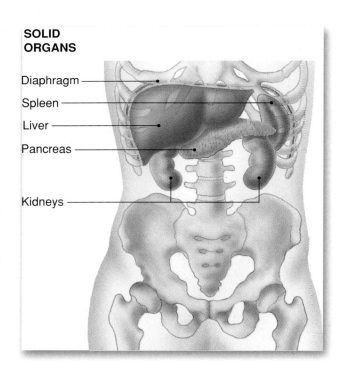

Diaphragm

Spleen

Liver

Pancreas

Kidneys

HOLLOW ORGANS

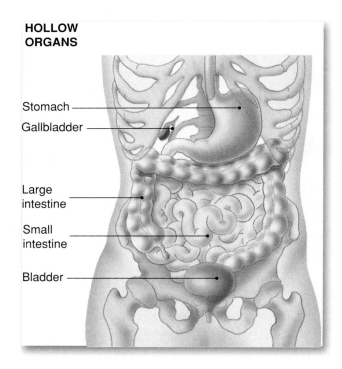

Stomach

Gallbladder

Large intestine

Small intestine

Bladder

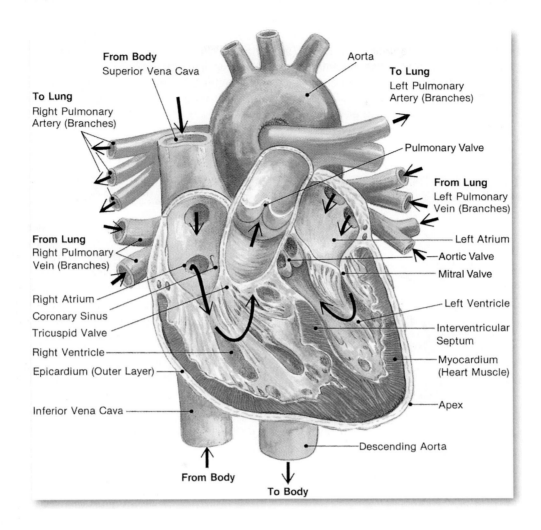

From Body
Superior Vena Cava

Aorta

To Lung
Right Pulmonary
Artery (Branches)

To Lung
Left Pulmonary
Artery (Branches)

Pulmonary Valve

From Lung
Left Pulmonary
Vein (Branches)

From Lung
Right Pulmonary
Vein (Branches)

Left Atrium

Aortic Valve

Mitral Valve

Right Atrium

Coronary Sinus

Tricuspid Valve

Left Ventricle

Interventricular
Septum

Right Ventricle

Epicardium (Outer Layer)

Myocardium
(Heart Muscle)

Inferior Vena Cava

Apex

Descending Aorta

From Body

To Body

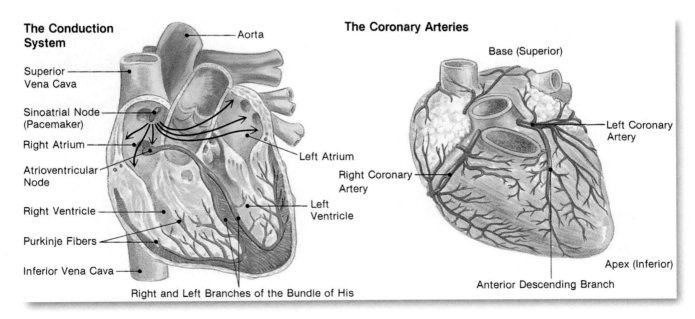

The Conduction System

Aorta

Superior Vena Cava

Sinoatrial Node (Pacemaker)

Right Atrium

Atrioventricular Node

Left Atrium

Right Ventricle

Left Ventricle

Purkinje Fibers

Inferior Vena Cava

Right and Left Branches of the Bundle of His

The Coronary Arteries

Base (Superior)

Left Coronary Artery

Right Coronary Artery

Anterior Descending Branch

Apex (Inferior)

The heart is a hollow, muscular organ that pumps 450 million pints of blood in the average lifetime. Its superior chambers, the atria, receive blood. Both atria fill and then contract at the same time. The inferior chambers are the ventricles. They pump blood out of the heart. Both ventricles fill and then contract at the same time. When the atria are relaxing, the ventricles are contracting.

The right side of the heart receives blood from the body and sends it to the lungs (pulmonic circulation). The heart's left side receives oxygenated blood from the lungs and sends it out to the body (systemic circulation).

The heartbeat originates at the sinoatrial node (pacemaker) and spreads across the atria to stimulate contraction. After a slight delay, the impulse is sent from the atrioventricular node, down the bundles of His, and out across the ventricles. This stimulates the ventricles to contract while the atria are relaxing.

The heart muscle (myocardium) receives its blood supply by way of the right and left coronary arteries. These vessels are the first branches of the aorta.

SCAN 4–3 Circulatory System: Blood Vessels

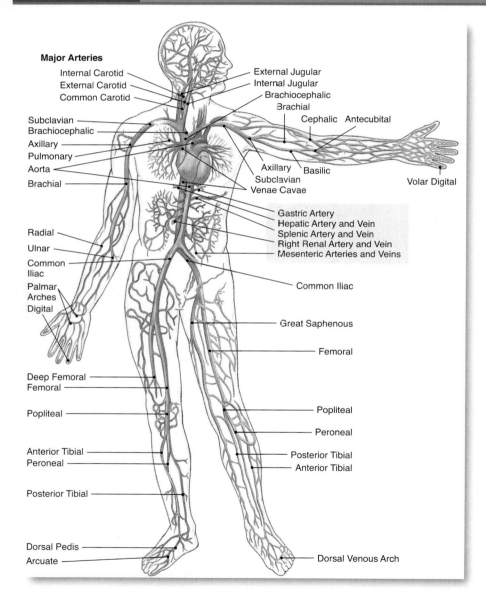

Major Arteries

Internal Carotid
External Carotid
Common Carotid
Subclavian
Brachiocephalic
Axillary
Pulmonary
Aorta
Brachial
Radial
Ulnar
Common Iliac
Palmar Arches
Digital
Deep Femoral
Femoral
Popliteal
Anterior Tibial
Peroneal
Posterior Tibial
Dorsal Pedis
Arcuate

External Jugular
Internal Jugular
Brachiocephalic
Brachial
Cephalic   Antecubital
Axillary   Basilic
Subclavian
Venae Cavae
Volar Digital
Gastric Artery
Hepatic Artery and Vein
Splenic Artery and Vein
Right Renal Artery and Vein
Mesenteric Arteries and Veins
Common Iliac
Great Saphenous
Femoral
Popliteal
Peroneal
Posterior Tibial
Anterior Tibial
Dorsal Venous Arch

Any blood vessel that carries blood away from the heart is an artery. Arteries have strong muscular walls and are very elastic, changing their diameter as the heart contracts to force blood into circulation. They decrease in diameter to become arterioles. These structures join with capillary beds. A capillary is thin-walled, being no thicker than the lining of an arteriole. Blood moves through the capillaries in a constant flow known as *perfusion*. During perfusion, oxygen and nutrients are given up to the body's tissues, and cellular carbon dioxide and wastes are picked up.

Any blood vessel that carries blood back to the heart is a vein. The small-diameter veins that leave capillary beds are called *venules*. These join with larger veins. The walls of the veins are not as thick or elastic as those of the arteries. Some veins have valves to prevent the backward flow of blood.

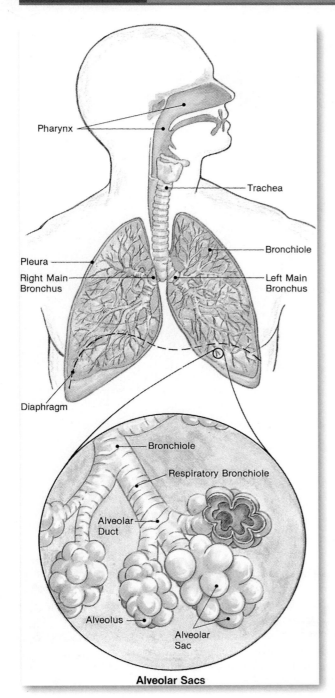

Pharynx

Trachea

Bronchiole

Pleura

Right Main
Bronchus

Left Main
Bronchus

Diaphragm

Bronchiole

Respiratory Bronchiole

Alveolar
Duct

Alveolus

Alveolar
Sac

Alveolar Sacs

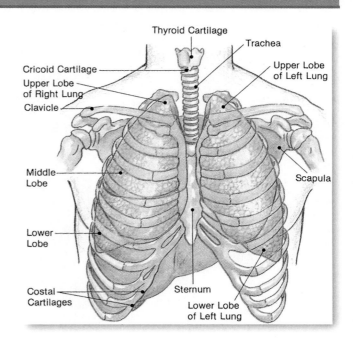

Thyroid Cartilage

Trachea

Cricoid Cartilage

Upper Lobe
of Left Lung

Upper Lobe
of Right Lung

Clavicle

Middle
Lobe

Scapula

Lower
Lobe

Costal
Cartilages

Sternum

Lower Lobe
of Left Lung

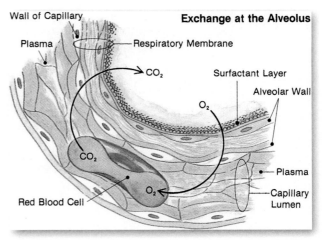

Wall of Capillary

Exchange at the Alveolus

Plasma

Respiratory Membrane

CO_2

Surfactant Layer

Alveolar Wall

O_2

CO_2

Plasma

Red Blood Cell

O_2

Capillary
Lumen

The airway consists of structures involved with the conduction and exchange of air. Conduction is the movement of air to and from the exchange levels of the lungs. Air enters through the nose (primary) and mouth (secondary) and travels down the pharynx to enter the larynx. After passing through the larynx, air enters the trachea. At its distal end, the trachea branches into the left and right primary bronchi. These bronchi branch into secondary bronchi, which then branch into the bronchioles. Some of the bronchioles end as closed tubes. Air movement in them helps the lungs expand. The rest of the bronchioles carry the air to the exchange levels of the lungs.

The respiratory bronchioles turn into alveolar ducts. These form alveolar sacs that are made up of the alveoli. Gas exchange takes place between the alveoli and the capillaries in the lungs.

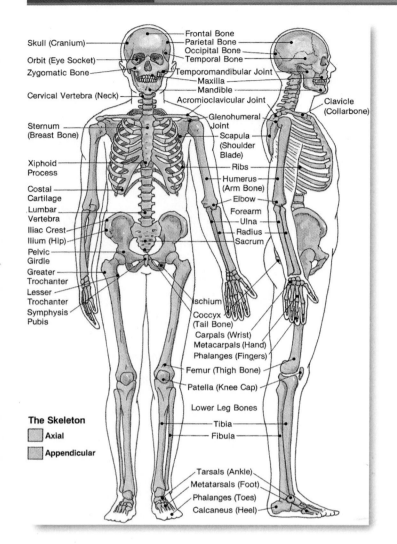

The Skeleton

- ▢ Axial
- ▢ Appendicular

Skull (Cranium)
Orbit (Eye Socket)
Zygomatic Bone
Cervical Vertebra (Neck)
Sternum (Breast Bone)
Xiphoid Process
Costal Cartilage
Lumbar Vertebra
Iliac Crest
Ilium (Hip)
Pelvic Girdle
Greater Trochanter
Lesser Trochanter
Symphysis Pubis

Frontal Bone
Parietal Bone
Occipital Bone
Temporal Bone
Temporomandibular Joint
Maxilla
Mandible
Acromioclavicular Joint
Glenohumeral Joint
Scapula (Shoulder Blade)
Ribs
Humerus (Arm Bone)
Elbow
Forearm
Ulna
Radius
Sacrum

Clavicle (Collarbone)

Ischium
Coccyx (Tail Bone)
Carpals (Wrist)
Metacarpals (Hand)
Phalanges (Fingers)
Femur (Thigh Bone)
Patella (Knee Cap)
Lower Leg Bones
Tibia
Fibula

Tarsals (Ankle)
Metatarsals (Foot)
Phalanges (Toes)
Calcaneus (Heel)

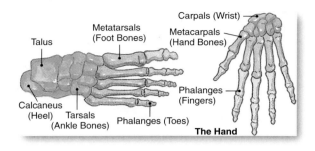

Carpals (Wrist)
Metatarsals (Foot Bones)
Metacarpals (Hand Bones)
Talus
Calcaneus (Heel)
Tarsals (Ankle Bones)
Phalanges (Toes)
Phalanges (Fingers)
The Hand

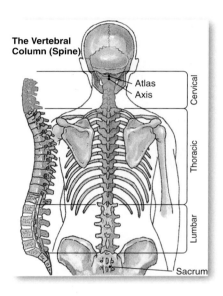

The Vertebral Column (Spine)

Atlas
Axis
Cervical
Thoracic
Lumbar
Sacrum

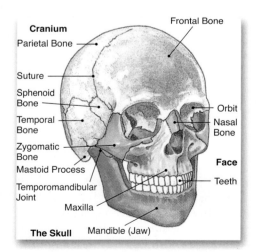

Cranium
Parietal Bone
Suture
Sphenoid Bone
Temporal Bone
Zygomatic Bone
Mastoid Process
Temporomandibular Joint
Maxilla
The Skull
Frontal Bone
Orbit
Nasal Bone
Face
Teeth
Mandible (Jaw)

The skeleton is a living framework made by the joining of bones. It serves to provide support, body movement powered by muscular contractions, protection for the vital organs and other soft structures, blood cell production, and storage for essential minerals. There are 206 bones in the adult body that form the two divisions of the skeletal system, the axial and appendicular skeletons. The axial skeletal is comprised of skull, vertebrae, rib cage, and sternum. The upper and lower extremities and the shoulder and pelvic girdles form the appendicular skeleton.

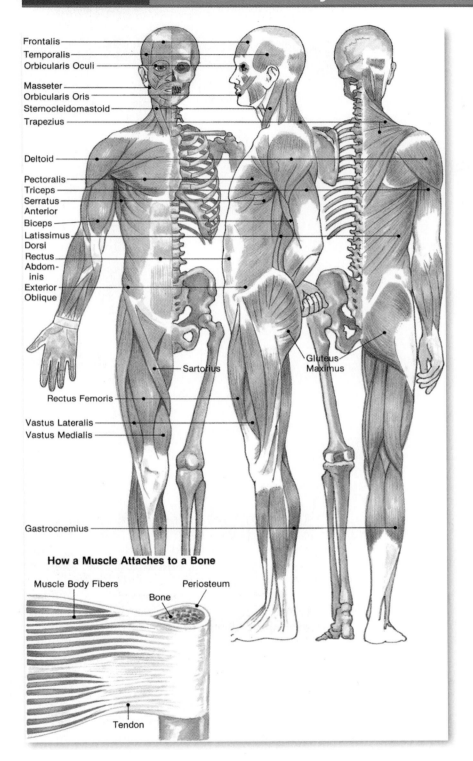

Frontalis
Temporalis
Orbicularis Oculi

Masseter
Orbicularis Oris
Sternocleidomastoid
Trapezius

Deltoid

Pectoralis
Triceps
Serratus
Anterior
Biceps
Latissimus
Dorsi
Rectus
Abdom-
inis
Exterior
Oblique

Sartorius

Rectus Femoris

Vastus Lateralis
Vastus Medialis

Gluteus
Maximus

Gastrocnemius

How a Muscle Attaches to a Bone

Muscle Body Fibers
Bone
Periosteum

Tendon

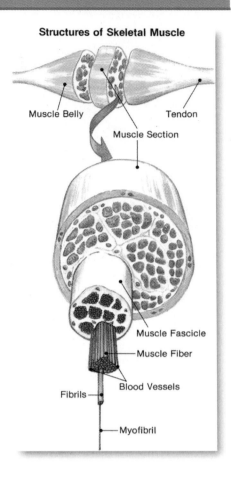

Structures of Skeletal Muscle

Muscle Belly
Tendon
Muscle Section

Muscle Fascicle
Muscle Fiber
Blood Vessels
Fibrils
Myofibril

The tissues of the muscular system comprise 40% to 50% of the body's weight. The skeletal muscles of the body are voluntary muscles, subject to conscious control. They exhibit the properties of excitability; that is, they will react to nerve stimulus. Once stimulated, skeletal muscles are quick to contract and relax and can quickly be ready for another contraction. There are 501 separate skeletal muscles that provide contractions for movement, coordinated support for posture, and heat production. Muscles connect to bones by way of tendons.

The Brain

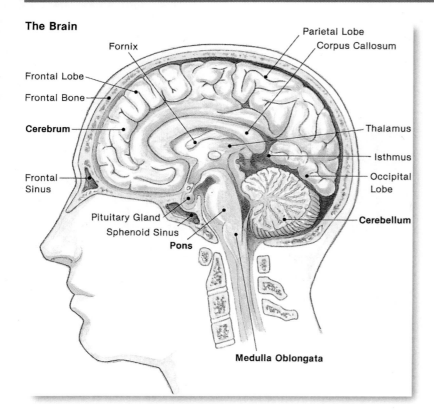

Fornix
Frontal Lobe
Frontal Bone
Cerebrum
Frontal Sinus
Pituitary Gland
Sphenoid Sinus
Pons
Medulla Oblongata
Parietal Lobe
Corpus Callosum
Thalamus
Isthmus
Occipital Lobe
Cerebellum

Divisions of the Spinal Cord

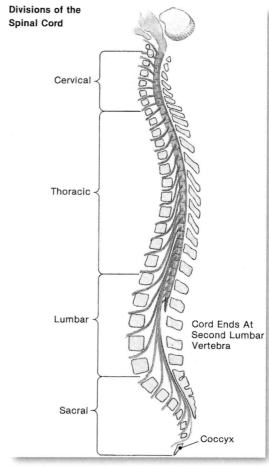

Cervical
Thoracic
Lumbar
Sacral
Cord Ends At Second Lumbar Vertebra
Coccyx

The Spinal Cord

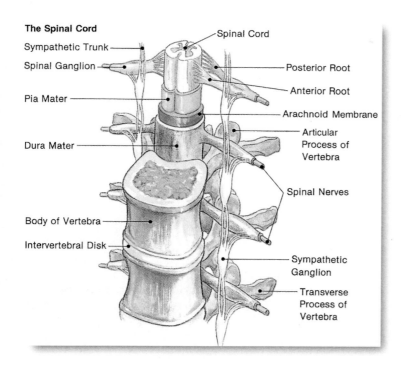

Sympathetic Trunk
Spinal Ganglion
Pia Mater
Dura Mater
Body of Vertebra
Intervertebral Disk
Spinal Cord
Posterior Root
Anterior Root
Arachnoid Membrane
Articular Process of Vertebra
Spinal Nerves
Sympathetic Ganglion
Transverse Process of Vertebra

The nervous system includes the brain, spinal cord, and nerves. Structures within the system may be classified according to divisions: central, peripheral, and autonomic. The central nervous system includes the brain and spinal cord. The sensory (incoming) and motor (outgoing) nerves make up the peripheral nervous system. The autonomic nervous system has structures that parallel the spinal cord and then share the same pathways as the peripheral nerves. This division is involved with motor impulses (outgoing commands) that travel from the central nervous system to the heart muscle, blood vessels, secreting cells of glands, and the smooth muscles of organs. The impulses will stimulate or inhibit certain activities.

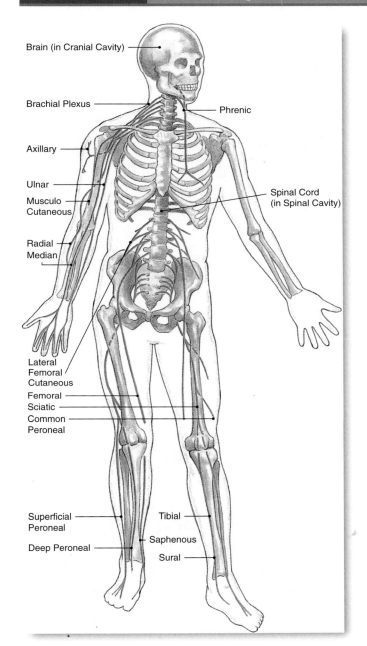

Brain (in Cranial Cavity)

Brachial Plexus

Phrenic

Axillary

Ulnar

Musculo Cutaneous

Spinal Cord (in Spinal Cavity)

Radial Median

Lateral Femoral Cutaneous

Femoral

Sciatic

Common Peroneal

Superficial Peroneal

Tibial

Saphenous

Deep Peroneal

Sural

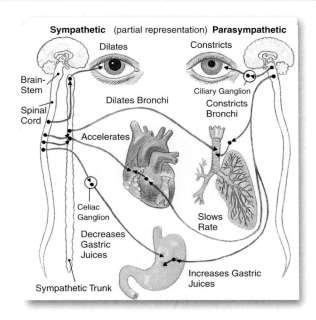

Sympathetic (partial representation) **Parasympathetic**

Dilates

Constricts

Brain-Stem

Ciliary Ganglion

Spinal Cord

Dilates Bronchi

Constricts Bronchi

Accelerates

Celiac Ganglion

Slows Rate

Decreases Gastric Juices

Increases Gastric Juices

Sympathetic Trunk

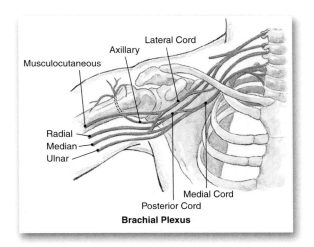

Lateral Cord

Axillary

Musculocutaneous

Radial

Median

Ulnar

Medial Cord

Posterior Cord

Brachial Plexus

Autonomic Nervous System

The autonomic nervous system affects the heart, blood vessels, digestive tract, salivary and digestive glands, pancreas, liver, spleen, anal sphincter, kidneys, urinary bladder, urinary sphincter, adrenal glands, thyroid gland, gonads, genitalia, nasal lining, larynx, bronchi, lungs, iris and ciliary muscles of the eyes, tear glands, and hair muscles. Impulses can increase or slow heart rate, stimulate dilation or constriction of blood vessels, cause glands to secrete or decrease secretion, initiate or inhibit contractions in the bladder, stimulate or decrease a wave of muscle contraction along the digestive tract, and many other essential body activities.

The Skin

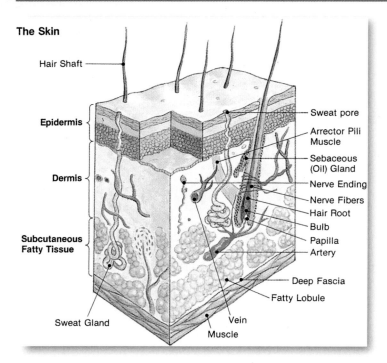

- Hair Shaft
- Epidermis
- Dermis
- Subcutaneous Fatty Tissue
- Sweat Gland
- Sweat pore
- Arrector Pili Muscle
- Sebaceous (Oil) Gland
- Nerve Ending
- Nerve Fibers
- Hair Root
- Bulb
- Papilla
- Artery
- Deep Fascia
- Fatty Lobule
- Vein
- Muscle

The Peritoneum

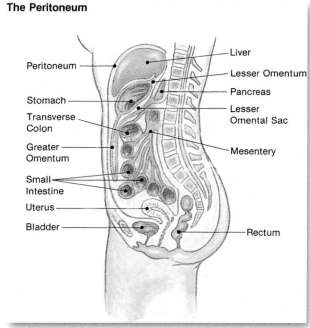

- Peritoneum
- Stomach
- Transverse Colon
- Greater Omentum
- Small Intestine
- Uterus
- Bladder
- Liver
- Lesser Omentum
- Pancreas
- Lesser Omental Sac
- Mesentery
- Rectum

Synovial Joint

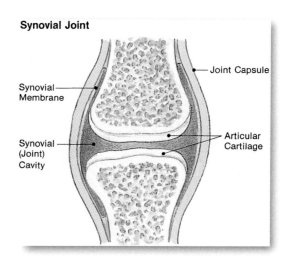

- Joint Capsule
- Synovial Membrane
- Synovial (Joint) Cavity
- Articular Cartilage

The Pleura

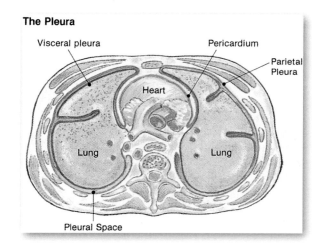

- Visceral pleura
- Pericardium
- Parietal Pleura
- Heart
- Lung
- Lung
- Pleural Space

Skin

The skin is the largest organ of the body. In the adult, the skin covers about 3,000 square inches (1.75 square meters) and weighs about six pounds. It is involved with protection, insulation, thermal regulation, excretion, and production of vitamin D.

Membranes

Membranes cover or line body structures to provide protection from injury and infection. There are four major classes of membranes. Mucous membranes line those structures that open to the outside world (such as the mouth, airway, digestive tract, urinary tract, and vagina). Serous membranes line the closed body cavities and cover the outsides of organs. The cutaneous membrane is the skin. Synovial membranes line joints to reduce friction during movement.

A serous membrane that covers an organ is called a *visceral layer*. The term *parietal layer* is used for the part of the serous membrane that lines a cavity. The serous membrane in the thoracic cavity is called *pleura*. In the abdominal cavity, it is called *peritoneum*. A double layer of peritoneum is called *mesentery*. The membrane that lines the sac surrounding the heart is called *pericardium*.

Liver, Stomach, and Pancreas

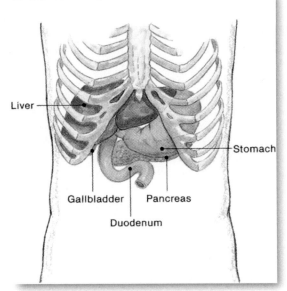

Liver
Stomach
Gallbladder
Pancreas
Duodenum

Small Intestine

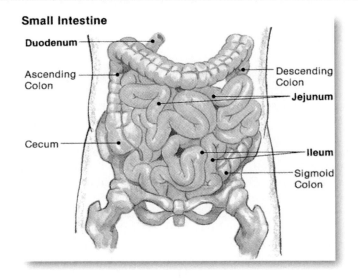

Duodenum
Ascending Colon
Descending Colon
Jejunum
Cecum
Ileum
Sigmoid Colon

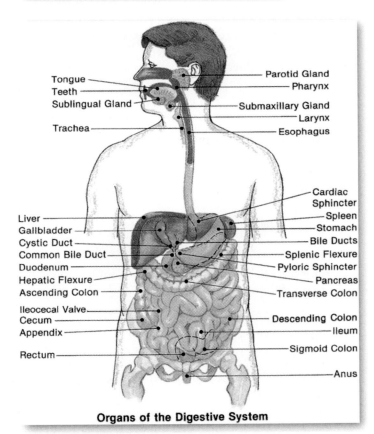

Tongue
Teeth
Sublingual Gland
Trachea
Parotid Gland
Pharynx
Submaxillary Gland
Larynx
Esophagus
Liver
Gallbladder
Cystic Duct
Common Bile Duct
Duodenum
Hepatic Flexure
Ascending Colon
Ileocecal Valve
Cecum
Appendix
Rectum
Cardiac Sphincter
Spleen
Stomach
Bile Ducts
Splenic Flexure
Pyloric Sphincter
Pancreas
Transverse Colon
Descending Colon
Ileum
Sigmoid Colon
Anus

Organs of the Digestive System

Large Intestine

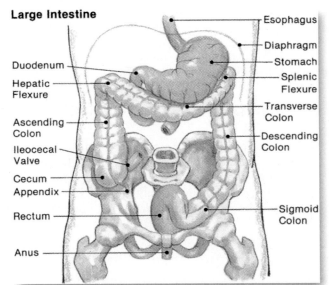

Duodenum
Hepatic Flexure
Ascending Colon
Ileocecal Valve
Cecum
Appendix
Rectum
Anus
Esophagus
Diaphragm
Stomach
Splenic Flexure
Transverse Colon
Descending Colon
Sigmoid Colon

The digestive system includes the digestive tract and various supportive structures and accessory glands. The tract begins at the oral cavity with the teeth and tongue. The salivary glands release saliva into the mouth to moisten food for swallowing. The tract continues down the throat to the esophagus through the cardiac sphincter and into the stomach. Acid and digestive enzymes are added to the food to produce chyme. The chyme passes through the pyloric sphincter to enter the small intestine. Digestive enzymes from the pancreas and bile from the liver are added to the chyme. The processes of digestion and absorption are completed in the small intestine. Wastes are carried through the ileocecal valve into the large intestine. The wastes are moved to the rectum, where they can be expelled through the anus.

Summary

Knowledge of the body's basic anatomy and general functions helps Emergency Medical Responders assess patients and communicate with other emergency care providers. When describing a patient and his or her associated signs or symptoms, always refer to the patient's right and the patient's left, with the body in the anatomical position. The anatomical position refers to the body standing upright, facing the viewer. The arms are down at the sides, and the palms are facing forward.

An imaginary vertical line, the midline, divides the body into halves. Medial means toward the midline, and lateral means away from the midline. Anterior is toward the front, and posterior is toward the back. Superior is toward the top of the head, and inferior is toward the feet. Proximal is toward the torso, and distal is away from the torso, both terms usually referring to the arms and legs. The terms *anterior, posterior, superior,* and *inferior* may be used for a body organ or gland. *Proximal* and *distal* may be used for any vessel, duct, or tube in the body.

When the patient is lying on his back, the body is supine. If face down, the patient's body is prone. The Emergency Medical Responder should use the term *lateral recumbent position* when the patient is lying on his side.

The body is divided into five regions (head, neck, torso, upper extremities, and lower extremities) and four cavities (cranial, thoracic, abdominal, and pelvic cavity).

The abdominal quadrants are centered around the navel: right upper quadrant (RUQ), left upper quadrant (LUQ), right lower quadrant (RLQ), and left lower quadrant (LLQ).

The major body systems include the circulatory system (heart, blood vessels, blood), respiratory system (nose, mouth, throat structures, lungs, respiratory muscles), digestive system (stomach, intestines, liver, gallbladder), urinary system (kidneys, ureters, bladder, urethra), reproductive system (uterus, ovaries, fallopian tubes, testicles, external genitalia), nervous system (brain, spinal cord, nerves), musculoskeletal system (bones, skeletal muscles, tendons and ligaments), skin (or integumentary system, including skin, hair, sweat glands, oil glands, and mammary glands), the special senses (eyes, ears, nose, mouth), and immune system, which protects the body from infection and certain diseases.

Remember and Consider

➤ It is important for the Emergency Medical Responder to learn to use the terms in this chapter. However, it is even more important that information pertaining to a patient be passed on accurately to other EMS personnel who will be providing patient care. So, if you are unable to remember the appropriate term in an emergency situation, use terms that are familiar to you and others.

➤ Use the terms *anterior, posterior, medial,* and *lateral.*

Investigate

➤ Outline your own major body cavities, and list what is found in each.

➤ Point to each of your abdominal quadrants. Name the organs found in each quadrant and describe their functions.

Quick Quiz

1. Which one of the following BEST describes the anatomical position?
   a. standing upright with arms at the sides
   b. lying supine with arms outstretched and palms up
   c. standing with hands at the sides and palms forward
   d. lying prone with arms held straight out, palms down

2. The navel is on the _____ aspect of the body.
   a. posterior
   b. anterior
   c. inferior
   d. superior

3. The spine can be felt (palpated) on the _____ aspect of the body.
   a. posterior
   b. anterior
   c. inferior
   d. superior

4. The imaginary line that bisects the body into two halves (left and right) is known as the:
   a. proximal break.
   b. inferior aspect.
   c. recumbent line.
   d. midline.

5. Any location on the body that is closer to the midline is referred to as:
   a. medial.
   b. recumbent.
   c. lateral.
   d. inferior.

6. The thumb is considered _____ to the palm.
   a. distal
   b. proximal
   c. lateral
   d. medial

7. A bruise that is on the anterior thigh just above the knee could be described as _____ to the knee.
   a. distal
   b. proximal
   c. lateral
   d. medial

8. The chin is _____ to the mouth.
   a. superior
   b. lateral
   c. inferior
   d. medial

9. The nose is _____ to the mouth.
   a. superior
   b. lateral
   c. inferior
   d. medial

10. A patient that is found lying face down is said to be in the _____ position.
    a. recumbent
    b. lateral
    c. supine
    d. prone

11. A patient with a suspected spine injury will likely be placed on a long spine board flat on his back or in a _____ position.
    a. recumbent
    b. lateral
    c. supine
    d. prone

12. The lateral recumbent position is also known as the _____ position.
    a. recovery
    b. lateral
    c. superior
    d. stroke

13. Which one of the following is NOT one of the major body regions?
    a. head
    b. upper extremities
    c. neck
    d. pelvis

14. The _____ cavity is also known as the thoracic cavity.
    a. pelvic
    b. chest
    c. abdominal
    d. cranial

15. The _____ separates the thoracic cavity from the abdominal cavity.
    a. pelvic wall
    b. midline
    c. diaphragm
    d. stomach

16. All of the following can be found in the abdominal cavity EXCEPT the:
    a. stomach.
    b. liver.
    c. spleen.
    d. heart.

17. The _____ cavity houses the bladder and part of the large intestine.
    a. pelvic
    b. abdominal
    c. thoracic
    d. cranial

18. The _____ is found in the upper right quadrant of the abdomen.
    a. spleen
    b. stomach
    c. kidney
    d. liver

19. An infection of the appendix would most likely cause pain in the:
    a. right upper quadrant (RUQ).
    b. left upper quadrant (LUQ).
    c. right lower quadrant (RLQ).
    d. left lower quadrant (LLQ).

20. The _____ is/are found in an area behind the abdominal cavity.
    a. kidneys
    b. bladder
    c. small intestine
    d. gall bladder

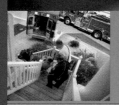

CHAPTER 5

Lifting, Moving, and Positioning Patients

Many Emergency Medical Responders are injured every year because they attempt to lift or move a patient or piece of equipment improperly. Injuries to the back are some of the most common and have the greatest potential to end what could otherwise be a long and rewarding career in EMS. One of the most important things you can do for yourself, your coworkers, and your patients is to learn how to lift and move patients and objects using proper body mechanics.

Just as important as knowing how to move patients properly is knowing when they should be moved. There are many factors the Emergency Medical Responder must consider before moving a patient, such as the safety of the scene, the patient's condition, and the number of rescuers.

This chapter discusses common situations when an Emergency Medical Responder should move a patient. It also describes some simple techniques of proper body mechanics that will make it possible for you to be an effective Emergency Medical Responder for many years to come.

OBJECTIVES

This chapter is based on the objectives of the U.S. DOT's First Responder National Standard Curriculum. Note that cognitive objectives are listed below and beside corresponding text throughout the chapter. You will also notice as you read each objective that the term Emergency Medical Responder is used. This is simply a name change and reflects the new name for the First Responder.

By the end of this chapter, you should be able to (from cognitive or knowledge information):

1–5.1 Define body mechanics. (p. 84)

1–5.2 Discuss the guidelines and safety precautions that need to be followed when lifting a patient. (pp. 84–85)

1–5.3 Describe the indications for an emergency move. (p. 86)

1–5.4 Describe the indications for assisting in non-emergency moves. (p. 88)

1–5.5 Discuss the various devices associated with moving a patient in the out-of-hospital arena. (pp. 97–104)

By the end of this chapter, you should be able to feel comfortable enough to (by changing attitudes, values, and beliefs):

1–5.6 Explain the rationale for properly lifting and moving patients. (pp. 83–85)

1–5.7 Explain the rationale for an emergency move. (p. 86)

By the end of this chapter, you should be able to show how to (through psychomotor skills):

1–5.8 Demonstrate an emergency move. (pp. 86–88)

1–5.9 Demonstrate a nonemergency move. (pp. 88–97)

1–5.10 Demonstrate the use of equipment utilized to move patients in the out-of-hospital arena. (pp. 97–104)

ADDITIONAL LEARNING TASKS

In an emergency situation, it is important to know how to safely move a patient in the most expedient way. In this chapter, you will also learn:

➤ The most common emergency moves to be used by Emergency Medical Responders and how to perform them.

➤ The most common nonemergency moves to be used by Emergency Medical Responders and how to perform them.

➤ The proper use and function of the recovery position.

 FIRST ON SCENE

Jesse Daniels had just put a new CD into the stereo when the front right tire on his car exploded, sending ropy pieces of black rubber in all directions. He grabbed the steering wheel with both hands and eased the small car completely off the road and onto the shoulder. He got out, swearing under his breath, and walked around to the front of the car to inspect the damage. The tire wasn't just flat. It was *gone*. A bare, bent wheel was the only thing that remained.

A man driving a pickup stopped in the roadway next to Jesse's car and shouted through the open passenger window, "Is everything okay?"

"Yeah. I just have to put the spare on," Jesse shouted back, knowing that he was definitely going to be late for his Emergency Medical Responder class at the community college.

"I'll pull over and help!" the man yelled back. Jesse smiled and started to say, "Thanks!" but the man and his pickup truck were suddenly gone in a deafening explosion of twisting metal, rushing air, and spinning chrome wheels. Jesse stumbled back, fell onto the ground, and watched in horror as a speeding semitrailer flashed larger than life just beyond the tips of his tennis shoes for a split-second before vanishing with the sound of locked-up tires roaring across the pavement.

Principles of Moving Patients

WHEN TO MOVE A PATIENT

FIRST ➤ In general, an Emergency Medical Responder should only move a patient when absolutely necessary. Your primary role is to assess the patient, provide basic emergency care, and continue to monitor the patient's condition until more advanced personnel arrive. Situations in which it may be necessary to move a patient include the presence of a dangerous environment where the patient is at risk for further injury; when you cannot adequately assess airway, breathing, and circulation (ABCs) or bleeding; or when you are unable to gain access to other patients who need life-saving care. You may also be called on to assist other EMS responders in lifting and moving patients. ■

Whenever possible, keep the patient at rest, even when the patient appears to be able to move. Remember that not all signs of an illness or injury show themselves immediately. Sometimes patients do not realize how sick or injured they are. In addition, some patients may not be straightforward in answering your questions or may even deny or hide the existence of an illness or injury.

BODY MECHANICS

body mechanics ■ the proper use of the body to facilitate lifting and moving and to minimize injury.

1–5.1 Define body mechanics.

1–5.2 Discuss the guidelines and safety precautions that need to be followed when lifting a patient.

FIRST ➤ **Body mechanics** is the proper use of your body to facilitate lifting and moving. These are important steps that Emergency Medical Responders must follow to lift efficiently and to prevent injury. ■

Before you lift or move a patient or an object, it is important to first plan what you will do and how you will do it (Figure 5.1) Estimate the weight of the patient or object and then, if needed, request additional help. It is also important to consider any physical limitations that may make lifting difficult or unsafe for you and those assisting you. Whenever possible, lift with a partner whose strength and height are similar to yours. Communicate with your partner and with the patient when you are ready to lift and continue to communicate throughout the process. Eye contact is an important component when coordinating a lift. To ensure good

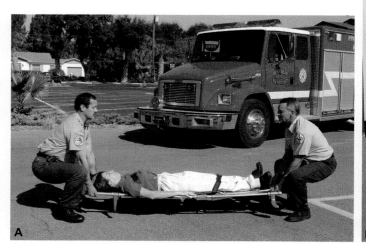
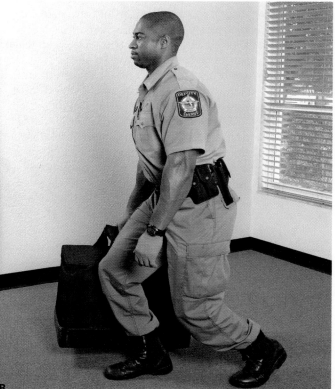

FIGURE 5.1 Plan ahead how you will lift a patient or an object and always use proper body mechanics.

communications, make sure you and your partner make eye contact before initiating any lift.

When you are ready to lift, follow these rules to minimize the chance of injury:

- Position your feet properly. They should be on a firm, level surface and positioned a comfortable width apart. Take extra care if the surface is slippery or unstable. It may be necessary to postpone the move until more help or equipment is on hand.
- Lift with your legs. Keep your back as straight as possible and bend at your knees. Try not to bend at the waist any more than you absolutely have to.
- When lifting with one hand, avoid leaning to either side. Bend your knees to grasp the object and keep your back straight.
- Minimize twisting during a lift. Attempts to turn or twist while you are lifting can result in serious injury.
- Keep the weight as close to your body as possible. The farther the weight is from your body, the greater your chance of injury.
- When carrying a patient on stairways, use a chair or commercial stair chair instead of a wheeled stretcher whenever possible. Keep your back straight, and let your legs do the lifting. If you are walking backward down stairs, ask someone to "spot" you, by walking behind you and placing a hand on your back to help guide and steady you (Figure 5.2).

Is It Safe ?

Sometimes the best decision is *not* to move the patient. If the patient is too heavy or in an awkward position, or you simply do not have enough people to help, consider a new plan and call for additional help. ∎

With the proper techniques, moving and lifting a patient can be done safely. Use proper body mechanics on every call.

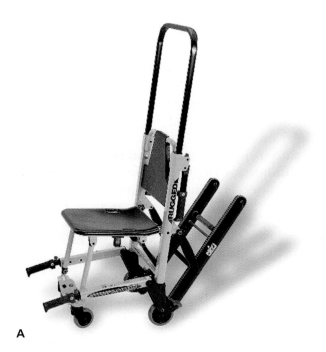

A

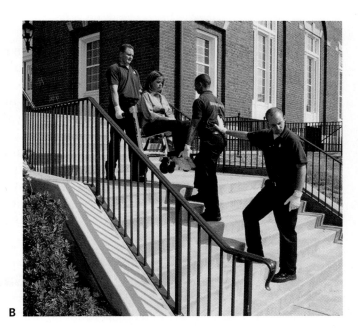

B

FIGURE 5.2 A. Example of a stair chair. (*Courtesy of Stryker EMS*) **B.** When you use a stair chair, have someone spot you as you walk backward down stairs.

MOVING AND POSITIONING PATIENTS
Emergency Moves

1–5.3 Describe the indications for an emergency move.

emergency move ■ a patient move that is carried out quickly when the scene is hazardous, care of the patient requires immediate repositioning, or you must reach another patient who needs life-saving care.

FIRST ▶ There are times when a patient must be moved immediately, even if you do not have the appropriate people or equipment to do so. These situations call for an **emergency move**. An emergency move should be considered in the following situations:

- The patient and/or the rescuers are in immediate danger. Situations that involve uncontrolled traffic, fire or threat of fire, possible explosions, impending structural collapse, electrical hazards, toxic gases, and other such dangers may make it necessary to move a patient quickly.
- Life-saving care cannot be given because of the patient's location or position. The inability to properly assess and care for problems with a patient's ABCs, or the inability to properly manage uncontrolled bleeding, makes it necessary to move a patient.
- You are not able to gain access to other patients who need life-saving care. This is seen most often in motor-vehicle crashes. ■

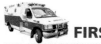

FIRST ON SCENE

Jesse climbed to his feet and watched the big rig slow to a crawl and pull off onto the shoulder several hundred feet down the highway. The twisted heap that once was a pickup truck sat smoking in the middle of the road just beyond it, the bed curled up over the top of the cab like a huge, metal scorpion. Jesse looked back up the highway and saw a car and another semi bearing down on the scene, heading right into the setting sun. He turned and sprinted as fast as he could down the shoulder of the road, past the parked semi, and up to a point where he was even with the wrecked pickup.

"Help me!" Incredibly the man in the pickup was alive and seemed fully conscious. Jesse could clearly see him in the deformed but still intact cab of the truck. "My legs are . . . uh . . . I think they're gone. What do I do?" The man kept looking over at Jesse and then back down into his own lap.

Jesse saw the other vehicles approaching rapidly. He began to yell and wave his arms, trying to get the drivers' attention. The car arrived seconds later, swerved around the wreckage and continued on without braking, throwing up bits of broken glass and metal as it sped by.

"Help me, please!" The man was now screaming over the deafening rumble of a rapidly approaching semi.

Emergency moves rarely provide any protection for a patient's injuries, and they may cause great pain for the patient. But because of the reasons listed above, an emergency move is justified; that is, the need to move the patient in order to ensure his safety or to provide life-saving care outweighs the risks associated with moving the patient quickly.

One of the greatest dangers in moving a patient quickly is the possibility of making a spine injury worse. If the patient is on the floor or ground, it is important to make every effort to pull the patient in the direction of the long axis of the body. This is the line that runs down the center of the body from the top of the head and along the spine. By pulling this way, you will provide as much protection to the spine as possible.

Drags One of the most common types of emergency move is the drag. In this type of move, the patient is pulled by the clothes, feet, or shoulders, or by using a blanket (Scan 5–1). Notice that drags provide little if any protection for the neck and spine.

In most cases, drags are initiated from the shoulders by pulling along the long axis of the body. This causes the remainder of the body to fall into its natural anatomical position, with the spine and all limbs in normal alignment. Never drag a patient sideways, with one arm or one leg unless absolutely necessary. A sideways drag can cause twisting motions of the spine that may aggravate existing injuries.

When using a drag to move a patient down stairs or down an incline, grab the patient under the shoulders and pull the patient

Is It Safe ?

Whenever walking backward down stairs to move a patient, it is best to have a second person walk behind you and act as a spotter. Have him place a hand on your back and talk you back down the stairs. ■

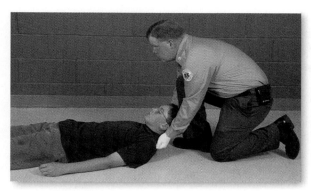

1 ■ **Clothes Drag.**

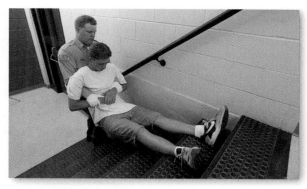

2 ■ **Incline Drag.** Always head first.

CAUTION: Always pull in the direction of the long axis of patient's body. Do not pull a patient sideways. Avoid bending or twisting the patient's trunk.

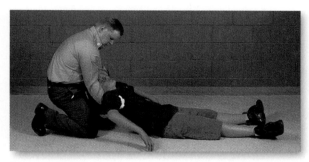

3 ■ **Shoulder Drag.**

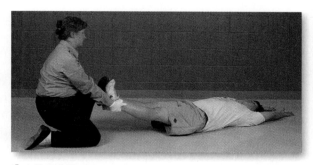

4 ■ **Foot Drag.**

CAUTION: Be careful. Try your best not to bump the patient's head as you drag him.

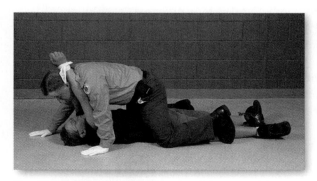

5 ■ **Firefighter's Drag.** Place patient on his back and secure his hands together with tape or roller gauze. Straddle the patient, facing his head. Crouch, pass your head through his trussed arms, and raise your body. Crawl on your hands and knees. Keep patient's head as low as possible.

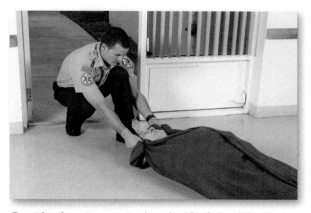

6 ■ **Blanket Drag.** Gather half of the blanket material up against patient's side. Roll patient toward your knees so that you can place the blanket under him. Gently roll patient back onto the blanket. During the drag, keep patient's head as low as possible.

head first as you walk backward. If possible, try to cradle the patient's head in your forearms as you drag.

Other Emergency Moves.   There are many other techniques that can be used to move a patient quickly. Some require only one rescuer (Scan 5–2). Others require two rescuers (Scan 5–3). Remember that any emergency move must be justified and should be carried out as quickly as possible.

━━━━━━━━━━━ **Geriatric Focus**

You must use extra caution when moving elderly patients. Their bones are much more brittle than those of younger patients and their joints—shoulders, elbow, and knees, for example—often have a limited range of motion.

Nonemergency Moves

nonemergency move ■ the preferred choice when the situation is not urgent, the patient is stable, and you have adequate time and personnel for a move.

1–5.4 Describe the indications for assisting in nonemergency moves.

FIRST ➤ A **nonemergency move** is the preferred choice when the situation is not urgent, the patient is stable, and you have adequate time and personnel for a move. Nonemergency moves should be carried out with the help of other trained personnel or bystanders. Take care to prevent additional injury to the patient, as well as to avoid patient discomfort and pain. ▪

Follow these rules when deciding to use a nonemergency move:

- Use a minimum of three rescuers whenever possible.
- Complete an initial assessment. The patient's ABCs should be intact and normal.
- Take care to avoid compromising a possible neck or spine injury. Avoid moving a patient who has neck pain, numbness, or weakness.
- Consider splinting suspected fractures, depending on the patient's condition.

The following are situations in which a nonemergency move may be appropriate:

- The patient is uncomfortable or his position is aggravating an injury.
- Emergency care requires moving the patient. This is usually seen in cases in which there are no suspected spinal injuries. Problems due to extreme heat or cold, such as heat cramps, heat exhaustion, hypothermia, and local cold injuries (frostbite and freezing) are good examples. Reaching a source of water for washing in cases of serious chemical burns also may be a reason to move a patient.
- The patient insists on being moved. If a patient will not listen to the reasons why he should not be moved and tries to move on his own, you may have to assist. You are not allowed to restrain patients. Sometimes a patient becomes so upset that stress worsens his condition. If this type of patient can be moved, and the move is short, you may have to make the move in order to keep him calm and relieve his stress. However, be cautious if the patient is intoxicated.

━━━━━━━━━━━ **Geriatric Focus**

When handling elderly patients, keep in mind that their skin may be easily injured. Care should be taken when gripping their arms or legs to prevent bruising and tearing.

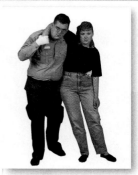

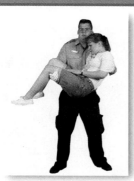

1 ■ **One-Rescuer Assist.** Place patient's arm around your neck, grasping her hand in yours. Place your other arm around patient's waist. Help her walk to safety. Be prepared to change technique if level of danger increases. Be sure to communicate with patient about obstacles, uneven terrain, and so on. *(© Michael A. Gallitelli)*

2 ■ **Cradle Carry.** Place one arm across patient's back with your hand under her arm. Place your other arm under her knees and lift. If your patient is conscious, have her place her near arm over your shoulder. *(© Michael A. Gallitelli)*

NOTE: The cradle carry places a lot of weight on the carrier's back. It is usually appropriate only for very light patients.

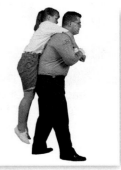

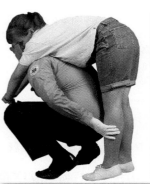

3 ■ **Pack Strap Carry.** Have the patient stand. Turn your back to her, bringing her arms over your shoulders to cross your chest. Keep her arms as straight as possible, with her armpits over your shoulders. Hold the patient's wrists, bend, and pull her onto your back. *(© Michael A. Gallitelli)*

4 ■ **Piggy Back Carry.** Assist the patient to stand. Place her arms over your shoulder so they cross your chest. Bend over and lift her. While she holds on with her arms, crouch and grasp each thigh. Use a lifting motion to move her onto your back. Pass your forearms under her knees and grasp her wrists. *(© Michael A. Gallitelli)*

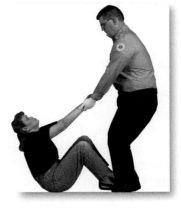

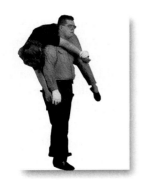

5 ■ **Firefighter's Carry.** Place your feet against patient's feet and pull her toward you. Bend at waist and flex knees. Duck and pull her across your shoulders, keeping hold of one of her wrists. Use your free arm to reach between her legs and grasp her thigh. Allow her weight to fall onto your shoulders. Stand up. Transfer your grip on her thigh to her wrist. *(© Michael A. Gallitelli)*

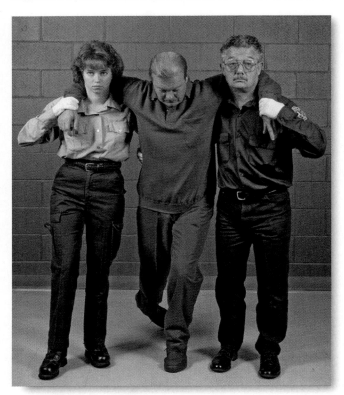

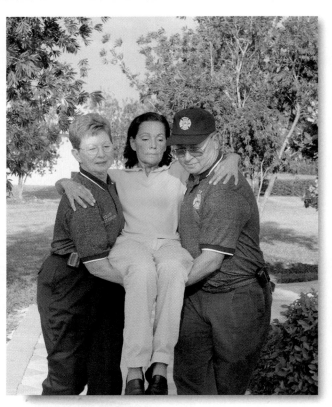

1 ■ **Two-Rescuer Assist.** Patient's arms are placed around shoulders of both rescuers. Each rescuer grips one of the patient's hands, places a free arm around the patient's waist, and helps him walk to safety.

2 ■ **Two-Rescuer Cradle Carry.** The rescuer's arms are clasped beneath the patient's legs and behind the back to support the patient in a seated position.

Direct Ground Lift

WARNING

It is poor practice to use only two rescuers for a direct ground lift. Two rescuers would not allow enough support for the patient or enough control during the move. If you must perform it, position your helper at the patient's thighs so one arm can be placed on the patient's back above her buttocks and the other arm under the patient's knees.

FIRST ➤ The direct ground lift is a three-rescuer nonemergency move that can be used to move a patient from the ground or floor to a bed or stretcher. This move is not recommended for use on patients with possible neck or spine injuries. Although it can be carried out by two people, three are recommended. ■

To perform a direct ground lift (Scan 5–4), the patient should be lying face up (supine), and the arms should be placed on the chest. You and your helpers should line up on one side of the patient. One rescuer should be at the patient's head, another at her midsection, and another at the lower legs. Each of you should drop to the knee closest to the patient's feet.

The rescuer at the head should place one arm under the patient's neck and grasp the far shoulder in order to cradle the head. The other arm should be placed under her back, just above the waist. The rescuer at her midsection should place one arm above and one arm below the buttocks. The rescuer at the patient's lower legs should place one arm under her knees and the other arm under her ankles.

First, on the signal of the rescuer at the head, everyone should lift the patient up to the level of their knees. Then, on signal, the rescuers should roll the patient

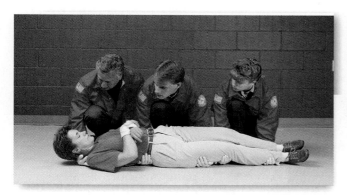

1 ■ Rescuers kneel on one side of the patient and position their hands to support and lift.

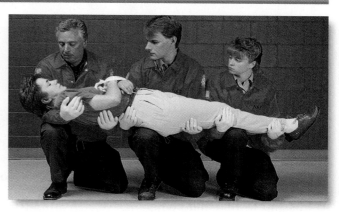

2 ■ Rescuers lift the patient to knee level at the direction of the rescuer at the head.

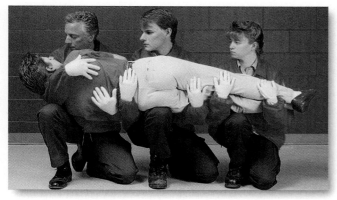

3 ■ Rescuers curl the patient to their chests.

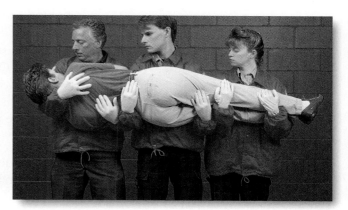

4 ■ Rescuers stand.

toward their chests. Finally, on signal, everyone should stand while holding the patient. You can now move her, reversing the process when it is time to place her in a supine position.

Extremity Lift

FIRST ➤ An extremity lift requires two people (Scan 5–5). This lift is ideal for moving a patient from the ground to a chair or the stretcher. It can also be used to move a patient from a chair to the stretcher. It should not be performed, however, if there is a possibility of head, neck, spine, shoulder, hip, or knee injury, or any suspected fractures to the extremities that have not been immobilized. ■

The patient should be placed face up, with knees flexed. You should kneel at the head of the patient, placing your hands under her shoulders. Have your helper stand at the patient's feet and grasp her wrists. Direct your helper to pull the patient into a sitting position, while you push the patient from the shoulders. (Do not have your helper pull the patient by the arms if there are any signs of suspected fractures.) Slip your arms under the patient's armpits and grasp the wrists. Once the patient is in a semisitting position, have your helper crouch down and grasp the patient's legs behind the knees.

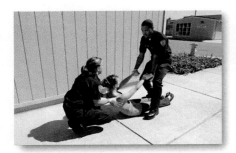

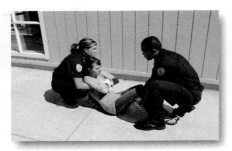

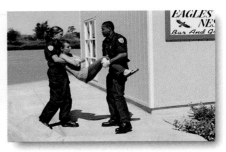

1 ▪ To get the patient into a sitting position, one rescuer pushes from behind while the other pulls from the wrists.

2 ▪ The rescuer at the head places arms under patient's armpits and grasps patient's wrists. While facing the patient, the rescuer at the feet grasps patient's legs behind the knees.

3 ▪ You can now carry the patient a short distance or place her on a stretcher or chair.

Direct your helper so that you both stand at the same time. For example, "Ready? Lift on three. One, two, three, lift." Then move as a unit when carrying the patient. Try to walk out of step with your partner to avoid swinging the patient. The rescuer at the head should direct the rescuer at the feet as to when to stop the carry and when to place the patient down in a supine or seated position.

Direct Carry Method   The direct carry is performed in order to move a patient with no suspected spine injury from a bed or from a bed-level position to a stretcher (Scan 5–6). First, position the stretcher perpendicular to the bed, with the head end of the stretcher at the foot of the bed. Prepare the stretcher by unbuckling straps and removing other items. Then, two rescuers should stand between the bed and the stretcher, facing the patient. The first rescuer should slide an arm under the patient's neck and cup the shoulder, while the second rescuer slides a hand under the patient's hip and lifts slightly. The first rescuer then slides his other arm under the patient's back, while the second rescuer places his arms underneath the patient's hips and calves. Finally, both rescuers should slide the patient to the edge of the bed, lift/curl him toward their chests, and rotate and place him gently onto the stretcher.

Draw Sheet Method   The other method of moving a patient with no suspected spine injury from a bed to a stretcher is the draw sheet method. It may be performed from the side of the bed or from either the head or the foot of the bed. Select a method that gives you the easiest access to the patient. Figure 5.3 illustrates how to do it from the side of the bed.

To perform the draw sheet method from the side of the bed, begin by loosening the bottom sheet of the bed and positioning the stretcher next to the bed. Then, adjust the height of the stretcher, lower the rails, and unbuckle the straps. Both rescuers should reach across the stretcher and roll the sheet against the patient. Grasp the sheet firmly at the patient's head, chest, hips, and knees. Finally, draw the patient onto the stretcher, sliding him in one smooth motion. When using the draw sheet method from the head or the foot of the bed, be sure to secure the stretcher so that it does not move while transferring the patient from the bed to the stretcher.

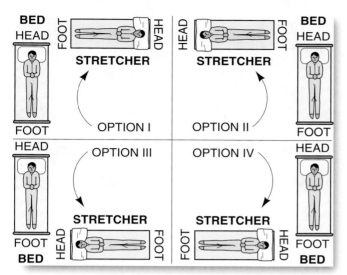

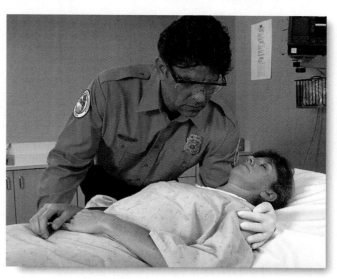

1 ■ Stretcher is placed at 90-degree angle to bed, depending on room configuration. Prepare stretcher by lowering rails, unbuckling straps, and removing other items. Both Emergency Medical Responders stand between stretcher and bed, facing patient.

2 ■ The Emergency Medical Responder standing at the patient's head cradles the patient's head and neck by sliding one arm under her neck and grasping her shoulder.

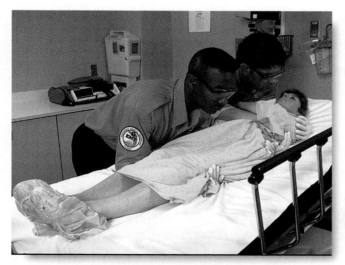

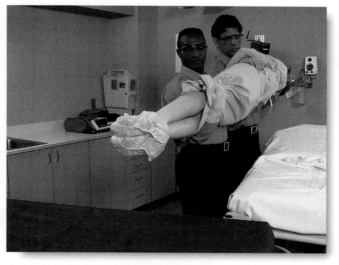

3 ■ The Emergency Medical Responder standing at the patient's feet slides a hand under the patient's hips and lifts slightly. Head-end Emergency Medical Responder slides the other arm under patient's back. Foot-end Emergency Medical Responder places arms under hips and calves.

4 ■ Emergency Medical Responders slide patient to edge of bed and bend toward her with their knees slightly bent. They lift and curl patient to their chests and return to a standing position. They rotate and slide patient gently onto stretcher.

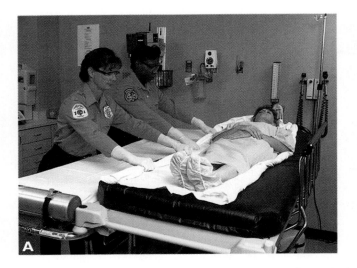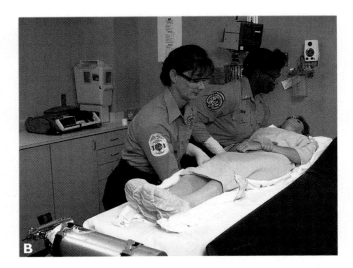

FIGURE 5.3 Draw sheet method of moving a patient from a bed to a stretcher.

Patient Positioning

Proper position of patients is one of the most important skills an Emergency Medical Responder can learn. Proper positioning is important for many reasons, including patient comfort and proper airway maintenance.

Recovery Position   An unresponsive patient with no suspected spine injury should be placed on his side in order to help maintain an open and clear airway. This position is commonly called the **recovery position** or *lateral recumbent position*. Unless the patient's condition suggests otherwise, place the patient on his left side. Because most stretchers secure against the driver's side wall in ambulances, this positioning will have him face the EMT for the ride to the hospital. Remember that patients with injuries, especially a suspected spine injury,

recovery position ■ the position in which a patient with no suspected spine injuries may be placed, usually on the left side. Same as *lateral recumbent position*.

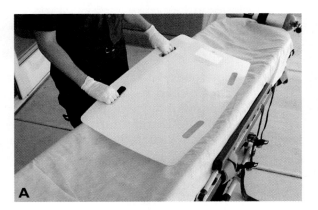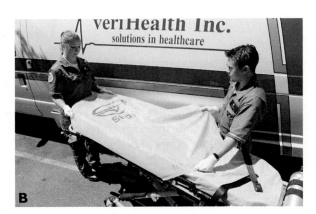

FIGURE 5.4 Devices such as **A.** slider boards and **B.** slide bags make the task of moving patients from stretcher to bed easier and safer for those facilitating the move.

should not be moved until additional EMS resources arrive to evaluate and stabilize them.

To place an unresponsive but uninjured patient in the recovery position, perform the following steps (Scan 5–7):

1. Kneel beside the patient on his left side. Raise the patient's left arm straight out above his head.
2. Cross the patient's right arm over his chest, placing his right hand next to his left cheek.
3. Raise the right knee until it is completely flexed.
4. Place your right hand on the patient's right shoulder and your left hand on the patient's flexed right knee. Using the flexed knee as a lever, pull toward you, guiding the patient's torso in a smooth rolling motion onto his side. The patient's head will rest on his left arm.
5. As best as you can, position the patient's right elbow and knee on the floor so that they act like a kickstand, preventing the patient from rolling completely onto his stomach. Place the patient's right hand under the side of his face. The arm will support the patient in this position. The hand will cushion his face and allow the head to angle slightly downward for airway drainage.

Many patients with no suspected spine injuries may be placed in a position of comfort. This may include patients with medical complaints such as chest pain, nausea, or difficulty breathing. Breathing is often aided by placing the patient in a semisitting (also called a *semi-Fowler's*) position, which is about a 45-degree angle.

Always position yourself appropriately to manage the patient's airway and monitor his mental status. Place the patient in the recovery position at the first sign of a decreased level of responsiveness.

Geriatric Focus

The elderly patient may become dizzy when his position is changed too quickly. Take care when moving him from a supine to a sitting position or from a sitting to a standing position. Move the patient gradually, while allowing him to get comfortable with the new position.

Log Roll When an unresponsive patient is face down (prone), you must assess breathing differently. Kneel down beside the patient's head and place your ear next to the patient's mouth and nose to listen and feel for breathing. If you hear and/or feel the movement of air, the patient has an airway and is breathing. The patient's condition may worsen, however, and ideally, you will want him on his back (supine) for further assessment and care.

To move a prone patient to a supine position and ensure stability of the head and spine where a trauma injury is suspected, perform a log roll. This move can be done with as few as two rescuers, but three is ideal to minimize twisting of the patient's spine during the procedure. Perform the following steps:

1. One rescuer should kneel at the top of patient's head and hold or stabilize the head and neck in the position found. Notice which way the patient's head is facing as you will most likely want to roll her in the opposite direction.
2. A second rescuer should kneel at the patient's side opposite the direction the head is facing. Quickly assess the patient's arms to ensure there are no

[handwritten margin note: Log roll every trauma pt - or even if your not sure if trauma]

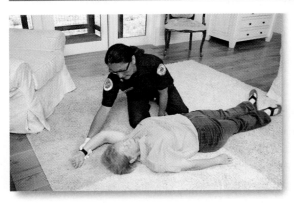

1 ■ Move the closest hand of the patient above her head.

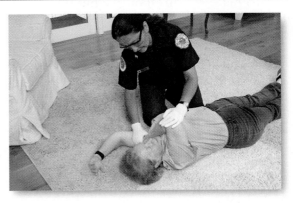

2 ■ Move the patient's far hand across to the opposite shoulder, next to the patient's cheek.

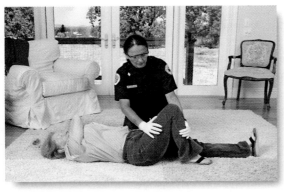

3 ■ Bring the patient's far leg to the flexed position.

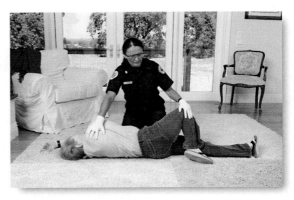

4 ■ Using the knee and shoulder, carefully pull the patient onto her side.

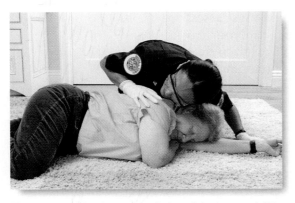

5 ■ Adjust the knee and shoulder to stabilize the patient. Then recheck the patient's ABCs.

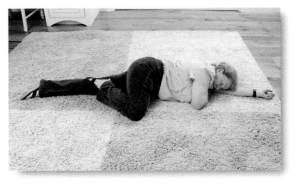

6 ■ Once properly positioned, the knee and elbow will support the patient.

obvious injuries. Raise and extend the patient's arm that is opposite the direction the head is facing. Position that arm straight up above her head. This allows for easy rolling to that side and provides support for the head during the roll. This is especially helpful if you must do the log roll alone.

3. The third rescuer should kneel at the patient's hips.
4. Rescuers should grasp the patient's shoulders, hips, knees, and ankles. If only one rescuer is available to roll the patient, he should grasp the heavy parts of the torso—the shoulders and hips.
5. The rescuer at the patient's head should signal and give directions: "On three, slowly roll. One, two, three, roll together." All rescuers should slowly roll the patient in a coordinated move and carefully keep her spine in a neutral, in-line position until she is supine. It is important to note that the rescuer holding the head should not initially try to turn the head with the body. Because the head is already facing sideways, allow the body to come into alignment with the head. Once the body and head are aligned, approximately half way through the roll, the rescuer at the head will then move with the body, keeping the head and body aligned until the patient is in the supine position.

Is It Safe ?

The most important person during a log roll is the person at the head. He must think ahead and position his hands in anticipation of the movement of the patient from face-down to face-up. Positioning the hands incorrectly will result in an awkward hand and body position of the rescuer and may result in excessive movement of the patient's neck. ◼

Sometimes the patient is already supine but must be placed on a blanket or spine board. If this is the case, then perform steps 1 through 5 above, maintaining control of the patient when she is rolled onto her side. Without removing your hands, continue with the following (Scan 5–8):

1. The rescuer at the patient's head should continue stabilization of the patient's head and neck until other rescuers position a blanket or long spine board (backboard) behind the patient.
2. At a signal from the rescuer at the head, they should slowly roll the patient in a coordinated move onto the blanket or spine board.
3. Finally, they should make sure the patient is positioned on the center of the spine board. If they must adjust the patient's position, they must keep her head and spine in neutral alignment.

Equipment

EMTs and advanced life support (ALS) personnel will often ask Emergency Medical Responders to assist with preparing the patient for transport and with lifting, moving, and loading

FIRST ON SCENE

Jesse could see the driver of the oncoming semi, immersed in a conversation on his cell phone, simply move the steering wheel to the left, guiding the huge truck onto the grassy center divide of the highway, where it passed the collision scene without so much as downshifting. Once the truck's flatbed trailer cleared the wreckage, it returned to the roadway and continued off into the distance.

"Please, please, help me!" The man, his face contorted with pain and terror, was now screaming at Jesse.

There were more oncoming vehicles, but at the moment they were nothing more than colorful specks on the distant horizon. Jesse ran to the pickup and was able to force the passenger-side door open, breaking it back onto the hinges. He reached over and released the driver's seat belt and found that the bench seat of the truck was covered with blood.

The man fell over onto the passenger side, grabbing for Jesse's arm. Jesse could see that both of his legs were severed, pinched between the truck's displaced engine and the now raised floor of the cab. He quickly glanced down the highway, saw the glint of the sun on a windshield, slid his hands under the man's arms, and began moving backward as fast as he could.

1–5.5 Discuss the various devices associated with moving a patient in the out-of-hospital arena.

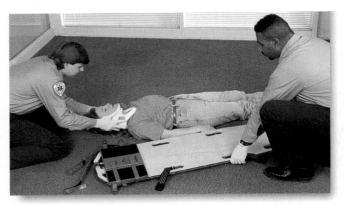

1 ■ Manually stabilize the patient's head and neck as you place the board parallel to the patient. Maintain manual stabilization throughout the log roll.

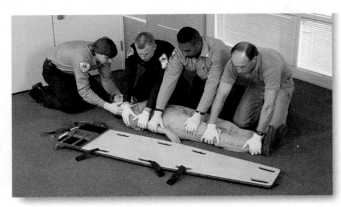

2 ■ Kneel at the patient's side opposite the board at the shoulder, waist, and knees. Reach across the patient and position your hands.

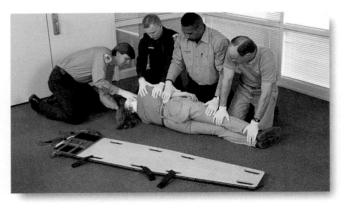

3 ■ On command from the rescuer at the head, roll the patient toward you as a unit. The spine board should be put in place.

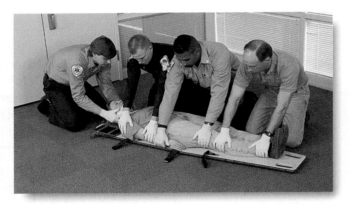

4 ■ Place the patient onto the board, rolling her as a unit.

patients into the ambulance. To help with these tasks, you must be familiar with the various carrying and packaging devices that are used. Many Emergency Medical Responder courses do not include information and practice on immobilization devices. Your instructor will teach you the procedures if you will be expected to perform them in your jurisdiction.

STRETCHERS

Typical equipment used for packaging and loading a patient into an ambulance includes a wheeled stretcher. This device is sometimes called a *stretcher, cot,* or *gurney*. It is used to transport a patient from the scene of the emergency to the ambulance and from the ambulance to the hospital. It is secured in the back of an ambulance by way of a simple locking mechanism. In addition, the head and the foot ends of many stretchers can be elevated to make the patient comfortable or to assist in caring for certain conditions such as shock.

There are many brands and types of wheeled stretchers. Some of them are (Scan 5–9):

- *Single-operator stretcher.* This type of stretcher allows a single operator to load the stretcher into the ambulance without the assistance of a second person. The undercarriage is designed to collapse and fold up as the stretcher is pushed into the ambulance.
- *Dual-operator stretcher.* This type of stretcher requires a second person to lift the undercarriage prior to pushing it into the ambulance.
- *Electric/pneumatic-lift stretcher.* This is the newest type of stretcher on the market and is equipped with a pneumatic or electric mechanism that will lift and lower the stretcher at the touch of a button. It minimizes the need for rescuers to lift a stretcher with a patient on it, thereby significantly reducing the risk of back injury.

Geriatric Focus

When transporting the elderly patient by mechanical means, such as a stair chair or stretcher, explain what you are doing and provide reassurance so that they will not become afraid of falling.

Other types of equipment used for packaging and loading the patient into an ambulance include the following (Scans 5–10 and 5–11):

- *Portable stretcher.* The type of stretcher is also known as a folding or flat stretcher. It is much lighter than a standard wheeled stretcher and makes the task of moving a patient down stairs or out of tight spaces much easier. Portable stretchers may be canvas, aluminum, or heavy plastic, and they usually fold, roll up, or collapse for easy storage. Aluminum and plastic stretchers are now commonly used because it is easy to disinfect them.
- *Stair chair.* The stair chair helps rescuers move seated medical patients down stairways and through tight places where a traditional stretcher will not fit. Newer brands are made of sturdy folding frames with either canvas or hard plastic seats and are easy to store. They have wheels that allow rescuers to roll them over flat surfaces. Some models have a tractor tread mechanism that allows them to easily slide down stairways just by tilting them.

Is It Safe ?

Scoop stretchers might not be appropriate for immobilization of the spine. The authors of this textbook have contacted several manufacturers of scoop stretchers, and all have indicated that the scoop stretcher is *not* recommended for use as a primary spinal immobilization device. However, it may be appropriate to place the patient on a scoop stretcher and then secure the scoop to a long spine board for additional support. Consult your local protocols for the proper use of the scoop stretcher.

- *Scoop (orthopedic) stretcher.* This device is typically made of hard plastic or aluminum. It is called a *scoop stretcher* because it splits vertically into two pieces, which can be used to "scoop" the patient up. Newer models are sturdier

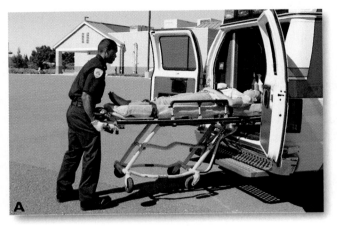
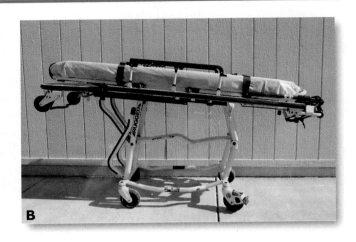

1 ■ **Single-Operator Stretcher.**

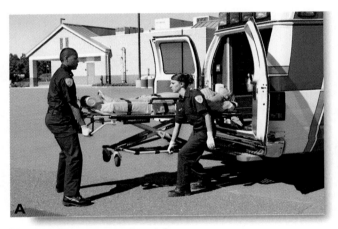
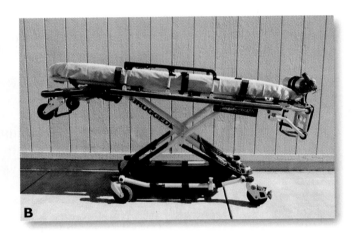

2 ■ **Dual-Operator Stretcher.**

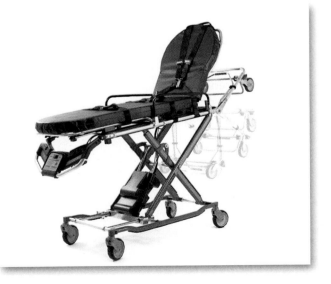

3 ■ **Electric/Pneumatic Lift Stretcher.** These eliminate the need for heavy lifting.
(© Ferno-Washington, Inc.)

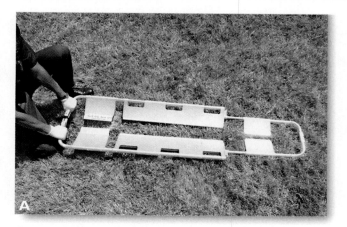

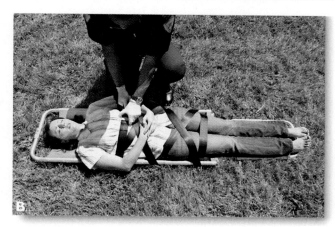

1 ■ Scoop Stretchers. A. These stretchers are ideal for moving patients in the position they are found. **B.** Once in place, the patient must be properly secured to the device before moving.

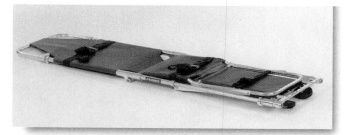

2 ■ Portable Stretcher. Beneficial for carrying supine medical patients down stairs.

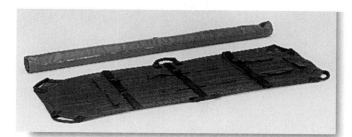

3 ■ Flexible Stretcher. Used in restricted areas or narrow hallways.

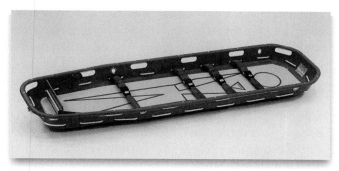

4 ■ Basket Stretcher. Used to transport over rough terrain.

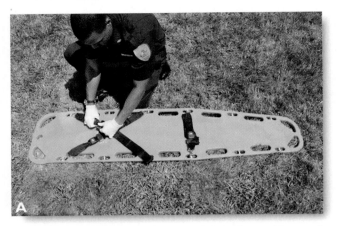

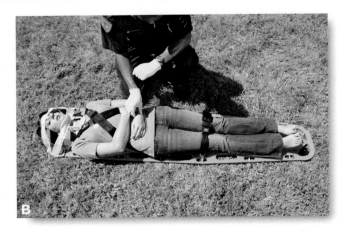

1 ■ **Long Spine Board. A.** This backboard is used to immobilize the spine of a supine patient. **B.** Long spine board with patient properly secured in place.

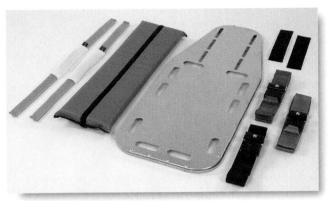

2 ■ **Short Spine Board.** This backboard is used to stabilize the spine while removing patient from vehicle.

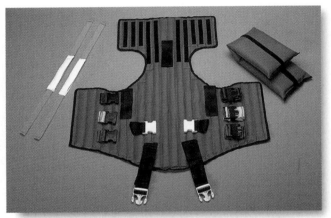

3 ■ **Vest-Type Extrication Device.** This device facilitates the extrication of a seated patient, while stabilizing the patient's head, neck, and spine.

and more rigid than older ones and provide more support to the spine. However, a scoop stretcher is commonly used for picking up and moving a patient with hip injuries or multiple injuries rather than for spine injuries. It is also used for transferring a patient from a bed or the floor to a wheeled stretcher or from the wheeled stretcher to the hospital bed. Follow your local protocols for using this device.

■ *Spine board.* Spine boards are also known as *backboards.* The long spine board is used for patients who are found lying down or standing and have a suspected spine injury. Short spine boards are becoming less common as they are being replaced by the vest-type extrication device. Short boards are used primarily for removing patients from vehicles when it is suspected that they have neck or spine injuries. Once secured to the short spine board, the patient may be moved from a sitting position in the vehicle to a supine position on a long spine board. Short boards are difficult to use in late model cars that have bucket seats because they do not fit the contour of the seat.

- *Vest-type extrication device.* The extrication vest is used to help immobilize and remove patients found in a seated position in a vehicle. It wraps around the patient's torso to stabilize the spine and has an extended section above the vest with side flaps for stabilizing the patient's head and neck. Rescuers secure the patient's head, neck, and torso with straps and padding. The vest has handles that aid in lifting the patient out of the vehicle and onto a long spine board.
- *Full-body immobilization device.* The most common type is the full-body vacuum splint. It consists of a large airtight bag filled with tiny beads. As the patient is placed on the device, it can be molded to fit the shape and contours of the patient's body. Once it is in place, a portable vacuum is activated to remove the air from the bag. The result is a hard cast-like splint that immobilizes the patient.
- *Basket stretcher.* This stretcher is typically used in more rural settings to move a patient from one level of ground to another or over rough terrain. The basket stretcher is also known as a *Stokes stretcher.*
- *Flexible stretcher.* This stretcher is made of rubberized canvas or other flexible material such as heavy plastic, often with wooden slats sewn into pockets. The flexible stretcher usually has three carrying handles on each side. Because of its flexibility, it can be useful in restricted areas or narrow hallways.
- *Pedi-board.* Special spinal immobilization boards are made to fit infants and children. The back of a child's head is larger proportionately than an adult's, so boards have a depression in the head end to fit. However, it is still necessary to pad the child's body from the shoulders to the heels to ensure his airway is in a neutral position while secured on the board.

CERVICAL COLLARS

When you package a patient on an immobilization device, you must first stabilize the head and neck by selecting and applying a cervical collar that is a size appropriate for your patient (Scans 5–12 and 5–13). Also called *extrication collars*, rigid cervical collars are applied to help maintain stability and alignment with the body in patients who have suspected neck and spine injuries (Scans 5–14 and 5–15). Your instructor will teach you the steps if Emergency Medical Responders are required to use collars in your jurisdiction. (Refer to Chapter 11 for care of patients with spine injuries.)

Regardless of whether or not you learn to size and place cervical collars during your training, it is vital to understand one important concept. Cervical collars will only minimize movement of the neck of a cooperative patient. A patient who is combative or otherwise uncooperative can still move his or her neck even with a cervical collar in place. Therefore, it is important to maintain manual stabilization of the head even after placement of a cervical collar.

There are many different makes and models of cervical collars on the market today. Some brands offer many sizes; others offer a "one-size-fits-all" adjustable collar. More than likely, you will not have a choice in the matter. Instead, you will be expected to use whatever collars are currently in use in your agency or region. Whatever the case, it is best to follow the manufacturer's suggested method for sizing and application. Your instructor will likely demonstrate the collars currently in use in your area.

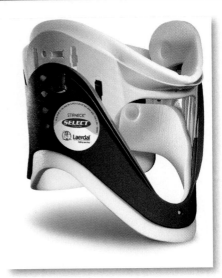

(Courtesy of Laerdal Medical Corporation)

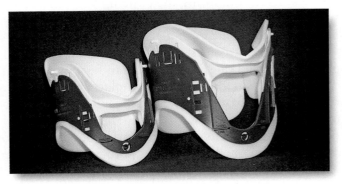

(Courtesy of Philadelphia Corporation)

Regardless of the brand or type of collar, the following guidelines can be used to ensure a proper fit for your patient:

- Once in place, check to see that the sides of the collar do not ride too far above or below the earlobes.
- Confirm the chin fits properly on the collar. The bony part of the chin should be well supported by the collar.
- The collar should be snug on all sides and not too tight or too loose.
- Consider using a different size or adjusting the collar if it does not fit properly.

 FIRST ON SCENE WRAP-UP

By the time the emergency crews arrived, summoned by the driver of the semi that had initially hit the pickup, several more cars and big rigs had sped through the collision scene. One even clipped the demolished pickup with a large chrome bumper, sending it skittering off the highway and into a ditch.

Jesse had pulled the injured man onto the side of the road. The semi driver who had hit the pickup came running up to the scene. Shaken and winded, he offered, "Can I help?" Grateful, Jesse showed him how to hold the man's head in a neutral, in-line position while Jesse applied pressure to the bleeding with his jacket.

Later, the paramedic who arrived with the ambulance credited Jesse's quick thinking and actions with ultimately saving the patient's life.

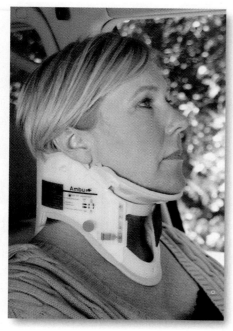

1 ■ When properly fitted, the sides of the collar should come very close to or slightly overlap the earlobe.

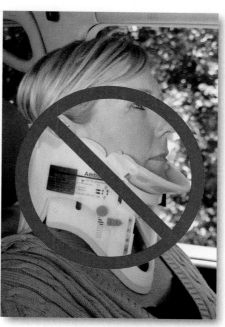

2 ■ A collar that is too big will extend way above the earlobes. Consider readjusting or selecting a smaller size collar.

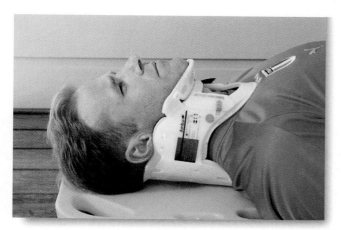

3 ■ When properly fitted, the patient's chin will fit completely and snugly within the saddle of the collar.

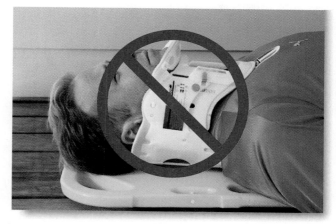

4 ■ A collar that is too big will extend well beyond the chin allowing for excessive movement. Consider readjusting or selecting a smaller size collar.

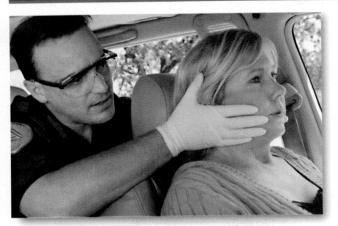

1 ■ Establish manual stabilization of the head while your partner selects a collar.

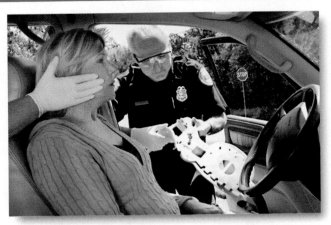

2 ■ Select an appropriate size collar or adjust the collar based on the patient's size. Follow the manufacturer's guidelines for size and adjustment selection.

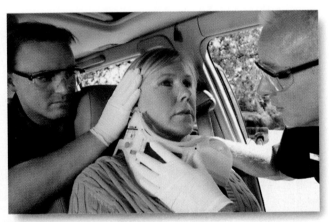

3 ■ Place the collar beneath the patient's chin and firmly against the lower jaw. The chin should fit well within the chin saddle of the collar.

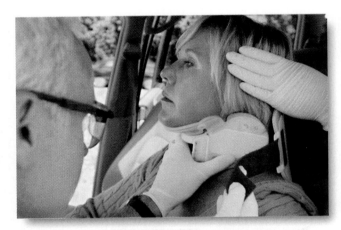

4 ■ Secure the collar in place by overlapping the Velcro closure at the side of the patient's neck. Confirm fit by looking at ears and chin.

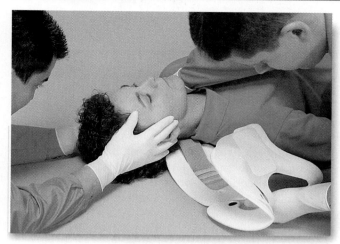

1 ■ Slide the back portion of the cervical spine immobilization collar behind the patient's neck. Fold the loop Velcro inward on the foam padding.

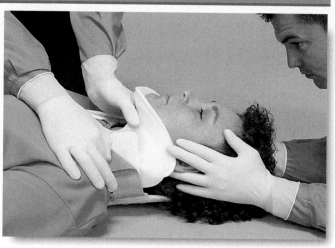

2 ■ Position the collar so that the chin fits properly. Secure the collar by attaching the Velcro.

Alternative Method

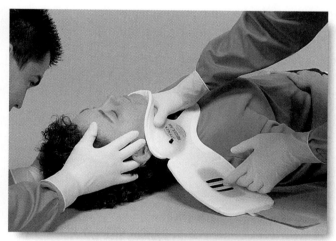

1 ■ An alternative method of applying the collar to a supine patient is to start by positioning the chin piece and then sliding the back portion of the collar behind the patient's neck.

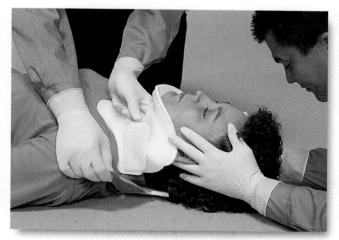

2 ■ Hold the collar in place by grasping the trachea hole. Attach the loop Velcro so it mates with (and is parallel to) the hook Velcro.

Summary

When you must move patients or equipment, use the proper body mechanics to prevent injury. However, in most instances, only attempt to move patients when it is absolutely necessary. Most of the time, it is possible to assess patients, care for them, and monitor their condition without significant movement. Do your best to keep your patients at rest.

Emergency moves are carried out quickly when the scene is hazardous, care of the patient requires immediate repositioning, or you must reach another patient who needs life-saving care. A heavy patient or one who is unresponsive or unable to move alone may be moved by using one of the drag methods. Always drag the patient along the long axis of the body, keeping his head as low as possible. The use of a drag may also be appropriate where there are possible spine injuries.

Nonemergency moves are the preferred choice when the situation is not urgent, the patient is stable, and you have adequate time and personnel for a move. Before performing a nonemergency move, complete a thorough patient assessment. Most nonemergency moves are *not* appropriate for patients with suspected spine injuries. It is best to splint any suspected fractures before these moves.

The direct ground lift is a nonemergency move that can be used for patients with no neck or spine injuries. You should have two, three, or more people to help. The patient must be supported at the head, neck, back, and knees. A rescuer should control and support the patient above and below the buttocks. Another rescuer should support the patient's knees and ankles. When moving the patient, you should keep the patient rolled toward your chest.

The extremity lift is a good nonemergency move, but it should *not* be used if the patient has possible head, neck, or spine injuries, is unresponsive, or has injuries to the upper or lower extremities (including the shoulder and hip). This lift requires two rescuers, with you lifting the patient at the shoulders and your helper lifting the patient at the knees.

Transfer patients from a bed to a stretcher using the direct carry method or the draw sheet method.

Sometimes it is necessary to position patients to ensure they can maintain an airway, breathe, and drain fluids. Use the recovery position for unresponsive patients who are breathing and have no spine injuries. Use a position of comfort or a semisitting position for responsive patients who have no spine injuries, such as those with chest pain, nausea, or difficulty breathing.

Emergency Medical Responders may be asked to assist with lifting, moving, and immobilizing patients. Many types of equipment are available, including wheeled, portable, scoop (orthopedic), basket, and flexible stretchers, full-body spinal immobilization devices, the stair chair, and short spinal immobilization devices, such as the extrication vest and short spine boards. There are also special immobilization devices for infants and children called pedi-boards.

Remember and Consider

Using poor body mechanics is dangerous, not only to you but also to your patient and coworkers. And remember that it is dangerous to push yourself past your physical limits.

➤ Learn and practice proper methods of lifting and moving patients until you are able to perform them comfortably.

➤ Never hesitate to ask for assistance from other EMS providers if a patient or equipment is too heavy for you to lift alone.

Investigate

Each EMS system has various types of equipment for packaging and carrying patients.

➤ Find out what kinds of patient carrying and immobilization devices are used on the ambulances in your community and become proficient in using them.

Quick Quiz

1. The term "body mechanics" is BEST defined as:
   a. properly using your body to facilitate a lift or move.
   b. using a minimum of three people for any lift.
   c. contracting the body's muscles to lift and move things.
   d. lifting with your back and not your legs.

2. An Emergency Medical Responder should immediately move a patient EXCEPT when the patient:
   a. has a blocked airway.
   b. is bleeding severely.
   c. has mild shortness of breath.
   d. is in cardiac arrest.

3. When lifting a patient, feet should be placed:
   a. one in front of the other.
   b. shoulder width apart.
   c. a comfortable distance apart.
   d. as close together as possible.

4. Good body mechanics means keeping your back _____ and bending at the knees when lifting a patient or large object.
   a. at a 45-degree angle
   b. straight
   c. curved
   d. slightly twisted

5. The load on your back is minimized if you can keep the weight you are carrying:
   a. as close to your body as possible.
   b. at least 6 inches in front of you.
   c. at least 18 inches in front of you.
   d. as low as possible.

6. What type of move is used when there is no immediate threat to the patient's life?
   a. emergency
   b. nonemergency
   c. rapid
   d. nonrapid

7. Which one of the following would be the BEST choice for a stable patient with a suspected spine injury?
   a. one-rescuer assist
   b. cradle carry
   c. two-rescuer assist
   d. shoulder drag

8. Which one of the following patients would BEST be served by placing in the recovery position?
   a. child who is unresponsive following a seizure
   b. adult in cardiac arrest and in need of CPR
   c. child who is face down and unresponsive in a pool
   d. adult victim of a vehicle collision

9. It is best if the rescuer at the _____ directs the actions of the other rescuers during a log roll.
   a. feet
   b. head
   c. legs
   d. torso

10. Which one of the following devices would be BEST suited to carry a responsive patient with no suspected spine injury down a flight of stairs?
    a. flexible stretcher
    b. wheeled stretcher
    c. scoop stretcher
    d. stair chair

Airway

6 Airway Management

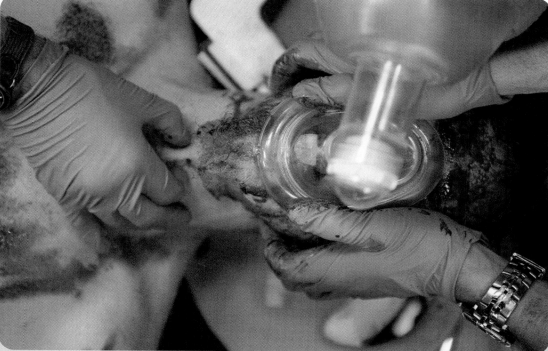
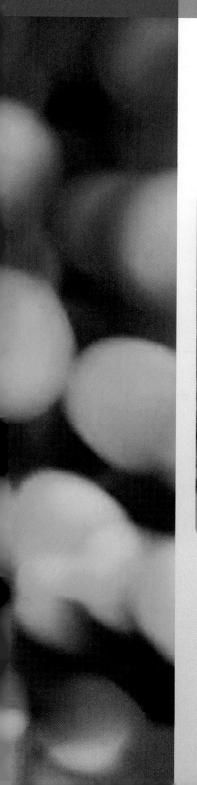

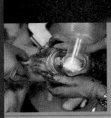

CHAPTER 6

Airway Management

Breathing is life. Each life-giving breath moves through the simple passages—the mouth, nose, and windpipe—that form the passageway into the lungs. Blood that circulates to the lungs drops off carbon dioxide and picks up oxygen. The heart then pumps the oxygenated blood to the rest of the body. When the blood returns to the heart with waste gases, it is pumped to the lungs to exchange those gases with oxygen. This continuous process is a simple one that we do not usually think about—until we cannot do it.

This chapter explains the process of breathing and how to recognize and provide emergency care to patients who are not breathing or who are not breathing adequately.

OBJECTIVES

This chapter is based on the objectives of the U.S. DOT's First Responder National Standard Curriculum. Note that cognitive objectives are listed below and beside corresponding text throughout the chapter. You will also notice as you read each objective that the term Emergency Medical Responder is used. This is simply a name change and reflects the new name for the First Responder.

By the end of this chapter, you should be able to (from cognitive or knowledge information):

2–1.1 Name and label the major structures of the respiratory system on a diagram. (pp. 117–118)

2–1.2 List the signs of inadequate breathing. (p. 119)

2–1.3 Describe the steps in the head-tilt, chin-lift. (p. 120)

2–1.4 Relate mechanism of injury to opening the airway. (p. 120)

2–1.5 Describe the steps in the jaw-thrust. (p. 121)

2–1.6 State the importance of having a suction unit ready for immediate use when providing emergency medical care. (p. 146)

2–1.7 Describe the techniques of suctioning. (pp. 146–148)

2–1.8 Describe how to ventilate a patient with a (pocket) resuscitation mask or barrier device. (pp. 122–125)

2–1.9 Describe how ventilating an infant or a child is different from ventilating an adult. (pp. 126–127)

2–1.10 List the steps in providing mouth-to-mouth and mouth-to-stoma ventilation. (pp. 122, 128)

2–1.11 Describe how to measure and insert an oropharyngeal (oral) airway. (pp. 139–141)

2–1.12 Describe how to measure and insert a nasopharyngeal (nasal) airway. (pp. 141–142)

2-1.13 Describe how to clear a foreign body airway obstruction in a responsive adult. (pp. 131–134)

2-1.14 Describe how to clear a foreign body airway obstruction in a responsive child with a complete obstruction or a partial obstruction and poor air exchange. (pp. 131–134)

2-1.15 Describe how to clear a foreign body airway obstruction in a responsive infant with a complete obstruction or a partial airway obstruction and poor air exchange. (pp. 134–135)

2-1.16 Describe how to clear a foreign body airway obstruction in an unresponsive adult. (p. 134)

2-1.17 Describe how to clear a foreign body airway obstruction in an unresponsive child. (p. 134)

2-1.18 Describe how to clear a foreign body airway obstruction in an unresponsive infant. (p. 135)

By the end of this chapter, you should be able to feel comfortable enough to (by changing attitudes, values, and beliefs):

2-1.19 Explain why basic life support ventilation and airway protective skills take priority over most other basic life support skills. (pp. 113, 115–116)

2-1.20 Demonstrate a caring attitude toward patients with airway problems who request emergency medical services. (pp. 127, 135–136, 142)

2-1.21 Place the interests of the patient with airway problems as the foremost consideration when making any and all patient care decisions. (pp. 133, 115–116, 127)

2-1.22 Communicate with empathy to patients with airway problems, as well as with family members and friends of the patient. (pp. 127, 135–136, 142)

By the end of this chapter, you should be able to show how to (through psychomotor skills):

2-1.23 Demonstrate the steps in the head-tilt, chin-lift. (p. 120)

2-1.24 Demonstrate the steps in the jaw-thrust. (p. 121)

2-1.25 Demonstrate the techniques of suctioning. (pp. 146–148)

2-1.26 Demonstrate the steps in mouth-to-mouth ventilation with body substance isolation (barrier shields). (pp. 124–125)

2-1.27 Demonstrate how to use a (pocket) resuscitation mask to ventilate a patient. (pp. 122–124)

2-1.28 Demonstrate how to ventilate a patient with a stoma. (p. 128)

2-1.29 Demonstrate how to measure and insert an oropharyngeal (oral) airway. (pp. 138–141)

2-1.30 Demonstrate how to measure and insert a nasopharyngeal (nasal) airway. (pp. 141–142)

2-1.31 Demonstrate how to ventilate infant and child patients. (pp. 126–127)

2-1.32 Demonstrate how to clear a foreign body airway obstruction in a responsive adult. (pp. 131–134)

2-1.33 Demonstrate how to clear a foreign body airway obstruction in a responsive child. (pp. 131–134)

2-1.34 Demonstrate how to clear a foreign body airway obstruction in a responsive infant. (pp. 134–135)

2-1.35 Demonstrate how to clear a foreign body airway obstruction in an unresponsive adult. (p. 134)

2-1.36 Demonstrate how to clear a foreign body airway obstruction in an unresponsive child. (p. 134)

2-1.37 Demonstrate how to clear a foreign body airway obstruction in an unresponsive infant. (p. 135)

ADDITIONAL LEARNING TASKS

This chapter explains the anatomy and function of the airway and the process of breathing. As you work through the chapter, you will come to understand better the reasons that airway and breathing are the first and most important steps in patient care. By the end of the chapter, you should be able to:

➤ State three reasons why we must breathe to stay alive.

When patients stop breathing, an Emergency Medical Responder only has a few minutes to assist them in starting the breathing process again. But if the delay is too long, patients will die. The time between breathing and not breathing is critical, and you need to understand what happens in those few minutes. Be able to:

➤ Explain the difference between clinical death and biological death and the approximate times for each.

When we breathe, pressure inside the lungs changes, causing air to flow in and out. Breathing in, or inhaling, is an active process that requires muscle contractions, but breathing out, or exhaling, is a passive process that works as muscles relax. The lungs function by pressure changes similar to blowing up a balloon and allowing it to deflate. Think about that process and be able to:

➤ Relate, in a very general way, changes in volume and pressure in the lungs to the process of breathing.

When Emergency Medical Responders physically help a patient breathe, they are ventilating the patient. Sometimes they ventilate too frequently or with too much pressure. When this occurs, the lungs get overfilled and the extra air may go into the stomach. You must recognize when this happens and know what to do about it. So, be able to:

➤ State two things to do when air gets in the patient's stomach (gastric distention) from assisted ventilations.

Sometimes, events or actions cause our airway to become blocked, and it becomes difficult or impossible to breathe. What are the causes? How can you tell if someone is having a breathing problem? What can Emergency Medical Responders do to help? You must be able to:

➤ List five factors that can cause airway obstruction.
➤ List three signs of partial airway obstruction.
➤ State when you should care for a partial airway obstruction as if it were a complete airway obstruction.
➤ Describe two things usually noticeable in a responsive patient with a complete airway obstruction.

In addition, for a patient with injuries, always consider the possibility of a spine injury. If there is any reason to suspect one, stabilize the injured patient's head and neck while opening the airway so you do not cause further spine damage. Be able to explain why and:

➤ Demonstrate the techniques used to manage the airway of patients with possible neck or spine injuries.

 FIRST ON SCENE

"Tami!" The neighbor's voice was full of panic. "Tami, are you home?"

Tami Perez, full-time mother and part-time volunteer firefighter, had been dozing in the backyard with a paperback novel shielding her eyes from the sun. "Yeah, Ruthie, I'm back here," she said, lifting the book up and squinting toward the back fence and her neighbor's red face.

"Tami. Quick. It's Jenna!" The neighbor stammered. "She fell off the pool slide onto the cement, and she's not moving."

Tami jumped up from her bright green lounge chair and raced to the gate separating the two backyards. Jim, Ruthie's husband and Jenna's stepfather, was kneeling over the motionless girl protectively.

"Nobody move her!" he said, probably louder than he had intended. "I think her neck might be hurt."

Tami looked past Jim and saw the girl lying awkwardly semiprone on the concrete with her chin propped against her chest.

"Ruthie, I need you to call 9-1-1 right now." Tami knelt next to the girl. "And Jim, we need to gently roll her over."

Breathing

WHY WE BREATHE

To maintain life, we breathe. The act of breathing is called **respiration**, during which oxygen is brought into the body. The body's cells, tissues, and organs need oxygen for life, and all life requires energy. The body uses oxygen to produce the energy needed to contract muscles, send nerve impulses, digest food, and build new tissues. In addition, the breathing process also removes carbon dioxide from cells and gives it off as waste.

The process of breathing maintains a constant exchange of carbon dioxide and oxygen. If breathing is not adequate or if it stops, carbon dioxide accumulates in the body's cells and becomes a deadly poison. A patient with an increase in carbon dioxide may present with the following signs and symptoms: rapid breathing to rid the body of the excess carbon dioxide; drowsiness as brain cells react to excess carbon dioxide; and hallucinations and loss of the ability to breathe, as brains cells begin to die. The patient is becoming **hypoxic**, will eventually lose consciousness, and if breathing is not restored, will go into a coma and die.

By regulating the levels of carbon dioxide in the blood and tissues, the respiratory system plays a key role in keeping a normal acid–base balance. This is measured using a pH scale. A low pH indicates too much acid and may be caused by a buildup of carbon dioxide, as may be seen in respiratory failure. Cells live and function within a narrow range of pH. If breathing is not adequate or if it fails, this balancing function stops. If blood pH level goes too far one way or the other on the scale, cells stop functioning and die. The brain is also very sensitive to improper levels of pH balance. Without proper pH, brain functions quickly cease, including the ones that control breathing.

Once breathing stops, the heart will soon follow. This is because the heart requires a continuous supply of oxygen to function. The moment both heartbeat and respirations stop is called **clinical death**. Over the next four to six minutes, oxygen is depleted and cells begin to die. This is the period when it is most critical for the patient to receive CPR. If the patient's cells do not receive oxygen within 10 minutes, they quickly die. The organ affected first, and the most critical one, is the brain. Biological death occurs during this 6- to 10-minute time frame (Figure 6.1). **Biological death** occurs when too many brain cells die. Clinical death can be reversed; biological death cannot.

HOW WE BREATHE

Breathing is automatic. Even though you can temporarily control depth and rate, that control is short term and is soon taken over by involuntary orders from the

respiration ■ the act of breathing; the exchange of oxygen and carbon dioxide that takes place in the lungs.

REMEMBER

The process of biological death may be delayed by factors such as cold, especially in cold-water drownings. This is because the body's metabolism and oxygen consumption by the cells is profoundly slowed by the cooling of the body. Always perform resuscitation procedures on cold-water drowning victims, even if they have been in the water longer than 10 minutes.

hypoxic ■ refers to an insufficient level of oxygen in the blood and tissues. The condition is called *hypoxia*.

clinical death ■ the moment when breathing and heart actions stop.

biological death ■ occurs approximately four to six minutes after onset of clinical death and results when there is an excessive amount of brain cell death.

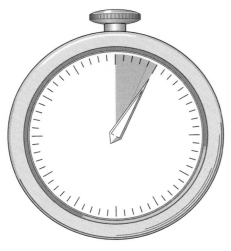

Clinical death—the moment breathing and heartbeat stop

Biological death—within 4–6 minutes

FIGURE 6.1 Without oxygen, brain cells begin to die within 10 minutes. Cell death may begin in as little as 4 minutes.

diaphragm (DI-ah-fram) ■ the dome-shaped muscle that separates the chest and abdominal cavities. It is the major muscle used in breathing.

respiratory centers of the brain. If you try to hold your breath, these centers will urge you to breathe, then take over and force you to breathe. If you try to breathe slow, shallow breaths while running, these brain centers will automatically adjust the rate and depth of breathing to suit the needs of your body. Asleep, or even unresponsive, if there is no damage to these respiratory centers and the heart continues to circulate oxygenated blood to the brain, breathing will be an involuntary, automatic function. The needs of your cells, not your will, are the determining factors in the control of breathing.

The lungs are elastic and expandable. This expansion is limited by the size of the chest cavity and the pressure within the cavity pushing back on the lungs. To inspire (inhale air), the size of the chest cavity must increase and the pressure inside the cavity must decrease. A simple law governs respiration: as volume increases, pressure decreases (Figure 6.2).

If you take the air out of a small balloon and place the same amount of air into a larger balloon, the final pressure inside the large balloon will not be as great as it was in the smaller one. Why? The larger balloon has a greater volume to be filled. The air from the small balloon will produce less pressure inside the large one.

FIRST ➤ The volume of the chest cavity is increased by muscle contraction. This may sound backward because contractions usually make things smaller. However, as the muscles between the ribs contract, they pull the front of the ribs up and out. When the **diaphragm** muscle contracts, it moves downward. Both actions result in an increase in the size and volume of the chest cavity.

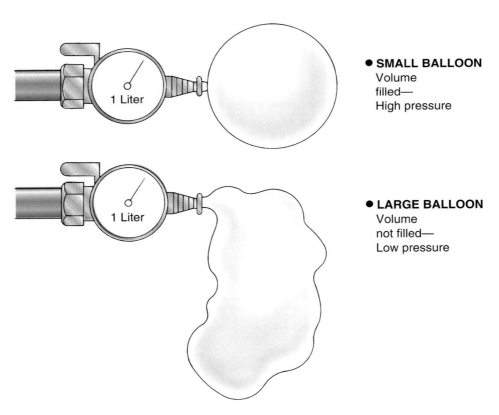

● **SMALL BALLOON**
Volume filled—
High pressure

● **LARGE BALLOON**
Volume not filled—
Low pressure

FIGURE 6.2 An equal amount of air delivered to each balloon will not produce the same pressure. An increase in volume means a decrease in pressure.

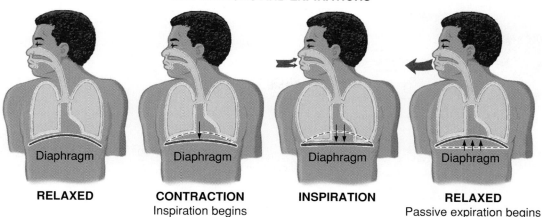

INSPIRATIONS AND EXPIRATIONS

| Diaphragm | Diaphragm | Diaphragm | Diaphragm |
| **RELAXED** | **CONTRACTION** Inspiration begins | **INSPIRATION** | **RELAXED** Passive expiration begins |

FIGURE 6.3 The respiratory cycle.

With each **inspiration**, the volume of the chest cavity increases, causing a decrease in the pressure within the lungs. (Figure 6.3 illustrates the breathing process.) When this occurs, the lungs expand automatically. As the lungs expand, the volume inside each lung increases. This means that the pressure inside each lung will decrease. As you know, air moves from high pressure to low pressure. (A punctured automobile tire demonstrates this principle.) So, when the pressure inside the lungs becomes less than the pressure in the atmosphere, air rushes into the lungs. It moves from high pressure (atmosphere) to low pressure (lungs). It will continue to do so until the pressure in the lungs equals the pressure in the atmosphere.

For **expiration** to occur, the process is reversed. The diaphragm muscle and the muscles between the ribs relax, which reduces the volume in the chest cavity. As the cavity gets smaller, pressure builds in the lungs until it becomes greater than the pressure in the atmosphere, when we must exhale. Air flows from high pressure (full lungs) to low pressure (atmosphere). ▪

inspiration ▪ refers to the process of breathing in, or inhaling. Opposite, *expiration*.

expiration ▪ refers to the passive process of breathing out, or exhaling. Opposite, *inspiration*.

Respiratory System Anatomy

FIRST ➤ Several important parts of the respiratory system have been discussed: the respiratory centers in the brain and the muscles of respiration, including the diaphragm and those between the ribs. Other major structures of the respiratory system include the upper and lower airways (Figure 6.4):

- *Nose.* The nose is the primary path for air to enter and leave the system.
- *Mouth.* The mouth is the secondary path for air to enter and leave the system.
- *Throat.* An air and food passage, the throat is also called the oral **pharynx**.
- *Epiglottis.* A leaf-shaped structure, the **epiglottis** covers the larynx when we swallow, which prevents food and fluids from entering the trachea.
- *Trachea.* The **trachea** is an air passage to the lungs. It is located below the larynx and is commonly called the *windpipe*.
- *Larynx.* An air passage at the top of the trachea, the **larynx** is also known as the *voice box* (the structure that contains the vocal cords).
- *Bronchial tree.* The bronchial tree is formed by tubes that branch from the trachea and take air to the lungs. Its two main branches are the right and left main stem bronchi, one for each lung. These branch into secondary bronchi in the lobes of the lungs. The secondary bronchi then branch into *bronchioles*, many of which have *alveoli*, the microscopic air sacs where the exchange of gases actually takes place.

2–1.1 Name and label the major structures of the respiratory system on a diagram.

pharynx (FAR-inks) ▪ the throat.

epiglottis (EP-i-GLOT-is) ▪ a flap of cartilage and other tissues located above the larynx. It helps close off the airway when a person swallows.

trachea (TRAY-ke-ah) ▪ the windpipe.

larynx (LAR-inks) ▪ the section of the airway between the throat and the trachea that contains the vocal cords. Also called *voice box*.

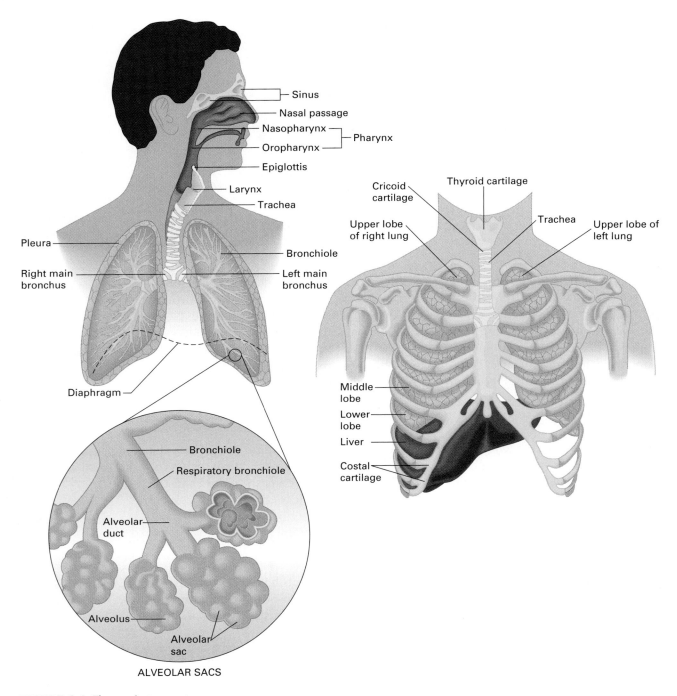

FIGURE 6.4 The respiratory system.

- *Lungs.* The lungs are elastic organs containing the bronchi, bronchioles, terminal bronchioles, and the alveoli.
- *Alveoli.* These are the small air sacs at the end of the terminal bronchioles where blood cells replenish their oxygen supply and release their accumulated carbon dioxide.

Respiratory Cycle

When our breathing muscles (the diaphragm and those between the ribs) contract and enlarge the chest cavity, air flows through the mouth and nose, into the throat, past the epiglottis, and into the trachea. Air then flows into the left and right main stem bronchi, then through the smaller bronchioles to the clusters of alveoli. The alveoli are surrounded by tiny blood vessels called *pulmonary capillaries*. Here is where oxygen and carbon dioxide exchange takes place. Oxygen travels through the walls of the alveoli and into the blood, which delivers it to the cells. Carbon dioxide travels from the blood through the alveoli walls where it is eliminated when we exhale.

PATIENT ASSESSMENT

Signs of Adequate Breathing

FIRST ➤ As you approach a patient and form a general impression of his condition, you can quickly determine if he is comfortable and breathing normally or if he is distressed and having trouble breathing. As you perform an initial assessment of the patient, you will:

- Look for adequate **tidal volume**. This is amount of air being moved in and out of the lungs with each breath. Tidal volume can be assessed by observing the even and effortless rise and fall of the chest with each breath.
- Listen for air entering and leaving the nose and mouth. The sounds should be quiet like a soft breeze (no gurgling, gasping, wheezing, or other unusual sounds).
- Feel for air moving into and out of the nose and mouth.
- Observe skin color. Although every person's skin is a different color, the skin should not be pale or **cyanotic** (tinted blue). Look for these signs, especially around the lips and eyes and in the nail beds, where it will be obvious if the patient is not breathing adequately.
- Observe the patient's level of responsiveness. A responsive patient who is not having difficulty breathing is almost always breathing adequately. ∎

Signs of Inadequate Breathing

FIRST ➤ A patient who has inadequate breathing will have the following signs and symptoms:

- Absent or shallow rise and fall of the chest.
- No air heard or felt at the nose or mouth.
- Noisy breathing or gasping sounds.
- Breathing that is irregular, too rapid, or too slow.
- Breathing that is too deep or labored, especially in infants and children.
- Use of **accessory muscles** in the chest, abdomen, and around the neck.
- Nostrils that flare when breathing, especially in children.
- Skin that is pale or cyanotic (tinted blue).
- Sitting or leaning forward in a tripod position in an effort to make breathing easier. ∎

Pulmonary Resuscitation

The term *pulmonary* refers to the lungs. *Resuscitation* is any effort to revive or to restore normal function. When you perform **pulmonary resuscitation**, you are providing artificial or assisted **ventilation** to the patient in an attempt to restore the normal delivery of oxygen into the blood and removal of carbon dioxide. This is also referred to as *rescue breathing*.

tidal volume ∎ the amount of air being moved in and out of the lungs with each breath.

cyanotic (sy-ah-OT-ik) ∎ bluish discoloration of the skin and mucous membranes; a sign that body tissues are not receiving enough oxygen. The condition is called *cyanosis (sy-ah-NO-sis)*.

2–1.2 List the signs of inadequate breathing.

accessory muscles ∎ muscles of the neck, chest, and abdomen that can assist during respiratory difficulty.

pulmonary resuscitation (PUL-mo-ner-e re-SUS-si-TAY-shun) ∎ a technique by which breaths are provided to a patient in an attempt to artificially maintain normal lung function. Also called *rescue breathing* or *artificial ventilation*.

ventilation ∎ the supplying of air to the lungs. See *pulmonary resuscitation*.

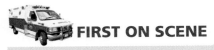

Because you provide air that has already been in your lungs to the patient, you might wonder if you are providing enough oxygen. The atmosphere contains about 21% oxygen. The air exhaled from your lungs can contain up to 16% oxygen. This is more than enough oxygen to keep most patients biologically alive until they can receive supplemental oxygen.

OPENING THE AIRWAY

As part of your initial assessment, make certain that the patient has an open airway and is breathing adequately. In an unresponsive patient, the muscles begin to relax, and the tongue may drop into the back of the throat and obstruct the airway. The simple act of tilting the head and lifting the chin could relieve this problem. If a patient is responsive and showing signs of obstruction (panicked appearance and hands at the throat), the problem is not likely to be the tongue. Immediately begin the steps to relieve airway obstructions (discussed later in this chapter).

Repositioning the Head

FIRST ➤ Simply repositioning the head may be enough to open the airway. If the patient is lying down with his head on several pillows or up against some object with head flexed forward, tilt the head back slightly by removing pillows or by repositioning the patient so that his head is not flexed forward. You may place one flat pillow beneath the patient's shoulders to help maintain the airway. Note that patients under the influence of alcohol or drugs often have trouble holding a head position that will keep the airway open. ▪

2–1.4 Relate mechanism of injury to opening the airway.

head-tilt, chin-lift maneuver ▪ technique used to open the airway of a patient with no suspected neck or spine injury.

jaw-thrust maneuver ▪ technique used to open the airway of a trauma patient with possible neck or spine injury.

2–1.3 Describe the steps in the head-tilt, chin-lift.

There are two methods of opening the airway. The first, the **head-tilt, chin-lift maneuver,** is used for ill or injured patients with no suspected spine injury. The second, the **jaw-thrust maneuver,** is used for patients who you suspect may have a spine injury.

Head-Tilt, Chin-Lift Maneuver

To perform the head-tilt, chin-lift maneuver, place one hand on the patient's forehead and two fingers of your other hand on the bone part of the patient's chin. Gently tilt the head back while lifting the chin. Be careful not to compress the soft tissues under the jaw. Lift up the patient's chin so the lower teeth are almost touching the upper teeth (Figure 6.5). This maneuver will move the tongue away from the back of the throat and allow air to flow freely as the patient breathes. It will also move the neck, which you do not want to do if the patient has a possible spine injury. In such cases, use the jaw-thrust maneuver.

Is It Safe ?

It is important to carefully consider the potential for spine injury before opening the patient's airway. For example, the absence of an obvious mechanism of injury does not automatically rule out spine injury. A patient found unresponsive in an alley could have been assaulted and therefore may have a neck or back injury. When in doubt, always take appropriate spinal precautions. ▪

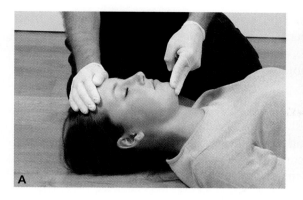
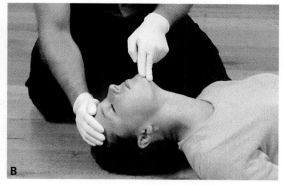

FIGURE 6.5 Use the head-tilt, chin-lift maneuver to open the airway if there are no spine injuries. **A.** First, position your hands. **B.** Then, tilt the patient's head back as far as it will comfortably go.

Jaw-Thrust Maneuver

This maneuver is the recommended method for opening the airway of patients with possible neck or spine injuries (Figure 6.6). Position yourself at the top of the patient's head. Reach forward and place one hand on each side of the chin behind the jaw, just below the ears. You may press your thumbs against the cheekbones for leverage. Push the jaw forward. Do not tilt or rotate the patient's head.

This method can also be used in conjunction with a **pocket face mask** when assisted ventilations are required.

2–1.5 Describe the steps in the jaw-thrust.

pocket face mask ▪ a device used to help provide ventilations. It has a chimney with a one-way valve and HEPA filter. Some have an inlet for supplemental oxygen.

Is It Safe ?

The Occupational Safety and Health Administration (OSHA) and the Centers for Disease Control and Prevention (CDC) guidelines state that EMS personnel can reduce the risk of contracting infectious diseases by using pocket face masks with one-way valves and high-efficiency particulate air (HEPA) filter inserts when ventilating patients. Always have one on hand. Also wear protective gloves during assessment and care of all patients. ▪

FIGURE 6.6 Use the jaw-thrust maneuver if there are possible neck or spine injuries. **A.** Side view and **B.** front view of the Emergency Medical Responder's hand position.

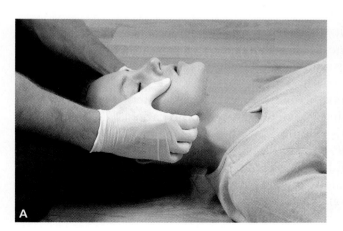
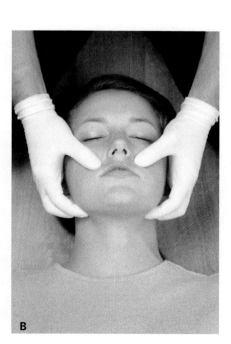

It is important to understand that if you are caring for a patient who has been injured and you are unable to effectively open the airway using the jaw-thrust maneuver, you must use the head-tilt, chin-lift maneuver instead. It is more important to establish an airway, and tilting the head back may be the only option.

RESCUE BREATHING

All Emergency Medical Responders should use barrier devices, such as pocket face masks or face shields, when providing artificial ventilations (rescue breaths). When you perform rescue breathing, you can come into direct contact with the patient's body fluids, such as respiratory secretions, saliva droplets, blood, or vomit. Take all steps necessary to ensure protection from infectious diseases. Always protect yourself.

One example of a barrier device is the pocket face mask. Pocket face masks are available in many sizes and should fit the patient and seal easily to the facial contours of the adult, child, or infant. Pocket face masks are typically made of durable plastic and have a replaceable one-way valve and filter. Some variations have an oxygen inlet to allow for the administration of supplemental oxygen.

Another example of a barrier device is the face shield, which is a durable plastic sheet with a built-in filter. When folded and stowed, it is small enough to be attached to a key ring, but it is large enough to cover the patient's lower face and act as a barrier to help prevent direct contact with body fluids.

NOTE

The mouth-to-mouth and mouth-to-nose procedures are no longer accepted as safe practices for Emergency Medical Responders. Laypeople learn these methods because they do not normally carry barrier devices and, usually, they would perform assisted ventilations only on their own family members. Even so, it is still common for all rescuers to learn how to deliver mouth-to-mouth and mouth-to-nose techniques because of the possibility of being in situations where there are no protective devices or where there are more patients than devices at the scene. Those who advocate rescue breathing without protective devices state that it is the rescuer's decision to provide ventilation without adequate rescuer protection.

NOTE

It is common for patients who are not breathing to vomit during the resuscitation effort. If you carry a suction device and are trained in its use, it is highly recommended that you have it out and available for use whenever you are providing rescue breaths for a patient. The proper use of suction is discussed later in this chapter. Always follow local protocols.

Mouth-to-Mask Ventilation

2–1.8 Describe how to ventilate a patient with a (pocket) resuscitation mask or barrier device.

The mouth-to-mask technique of providing assisted ventilations is the recommended method when there is only a single rescuer present. A pocket face mask allows you to provide ventilations without having to make direct skin-to-skin contact. The mask should have a one-way valve in the stem to minimize the chances of the rescuer breathing in exhaled air from the patient. The pocket face mask that you use should also come with the disposable filter called a *high-efficiency particulate air (HEPA) filter* (Figure 6.7). It snaps inside the pocket face mask and traps air droplets and secretions that may contain dangerous pathogens.

The pocket face mask is made of soft plastic material that can be folded and carried in your pocket. It is available with or without an oxygen inlet. You provide mouth-to-mask ventilations through a chimney on the mask (Figure 6.8). If the

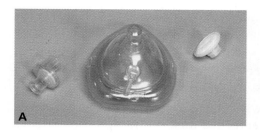

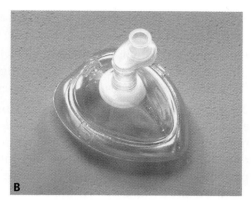

FIGURE 6.7 Pocket face mask with one-way valve and HEPA filter, **A.** unassembled and **B.** assembled.

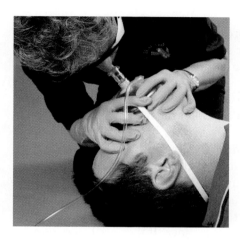

FIGURE 6.8A Place yourself beside the patient's head and apply the mask.

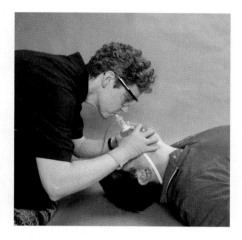

FIGURE 6.8B ALTERNATIVE: Position yourself directly above (at the top of) the patient's head and apply the mask.

mask has a second port for oxygen, you can simultaneously ventilate the patient with air from your lungs and with additional oxygen from an oxygen source.

Another advantage of the pocket face mask is that it allows you to use both hands to maintain a proper head-tilt or jaw-thrust and still hold the mask firmly in place. It is relatively easy to keep a good seal between the face mask and a patient's face with this device. The pocket face mask also can be used with or without an airway adjunct (discussed later in the chapter).

FIRST ➤ To provide mouth-to-mask ventilations, make sure you are wearing appropriate PPE. Then follow these steps:

1. Kneel beside the patient and confirm unresponsiveness.
2. Open the airway using the most appropriate maneuver.
3. Check for breathing.
   — Look for chest movements. Does the chest rise and fall evenly?
   — Listen for air flow from the mouth or nose. Are there unusual sounds (gurgling, crowing, snoring)?
   — Feel for air exchange against your cheek at the patient's mouth and nose.
   — Observe skin color. Is it pale or bluish (cyanotic)?
4. Take no more than 10 seconds to determine if the patient is breathing adequately. If not breathing adequately, then attach the one-way valve to the face mask. Position the mask on the patient's face so that the apex (upper tip of the triangle)

REMEMBER

If your patient is an unresponsive infant or child and you are alone, provide two minutes of rescue support and then call 9-1-1. If you are working with a partner or others are around, have one of them call 9-1-1 while you begin care.

is over the bridge of the patient's nose and the base of the mask is between the lower lip and the chin.

5. Firmly hold the mask in place while keeping the airway open. To accomplish this, place both thumbs and index fingers on the cone of the mask to form a "C" around both sides. Apply even pressure on both sides of the mask.

6. Take a normal breath and breathe slowly into the one-way valve, delivering each breath over one second. Air will enter the airway through the patient's nose and slightly open mouth. Watch for the patient's chest to rise. Remember that there is no need to remove your mouth to allow the patient to exhale. The patient's exhaled air will escape through separate vents in the one-way valve.

   If air does not enter on the initial breath, reposition the patient's head and try again. If air still does not enter, perform the steps for clearing an obstructed airway (explained later in the chapter).

7. If the initial breath is successful, continue providing rescue breaths as appropriate. One breath every five to six seconds for an adult and every three to five seconds for an infant or child, or 10–12 times a minute for adults and 12–20 times a minute for infants and children. ■

REMEMBER

Deliver one breath every five to six seconds for adults, and one breath every three to five seconds for infants and children.

An alternative method for ventilating with a pocket mask is to kneel at the top of the patient's head. Place both thumbs and index fingers on the cone of the mask to form a "C" around both sides. Place the third, fourth, and fifth fingers of each hand under the jaw to form an "E" on both sides of the patient's jaw. Apply even pressure on both sides of the mask while maintaining a head tilt.

It may be difficult to get a good mask-to-face seal when dentures are removed, and loose dentures can cause an airway obstruction and interfere with your efforts to ventilate a patient. If dentures are secure, leave them in place. If they are loose, remove them. Make sure you position the mask properly and open the airway appropriately.

The best signs of adequate mouth-to-mask ventilations are obvious chest rise and fall with each ventilation.

If you find that your efforts to ventilate the patient are *not* adequate, you must make adjustments, such as increasing the volume, changing the rate of ventilations, or adjusting the seal between the mask and the patient's face.

Mouth-to-Barrier Ventilation
To use a face shield when performing mouth-to-barrier ventilation, first make sure you are wearing appropriate BSI equipment. Then follow these steps:

1. Kneel beside the patient and confirm unresponsiveness.
2. Open the airway using the most appropriate maneuver.
3. Check for breathing:
   — Look for chest movements. Does the chest rise and fall evenly?
   — Listen for air flow from the mouth or nose. Are there unusual sounds (gurgling, crowing, snoring)?
   — Feel for air exchange against your cheek at the patient's mouth and nose.
   — Observe skin color. Is it pale or bluish (cyanotic)?

4. Take no more than 10 seconds to determine if the patient is breathing adequately. If the patient is not breathing adequately, properly position a protective face shield over the patient's mouth and hold it in place with your fingers.
5. Keep the airway open as you pinch the nose closed with the thumb and forefinger of the hand on the patient's forehead.
6. Open your mouth wide and take a normal breath.

7. Place your mouth over the face shield opening. Make a tight seal by pressing your lips against it.

8. Exhale slowly into the patient's airway until you see the chest rise. If this first attempt to provide a breath fails, reposition the patient's head or open the airway using the head-tilt, chin-lift maneuver and try again.

9. Break contact with the face shield to allow the patient to exhale. Quickly take in another breath and ventilate the patient again. You will give two initial breaths.

10. If the patient does not begin breathing adequately on his own, check for a pulse. If the patient has a pulse but is not breathing, continue with rescue breaths at a rate of one breath every five to six seconds for adults and one breath every three to five seconds for infants and children.

Constantly monitor the status of the pulse. If there is no pulse, begin CPR. If the patient has a pulse, continue rescue breathing until the patient begins to breathe on his own, someone with more training takes over, or until you are too exhausted to continue.

If you are following the correct procedures and the patient's airway is not obstructed, you should be able to feel resistance to your ventilations as the patient's lungs expand, see the chest rise and fall, hear air leaving the patient's airway as the chest falls, and feel air leaving the patient's mouth as the lungs deflate. Monitor the patient to determine if he has begun to breathe unassisted.

The most common problems with the mouth-to-barrier technique are:

- Failure to form a tight seal over the face shield opening and the patient's mouth (often caused by failing to open your mouth wide enough to make an effective seal, as well as pushing too hard in an effort to form a tight seal).
- Failure to pinch the nose completely closed.
- Failure to tilt the head back far enough to open the airway.
- Failure to open the patient's mouth wide enough to receive ventilations.
- Failure to deliver enough air during a ventilation.
- Providing breaths too quickly.
- Failure to clear the airway of obstructions.

Two additional problems—air in the patient's stomach and vomiting—are covered later in this chapter.

Mouth-to-Nose Ventilation

Patients may have injuries to the mouth and/or jaw, missing teeth or dentures, or airway obstructions that will make the previous techniques ineffective. For these patients, use the mouth-to-nose technique. (Depending on the location of the obstruction, mouth-to-nose ventilation may not work if mouth-to-mask or mouth-to-barrier ventilation has failed, but it should be tried.)

Most of this procedure is the same as mouth-to-barrier ventilation. The differences in the mouth-to-nose technique are that you will:

- Use your thumb to seal the mouth shut. Do not pinch the nose.
- Seal your mouth around the patient's nose.
- Deliver ventilations through the nose, so be sure to keep the patient's mouth closed.
- Break contact with the nose and open the mouth slightly to allow the patient to exhale. Keep your hand on the patient's forehead to keep the airway open.

Like mouth-to-mouth ventilation, mouth-to-nose ventilation exposes the rescuer to potentially infectious body fluids.

REMEMBER

You may use the jaw-thrust maneuver with the mouth-to-nose technique. To do so, seal the patient's mouth with your cheek.

stoma (STO-mah) ■ any permanent opening that has been surgically made; the opening in the neck of a neck breather.

2–1.9 Describe how ventilating an infant or a child is different from ventilating an adult.

gastric distention ■ inflation of the stomach.

Special Patients

Among your patients will be infants and children, elderly patients, patients with a **stoma** (neck breathers), and trauma victims (some with possible neck and spine injuries).

Infants (Birth–One Year) and Children (One Year to the Onset of Puberty)   The airways of infants and children have several physical characteristics that are different from adults. In the infant and child, the:

- Mouth and nose are much smaller and more easily obstructed.
- Tongue takes up more space in the mouth and throat.
- Trachea (windpipe) is smaller and more easily obstructed by swelling. It also is softer, more flexible, and can become obstructed by tilting the head back too far (hyperextension).
- Chest muscles are not as well developed, causing the infant and child to depend more on the diaphragm for breathing.
- Chest cavity and lung volumes are smaller, so **gastric distention** (air getting into the stomach) occurs more commonly.

You must recognize and aggressively care for airway and respiratory problems in infants and children. Respiratory distress and failure can quickly lead to cardiac arrest in these patients.

FIRST ➤ When assisting ventilations for an infant (Figure 6.9) or small child, make sure you are wearing appropriate BSI equipment. Then perform the following steps:

1. Kneel or stand beside the patient and confirm unresponsiveness.
2. Open the airway using the most appropriate maneuver.
3. Check for breathing, but take no more than 10 seconds.
   — Look for chest movements. Does the chest rise and fall evenly?
   — Listen for air flow from the mouth or nose. Are there unusual sounds (gurgling, crowing, snoring)?

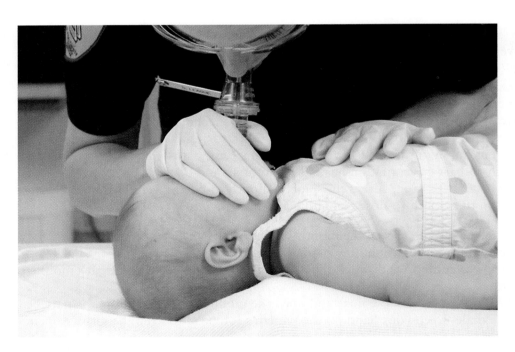

FIGURE 6.9 Mask-to-mouth ventilation of an infant.

- — Feel for air exchange against your cheek at the patient's mouth and nose.
- — Observe skin color. Is it pale or bluish (cyanotic)?

4. If the patient is not breathing adequately, give two breaths.

- — If air enters, check the pulse. If no pulse, start CPR. If there is a pulse and you are alone, provide rescue breaths for two minutes. Then alert the EMS dispatcher or have someone else call 9-1-1. If there are others with you, send them to call 9-1-1 immediately.
- — If air does not enter on the initial breath, reposition the head and try again. If air still does not enter, perform the steps for an obstructed airway (later in this chapter).

5. Position an appropriate size pocket face mask or face shield on the patient.

6. Assist ventilations with gentle but adequate breaths. The volume of breath for the infant or child is determined by ventilating until you see the chest rise. Watch for the chest to rise with each breath.

7. Allow the patient to exhale.

8. Give ventilations at a rate of one breath every three to five seconds for infants and children and deliver each breath over one second. ■

REMEMBER

Some guidelines allow adult masks to be inverted for use on children.

NOTE

If there is no reason to suspect spine injury, it is helpful to place a folded towel or similar object under an infant's shoulders to help maintain an open airway.

Terminally Ill Patients   Many terminally ill patients choose to spend their remaining time at home with family and friends. Many others enter a hospice program, which supports and advises the patient and family or makes arrangements with doctors for advance directives such as DNR orders. For guidelines on how to care for hospice or DNR patients, check your jurisdiction for training programs and follow your local protocols.

Geriatric Focus

Elderly patients may require special care because of changes in their bodies that are normal for aging. First, the lungs may have lost some elasticity, and the rib cage may be more rigid and more difficult for you to expand when assisting ventilations. The jaw joints and neck may be stiff and arthritic, which can make it difficult to open the airway, but you will be able to get sufficient air in the patient with the usual maneuvers. With the mouth-to-mask technique, air will still enter the nose, even if the mouth will not open, but your ventilations may have to be a little more forceful. Patients who have lost their teeth and do not use dentures have receding chins and sunken cheeks that make it difficult to seal a mask to the face. Always be aware of resistance to your ventilations and the rise and fall of the patient's chest.

Second, realize that the elderly patient's bones may be more brittle than the bones of younger patients. If elderly patients have fallen, they are more likely to suffer spine injury. When such injuries are possible or when you are in doubt, use the jaw-thrust maneuver to open the airway.

Finally, you may be faced with bystanders who say such things as "He's so old. Let him die in peace." It is not their right to make that decision. You are charged with the responsibility of assisting all patients who need care, unless direct orders stating otherwise have been given to you by a physician. What bystanders tell you may not be what the patient wants. Any time there is conflict in care priorities, contact medical direction.

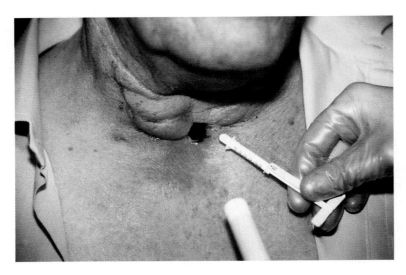

FIGURE 6.10 A typical neck stoma. (© *Shout Pictures/Custom Medical Stock Photo*)

laryngectomy (lar-in-JEK-to-me)
■ the total or partial removal of the larynx.

2–1.10 List the steps in providing mouth-to-mouth and mouth-to-stoma ventilation.

Stomas   Some people have had a surgical procedure called a **laryngectomy** to remove part or all of the larynx (voice box). An opening called a stoma is made from outside the neck to the trachea (windpipe) to create an adequate airway for breathing. These patients breathe through that opening (Figure 6.10), not through the nose or the mouth.

FIRST ➤ The opening in the neck is called a stoma. Because the patient no longer takes air into the lungs by way of the nose and mouth, you will have to use the mouth-to-mask-to-stoma technique to assist ventilations. Always look to see if there is a stoma. If so, ventilate the patient through the stoma. Currently, there is no specific mask for ventilating these patients, but an infant-size mask often fits, allowing you to establish a seal around the stoma. You may also assist ventilations with a protective face shield or by attaching a bag-valve resuscitator directly to the patient's stoma tube if one is in place in the stoma opening. Follow the protocols of your jurisdiction. Remember, direct contact increases the risk of infection. ■

When ventilating a stoma patient (Figure 6.11), take appropriate BSI precautions. Then perform the following steps:

1. Keep the patient's head in a neutral or normal position. Do not tilt the head.
2. Ensure the stoma is free and clear of any obstructions such as mucus or vomit. Do not remove the breathing tube if one is in place.
3. Use the same procedures as you would for mouth-to-mask or mouth-to-barrier resuscitation, *except:*
   — Do not pinch the patient's nose closed.
   — Place the mask or face shield on the neck over the stoma.

If the chest does not rise, the patient may be a partial neck breather. This means that the patient takes in and expels some air through the mouth and nose. In such cases, you will have to pinch the nose closed, seal the mouth with the palm of your hand, and ventilate through the stoma.

Crash Victims   Opening the airway and assisting ventilations are easier for you to perform when the patient is lying down. This means that a collision victim who is

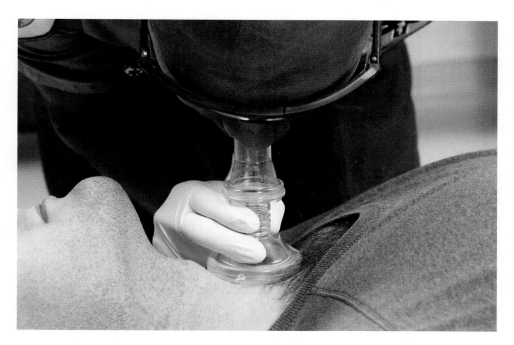

FIGURE 6.11 Performing mask-to-stoma ventilation.

not breathing but who is still in his vehicle must be repositioned. There is always a risk of causing further spine injury if you move the patient, but you must be realistic. If you wait for other EMS personnel to arrive, or if you take time to put on a rigid cervical collar and secure the patient to a spine board, the patient will likely not survive due to a lack of oxygen to the brain. Airway and breathing are always the first priorities of patient care.

Without risking your own safety, reach the victim as quickly as possible. Look, listen, and feel for breathing before moving him. If the patient is breathing, the airway is open and you do not have to move him. If you believe the mechanism of injury may have caused damage to the spine or neck and the patient is not breathing, stabilize the head and open the airway with the jaw-thrust maneuver. Then check again for breathing. If the patient is breathing, keep the airway open while maintaining the head and neck in a neutral position. Monitor breathing until assistance arrives. If the patient is not breathing and his position does not allow you to maintain an airway while you assist ventilations, you will have to reposition him.

Your instructor will show you methods to practice so you can reposition a patient with maximum head stabilization and as little spinal movement as possible. If you have help, using both hands and forearms, hold the patient's head and neck in line with the rest of the spine and work swiftly with your helpers to lay the patient flat.

Air in the Stomach and Vomiting

A common problem with assisted ventilations is that overinflating the lungs or breathing too quickly will force air into the patient's stomach. Remember to carefully watch the chest rise as you ventilate. It will only rise so far. Do not keep ventilating when it stops rising. When the chest rises completely, allow the patient to exhale. Forcing more air than the lungs can hold during ventilation can cause or worsen inflation of the stomach. Air in the stomach will cause the abdomen to distend. This condition is called *gastric distention*.

Watch for gastric distention when you ventilate a patient. Excessive distention will force the patient's diaphragm upward into the chest cavity, which will reduce the ability for the lungs to expand normally. Reduced lung capacity restricts ventilations and reduces oxygen flow to the body. Gastric distention can also cause extra pressure in the stomach, which can result in the patient vomiting.

Do not worry about slight bulging or distention, but you will have to make adjustments if you notice extensive bulging. In cases of air in the stomach where you see a noticeable bulge, reduce the force of your ventilations and:

- Reposition the patient's head to ensure an open airway.
- Be prepared for vomiting. If the patient begins to vomit, turn the patient (not just the head) to one side so the vomit will flow out of the airway and not back into it. (Vomit can obstruct the airway and damage the lungs.) Have suction equipment on hand if you carry it on your unit.
- Stabilize the head and move the patient as a unit if you suspect neck or spine injuries. If the patient is an unresponsive medical patient with no indication of injury, place him in the recovery position.
- Do not push on the stomach to release the air. This may cause vomiting, which can block the airway or enter the lungs. Even if the patient is on his side when he vomits, the vomit will not simply flow out. With your gloved hand, clear his mouth with gauze and finger sweeps or use suctioning equipment.

Airway Obstruction

CAUSES OF AIRWAY OBSTRUCTION

FIRST ➤ Many factors can cause the airway to become partially or completely obstructed, including a foreign object lodged in the airway or excess saliva or blood accumulating in the mouth.

The following are examples of upper airway obstructions that you may be able to relieve (Figure 6.12):

- *Obstruction by the tongue.* Common in unresponsive patients, the tongue falls back in the throat to block the airway.
- *Obstruction by the epiglottis.* The patient attempts to force inspirations when he is having difficulty breathing. This effort may create a negative pressure that can force the epiglottis and tongue to block the airway.
- *Foreign objects (also called mechanical obstructions).* Objects and other matter, such as pieces of food, ice, toys, dentures, vomit, and liquids pooling in the back of the throat can block the airway.

The following obstructions may be impossible for you to relieve, but you must still attempt to assist ventilations:

- *Tissue damage.* Tissue damage can be caused by punctures to the neck, crush wounds to the neck and face, upper-airway burns from breathing hot air (as

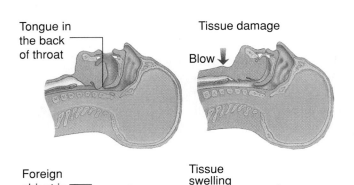

Tongue in the back of throat

Tissue damage

Blow ↓

Foreign object in throat

Tissue swelling

FIGURE 6.12 Possible causes of airway obstruction.

in fires), poisons, and severe blows to the neck. The tissues of the throat and windpipe become swollen and make it difficult for air to flow through the airway.

- *Allergic reactions.* The tissues of the oral pharynx, tongue, and/or the epiglottis become swollen in response to the patient's exposure to something he or she is allergic to, such as a bee sting or a certain food.
- *Infections.* Pharyngeal and epiglottic (ep-i-GLOT-ik) infections can produce airway obstruction. ■

Signs of Partial Airway Obstruction
A patient who is having difficulty breathing may have only a partial obstruction and may still be able to move some air.

FIRST ➤ The signs of partial airway obstruction include the following:

- Noisy breathing, such as:
  — *Snoring* is usually caused by the tongue partially or intermittently obstructing the back of the throat.
  — *Gurgling* is usually caused by fluids or blood in the airway or by a foreign object in the trachea.
  — *Crowing* is usually caused by spasms of the larynx (voice box).
  — *Wheezing* is usually due to swelling or spasms along the lower airway caused by asthma, but it does not always mean there is an airway problem. Wheezing may sound serious but is not usually associated with airway obstruction. It is more common during exhalation.
  — *Stridor* is a high-pitched harsh sound usually caused by swollen tissue in the throat or larynx (voice box) and typically heard when the patient inhales.
- Breathing is present, but skin is pale or blue at the lips, earlobes, fingernail beds, or tongue. The usual presentation in a responsive patient is fear, panic, or agitation. Nothing invokes terror in a person like a threatened airway or the inability to breathe. ■

If a responsive patient is experiencing a partial airway obstruction, encourage him to cough. A forceful cough indicates that he has enough air exchange, and coughing may dislodge and expel foreign materials. Do not interfere with the patient's own efforts to clear the airway.

If the patient has poor air exchange and cannot cough or only coughs weakly, begin care as if there is a complete airway obstruction. (Care steps follow later in the chapter.) Do the same if the patient has poor air exchange at first assessment or when good air exchange becomes poor air exchange.

Signs of Complete Airway Obstruction
When the airway is completely obstructed, the responsive patient will be unable to speak and cough. The patient often will grasp her neck and open her mouth, which is the universal sign of choking (Figure 6.13). The unresponsive patient will not have any of the typical chest movements or the other signs of good air exchange.

CLEARING A FOREIGN BODY AIRWAY OBSTRUCTION

Responsive Adult or Child Patient
Ongoing research conducted by the American Heart Association suggests that the use of **abdominal thrusts** is still the most effective method for clearing the airway of an adult or child who is choking. A slightly different technique is used to clear the airway of an infant.

2–1.13 Describe how to clear a foreign body airway obstruction in a responsive adult.

2–1.14 Describe how to clear a foreign body airway obstruction in a responsive child with a complete obstruction or a partial obstruction and poor air exchange.

abdominal thrusts ■ manual thrusts delivered to create pressure that can help expel an airway obstruction in an adult or child. Also known as *Heimlich maneuver.*

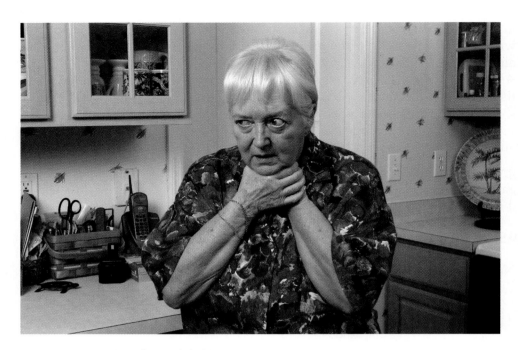

FIGURE 6.13 Universal sign of choking.

Is It Safe ?

The American Heart Association (AHA) does not recommend abdominal thrusts for infants. This is due in part to the unique placement of the underlying internal organs in an infant. The risk of causing damage to them is too great. A slightly different technique is used instead and is described later in this chapter.

Abdominal thrusts are achieved by having the rescuer stand behind the patient, place one fist just above the navel, grasp that fist with the other hand, and provide inward and upward thrusts. These thrusts push up on the diaphragm muscle, creating pressure inside the chest cavity and forcing air out of the lungs. As the air is forced out of the lungs, it pushes the foreign object out ahead of it.

Perform the following steps for removal of a foreign body airway obstruction for a responsive adult or child patient (Scan 6–1):

1. Determine that there is complete obstruction or a partial obstruction with poor air exchange. Ask, "Are you choking?" or "Can you speak?" Look and listen for signs of complete obstruction or poor air exchange. Tell the patient you will help.
2. Position yourself behind the patient and with the index finger of one hand, locate the navel.
3. Make a fist with the other hand and place it against the abdomen thumb side in, just above the navel.
4. Grasp the fist with the first hand and give up to five abdominal thrusts in rapid succession. Watch and listen for evidence that the object has been removed. The patient will begin to cough or speak if the object is removed.

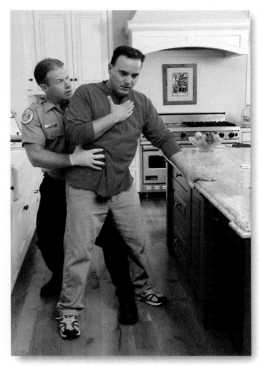

1 ■ Stand behind the patient. Place one leg between the patient's legs to obtain a stable stance.

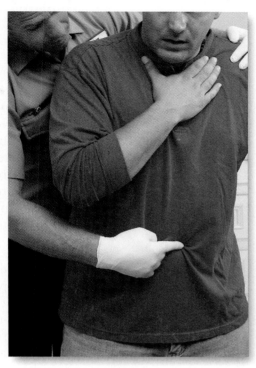

2 ■ Reach around with one hand to locate the patient's navel.

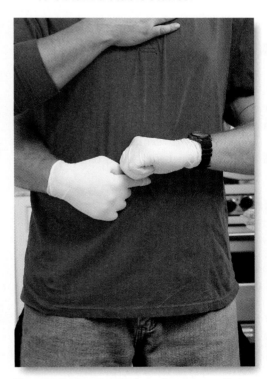

3 ■ With the other hand, make a fist and place it just above the patient's navel.

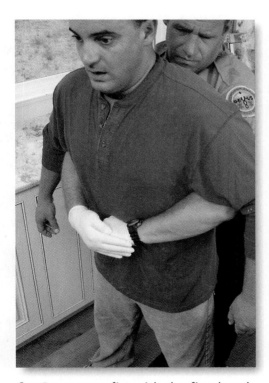

4 ■ Grasp your fist with the first hand and pull in and up with swift firm thrusts.

5. If the patient's airway remains obstructed, repeat the thrusts until the airway is cleared or until the patient loses responsiveness.
6. If the patient becomes unresponsive before you are able to clear the airway obstruction, direct someone to call 9-1-1 and begin CPR.

Unresponsive Adult or Child

2–1.16 Describe how to clear a foreign body airway obstruction in an unresponsive adult.

2–1.17 Describe how to clear a foreign body airway obstruction in an unresponsive child.

The following guidelines for the care of an unresponsive patient apply to adults and children (one year up to the onset of puberty). When you suspect a patient may be suffering from an airway obstruction, move swiftly to clear the airway. For unresponsive patients, act quickly to determine if you are able to provide adequate ventilations. Because the tongue is the most common cause of airway obstruction for these patients, make certain to open the airway using the most appropriate maneuver, *prior* to attempting ventilation. Once you have confirmed that you are unable to ventilate, begin CPR. The specific techniques for performing CPR are explained in Chapter 8.

Perform these steps when caring for an unresponsive patient with an airway obstruction:

1. Take the appropriate BSI precautions.
2. With the patient lying face up (supine), tap and shout to assess responsiveness.
3. If unresponsive, direct someone to activate 9-1-1. Then open the airway using the most appropriate technique for the patient's size and condition.
4. Place your ear next to the patient's nose and mouth and assess for the presence of breathing by looking, listening, and feeling for air exchange for no more than 10 seconds.
5. If there are no signs of breathing, attempt to provide two slow breaths. If you are unable to achieve adequate chest rise, reposition the head and try again.
6. If after two attempts you are unable to achieve adequate chest rise, begin CPR.

chest thrusts ■ manual thrusts delivered to create pressure that can help expel an airway obstruction in an infant or in pregnant or obese patients.

CLEARING A FOREIGN BODY AIRWAY OBSTRUCTION IN AN INFANT

The steps for caring for an infant (younger than one year of age) are slightly different from those used for adults and children. For the responsive infant, a combination of **chest thrusts** and back slaps are used to remove the foreign object.

Responsive Infant

Perform these steps when caring for a responsive infant with an airway obstruction:

1. Take appropriate BSI precautions.
2. Pick up the infant and support him between the forearms of both arms. Support the infant's head as you place him face down on your forearm. Use your thigh to support your forearm. Remember to keep the infant's head lower than the trunk.
3. Rapidly deliver five back blows between the shoulder blades (Figure 6.14). If this fails to expel the object, proceed to Step 4.

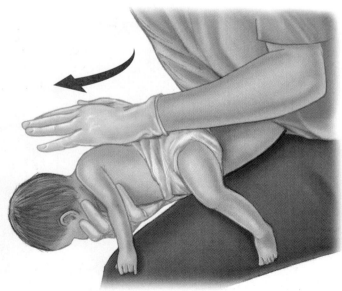

FIGURE 6.14 For back slaps, support the infant face down on your forearm.

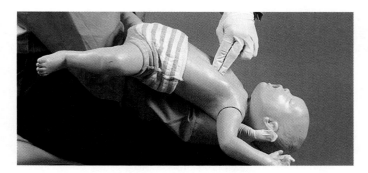

FIGURE 6.15 Chest thrusts on an infant.

4. While supporting the infant between your arms, turn him over onto his back, again keeping the head lower than the trunk. Use your thigh to support your forearm.
5. Locate the compression site and deliver five chest thrusts with the tips of two or three fingers along the midline of the breastbone (Figure 6.15).
6. Continue with this sequence of back slaps and chest thrusts until the object is expelled or the infant loses responsiveness.
7. If the infant becomes unresponsive before you can expel the object, begin CPR.

Unresponsive Infant
Perform these steps when caring for an unresponsive infant with an airway obstruction (Scan 6–2):

1. Take the appropriate BSI precautions.
2. With the infant lying face up (supine), tap and shout to assess responsiveness.
3. If the infant is unresponsive, direct someone to activate 9-1-1. Then open the airway by placing the infant's head in a neutral or "sniffing" position. If you are alone, provide two minutes of rescue support before stopping to call 9-1-1.
4. Place your ear next to the infant's nose and mouth and assess for the presence of breathing by looking, listening, and feeling for air exchange, but for no more than 10 seconds.
5. If there are no signs of breathing, attempt to provide two slow gentle breaths. If you are unable to achieve adequate chest rise, reposition the head and try again.
6. If after two attempts, you are unable to achieve adequate chest rise, begin CPR.

SPECIAL CONSIDERATIONS

Obese and Pregnant Patients
Some choking patients present specific challenges that must be overcome if you are going to have any chance of clearing the airway. For example, a patient's large size may prevent you from getting your arms completely around him, making it impossible to provide adequate abdominal thrusts. Providing abdominal thrusts to a pregnant woman can cause serious injury to the developing fetus. For these two responsive

2–1.15 Describe how to clear a foreign body airway obstruction in a responsive infant with a complete obstruction or a partial airway obstruction and poor air exchange.

WARNING

Back slaps are recommended for conscious infants who have complete airway obstructions. Do not use this procedure on children or adults.

2–1.18 Describe how to clear a foreign body airway obstruction in an unresponsive infant.

REMEMBER

Chest thrusts must be used for infants, obese patients, and women in the later stages of pregnancy.

FIRST ON SCENE

Jim thought for a second, his eyes moving from his unconscious stepdaughter to Tami's face. When he finally agreed to let Tami provide emergency care, Tami instructed him on how to help her roll the girl over while keeping her head and neck in a neutral, in-line position.

As soon as Jenna's chin moved from her chest, the child inhaled noisily and began breathing again. Jim closed his eyes and took several deep breaths before opening them again. "Thank you," he said quietly.

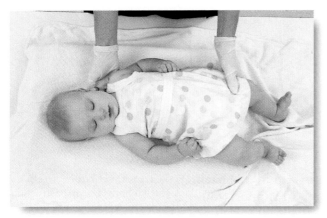

1 ■ Place the infant supine on a firm surface.

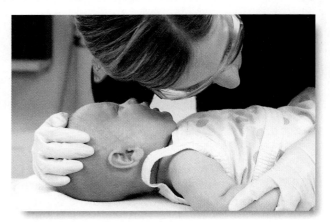

2 ■ Assess breathing for no more than 10 seconds.

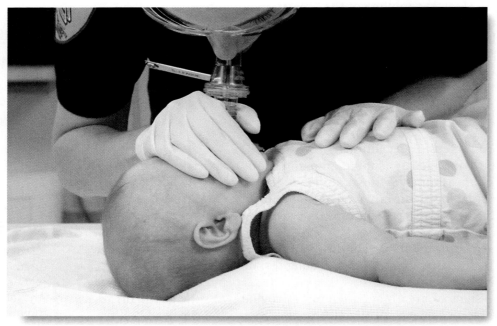

3 ■ Attempt to ventilate the infant.

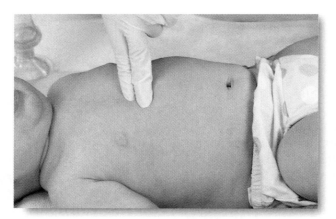

4 ■ If unable to ventilate, start CPR beginning with chest compressions.

patients, attempt to provide chest thrusts as an alternative to abdominal thrusts. For the obese patient, the chest area is typically smaller in diameter than the abdomen, making it more likely that you can provide adequate and successful thrusts. For the pregnant patient, chest thrusts provide a suitable alternative and eliminate the possibility of injuring the developing fetus (Figure 6.16).

Perform the following steps to provide chest thrusts:

1. Determine that there is complete obstruction or a partial obstruction with poor air exchange. Ask, "Are you choking?" or "Can you speak?" Tell the patient you will help.
2. Position yourself behind the patient and place the thumb side of one fist on the center of the breastbone.
3. Grasp the fist with the other hand and give up to five chest thrusts in rapid succession. Watch and listen for evidence that the object has been removed. The patient will begin to cough or speak if it has been.
4. If the patient's airway remains obstructed, repeat the thrusts until the airway is cleared or until the patient loses responsiveness.
5. If the patient becomes unresponsive before you are able to clear the airway obstruction, direct someone to call 9-1-1 and begin CPR.

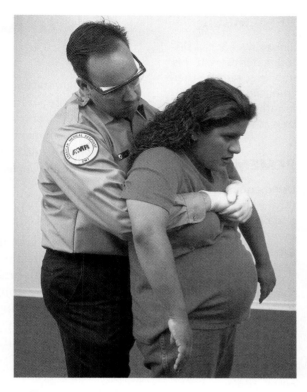

FIGURE 6.16 Chest thrust to a pregnant patient.

Finger Sweeps

A finger sweep is the technique of using your finger to sweep through the patient's mouth in an attempt to remove a foreign object. It is important to know that you should only perform finger sweeps if you can see an object in the patient's mouth (Figure 6.17). Be careful not to accidentally force the object back down the patient's throat in your attempt to sweep it out.

In most cases, a responsive patient has a **gag reflex**. Probing the mouth with your finger may stimulate the gag reflex and cause vomiting. If this occurs, the patient may inhale the vomit, resulting in the potential for serious illness later. Therefore, only attempt finger sweeps on unresponsive patients and only when you can actually see the object you are going after.

WARNING

Do not use the finger sweep technique on responsive patients or on unresponsive patients who have a gag reflex.

gag reflex ■ a retching action, hacking, or vomiting that is induced when something touches a certain level of the patient's throat.

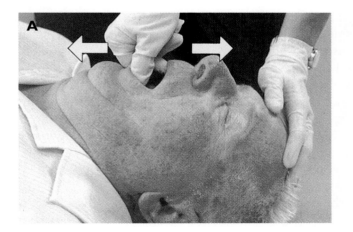 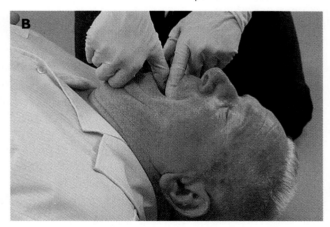

FIGURE 6.17 **A.** Open the mouth with the crossed-finger technique, and **B.** then use a finger sweep to remove foreign objects.

oropharyngeal (or-o-fah-RIN-je-al) airway (OPA) ▪ a curved breathing tube inserted into the patient's mouth. It will hold the base of the tongue forward. Also called *oral airway*.

nasopharyngeal (na-zo-fah-RIN-je-al) airway (NPA) ▪ a flexible tube that is lubricated and then inserted into a patient's nose to the level of the nasopharynx (back of the throat) to provide an open airway. Also called *nasal airway*.

bag-valve mask (BVM) ▪ an aid for pulmonary resuscitation; made up of a face mask, self-refilling bag, and valves that control the one-way flow of air.

Aids to Resuscitation

NOTE

Some jurisdictions and agencies do not require or allow Emergency Medical Responders to use special equipment called "airway adjuncts" for airway management or resuscitation. This part of the chapter is provided for those who must learn such skills to meet the requirements of their EMS agency or system. These skills must be learned and practiced on manikins under your instructor's supervision. Students who must learn to administer supplemental oxygen should refer to Appendix 2.

The use of basic airway adjuncts can help the Emergency Medical Responder provide more effective airway management. There are a variety of such devices in use in EMS systems across the United States. Some of them are used by both EMTs and Paramedics with more advanced training and are not within the scope of the typical Emergency Medical Responder training course. Three types of equipment are commonly used by Emergency Medical Responders. They are the **oropharyngeal airway (OPA), nasopharyngeal airway (NPA)**, and the **bag-valve mask (BVM).** As you learn to use these devices, it is important to understand that they are only adjuncts or aids that assist you in managing a patient's airway and breathing status.

The OPA and NPA help the Emergency Medical Responder maintain an open airway for the patient, allowing more effective ventilations to be delivered to the patient. With less risk of being exposed to the patient's body fluids, the BVM allows the Emergency Medical Responder to deliver better ventilations for those patients who are not breathing adequately on their own. The OPA and NPA are often used together with the BVM to provide the best possible ventilations.

One disadvantage of all adjunct equipment is that it can delay the beginning of resuscitation if it is not readily available. Your pocket face mask and airway adjuncts should always be handy. Never delay the start of ventilations or CPR while you try to find, retrieve, or set up airway adjunct equipment.

OROPHARYNGEAL AIRWAYS

Oro- refers to the mouth. *Pharyngeo-* refers to the throat. An oropharyngeal airway (OPA) is a device, usually made of plastic, that can be inserted into a patient's mouth. It has a flange that rests against the patient's lips. The lower portion curves back into the throat and rests against the patient's tongue, restricting its movement and minimizing the chance that it will block the airway. Once a patient's airway is opened manually—by using the head-tilt, chin-lift or jaw-thrust maneuver—an OPA may be inserted to help keep it open.

OPAs should only be used in unresponsive patients who do *not* have a gag reflex. These devices can stimulate a patient's normal gag reflex, causing him to vomit. If the unresponsive patient vomits, he can aspirate or breathe the vomit back into his airway and lungs, causing a blockage and possibly a serious infection. If the patient is responsive, even if disoriented or confused, or unresponsive with a gag reflex, do not insert an OPA. Do not continue to insert or leave the airway in the patient's mouth if you meet any resistance or if the patient begins to gag as you insert it.

You may already see that the rules for deciding whether or not to use an OPA can be something of a "catch-22" (a contradictory message). You are not supposed to use an OPA on a patient with a gag reflex, yet you will not know if the patient has one unless you attempt to insert the OPA first. To resolve this dilemma, you must be very focused as you insert the OPA in an unresponsive patient. Expect that he may have a gag reflex, and at the first indication that he does, remove the airway.

If you carry a suction unit and are trained to use it, have it ready for any patient who is unresponsive and may need an airway. You do not want to be caught unprepared when your patient vomits.

Measuring the Oropharyngeal Airway

There are numerous sizes of OPAs designed to fit infants, children, and adults (Figure 6.18). To use this device effectively, you must be able to select the correct size for the patient. Before inserting an airway, hold the device against the patient's face and measure to see if it extends from the center of the mouth to the angle of the lower jaw. The airway may also be sized by holding it at the corner of the patient's mouth and seeing if it will extend to the tip of the earlobe on the same side of the face. If the airway is not the correct size, do not use it on the patient. Instead, select another airway and re-measure to ensure the correct size before inserting.

An airway that is the wrong size has the potential to cause more harm than good. If the airway is too long, it might extend too far into the throat and block the airway. If the device is too short, it will not restrict the movement of the tongue as it should, thus allowing the tongue to block the airway.

Inserting the Oropharyngeal Airway

To insert an OPA, you should (Scan 6–3):

1. Take the appropriate BSI precautions.
2. With the patient on his back, manually open the airway using the head-tilt, chin-lift or jaw-thrust maneuver.
3. Select the appropriate size airway by measuring from the middle of the mouth to the angle of the jaw or from the corner of the mouth to the earlobe.
4. Insert the airway by positioning it so that its tip is pointing toward the roof of the patient's mouth.
5. Insert the airway and slide it along the roof of the mouth, being certain not to push the tongue back into the throat as you insert the airway.
6. Once the airway is about halfway in, rotate it 180 degrees so that the tip is positioned at the base of the tongue. Allow the flange to rest against the outside of the lips.
7. Monitor the airway constantly. Check to see that the flange of the airway is against the patient's lips. If the airway is too long, it will keep slipping out of the mouth and the flange will not rest on the lips. If the airway is too short, the patient's mouth may remain slightly open in an awkward position.
8. Ventilate the patient with the most appropriate technique.
9. Continue to closely monitor the patient's airway. If the patient becomes responsive, he may attempt to remove, displace, or cough up the airway. You must be ready to assist or remove it for him.

An alternative method for inserting an OPA is to insert it sideways into the mouth until it is approximately halfway in. Then simply rotate it 90 degrees. Just as with the first method, make certain that the tip of the airway is positioned at

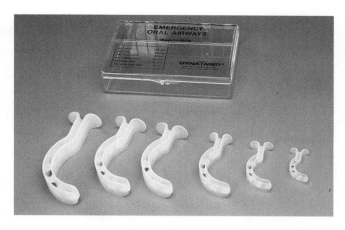

FIGURE 6.18 Various sizes of oropharyngeal airways (OPAs).

2–1.11 Describe how to measure and insert an oropharyngeal (oral) airway.

WARNING

If there is any possibility of spine injury in your patient, open the airway with the jaw-thrust maneuver while you stabilize the patient's head.

REMEMBER

You must still manually maintain the patient's airway when using an OPA.

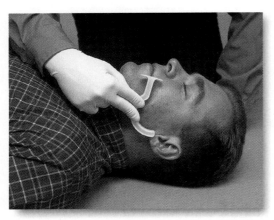

1 ■ Measure from the corner of the patient's mouth to the tip of the earlobe.

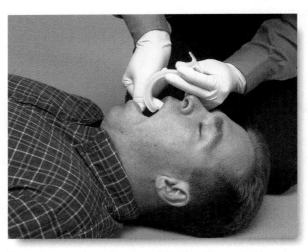

2a ■ Insert the airway with the tip pointing to the roof of the patient's mouth.

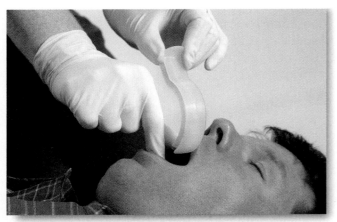

2b ■ An alternative method is to insert the airway sideways and then rotate it 90 degrees.

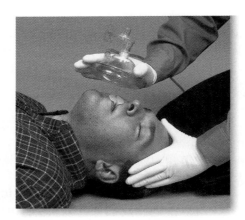

3 ■ After proper insertion, the patient is ready for ventilation.

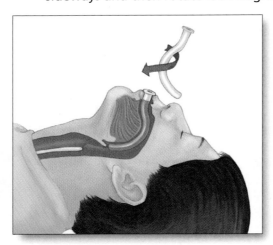

4 ■ Rotate the airway 180 degrees into position. When the airway is properly positioned, the flange rests against the patient's mouth.

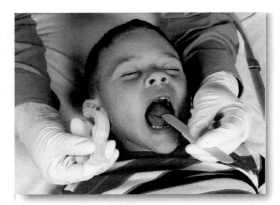

Insertion of an oropharyngeal airway into a child, using a tongue depressor.

WARNING: Never practice the use of airways on anyone. Manikins should be used for developing airway skills.

the base of the tongue. This method is less likely to cause trauma to the roof of the patient's mouth during insertion. As with all other skills, follow both your instructor's preference and local protocols.

Inserting the Oropharyngeal Airway in an Infant or Child

To minimize injury to the roof of the mouth of the infant or child while inserting an OPA, the following method is recommended:

1. Use a tongue blade to gently place downward pressure on the tongue.
2. Insert the OPA with the tip pointing toward the tongue and throat, in the same position it will be in after insertion, rather than upside down.

The OPA is inserted in this way because the infant's or child's mouth is smaller than an adult's and the upper portion of the oral cavity is more easily injured. Rotating the airway can damage the soft palate or the uvula.

> **NOTE**
>
> The OPA is an adjunct. It does not maintain an open airway position by itself. You must still manually maintain the appropriate head position at all times.

NASOPHARYNGEAL AIRWAYS

The nasopharyngeal airway (NPA) is a soft flexible tube that is inserted into the nose in order to create a clear and open path for air. It is the preferred choice when the patient is not totally unresponsive or has a gag reflex. NPAs are the next choice of airway adjunct (after OPAs) because they are less likely to stimulate a gag reflex and, therefore, do not have to be removed if the patient becomes responsive.

An NPA is easy to insert because you do not have to reposition the patient's head or pry open the mouth. If there is any injury to the mouth, teeth, or oral cavity, the NPA will still provide an open airway for the patient. The only precaution is for patients with possible skull or facial fractures. If there is any indication of head or facial injury, do not insert the NPA. If a facial or skull fracture exists, inserting the NPA may cause it to enter the cranial cavity through the unseen fracture. This could cause direct damage to the brain.

Measuring the Nasopharyngeal Airway

There are numerous sizes of NPAs designed to fit infants, children, and adults (Figure 6.19). To use an NPA effectively, you must be able to select the correct size for the patient. Begin by selecting an airway that is approximately the same diameter as the patient's nostril opening. You can also use the patient's little finger as a guide.

2–1.12 Describe how to measure and insert a nasopharyngeal (nasal) airway

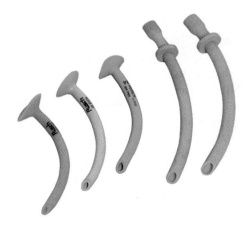

FIGURE 6.19 Various types of nasopharyngeal airways (NPAs).

(The little finger is often the approximate size of the patient's nostril opening.) Next, make sure that the tube length is appropriate by measuring from the tip of the patient's nose to the earlobe. If the airway is not the correct size, do not use it on the patient. Instead, select another airway and re-measure to check correct size before inserting.

Is It Safe ?

Remember that the main contraindication for the use of an NPA is the presence of facial trauma. Inserting an NPA in a patient with a facial fracture could result in the NPA being inserted into the cranial cavity. Carefully consider the mechanism of injury, and assess your patient for signs of facial injury prior to insertion. ▪

Inserting the Nasopharyngeal Airway

Perform the following steps to insert an NPA (Scan 6–4):

1. Take the appropriate BSI precautions.
2. Select the largest diameter NPA that will fit into the patient's nostril without force. Then measure the length from the tip of the patient's nose to the earlobe.
3. Use a water-based lubricant on the outside of the tube before you insert it. Do not use petroleum jelly or any other nonwater-based lubricant.
4. Keep the patient's head in a neutral position while you gently push the tip of the nose upward. Insert the airway straight back through the nostril. If the airway has a beveled (angled) end, that end should point toward the septum (the midline of the nose). Gently advance the airway until the flange rests firmly against the patient's nostril. Never force the airway. If the airway will not advance into the nostril easily, remove it, and try it in the other nostril. If the airway will not advance into the other nostril, make another attempt with an airway that is slightly smaller in diameter.

REMEMBER

If you meet resistance while inserting the NPA, attempt insertion in the opposite nostril.

> **NOTE**
>
> Most NPAs are made with the bevel facing to the left; therefore, they are meant to fit into the right nostril. Before inserting the NPA into the left nostril, use a pair of scissors to carefully snip the end of the airway to change the bevel from the left to the right. Then lubricate and insert. It is not recommended to insert an NPA against its natural curvature because it is likely to rotate on its own after being inserted.

▰ ◢ ▰ Geriatric Focus

The elderly patient is prone to nosebleeds for two reasons. First, they have thin, easily damaged mucosa. Second, many of them are on "blood thinners," such as Coumadin. Take this into consideration when placing an NPA. Ensure the airway is adequately lubricated and avoid forcing it past any obstruction. Frequently, a rotational maneuver is very successful when inserting an NPA in the elderly.

BAG-VALVE MASK VENTILATION

> **NOTE**
>
> Most EMS systems recommend that an OPA or NPA should be inserted before attempting to ventilate the patient with a BVM.

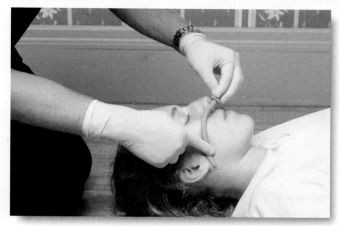

1 ▪ Measure the NPA from the patient's nostril to the earlobe, or to the angle of the jaw.

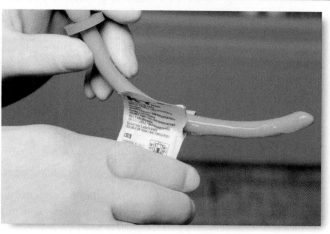

2 ▪ Apply a water-based lubricant before insertion.

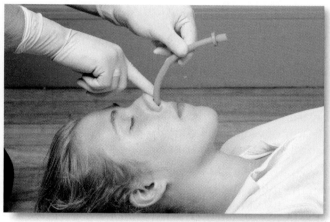

3 ▪ Gently insert the airway, advancing it until the flange rests against the nostril.

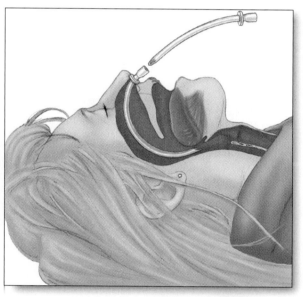

4 ▪ Nasopharyngeal airway, properly inserted.

The BVM is one of the most commonly used devices for ventilating a nonbreathing patient. Some EMS systems also use the BVM to ventilate patients with inadequate respirations (for example, in drug overdose). The BVM is available in sizes for infants, children, and adults. It also acts as an effective infection-control barrier between you and your patient.

The BVM delivers room air (21% oxygen) to the patient when it is squeezed through the unit to the patient's lungs. (In contrast, a pocket face mask will deliver between 10% and 16% oxygen from your exhaled air.) The BVM can be connected to an oxygen supply source to enrich room air and deliver a concentration of up to 100% oxygen.

There are many brands of BVMs available, but all have the same basic parts: a self-refilling bag, valves that control the one-way flow of air, and a face mask. There is a standard 15/22 mm respiratory fitting, so a variety of respiratory equipment and face masks can be used with it. The BVM must be made of material that can be easily cleaned and sterilized. Many EMS systems now use disposable units (Figure 6.20).

The principle behind the operation of the BVM is simple. When you squeeze the bag, air is delivered to the patient through a one-way valve. When you release the bag, fresh air enters the bag from the rear while the exhaled air from the patient flows out near the mask. The exhaled air does not go back into the bag.

There are times when the BVM will not deliver air to the patient's lungs. Sometimes the problem occurs because the patient has an airway obstruction that must be cleared. More often, the problem is caused by an improper seal between the patient's face and mask. If this occurs, you should reposition your fingers and check placement of the mask.

Geriatric Focus

Because the elderly often have recessed chins due to loss of teeth, two hands are frequently required to maintain the mask-to-face seal. Therefore, two rescuers are required to perform BVM ventilation.

Two-Rescuer BVM Ventilation

For the best possible results, the BVM should be used with two rescuers. One rescuer can use two hands to maintain a good mask seal, while the second rescuer squeezes the bag. Note also that for trauma patients who must have their airway opened by the jaw-thrust maneuver, the two-rescuer method is more effective. The rescuer holding the mask in place can more easily perform the jaw-thrust while the other rescuer provides effective ventilations.

> **NOTE**
>
> In some instances as a single rescuer, it may be more effective to provide assisted ventilations using the mouth-to-mask technique than attempting to use a BVM by yourself.

Perform the following steps to provide ventilations using the two-rescuer BVM technique (Scan 6–5):

1. Take the appropriate BSI precautions.
2. Ensure an open airway and position yourself at the patient's head. Clear the airway if necessary.
3. Insert an appropriate airway adjunct.
4. Rescuer 1 should kneel at the top of the patient's head, holding the mask firmly in place with both hands.
5. Rescuer 2 should kneel beside the patient's head and connect the bag to the mask (if not already done). He should then squeeze the bag once every five seconds for an adult (once every three seconds for a child or an infant). Ensure adequate rise and fall of the chest each time the bag is squeezed.

The BVM also can be used effectively during two-rescuer CPR by a skilled operator. The ventilator squeezes the bag and provides two back-to-back ventilations following each cycle of compressions.

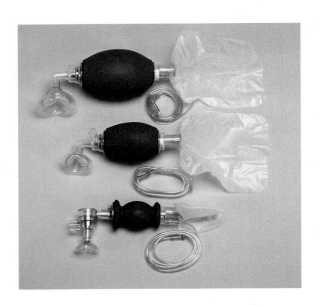

FIGURE 6.20 Disposable bag-valve mask (BVM) ventilators.

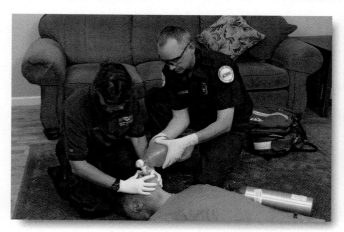

1 ■ Proper technique for using the BVM with two rescuers.

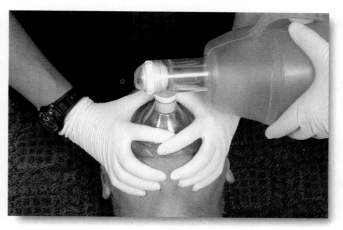

2 ■ Proper hand position for BVM ventilation with two rescuers.

One-Rescuer BVM Ventilation

For a single rescuer alone, the BVM can be difficult to operate. This is especially true if you have small hands or do not use a BVM on a regular basis. The most difficult part is maintaining an adequate mask-to-face seal with one hand. If you are assigned a BVM for use in the field, practice using it in the classroom until your technique is well developed.

> **NOTE**
>
> Some EMS systems have decided that one-rescuer BVM ventilation skills are poorly maintained, and thus have selected the pocket face mask as the preferred ventilation-assist device for Emergency Medical Responders.

Perform the following steps to ventilate a patient using the BVM as a single rescuer (Scan 6–6):

1. Take the appropriate BSI precautions.
2. Ensure an open airway and position yourself at the patient's head. Clear the airway if necessary.
3. Insert an appropriate airway adjunct.
4. Use the correct mask size for the patient. Place the apex, or top, of the triangular mask over the bridge of the nose. Rest the base of the mask between the patient's lower lip and the projection of the chin.
5. With one hand, hold the mask firmly in position.
6. With your other hand, squeeze the bag at the appropriate rate, delivering each breath over approximately one second. Observe for adequate rise and fall of the patient's chest.

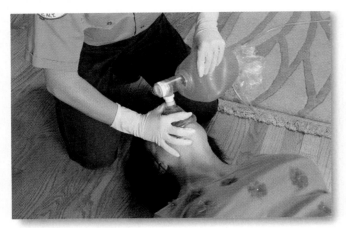

1 ■ Proper technique for using the BVM with one rescuer.

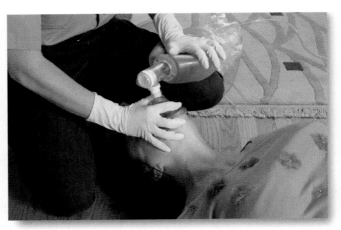

2 ■ An alternative is to press the bag against your leg.

Suction Systems

2–1.6 State the importance of having a suction unit ready for immediate use when providing emergency medical care.

To clear blood, mucus, and other body fluids from a patient's airway, an Emergency Medical Responder usually will position the patient on his side (recovery position) or use finger sweeps appropriately. However, a suction device can assist in keeping a patient's airway clear. There are several types of portable suction units available, including manually powered, oxygen- or air-powered, and electrically powered units (Scan 6–7).

All types of suction units must have thick-walled, nonkinking, wide-bore tubing; a nonbreakable collection container (bottle); and sterile, disposable, semirigid but flexible or rigid suction tips. The longer, flexible suction tips are usually called *catheters*. Rigid suction tips are sometimes referred to as *tonsil suction tips*. In all units, vacuum flow must be adequate for mouth, throat (pharyngeal), and stoma suctioning.

REMEMBER

A manually powered suction unit may have a rubber bulb or a hand- or foot-operated device to produce the vacuum. Follow manufacturer guidelines for operating the device.

GENERAL GUIDELINES FOR SUCTIONING

- Always use appropriate BSI precautions, including a mouth and eye shield because the potential for being sprayed with body fluids such as vomit, blood, and saliva are high.
- Keep your suctioning time to a minimum. Remember that while you are suctioning, you are not ventilating. Also, suction removes valuable oxygen along with dangerous fluids. One suggested guideline is to suction for no more than 15 seconds for adults, 10 seconds for children, and 5 seconds for infants.
- If there is lots of fluid in the patient's airway, it may be helpful to roll him onto his side and then suction. You may need to suction, ventilate, and then suction again in a continuous sequence as long as necessary.
- Measure the suction catheter before inserting it into the patient's mouth as you would for an OPA. Prior to inserting into the nose, measure the catheter as you would for an NPA.
- Activate the suction unit only after it is completely inserted and as you withdraw the catheter.

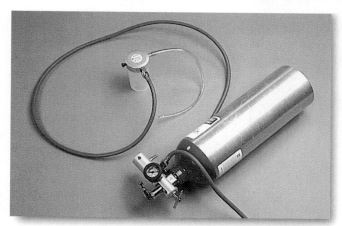

1 ■ An oxygen-powered portable suction unit.

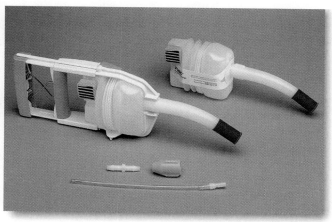

2 ■ Manually operated suction device (V-VAC).

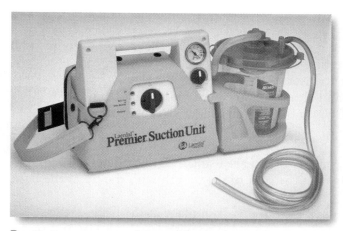

3 ■ Battery-powered portable suction unit.

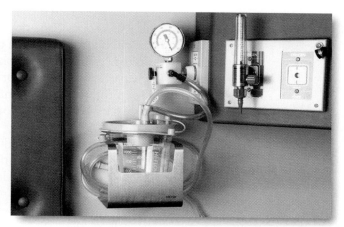

4 ■ Mounted suction unit installed in an ambulance patient compartment.

- Twist and turn the tip of the catheter as you are removing it from the mouth, nose, or stoma.
- When suctioning the mouth, concentrate on the back corners of the mouth, where most fluids tend to accumulate. *Do not* place the tip directly over the back of the tongue, because this will likely stimulate the gag reflex.

SUCTIONING TECHNIQUES

There are many variations to the techniques used to suction the mouth, nose, or stoma. One example is given as follows and in Figure 6.21. However, you *must* follow your own local protocols.

2-1.7 Describe the techniques of suctioning.

1. Before suctioning any patient, be sure to take the appropriate BSI precautions.
2. Attach the catheter and activate the unit to ensure that there is suction.

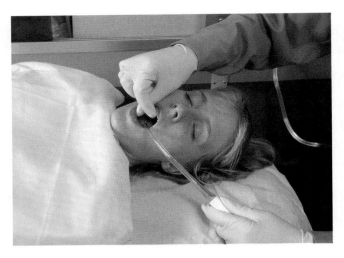

FIGURE 6.21A Apply suction only after the catheter has been inserted into the mouth. Do not lose sight of the tip while suctioning.

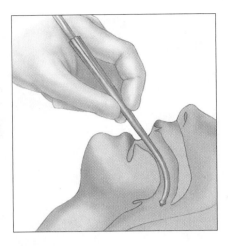

FIGURE 6.21B Keep the convex side of the catheter against the roof of the mouth. Insert no farther than you can see.

3. Position yourself at the patient's head. If possible, turn the patient onto his side. Follow guidelines for protection of the spine.

4. Measure the catheter prior to insertion.

5. Open the patient's mouth and clear obvious matter and fluid from the oral cavity by letting the mouth drain or by using finger sweeps with a gloved hand.

6. Insert the tip of the catheter to the appropriate depth. Usually, the tip is inserted to the base of the tongue. If you are using a rigid catheter, place the convex (curved-out) side against the roof of the mouth with the tip at the base of the tongue.

7. Apply suction *only* when the tip or catheter is in place at the back of the mouth or base of the tongue and as you begin to withdraw it. Twist and turn it from side to side and sweep the mouth. This twisting action prevents the end of the catheter from grabbing the soft tissue inside the mouth.

8. Remain alert for signs of a gag reflex and vomiting.

FIRST ON SCENE WRAP-UP

A few minutes later, just as Jenna was beginning to blink her eyes and look around, a team of firefighter Emergency Medical Responders appeared in the backyard, followed closely by an ambulance crew. The ambulance crew performed an initial assessment and began oxygen therapy, while the firefighters helped secure the girl to a long spine board, move her to the wheeled stretcher, and get her into the ambulance.

"She has good sensation and motor function in her extremities," one of the EMTs said to Tami. "I think she probably just got a good bump on the head. It could have been a lot worse."

"Tell me about it," Tami said and waved reassuringly at Jim and Ruthie as they got into their car to follow the ambulance.

Summary

We breathe to bring in oxygen, remove carbon dioxide, and help regulate the pH level of our blood—a process called respiration. The major muscle of breathing, the diaphragm, and the muscles between our ribs contract to increase the volume of the chest cavity. This increase in volume causes a vacuum inside the chest cavity and fills the lungs with air. When we exhale, changes in chest size and pressure cause air in the lungs to flow out. This is an involuntary, automatic process, which is mainly controlled by the respiratory centers of the brain.

Clinical death occurs when an individual stops breathing and the heart stops beating. Biological death begins approximately four to six minutes later when a significant number of brain cells have died. Without oxygen, brain death can occur within 10 minutes.

In addition to the respiratory centers in the brain, the diaphragm muscle, and the muscles between the ribs, the respiratory system includes the nose and mouth, pharynx (throat), larynx (voice box), epiglottis, trachea (windpipe), bronchial tree, and the alveoli deep within the lungs.

To assess normal breathing, look for adequate rise and fall of the chest, listen and feel for air movement, and observe skin color for a pale or bluish tint. Suspect problems when you notice changes in breathing effort, breathing rate, and depth, or changes in skin color.

Opening the airway is the first important step in patient care. Simply repositioning the patient's head may solve many breathing problems. The head-tilt, chin-lift maneuver is used to open the airway of patients with no neck or spine injuries. The jaw-thrust maneuver is used when there are possible neck or spine injuries. Only a slight head-tilt with chin-lift, or sniffing position, is used for children. The infant's head is kept in the neutral position to maintain the airway.

Mouth-to-mask ventilation is the recommended procedure for performing assisted ventilations for a single rescuer. It is preferred that you use a pocket face mask with one-way valve and HEPA filter. Mouth-to-barrier ventilation is another way to assist ventilation that helps to provide protection from infectious disease. Mask-to-stoma ventilation is used for patients who have a stoma. Methods that do not use a mask or some other barrier increase the risk of infectious disease transmission.

The bag-valve mask (BVM) is an excellent choice for ventilating any patient with inadequate breathing. It can be used by one or two rescuers but is best used when two rescuers are available. It can also be used with or without supplemental oxygen.

Watch for gastric distention when you perform assisted ventilations. Reposition the head and adjust your ventilations to minimize gastric distention. Be on guard for vomiting.

When you begin artificial ventilation, start with two adequate breaths. Assist ventilations for the nonbreathing adult at a rate of one breath every five to six seconds. This rate can also be expressed as 10 to 12 breaths per minute. For infants and children, the rate is one breath every three to five seconds or 12 to 20 breaths per minute.

A variety of problems can cause partial or complete airway obstruction. These include the tongue, foreign objects, tissue damage, tissue swelling, and disease. In addition to the signs of inadequate breathing, signs of partial airway obstruction include snoring, gurgling, crowing, wheezing, and stridor sounds. For complete airway obstruction, there will be no chest movements, no sounds of respiration, and no air exchange felt at the nose and mouth.

Encourage patients with a partial obstruction to cough forcefully. If they cannot cough forcefully, or if there is poor air exchange, provide care as if there is a complete airway obstruction. To clear a complete airway obstruction in a responsive adult or child, deliver abdominal thrusts just above the navel in rapid succession. For patients who are obese or pregnant, attempt chest thrusts instead of abdominal thrusts. For infants (younger than one year of age), deliver a combination of back blows and chest thrusts until the object is removed.

Airway adjuncts, such as the oropharyngeal airway (OPA) and the nasopharyngeal airway (NPA), help manage the patient's airway while ventilations are provided. Measure the OPA by one of two methods: from the center of the mouth to the angle of the jaw, or from the corner of the mouth to the earlobe. Begin inserting the OPA upside down in adults and turn it to the correct position to seat it properly in the oral cavity. For infants and children, insert the OPA in the right-side-up position. Turning the airway in pediatric patients may damage the oral cavity. The NPA should be slightly smaller in diameter than the patient's nostril and at least as long as the distance between the tip of the nose and the earlobe. Lubricate the NPA with a water-soluble gel before inserting it. Reassess the patient's airway after inserting any airway adjunct.

Remember and Consider

Making sure that a patient has an open airway and knowing how to maintain and manage it is the most important care you can provide. All other patient care activities are secondary. The steps for opening an airway are simple and easy to perform. However, the skills required to maintain and manage an airway take practice. Practicing airway maintenance and management skills helps you develop an ability and proficiency that will help you act quickly in a stress-filled emergency.

➤ Consider practicing the two ways to open an airway on someone with whom you are training.

➤ Consider the rationale for when to use a head-tilt, chin-lift rather than a jaw-thrust maneuver.

You will practice measuring and inserting NPAs and OPAs on manikins in class. You will also practice using pocket face masks and possibly BVMs, too. Go back to your station and check the response units and airway kits for airways and masks.

➤ What kinds and sizes of airways do you have? Where are they located? Are they easy to get to?

➤ What kinds of pocket face masks do you have? Which one is easiest for you to use? Have you tried using one on a person or just a manikin?

➤ Ask a member of your family, a friend, or other EMS company member if you can position a pocket face mask on his or her face so you can get used to the placement and grip. Ask the person to breathe in and exhale normally. Check the mask-face seal. Does air leak out around the cheeks, or does it exit through the one-way valve only? If you feel you have to press hard to get a seal, then you may not have the mask in the correct

position. Reposition it until you get a good seal. Be sure to thoroughly wash and dry the mask after practice.

Remember the signs of an obstructed airway and how to manage the patient in all three situations: responsive, becomes unresponsive, is unresponsive when you arrive.

➤ What do you do if you cannot get air into the unresponsive patient with your first or second breath? What if you are doing abdominal thrusts on a responsive patient and he becomes unresponsive?

➤ Have you ever had to perform abdominal thrusts on a real person? Ask other EMS personnel to share their experiences with you.

➤ Ask people you know who are different sizes (tall and short) and various girths (slender and stout) if you can practice locating the correct hand positions on them. Where do you place yourself or the patient when he is much taller or shorter than you or when his girth is larger than your arms can reach? Is it more difficult to find the correct position on the abdomen when someone is obese?

NOTE

Do not practice manual thrusts on a real person, only on manikins. Even though obstructed airway procedures do not require extremely forceful thrusts, they can cause discomfort or injury. Therefore, although you can practice positioning on people of different sizes, perform the complete maneuver only on manikins.

Investigate

➤ How does your company's suctioning unit work? Is the suction unit a portable battery-operated one or a hand-operated unit, or do you have both kinds? Do you know how to assemble and disassemble them? Where are the replacement parts and tubing kept? Where do you dispose of the contents? Do you have labels for the collection containers in case the hospital wants the contents? What would you put on a label?

➤ Will you be able to manage a patient with a stoma? Do you know anyone with a stoma? Where can you get information on stoma patients? Check the Internet for Web pages and local directories for phone numbers of the American Heart Association, the American Lung Association, or your local health department. These resources will give you additional information. Local agencies will probably have speakers willing to give a presentation or show a film

at your department on how to manage patients with stomas.

➤ How often do you practice your ventilation skills? Do you know that motor skills will rapidly deteriorate if you do not use them regularly? Practice makes you more confident, and in order to be able to assist ventilations quickly and accurately, you must practice them frequently. There are many steps to perform when you assist ventilations, but once you are familiar with them and develop an automatic response, they flow in a logical sequence. Check with your agency or company and find out how often it holds drills. Do you have manikins at your station? Find out if you can get them out and practice on them when you are on duty. Even without the actual manikins, you can review the pictures in the text and mentally picture yourself performing each step. Go through the motions even without the manikin.

Quick Quiz

1. Pulmonary resuscitation is:
   a. any effort to restart normal heart rhythms.
   b. any effort to revive or restore normal breathing.
   c. the use of mechanical devices to restart breathing.
   d. the ability to restore normal heart rhythm and breathing.

2. When performing the head-tilt, chin-lift maneuver on an adult, tilt the head:
   a. as far back as possible.
   b. into the sniffing position.
   c. to get the tongue to close the epiglottis.
   d. so that upper and lower teeth are touching.

3. The recommended method for opening the airway of a patient with a possible neck or spine injury is the _____ maneuver.
   a. jaw-thrust
   b. mouth-to-nose
   c. abdominal thrust
   d. head-tilt, chin-lift

4. Clinical death occurs when the patient's:
   a. brain cells begin to die.
   b. breathing has stopped for four minutes.
   c. pulse has been absent for five minutes.
   d. cardiac and respiration function have stopped.

5. A pocket face mask allows the rescuer to provide ventilations WITHOUT:
   a. having to hold the mask firmly in place.
   b. delivering his own breaths to the patient.
   c. direct contact with the patient's mouth and nose.
   d. worrying about keeping the head and spine in line.

6. During pulmonary resuscitation, you should check for adequate breathing by:
   a. looking for chest rise and fall.
   b. listening for airflow from the mouth and nose.
   c. observing skin color, such as paleness or cyanosis.
   d. looking for chest rise and fall, listening for airflow, and observing skin color.

7. If an infant becomes unresponsive before you can clear an airway obstruction, you should first:
   a. place the infant face down and lift her chest with your hands.
   b. place her on a firm surface and begin chest compressions.
   c. hold her face up and deliver chest thrusts.
   d. turn her face down and deliver back slaps.

8. For suctioning a patient, the appropriate body substance isolation precautions include:
   a. pocket face mask.
   b. oropharyngeal airway.
   c. eye and face protection.
   d. folded towel under his shoulders.

9. Which one of the following improves ventilations delivered by way of a bag-valve mask?
   a. inserting an oropharyngeal airway
   b. applying suction for four to six minutes
   c. alternating chest thrusts and squeezing the bag
   d. combining finger sweeps with a mouth-to-mouth technique

10. Which one of the following is recommended for clearing an airway obstruction in an unresponsive 10-month old baby?
    a. abdominal thrusts
    b. chest thrusts
    c. back slaps and finger sweeps
    d. abdominal thrusts and finger sweeps

11. The primary muscle of respiration is the:
    a. trachea.
    b. esophagus.
    c. diaphragm.
    d. pharynx.

12. The _____ prevents food and other material from entering the trachea.
    a. tongue
    b. alveoli
    c. pharynx
    d. epiglottis

13. Deep within the lungs, the _____ are the tiny balloon-like structures where gas exchanges take place.
    a. alveoli
    b. bronchioles
    c. trachea
    d. epiglottis

14. All of the following are signs of inadequate breathing EXCEPT:
    a. poor chest rise.
    b. pale or bluish skin color.
    c. use of accessory muscles.
    d. good chest rise and fall.

15. When caring for an unresponsive medical patient, tilting the head back improves the airway by:
    a. lifting the tongue from the back of the throat.
    b. shifting the epiglottis from front to back.
    c. allowing fluids to flow more easily.
    d. opening the mouth.

16. An airway stoma is found on the:
    a. chest.
    b. arm.
    c. neck.
    d. cheek.

17. Noisy breathing is a sign of _____ airway obstruction.
    a. bilateral
    b. complete
    c. adequate
    d. partial

18. You have just made two attempts to ventilate an unresponsive child with an airway obstruction. Your next step is to:
    a. begin chest compressions.
    b. continue to ventilate.
    c. perform five chest thrusts.
    d. provide back slaps.

MODULE **3**

Patient Assessment

7 Assessment of the Patient

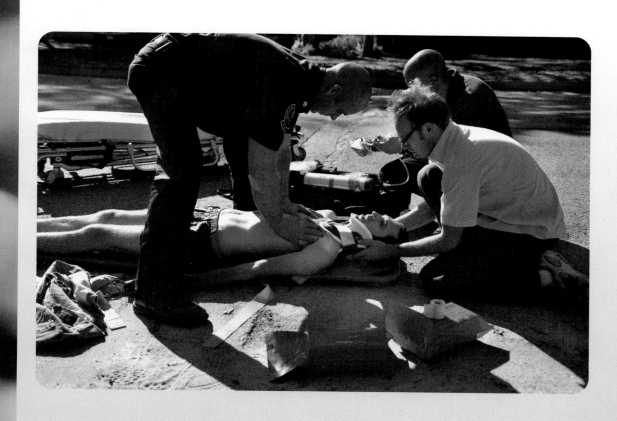

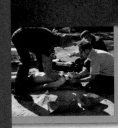

Assessment of the Patient

An Emergency Medical Responder may be active in a small part of the initial care of one patient or have responsibilities that involve all aspects of emergency care for another. Whatever your role, it is always true that your patient assessment skills are the foundation for the care you provide.

Patients cannot receive the care they need until their problems are identified. You must assess each patient in order to detect possible illness or injury and determine the direction of the emergency care needed. This assessment must be done in a specific and orderly fashion to minimize the chance of overlooking an important sign or symptom.

Remember that a good patient assessment almost always leads to appropriate patient care. A poor assessment almost always results in poor patient care. This chapter assists you in learning how to perform a thorough and methodical patient assessment.

OBJECTIVES

This chapter is based on the objectives of the U.S. DOT's First Responder National Standard Curriculum. Note that cognitive objectives are listed below and beside corresponding text throughout the chapter. You will also notice as you read each objective that the term Emergency Medical Responder is used. This is simply a name change and reflects the new name for the First Responder.

By the end of this chapter, you should be able to (from cognitive or knowledge information):

3-1.1 Discuss the components of scene size-up. (pp. 163–167)

3-1.2 Describe common hazards found at the scene of a trauma and a medical patient. (p. 165)

3-1.3 Determine if the scene is safe to enter. (p. 165)

3-1.4 Discuss common mechanisms of injury/nature of illness. (pp. 166, 178)

3-1.5 Discuss the reason for identifying the total number of patients at the scene. (pp. 166–167)

3-1.6 Explain the reason for identifying the need for additional help or assistance. (pp. 166–167)

3–1.7 Summarize the reasons for forming a general impression of the patient. (pp. 168–170)

3–1.8 Discuss methods of assessing mental status. (pp. 170, 172)

3–1.9 Differentiate between assessing mental status in the adult, child, and infant patient. (pp. 175–176)

3–1.10 Describe methods used for assessing if a patient is breathing. (pp. 172, 174)

3–1.11 Differentiate between a patient with adequate and inadequate breathing. (pp. 172, 174, 187–188; see also Chapter 6)

3–1.12 Describe the methods used to assess circulation. (pp. 174, 185–186)

3–1.13 Differentiate between obtaining a pulse in the adult, child, and infant patient. (p. 174)

3–1.14 Discuss the need for assessing the patient for external bleeding. (pp. 174–175)

3–1.15 Explain the reason for prioritizing a patient for care and transport. (p. 175)

3–1.16 Discuss the components of the physical exam. (pp. 176–178)

3–1.17 State the areas of the body that are evaluated during the physical exam. (pp. 192–196)

3–1.18 Explain what additional questions may be asked during the physical exam. (pp. 183–184)

3–1.19 Explain the components of the SAMPLE history. (p. 183)

3–1.20 Discuss the components of the ongoing assessment. (pp. 198–199)

3–1.21 Describe the information included in the hand-off report. (p. 199)

By the end of this chapter, you should be able to feel comfortable enough to (by changing attitudes, values, and beliefs):

3–1.22 Explain the rationale for crew members to evaluate scene safety prior to entering. (pp. 163–167)

3–1.23 Serve as a model for others by explaining how patient situations affect your evaluation of the mechanism of injury or nature of illness. (pp. 166, 178)

3–1.24 Explain the importance of forming a general impression of the patient. (pp. 168–170)

3–1.25 Explain the value of an initial assessment. (pp. 168–176)

3–1.26 Explain the value of questioning the patient and family. (pp. 181–184)

3–1.27 Explain the value of the physical exam. (pp. 176–179, 190–198)

3–1.28 Explain the value of an ongoing assessment. (pp. 198–199)

3–1.29 Explain the rationale for the feelings that these patients might be experiencing. (pp. 177, 181–184)

3–1.30 Demonstrate a caring attitude when performing patient assessments. (pp. 181–184)

3–1.31 Place the interests of the patient as the foremost consideration when making any and all patient-care decisions during patient assessment. (pp. 181–184)

3–1.32 Communicate with empathy during patient assessment to patients as well as with family members and friends of the patient. (pp. 181–184)

By the end of this chapter, you should be able to show how to (through psychomotor skills):

3–1.33 Demonstrate the ability to differentiate various scenarios and identify potential hazards. (pp. 163–167)

3–1.34 Demonstrate the techniques for assessing mental status. (pp. 170, 172, 175–176)

3–1.35 Demonstrate the techniques for assessing the airway. (pp. 172, 174)

3–1.36 Demonstrate the techniques for assessing if the patient is breathing. (pp. 172, 174, 187–188; see also Chapter 6)

3–1.37 Demonstrate the techniques for assessing if the patient has a pulse. (pp. 174, 175, 185–186)

3–1.38 Demonstrate the techniques for assessing the patient for external bleeding. (pp. 174–175)

3–1.39 Demonstrate the techniques for assessing the patient's skin color, temperature, condition, and capillary refill (infants and children only). (pp. 175, 188–189)

3–1.40 Demonstrate questioning a patient to obtain a SAMPLE history. (p. 183)

3–1.41 Demonstrate the skills involved in performing the physical exam. (pp. 176–178)

3–1.42 Demonstrate the ongoing assessment. (pp. 198–199)

In addition to the objectives listed in the previous section, you should be able to:

- State the three things you must say to a responsive patient on your arrival at the scene.
- Describe the personal protective equipment (PPE) you should wear during the assessment of a patient.
- Describe how to ensure an open airway.
- Differentiate between a sign and a symptom.
- Define and describe how to obtain accurate vital signs, and describe the characteristics you should be assessing for each vital sign.
- Define the term *baseline vital signs* and explain why they are important when obtaining additional sets of vital signs.
- Distinguish between a stable and an unstable patient.
- List examples of significant mechanisms of injury.
- List, in correct order, the steps of the focused history and physical exam for a trauma patient with no significant mechanism of injury (MOI).
- List, in correct order, the steps of the rapid trauma assessment for a trauma patient with a significant MOI.
- List, in correct order, the steps of the focused history and physical exam for a responsive medical patient.
- List, in correct order, the steps of the rapid physical exam for an unresponsive medical patient.
- List 10 Emergency Medical Responder rules that apply to patient assessment.
- Describe the detailed physical exam and the ongoing assessment.

NOTE

Patient assessment procedures can bring you into contact with a patient's blood and body fluids. Always take appropriate BSI precautions whenever you care for a patient. Disposable gloves should always be worn during assessment and emergency care. Eye protection may also be required, depending on the type of emergency and patient condition. Wear any other items of personal protection required for your safety and that of your patients. Follow OSHA, CDC, and local guidelines to help prevent the spread of infectious diseases. Review the personal safety and protection information in Chapter 3.

FIRST ON SCENE

"Attention all employees." The voice from the overhead paging system in the Booker Manufacturing warehouse halted the bustle of the shipping staff. They all turned to look up at the loudspeaker. "Will all third-shift MERT members please respond to the number seven loading dock for a medical emergency."

Two of the warehouse employees removed their leather gloves and face shields and quickly walked to a white locker with "MERT" stenciled on its side in wide red letters. They opened the cabinet, removed two nylon bags, and hurried toward the loading docks at the south end of the building.

"I'll be the patient-care person if you'll do scene control," Jared Sutter, the taller of the two, said.

"Okay," Ray Johnson replied, fishing a pair of gloves from his bag and putting them on. Ray was actually relieved to be with an experienced MERT member. He was new to the team, and the patient assessment process was still a little confusing to him.

As the two passed the dock manager's small office and turned left, they were met by a forklift operator whose name, according to his embroidered shirt, was Tariq. "I'm glad you're here," he spoke quickly. "It's one of the truck drivers. I think he's having a heart attack."

Overview of Patient Assessment

Many EMS systems use an assessment-based approach to providing care to patients. This is to say that Emergency Medical Responders and other EMS personnel are trained to identify, prioritize, and care for major **signs** and **symptoms**. What they will not do is try to diagnose a patient's specific problems. For example, an Emergency Medical Responder will do what he can to make sure a patient with difficulty breathing has an open airway and supplemental oxygen. What he will *not* do is waste critical time attempting to figure out the underlying cause of the patient's difficulty. Once all life threats have been cared for, the Emergency Medical Responder will complete a more thorough assessment of the patient, try to identify any less obvious signs and symptoms, and gather a pertinent medical history.

SCENE SAFETY

The components of **patient assessment** and the order in which they are performed may vary from patient to patient based on each patient's problem. But before you study those components, you must address issues relating to the safety of the scene.

The conditions at a safe scene allow for rescuers to safely access and provide care to patients. An unsafe scene is one that contains hazards that are either immediate or potential. An example may be a motor-vehicle crash site. It is not unusual to find vehicles or objects that can move or shift position (an overturned car and broken glass are examples of immediate hazards). In addition, fire could break out or fuel and other fluids could leak and increase the danger, causing the scene to become even more unsafe. These are examples of potential hazards.

ASSESSMENT COMPONENTS

For most patients, an Emergency Medical Responder's assessment should begin as follows:

1. Perform a **scene size-up** so that you can ensure your own safety and the safety of your patient.
2. Perform an **initial assessment** to identify and care for any immediate life threats.

The initial assessment is a set of procedures meant to detect and correct life-threatening problems. The remaining components of patient assessment change slightly with each of the four types of patient: **medical patients**—responsive and unresponsive, and **trauma patients**—those who have a significant **mechanism of injury (MOI)** and those who do not.

At times, the type of patient you are caring for is not so clearly defined. For example, a patient experiencing a medical problem may fall and injure himself, or a medical problem may have actually caused a car crash. Your patient assessment will need to include elements for both medical and trauma emergencies. What should guide your assessment should be the more serious of the patient's problems.

Medical Patients

For a responsive medical patient, you will (Scan 7–1):

- Perform a scene size-up and an initial assessment.
- Perform a **focused history and physical exam** based on the patient's chief complaint.

---

signs ■ objective indications of illness or injury that can be seen, heard, felt, and smelled by another person.

symptoms ■ subjective indications of illness or injury that cannot be observed by another person but are felt and reported by the patient.

WARNING

A patient who appears to be stable can become unstable without warning.

patient assessment ■ the gathering of information to determine a possible illness or injury. It includes interviews and physical examinations.

scene size-up ■ an overview of the scene to identify any obvious or potential hazards; consists of taking BSI precautions, determining the safety of the scene, identifying the mechanism of injury or nature of illness, determining the number of patients, and identifying additional resources.

medical patient ■ one who has or describes symptoms of an illness; a patient with no injuries.

trauma patient ■ one who has a physical injury caused by an external force.

mechanism of injury (MOI) ■ the force or forces that may have caused injury.

focused history and physical exam ■ part of patient assessment that includes the patient history, a physical examination, and vital signs.

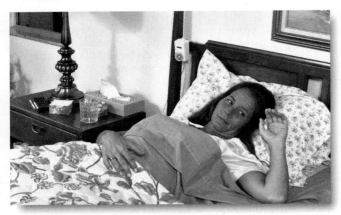

1 ■ Size up the scene. Enter only if it is safe to do so.

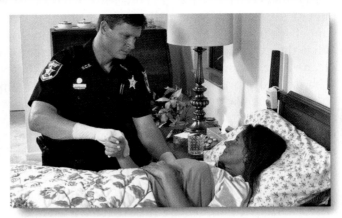

2 ■ Perform an initial assessment. Care for immediate life threats first.

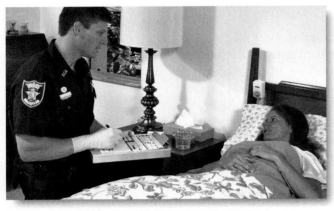

3 ■ Perform a focused history and physical exam based on the patient's chief complaint. Obtain baseline vital signs.

4 ■ Perform ongoing assessments as often as necessary, depending on the patient's condition.

baseline vital signs ■ the first determination of vital signs; used to compare with all further readings of vital signs in order to identify trends.

detailed physical exam ■ a complete head-to-toe exam.

ongoing assessment ■ the last step in patient assessment, which is used to detect changes in a patient's condition; includes repeating initial assessment, reassessing and recording vital signs, and checking interventions.

nature of illness (NOI) ■ what is medically wrong with the patient; a complaint not related to an injury.

vital signs ■ objective signs that include assessment of the patient's pulse, respirations, skin, blood pressure, and pupils.

- Obtain **baseline vital signs**.
- Perform a complete **detailed physical exam** as needed.
- Perform an **ongoing assessment**, including a reassessment of the patient's vital signs in order to identify any changes in the patient's condition.

For an unresponsive medical patient, you will (Scan 7–2):

- Perform a scene size-up and an initial assessment. Care for immediate life threats first.
- Perform a rapid physical exam to look for signs of illness.
- Obtain baseline vital signs.
- Attempt to interview the patient's family or bystanders to determine the patient's chief complaint and **nature of illness (NOI)**.
- Perform a complete detailed physical exam as needed.
- Perform ongoing assessments, including a reassessment of **vital signs** in order to identify any changes in the patient's condition.

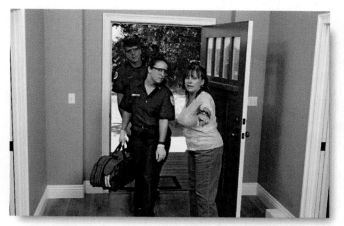

1 ■ Size up the scene. Enter only if it is safe. If it is not, contact dispatch for additional resources.

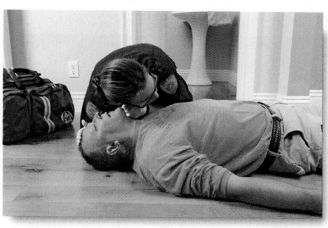

2 ■ Perform an initial assessment. Care for immediate life threats first.

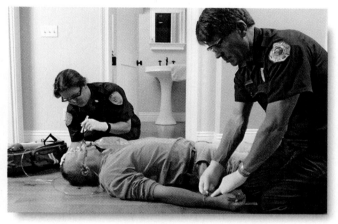

3 ■ Perform a rapid physical exam to look for signs of illness. Obtain baseline vital signs.

4 ■ Perform ongoing assessments as often as necessary, depending on the patient's condition.

Trauma Patients

For a trauma patient with no significant mechanism of injury (MOI), you will (Scan 7–3):

- Perform a scene size-up and an initial assessment. Include a scan of the scene to determine the mechanism of injury (MOI).
- Conduct a physical exam based on the patient's chief complaint.
- Obtain baseline vital signs.
- Perform a complete detailed physical exam as needed.
- Perform ongoing assessments, including a reassessment of vital signs in order to identify any changes in the patient's condition.

For a trauma patient with a significant MOI, you will (Scan 7–4):

- Perform a scene size-up. Include a scan of the scene and make note of the MOI.
- Perform an initial assessment. Manually stabilize the patient's head and neck. Care for any life threats as you detect them.

No Significant Mechanism of Injury

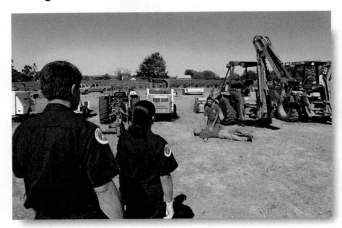

1 ■ Perform a scene size-up first.

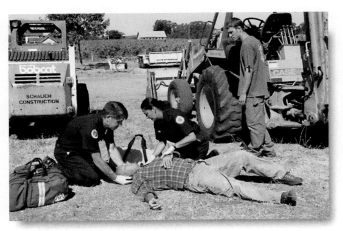

2 ■ Perform an initial assessment.

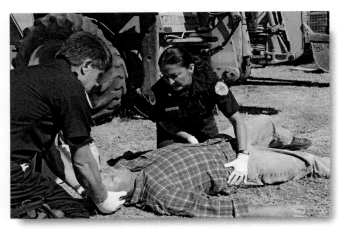

3 ■ Examine the patient based on his complaints. Obtain a medical history, take baseline vital signs, and perform a detailed physical exam as needed.

4 ■ Perform ongoing assessments as often as necessary, depending on the patient's condition.

rapid trauma assessment ■ a quick, safe head-to-toe exam of the trauma patient.

■ Perform a **rapid trauma assessment** to look for obvious serious injuries. Simultaneously, begin to question family and bystanders about the incident.
■ Obtain baseline vital signs.
■ Perform a complete detailed physical exam if time allows.
■ Perform ongoing assessments, including a reassessment of vital signs in order to identify any changes in the patient's condition.

ASSESSMENT-BASED CARE

FIRST ➤ A typical patient assessment contains seven major components. Although only some portions of them apply to the Emergency Medical Responder, you should be familiar with all of them in order to communicate with other EMS responders properly. The seven components are (Figure 7.1):

Significant Mechanism of Injury

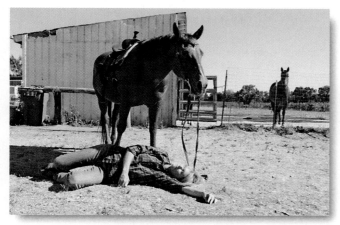

1 ▪ Size up the scene. Determine the mechanism of injury. Enter only if it is safe to do so.

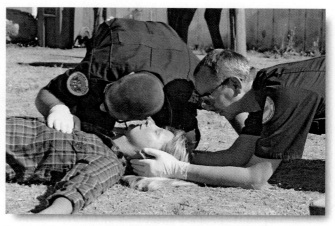

2 ▪ Perform an initial assessment. Manually stabilize the patient's head and neck. Simultaneously, as you check for an open airway, adequate breathing, and serious bleeding, gather a patient history.

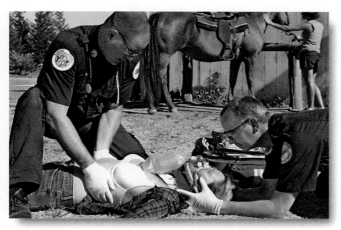

3 ▪ Perform a rapid trauma assessment to detect any serious injuries. Take baseline vital signs. Perform a detailed physical exam.

4 ▪ Perform an ongoing assessment.

▪ *Scene size-up.* This component is an overview of the scene to identify any obvious or potential hazards.
▪ *Initial assessment.* This is a quick assessment of the patient's ABCs in order to detect and correct any immediate life-threatening problems.
▪ *Focused history and physical exam or rapid trauma assessment.*
  — *Trauma patient.* For the injured patient, this is a physical exam based on information obtained from the patient and the MOI. Vital signs are taken, and, if possible, a patient history from the patient, family, or bystanders is obtained.
  — *Medical patient.* For the patient who is ill, this component is made up of a history, any required physical exam, and vital signs.

Patient Assessment

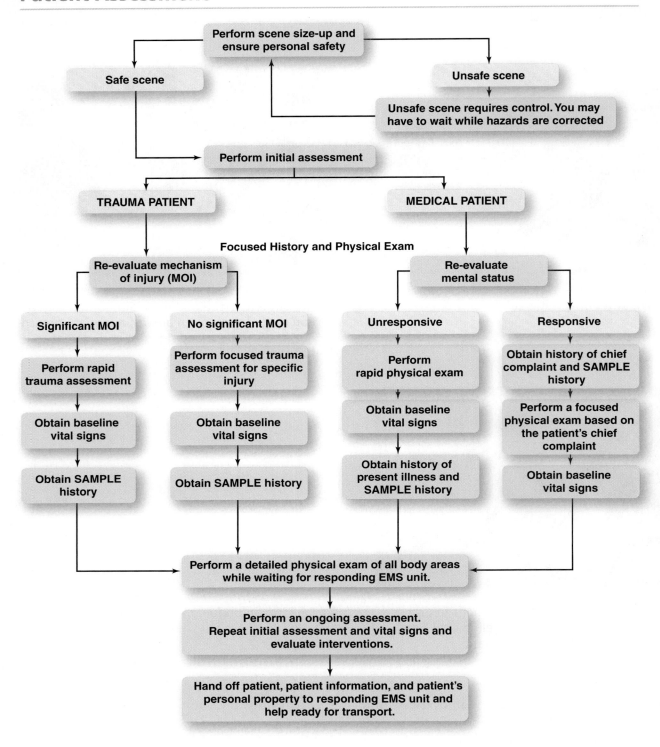

FIGURE 7.1 Patient assessment algorithm.

- *Detailed physical exam.* When time and the patient's condition permit, this careful head-to-toe exam is called for in all patients.
- *Ongoing assessments.* Monitoring the patient to detect any changes in his condition, this component repeats the initial assessment (usually done en route to the hospital), corrects any additional life-threatening problems, repeats vital signs, and evaluates and adjusts as needed any **interventions** performed, such as repositioning the patient or increasing supplemental oxygen. You will find that the condition of your patient will improve, stay the same, or get worse.
- *Communications.* Patient information is related to the higher-level providers who will be taking over patient care.
- *Documentation.* All required written reports and forms are accurately and completely filled out. ▪

interventions ▪ actions taken to correct or stabilize a patient's illness or injury.

FIRST ➤ The typical Emergency Medical Responder program stresses five major parts of patient assessment. They include:

- Scene size-up.
- Initial assessment.
- Focused history and physical exam.
- Detailed physical exam (head-to-toe exam).
- Ongoing assessments. ▪

Although the responsibilities of the Emergency Medical Responder may differ from one EMS system to another, most use an assessment-based approach to patient care. After ensuring one's own personal safety, an Emergency Medical Responder's first concern is to safely detect and begin to correct life-threatening problems in his patient. The second concern is to safely identify and provide care for problems that are serious or may become serious. The third concern is to safely monitor the patient to quickly detect any changes in his condition.

Scene Size-Up

Safety is a primary goal of the scene size-up. The scene size-up actually begins with the information you receive from dispatch before you arrive at the emergency scene. While en route, bring to mind the dispatcher's description of the emergency. Think about the types of injuries or hazards you may find at that particular scene, or the signs and symptoms you may see in a patient with that particular emergency.

FIRST ➤ When you arrive on scene, take appropriate BSI precautions and make sure the scene is safe to enter. When the scene is safe to enter, remain cautious and continue to evaluate scene safety throughout the call. Next, look for the MOI at calls involving a trauma patient (Figure 7.2). Identify the nature of illness (NOI) at medical emergencies (Figure 7.3). Note the number of patients, and anticipate any additional resources that may be needed.

To recap, every patient assessment begins with scene size-up, which includes (Scan 7–5):

3–1.1 Discuss the components of scene size-up.

- Take BSI precautions.
- Determine if the scene is safe for you, other responders, the patient, and bystanders.

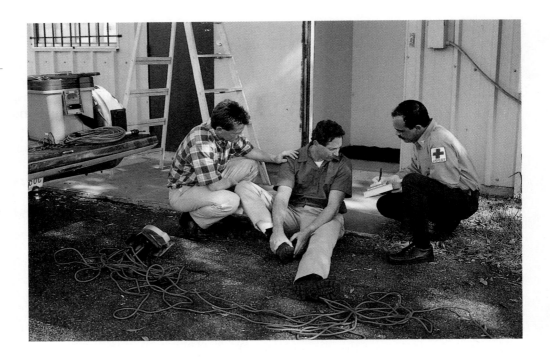

FIGURE 7.2 Clues to the trauma patient's injuries may be gathered on arrival at the scene.

- Identify the MOI or NOI.
- Determine the number of patients.
- Identify any additional resources needed. ▪

TAKE BSI PRECAUTIONS

(You may want to review Chapter 3 on personal safety and protection at this time.) Always take appropriate BSI precautions when assessing and caring for patients. At the very least, this includes wearing disposable synthetic gloves. Wear eye protection, and use additional personal protective equipment as needed, depending on the patient's problem. Remember, BSI precautions are meant to protect both you and your patient, so take precautions before you make contact.

FIGURE 7.3 The medical patient's chief complaint may be apparent as you approach.

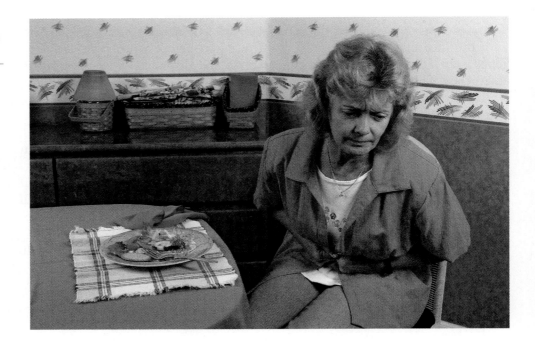

Trauma Patient

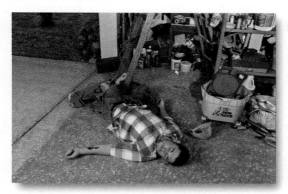

As you approach the trauma patient:

- Take the appropriate BSI precautions.
- Determine if the scene is safe for you, the patient, and any bystanders.
- Identify and evaluate the mechanism of injury.
- Determine the number of patients.
- Decide if additional resources are needed, such as an ambulance, fire department, law enforcement, helicopter, or utility company.
- Consider the need for spinal immobilization.

Medical Patient

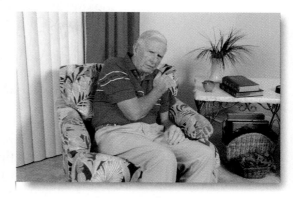

As you approach the medical patient:

- Take the appropriate BSI precautions.
- Determine if the scene is safe for you, the patient, and bystanders.
- Identify and evaluate the nature of illness.
- Determine the number of patients.
- Decide if additional resources are needed, such as an ambulance, fire department, law enforcement, helicopter, or utility company.

ENSURE SCENE SAFETY

A dangerous and sometimes fatal mistake that responders make is entering an unsafe or hazardous scene. Never assume that any scene is safe. Take the time to stop and carefully assess the scene for yourself. If the scene is unsafe, do not enter it. For example, if a scene has the potential for violence and you are not a law enforcement officer, do not enter until law enforcement indicates it is safe for you to do so. If there is the potential for a hazardous materials release, remain a safe distance away. If it is unsafe for you to enter the scene, appropriately trained and equipped hazardous materials team members will bring patients to you after they have been properly decontaminated.

Examples of unsafe scenes include those involving crash/rescues, the release of toxic substances, violence or crime, any weapon, and unsafe surfaces. Also look for signs of domestic disturbances, electrical hazards, potential for fire or explosions, and guard dogs and vicious, wild, or unusual animals. Use all your senses to detect unsafe scenes. Remain at a safe distance to keep yourself and others away from harm.

An important rule to remember is: *Do not add more victims to the scene.* Every year many rescuers are injured and some are killed by vehicles passing the emergency scene. In some cases, rescuers are not visible or are too close to traffic. To ensure safety at an emergency scene, use adequate lighting and properly position emergency vehicles. Also remember that weather conditions, such as icy roads, should be of concern to rescuers. Learn to always relate scene size-up findings to scene safety. The better your scene size-up, the better your ability to recognize and deal with unsafe scenes.

3–1.2 Describe common hazards found at the scene of a trauma patient and a medical patient.

3–1.3 Determine if the scene is safe to enter.

IDENTIFY MECHANISM OF INJURY OR NATURE OF ILLNESS

During the scene size-up, identify the mechanism of injury (MOI) for a trauma patient and the nature of illness (NOI) for a medical patient. Information may be obtained from the patient, from family members or bystanders, and by carefully looking at the scene for clues.

The MOI is made up of the combined forces that caused the injury. Did this patient fall? Is there a penetrating wound? Was he involved in a motor-vehicle collision? A damaged steering wheel of a vehicle, for example, should lead you to consider the possibility of a chest injury. A cracked windshield could be an indication of a head injury. Consider spine injuries in a patient who experienced a fall.

Identifying the NOI is similar to identifying a MOI. In most instances, the NOI will be directly related to the patient's chief complaint. Common NOIs include chest pain, difficulty breathing, and altered mental status. Look at the patient and the area in which he is found for clues to his problem. Does the patient look as if he is in distress? Does his position suggest where there might be pain or discomfort? Are there medications, or is there home oxygen equipment in view? Do you detect any odors, such as vomit or urine? Although diagnosing why the patient is having a particular medical problem is not necessary, the NOI will guide you in the appropriate direction for care.

Both the MOI for trauma patients and the NOI for medical patients will allow you to consider what complications may have not yet developed. For example, if the patient is complaining about chest pain, consider the possibility of a heart problem and the potential for cardiac arrest. Be prepared.

Your size-up of the MOI and NOI is meant to help you recognize obvious life-threats to your patient and give you a general overview of the patient's condition. Later, when you are at the patient's side, you will be able to assess the MOI and NOI more thoroughly. Be prepared to change your impression of the patient's condition as you gather more information.

Geriatric Focus

It is important to recognize that the elderly may suffer severe injuries from less significant mechanisms of injury than younger patients. Therefore, when caring for the elderly trauma victim, you should maintain a high index of suspicion, regardless of the apparent mechanism.

DETERMINE NUMBER OF PATIENTS AND ADDITIONAL RESOURCES

3-1.5 Discuss the reason for identifying the total number of patients at the scene.

3-1.6 Explain the reason for identifying the need for additional help or assistance.

The final part of the scene size-up is to determine the number of patients and whether or not you have sufficient resources to handle the call. It is important to account for all patients involved. How many people were in the vehicle? Did someone walk away from a crash scene? Did a patient get thrown from the vehicle?

Once you are certain of the number of patients involved in the emergency, you must determine if additional resources are needed. More than one EMT unit may be required to handle several patients. In fact, you may require additional resources even on calls with only one patient. You may need additional lifting help if a heavy patient must be carried down stairs. You may require a fire services response to help with extrication (to disentangle and free patients from entrapment) or to make a collision scene safe. Or the patient may require air transport to a specialty medical facility such as a regional trauma center.

An important part of scene size-up is recognizing the need for additional resources and calling for them early. If you put off calling for assistance, you may become so involved in patient care that you forget to call until it is too late.

ARRIVING AT THE PATIENT'S SIDE

On arrival at the patient's side, begin by identifying yourself, even when initially it appears that the patient may be unresponsive. If you wear a uniform, such as that of a law enforcement officer or firefighter, most bystanders and patients will allow you to take charge of the scene without question. If you do not wear a uniform, verbally identifying yourself is critical in allowing you to go about your duties. Simply state your name and then the following: "I am an Emergency Medical Responder, and I've been trained to provide emergency medical care." Although many people may not know what an Emergency Medical Responder is, the statement should allow you access to the patient and the cooperation of bystanders.

Your next statement should be to the patient: "May I help you?" As noted in Chapter 2, by answering "yes" to this question, the patient is giving you expressed consent to begin assessment and care. The patient may not answer "yes" to your question, but instead may simply remain still and allow you to provide care. A patient who is alert and does not refuse your care is said to be providing consent.

Geriatric Focus

Address the elderly with respect by using their last name if you know it or by asking them their name and then addressing them with Mr. or Mrs. Never use terms of endearment, such as "grandpa," "dear," or "honey," and especially avoid the use of ageism, which is reflected in terms such as "gramps" or "pop."

Sometimes a patient's fear may be so great that he is confused and will answer "no" or "just leave me alone." Gaining the patient's confidence by talking with him is usually easy. If the patient is unresponsive or unable to give expressed consent, implied consent allows you to care for the patient. This means that if the patient were able to do so, it is assumed that he would consent to care. (Review Chapter 2 for a more detailed discussion of consent.)

Remember, on arrival and after conducting a scene size-up, you must:

1. State your name.
2. Identify yourself as a trained Emergency Medical Responder. Let the patient and bystanders know that you are with the Emergency Medical Services system.
3. Ask the patient if you may help.

If someone is already providing care to the patient when you arrive, identify yourself as an Emergency Medical Responder. If the person's training is equal to or at a higher level than your own, ask if you may assist. You should still identify yourself to the patient and ask if he wants you to help.

If you have more training than the person who has begun care, respectfully ask to take over responsibility for the patient. Compliment him on what he has done so far and ask him to assist you. Do not criticize or argue with anyone who may have initiated care. Unless you are a law enforcement officer, or there are specific emergency care laws in your state, you may not order the first provider to relinquish care of the patient to you. Check your local laws and protocols.

"Darn it, Tariq!" the driver said loudly. "I told you it's not a heart attack! I think I pulled a muscle in my chest." The older man was sitting on a pallet of low boxes with his hand pressed to the center of his chest.

"Hello, sir," Jared said as he knelt beside the patient. "I'm Jared. This is Ray. We're Emergency Medical Responders with the company's MERT team. Do I have permission to make sure that you're okay?"

The driver sighed, rolled his eyes, and said, "Yes, but I'm fine."

"Great," Jared smiled. "That makes it a good day for both of us, doesn't it? What's your name?" He then touched the driver's wrist with his gloved hand and paused to feel for a pulse.

"Craig," the driver said between rapid breaths. At first, Craig's pulse was weak and somewhat irregular, and Jared noticed that the driver was growing pale and anxious. After a moment, though, his pulse took on a more regular rhythm, and his color returned.

Initial Assessment

The initial assessment is designed to help the Emergency Medical Responder detect and correct all immediate threats to life. Immediate life threats typically involve the patient's ABCs, and each is corrected as it is found. The initial assessment is begun as soon as you reach the patient.

FIRST ➤ The initial assessment has six components (Scans 7–6 to 7–8). They are:

- Form a general impression of the patient.
- Assess the patient's mental status. Initially, this may mean determine if the patient is responsive or unresponsive.
- Assess the patient's airway
- Assess the patient's breathing.
- Assess the patient's circulation (pulse and bleeding).
- Make a decision on the priority or urgency of the patient for transport. ■

FIRST ➤ While conducting the initial assessment, you will look for life-threatening problems in three major areas. Those areas are:

- *Airway.* Is the patient's airway open?
- *Breathing.* Is the patient breathing adequately?
- *Circulation.* Does the patient have an adequate pulse to circulate blood? Is there serious bleeding? Did the patient lose a large quantity of blood prior to your arrival? ■

ABCs ■ the patient's airway, breathing, and circulation as they relate to the initial assessment.

This assessment and the actions taken are known as the **ABCs** of emergency care, which stand for:

A — Airway
B — Breathing
C — Circulation

During the initial assessment, if a life-threatening problem is detected, it may be necessary to start simultaneous actions focused on the ABCs of emergency care. For example, a trauma patient may require manual stabilization of his head and neck at the same time you are opening his airway, providing ventilations, and controlling bleeding. A medical patient may require you to assess his mental status at the same time you are taking a pulse and assessing his breathing. Simultaneous actions may prove to be very challenging. It is essential that you know how to assess a patient's ABCs, as well as how to provide the care related life-threatening problems require.

FORM A GENERAL IMPRESSION

3–1.7 Summarize the reasons for forming a general impression of the patient.

As you approach your patient and perform your initial assessment, you also will be forming a general impression of the patient and the patient's environment. Your general impression is your first "informal" assessment of the patient's overall condition.

No Significant Mechanism of Injury

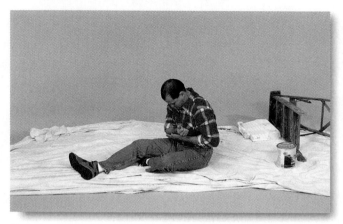

1 ▪ Form a general impression of the patient.

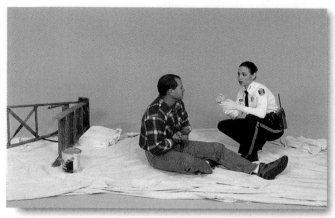

2 ▪ Assess the patient's mental status. Initially, this may be to determine if the patient is responsive or unresponsive.

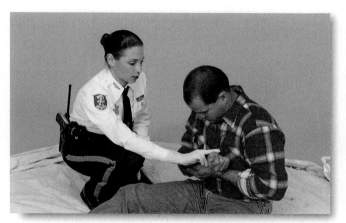

3 ▪ Assess the patient's airway, breathing, circulation, and evidence of bleeding.

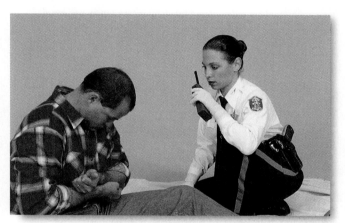

4 ▪ Make a decision on the priority or urgency of the patient for transport.

The general impression will help you decide the seriousness of the patient's condition based on his level of distress and mental status. You may also be given information by the patient or bystanders at this time, such as the reason why EMS was called. In most cases, the reason EMS was called can be determined by identifying the patient's **chief complaint.**

Emergency Medical Responders have always formed a general impression when they first see a patient, even if they are not immediately aware of doing so. With experience, you may form one on intuition alone. You may notice if the patient looks very ill, pale, or cyanotic (blue coloring to the skin). You may notice unusual details such as odors, temperature, and living conditions. You may immediately see serious injuries or that the patient looks quite stable. This impression forms an early opinion of how seriously ill or injured the patient is.

chief complaint ▪ the reason EMS was called in the patient's own words.

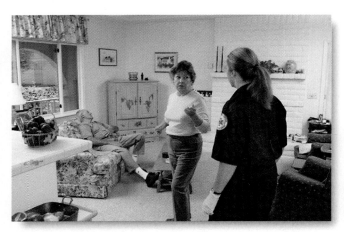

1 ■ As you approach, form a general impression of the patient.

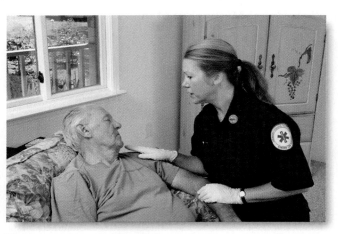

2 ■ Assess the patient's mental status. Initially, this may be to determine if the patient is responsive or unresponsive.

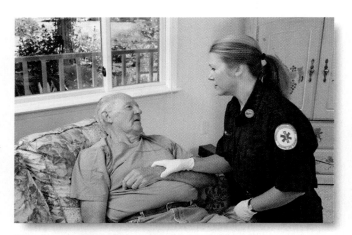

3 ■ Assess the patient's airway, breathing, and circulation.

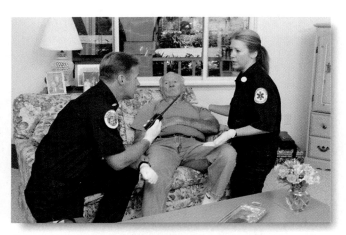

4 ■ Make a decision on the priority or urgency of the patient for transport.

Your decision to request immediate transport or to continue assessing the patient may be based solely on your general impression.

ASSESS MENTAL STATUS

3–1.8 Discuss methods of assessing mental status.

Your actual assessment of a patient begins by determining the patient's level of responsiveness. If you do not suspect trauma, especially spine injury, check for responsiveness by gently squeezing the patient's shoulder and shouting, "Are you okay?" Speak loudly enough to wake the patient if he is merely sleeping.

Classify the patient's mental status by using the **AVPU scale**, the letters of which stand for *alert, verbal, painful,* and *unresponsive.*

AVPU scale ■ a memory aid for the classifications of mental status, or levels of responsiveness. The letters stand for *alert, verbal, painful,* and *unresponsive.*

A — *Alert.* The alert patient will be awake, responsive, oriented, and talking with you.

V — *Verbal.* This is a patient who appears to be unresponsive at first, but who will respond to a loud verbal stimulus from you.

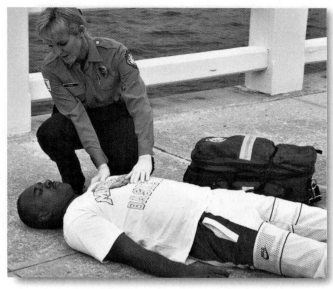

1 ■ As soon as you approach the patient, establish his level of responsiveness.

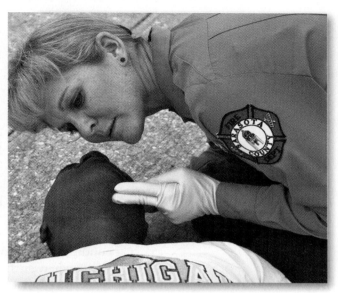

2 ■ Ensure an open airway. Then look, listen, and feel for breathing.

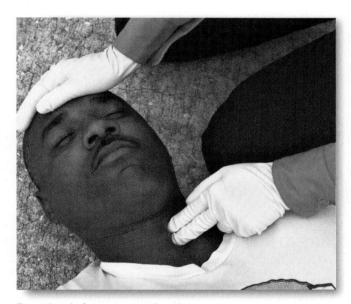

3 ■ Check for a carotid pulse.

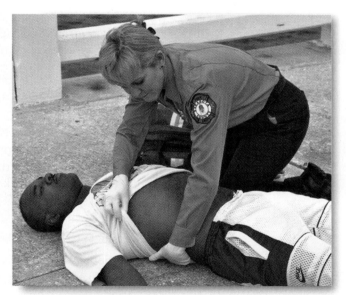

4 ■ Look for and control all major bleeding. Then make a decision on the priority or urgency of the patient for transport.

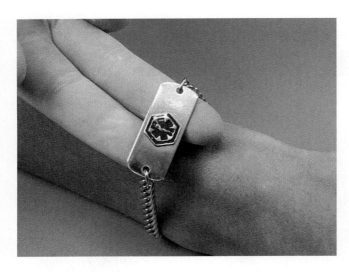

FIGURE 7.4 Example of a medical identification bracelet.

P — *Painful.* If the patient does not respond to verbal stimuli, he may respond to painful stimuli, such as a sternal (breastbone) rub or a gentle pinch to the shoulder. Be careful not to injure the patient when applying painful stimuli. Never forcefully pinch the skin. Never stick the patient with a sharp object.

U — *Unresponsive.* If the patient does not respond to either verbal or painful stimuli, he is said to be unresponsive

Notice that the term *verbal* does not mean the patient is answering your questions or initiating a conversation. Instead, the patient may speak, or he may grunt, groan, or say "huh," or he may simply look at you in response to your verbal stimulus. It is possible that the patient may have a medical condition such as a stroke or a problem associated with trauma such as a head injury. Either of these examples may cause the patient to lose the ability to speak. In rare cases, a pre-existing condition may have rendered the patient unable to speak prior to the emergency. Often, when such a condition is present, the patient will have a medical identification card or jewelry, such as a bracelet or necklace (Figure 7.4). Check with bystanders. They may know the patient and be able to alert you to the problem.

Geriatric Focus

The presence of dementia in the elderly patient can make it very difficult to accurately assess mental status. You must take extra time to ask family members and/or caregivers if the patient's mental status is normal for him or if it is different in some way. With dementia, the patient may appear alert and oriented one minute and completely confused the next. Be aware of the effects of dementia, and learn to rely on family and caregivers to help establish a normal mental status baseline for the patient.

Try to assess mental status without moving the patient. But if the patient is unresponsive, you may need to reposition him to check for breathing, pulse, and serious bleeding, or to perform CPR. Follow the procedures shown in Scan 7–9.

Always suspect the presence of neck or spine injuries in the unresponsive trauma patient. Moving this type of patient may cause additional injuries, but it may be necessary to check for life-threatening problems. (Moving a patient safely was covered in Chapter 5.)

ASSESS AIRWAY AND BREATHING

3–1.10 Describe methods used for assessing if a patient is breathing.

If the patient is unresponsive, stabilize his head and neck and use the jaw-thrust maneuver to ensure an open airway. If you do not suspect a spine injury, position the patient flat on his back and yourself by his side. Use the head-tilt, chin-lift maneuver to open the airway. Remember, for patients with suspected spine injury, use the jaw-thrust.

3–1.11 Differentiate between a patient with adequate and inadequate breathing.

Then check for adequate breathing. With the airway open, place your ear over the patient's nose and mouth, and watch the chest for movement. If the patient is breathing, you will hear and feel the exhaled air on your ear, and you will see the chest rise and fall with each respiration. Listen to the quality of the breaths. Are there any noises that indicate a possible obstruction?

WARNING: This maneuver is used to initiate basic life support when you must act alone. For all other situations, use a two- to three-rescuer log roll.

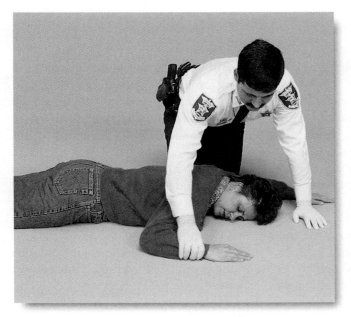

1 ■ Straighten the legs and reposition the arms.

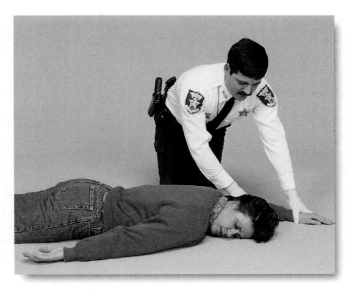

2 ■ Place the arms close to the patient's side. They will help splint the torso as you roll the patient.

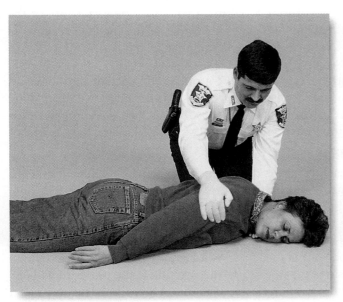

3 ■ Cradle the head and neck, and then grasp the distant shoulder. Move the patient as a unit onto her side.

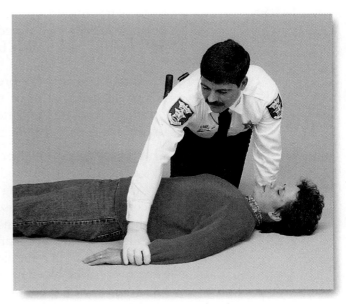

4 ■ Move the patient onto her back.

Determining breathing status should take no more than 10 seconds. The patient is not breathing if there is no chest movement, even if you hear noises coming from the patient's mouth. Sporadic respirations are called *agonal respirations*. They typically occur just prior to death.

If the patient is not breathing adequately, you must check for the presence of a pulse. Depending on what you find, you may need to take immediate action to correct the problem. (The procedures to follow are covered in Chapter 6.)

ASSESS CIRCULATION

Check for a Pulse

If the patient is not breathing, check for a **carotid pulse** at the neck to determine if blood is circulating (Scan 7–8.3). The pulse at the neck is considered more reliable than the pulse at the wrist. If the patient is breathing, you may either check for a carotid pulse or a **radial pulse** (the pulse at the wrist). The radial pulse may be absent if the patient is in shock. If you check the radial pulse first and find it absent, then check the carotid pulse.

To assess the carotid pulse, first locate the patient's thyroid cartilage (Adam's apple). Place the tip of your index and middle fingers directly over the midline of this structure. Now, slide your fingertips to the side of the neck closest to you. Do not slide your fingertips to the opposite side of the patient's neck because this may apply improper pressure and close the airway. Do not attempt to take a carotid pulse on both sides of the neck at the same time. This may interfere with circulation to the brain. You should detect a pulse in the groove between the trachea and the large muscle on the side of the neck. Only moderate pressure is needed to feel it. Take the carotid pulse for 5 to 10 seconds. Frequent practice will make this skill easy to master.

Geriatric Focus

The elderly often have an irregular pulse. This is rarely a life-threatening condition. However, the speed of the pulse, both too fast and too slow, can be life-threatening and therefore the rate is more important to notice than the regularity.

It is not important during the initial assessment to count the exact rate of the pulse. You only want to confirm the presence of a pulse. If the pulse is very rapid or weak, the patient may be in shock. If there is no pulse, alert dispatch and begin CPR.

If the patient is not breathing but does have a pulse, the patient may have an airway obstruction or he may be in respiratory arrest. You must take immediate action to ventilate the patient before the heart stops. If the chest does not rise during ventilations, the patient may have an airway obstruction. (See Chapter 6.)

Check for Serious Bleeding

The next step in the initial assessment is checking for serious bleeding. Although any uncontrolled bleeding may eventually become life threatening, you will only be concerned with profuse bleeding during the initial assessment. Blood that is bright red and spurting may be coming from an *artery*. Because blood in arteries is under a great deal of pressure, large amounts of blood may be lost in a short period of time. Flowing blood that is darker in color is most likely coming from a *vein*. Even if the bleeding is slow, it may be life threatening if the patient has been bleeding for a long period of time. Look at the amount of blood that has been lost on the ground, in clothing, and in the hair. Your concern is for the total amount of blood that has been lost, not just how fast or slow the bleeding is. (Methods of controlling serious bleeding are covered in Chapter 10.)

3–1.12 Describe the methods used to assess circulation.

3–1.13 Differentiate between obtaining a pulse in the adult, child, and infant patient.

carotid pulse ■ the pulse that can be felt on either side of the neck.

radial pulse ■ the pulse that can be felt on the thumb side of the wrist.

REMEMBER

If the patient's pulse is irregular, count the pulse rate for a full minute.

3–1.14 Discuss the need for assessing the patient for external bleeding.

Assessment of circulation may be altered slightly when you immediately see profuse bleeding. In this case, attempt to control the bleeding as soon as it is discovered. Do what you can to control it, but never neglect the patient's airway and breathing status.

> **NOTE**
>
> In some EMS systems, assessing circulation also includes checking skin signs—color, temperature, and moisture. An abnormal finding such as pale, cool, moist skin could indicate a serious circulation problem, such as shock.

DETERMINE PATIENT PRIORITY

Information you give to dispatch will help determine the priority of the patient for transport. A high-priority patient should be transported immediately, with little time spent on the scene. High-priority conditions include a poor general impression, unresponsiveness, breathing difficulties, severe bleeding or shock, complicated childbirth, chest pain, and any severe pain.

3–1.15 Explain the reason for prioritizing a patient for care and transport.

SPECIAL CONSIDERATIONS FOR INFANTS AND CHILDREN

Your assessment of an infant or child will differ from that of an adult in a few ways. It is important for you to realize that children are not little adults. They react to illness and injury differently. For example:

3–1.9 Differentiate between assessing mental status in the adult, child, and infant patient.

- Infants and children are often shy and distrustful of strangers. When checking the mental status of a responsive infant, talk to him and flick the bottom of his feet. A responsive infant or a child who pays no attention to you or what you are doing may be seriously ill.
- Opening the airway of an infant involves moving the head into a neutral position, not tilting it back as with an adult. Opening the airway of a child requires only slight extension.
- Breathing and pulse rates are faster in infants and children than in adults. The pulse to check in an infant or a small child is the **brachial pulse**. It is taken at the brachial artery in the upper arm, not at the neck or wrist.

brachial pulse ■ the pulse that can be felt in the medial side of the upper arm between the elbow and shoulder.

An additional part of checking an infant's or a child's circulation is **capillary refill**. When the end of a child's fingernail is gently pressed, it turns white because blood flow is restricted. When the pressure is released, the nail bed turns pink again, usually in less than two seconds. This is a good way to evaluate the circulation of blood in an infant or a child. If it takes longer than two seconds for the nail bed to become pink again or if it does not return to pink at all, there may be a problem with circulation, such as shock or blood loss. If the infant's nail beds are too small, you may perform the same test on the top of his foot or back of his hand. To judge the amount of time it takes for the blood to flow back, count, "one-one thousand, two-one thousand," or simply say "capillary refill."

capillary refill ■ the return (refill) of blood into the capillaries after it has been forced out by fingertip pressure. Normal refill time is two seconds or less.

Usually, when adult patients have a serious problem, they become worse gradually. The downward trend often can be spotted in time to take appropriate action. However, an infant's or child's body can compensate so well for a problem such as blood loss that he may appear stable for some time, and then suddenly become much worse. Children can actually maintain a near-normal blood pressure up to the time when almost half of their total blood volume is gone. That is why blood pressure is not a reliable assessment of a child's circulation. Checking capillary refill time is more reliable.

It is vital for the Emergency Medical Responder to recognize the seriousness of a child's illness or injury early, before it is too late. You will learn about other considerations in approaching and assessing infants and children in Chapter 13.

ALERT DISPATCH

Depending on what you find once you arrive on scene, it may be necessary to contact EMS dispatch and update them with details about the scene. For instance, you may want to confirm the location, ask for additional resources, or confirm the number of patients.

The information you give dispatch can determine the type and level of response sent. Many EMS dispatch centers are now using an emergency medical dispatch system, or *priority dispatching*. This system determines if basic life support (BLS) or advanced life support (ALS) is needed, or a combination of both. It also determines the response mode used, such as "cold" (Code 2) with no lights or siren or "hot" (Code 3) with lights and siren.

If you have called for additional resources, such as an ambulance or helicopter, it may be helpful to give them an update of the patient's condition. Your update should include information about the patient such as mental status, age and gender, chief complaint, airway and breathing status, circulation status, and interventions and their results.

Focused History and Physical Exam

3–1.16 Discuss the components of the physical exam.

A focused history and physical exam should be performed after the initial assessment. It assumes that life-threatening problems have been found and corrected. If you have a patient with a life-threatening problem that you must continually care for (performing CPR on a cardiac arrest patient, for example), you may not get to this assessment component.

The main purpose of the focused history and physical exam is to discover and care for the patient's specific injuries or medical problems. It is a systematic approach to patient assessment. It also may assure the patient, family, and bystanders that there is concern for the patient and that something is being done for the patient immediately.

The focused history and physical exam includes a physical examination that focuses in on a specific injury or medical complaint, or it may be a rapid exam of the entire body. It also includes obtaining a patient history and taking vital signs. The order in which these steps are accomplished is based on the patient's type of emergency (Table 7–1).

FIRST ➤ Some important terms associated with patient assessment are introduced in the following list. Each term is discussed in greater detail later in the chapter. They include:

patient history ■ information relating to a patient's current complaint or condition, as well as information about past medical problems that could be related.

■ *Patient history.* A **patient history** includes any information relating to the patient's current complaint or condition, as well as information about past medical problems that could be related.
■ *Rapid assessment.* This is a quick, less detailed head-to-toe assessment of the most critical patients.

TABLE 7-1 Focused History and Physical Exam

TRAUMA PATIENT	MEDICAL PATIENT
Significant Mechanism of Injury	**Unresponsive Medical Patient**
• Perform a rapid trauma assessment.	• Perform a rapid physical exam.
• Take vital signs.	• Take vital signs.
• Gather patient history.	• Gather patient history.
No Significant Mechanism of Injury	**Responsive Medical Patient**
• Perform a focused trauma assessment.	• Gather patient history.
• Take vital signs.	• Perform focused physical exam.
• Gather patient history.	• Take vital signs.

- *Focused assessment.* This is an exam conducted on stable patients. It focuses on a specific injury or medical complaint.
- *Vital signs.* These include pulse, respirations, skin signs, and pupils. In some areas, Emergency Medical Responders also include assessment of blood pressure. The first set of vital signs taken on any patient is referred to as the *baseline vital signs.* All subsequent vital signs should be compared to the baseline set to identify developing trends.
- *Symptoms.* Reported by the patient, symptoms such as chest pain, dizziness, and nausea are felt by the patient. They are also called *subjective findings.*
- *Signs.* These are what you see, feel, hear, and smell as you examine the patient, such as cool clammy skin or unequal pupils. They are also called *objective findings.*

Objective findings can be seen, felt, or in some way measured scientifically. *Subjective findings* are influenced by the person, who in this case is the patient, family members, or bystanders reporting the symptoms. The objective portion of patient assessment is considered part of the science of medicine; the subjective portion as part of the art of medicine.

Many of the signs and symptoms you will find during the physical exam are the result of the body's attempt to compensate for the stress it is under. For example, to compensate for blood loss, the body will increase pulse and breathing rates and close down, or constrict, blood vessels in the extremities, all of which results in pale, cool, clammy skin. These actions are attempts by the body to circulate an adequate amount of oxygenated blood to the vital organs. Adequate flow of oxygenated blood to all cells of the body is called **perfusion**. Inadequate blood flow can lead to shock.

perfusion ▪ the adequate flow of oxygenated blood to all cells of the body.

Is It Safe ?

By stopping to care for an injury that is not life threatening, you may delay or forget the remainder of the exam and miss a more important problem.

Abnormal findings during your exam indicate a problem that should not be ignored. However, unless the problem is likely to get worse, do not interrupt a focused history and physical exam. You can stop bleeding from getting worse, but there is little you can do to stop a broken leg from getting worse. It is important to complete your examination.

EXAMINING A TRAUMA PATIENT

A trauma patient is one who has received a physical injury of some type. Your assessment of a trauma patient will consist of a physical exam, vital signs, and patient history. The type of physical exam you perform and the order in which you do the various steps will be based on the MOI.

The trauma patient is classified as either having no significant MOI (probably not causing a serious injury) or having a significant MOI (probably causing a serious injury). The assessment is different for each type of patient.

focused trauma assessment
■ an examination of the area the patient tells you is injured.

To assess a trauma patient with no significant MOI, perform a **focused trauma assessment** on the area that the patient tells you is injured (Scan 7–10). Obtain vital signs and gather a patient history. Provide continued care during the ongoing assessment. (There is usually no need to perform a detailed physical exam on a patient with no significant MOI.)

To detect and care for serious injuries in a patient with a significant MOI, perform a rapid trauma assessment of the entire body (Scan 7–11). Obtain vital signs and gather a patient history. Then, if time permits, perform a detailed physical exam. Provide continued care during the ongoing assessments.

3–1.4 Discuss common mechanisms of injury/nature of illness.

Significant mechanisms of injury for an adult include:

- Ejection from a vehicle.
- Death of one or more passengers in the same vehicle as the patient.
- Falls greater than 20 feet.
- Rollover vehicle collision.
- High-speed vehicle collision.
- Vehicle-pedestrian collision.
- Motorcycle crash.
- Unresponsiveness or altered mental status.
- Penetrations of the head, neck, chest, or abdomen.
- Amputations proximal to the wrist or ankle.

Significant mechanisms of injury for a child include:

- Falls of more than 10 feet or two to three times the height of the pediatric patient.
- Bicycle collision.
- Medium-speed vehicle collision.

NOTE

Many years of careful medical studies have demonstrated that people are more likely to be seriously injured in falls that are three times the patient's height. Injuries may be serious in shorter falls, often depending on the nature of the surface on which the patient lands and how the patient strikes the surface. Based on research, Emergency Medical Responders should consider all falls as potentially serious.

EXAMINING A MEDICAL PATIENT

The focused history and physical exam for a medical patient and a trauma patient are similar, but the order and emphasis are different. For a medical patient, you are more concerned with the medical history of the patient. For the unresponsive

No Significant MOI

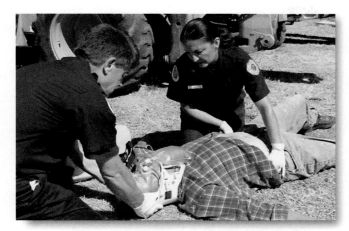

1 ■ Examine the area that the patient tells you is injured.

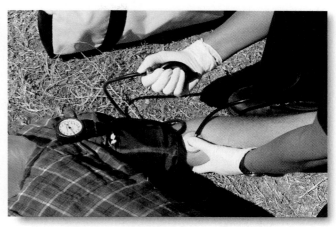

2 ■ Obtain baseline vital signs.

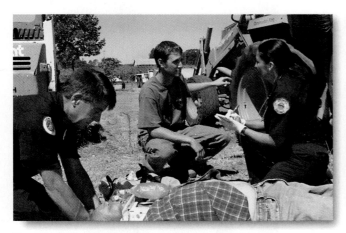

3 ■ Gather a patient history.

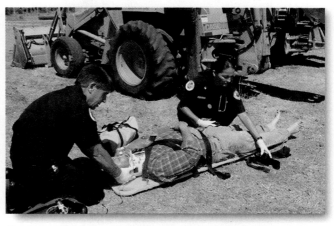

4 ■ Provide appropriate care for the injury.

medical patient, perform a **rapid physical exam** to determine if there are any obvious signs of illness. Obtain baseline vital signs. Gather a patient history, if possible. Provide care as needed.

For the responsive medical patient (Scan 7–12), gather a patient history, observing signs and symptoms while asking about the history of the illness. The patient's chief complaint helps direct the questioning. Perform a **focused physical exam** based on the patient's problem areas. Obtain baseline vital signs. Provide care as needed. Provide continued care during the ongoing assessments.

Medical patients rarely require a detailed physical exam, and if one is necessary, there is usually a significant MOI or the rescuer believes there is a potential for injuries, such as when a medical patient has fallen.

rapid physical exam ■ a quick head-to-toe assessment of the most critical patients.

focused physical exam ■ an examination conducted on stable patients, focusing on a specific injury or medical complaint.

Significant MOI or Unresponsive Medical Patient

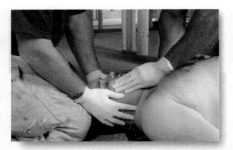

1 ■ First, have your partner stabilize the patient's head and neck. Then check the head (scalp and face).

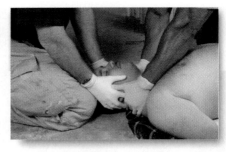

2 ■ Check the patient's neck. Apply a cervical collar, if you are trained to do so.

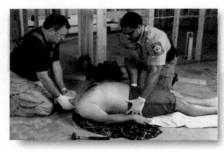

3 ■ Check the chest.

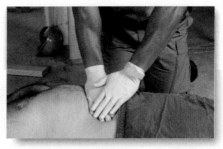

4 ■ Check each quadrant of the abdomen.

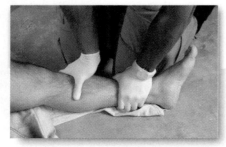

5 ■ Check the pelvis, pressing gently down and inward.

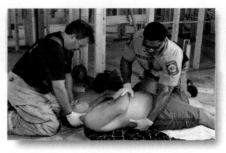

6 ■ Check the back and buttocks by sliding your hands under the patient. (If you have to reposition the arms to check his back, first make sure that there are no injuries to his arms.)

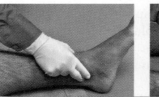

7 ■ Check the extremities, legs first and then the arms.

8 ■ Check for circulation, sensation, and motor function in each extremity.

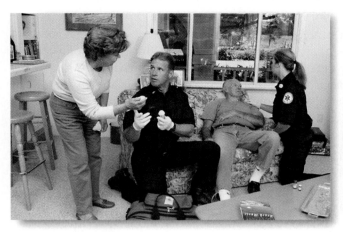

1 ■ Gather a patient history.

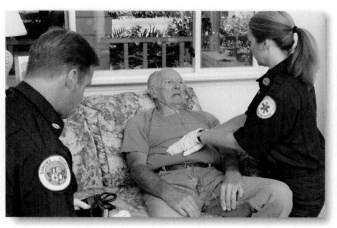

2 ■ Perform a focused physical exam based on the patient's problem areas.

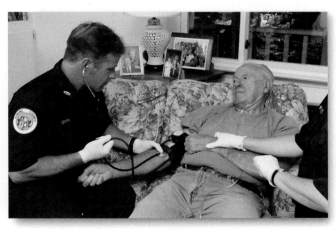

3 ■ Obtain baseline vital signs.

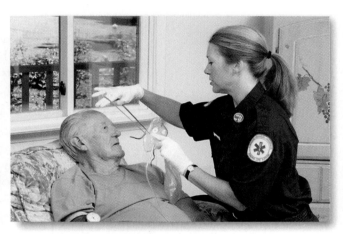

4 ■ Provide the appropriate care as indicated.

NOTE

The patient history and physical exam can be performed simultaneously. There is no need to wait to take vital signs until the history has been completed. You may obtain the history while performing the physical exam of the patient or while controlling bleeding from a wound. You can do both at the same time.

PATIENT HISTORY

Patient Interview

An alert patient is your best source of information. Direct your questions to him. Ask questions clearly at a normal rate and in a normal tone of voice. Avoid leading questions. Do not falsely reassure the patient. Do not say things such as "Everything will be fine" or "Take it easy, everything's okay." The patient knows this is not true and will lose confidence in you if you attempt to provide false reassurance. Phrases such as "I'm here to help you" or "I'm doing everything I can to help you" are more appropriate.

FIRST ➤ When interviewing a patient who is alert, ask the following questions:

1. *What is your name?* This is an essential piece of information. It shows your patient that you are concerned for him as a person. Remember his name and use it often. Also, if your patient's mental status decreases, you can call him by name to elicit a response.

2. *How old are you?* As an Emergency Medical Responder, you do not need to know more than the general age of your adult patient. But the age of a child is important because it may determine what type of care is provided. Ask all children their age. It may be appropriate to ask an adolescent his age in order to be certain that he is a minor. Also ask minors: *How can I contact your parents?* Children may already be upset at being hurt or ill without a parent being there to help them. Always reassure them that someone will contact their parents.

3. *What is wrong?* This usually is the patient's chief complaint. No matter what is wrong, ask if there is any pain. When an extremity is involved, ask if there is numbness, tingling, or a burning sensation in the limb. Any of these could indicate possible nerve or spine injury. As you learn more about various illnesses and injuries, you will also learn additional questions to ask.

4. *How did it happen?* When caring for trauma patients, knowing how the patient was injured will help direct you to problems that may not be noticeable or obvious to you or the patient. If your patient is lying down, determine if he got into that position himself or was knocked down, fell, or was thrown. Do this for patients with medical problems as well. Remember, the injury to the patient may be the result of a medical problem. This information may indicate the possibility of a spine injury or internal bleeding.

5. *How long have you felt this way?* You want to know if the patient's problem occurred suddenly or if it has been developing for the past few days or over a period of time.

6. *Has this happened before?* It is especially important to ask this question of medical patients. You want to know if this is the first time or if it is a recurring, or chronic, problem. This question is not usually asked of trauma patients, unless you suspect a recurring problem. If your patient has been hit by a car, it is not necessary to ask him if this has happened before.

7. *Are there any current medical problems?* Has the patient been feeling ill lately or has he seen or is he being treated by a doctor for any problems?

8. *Are any medications being taken?* Your patient may not be able to tell you the exact name of a medication he is taking, especially if he is taking several. He may be able to tell you just general medication categories, such as "heart pills" or "water pills." Ask not only about prescription medications, but also about over-the-counter medications. Routine use of simple medications such as aspirin may alter the treatment the patient receives at the hospital.

   Do not use the terms *drugs* or *recreational drugs* in general. They imply misuse or abuse. Some patients may think that you are trying to gather criminal evidence and become uneasy. Instead, ask the patient if he can think of anything else that he might be taking. If you still feel that the patient has not given all the information needed, explain your feelings to the EMTs who take over patient care. Be certain that your concern is stated in both your patient assessment notes and the patient assessment record used by the EMTs.

9. *Do you have any allergies?* Allergic reactions can vary from simple hives or itching to life-threatening airway problems and shock. Knowing that the patient is allergic to a substance will enable you to keep it away from him. Be sure to ask

specifically about allergies to medications, adhesive tape, and latex (as used in gloves) because the patient may come in contact with any of these during care.

10. *When did you last eat?* This is an important question if your patient is a candidate for surgery. It also is important information when dealing with a patient who is having a diabetic emergency. ■

Geriatric Focus

Just as it may be difficult to accurately assess mental status in an elderly patient with dementia, obtaining a thorough and accurate history can prove just as challenging. It will become important to rely on family members and caregivers to confirm the information that the patient is telling you or to simply fill in the gaps left by the patient's own history. Hearing loss also can make it challenging to obtain a history. You may have to speak louder than usual, and it will also help if you speak slowly and clearly.

To obtain a patient history, many EMS systems use the acronym **SAMPLE history** as a memory aid for the questions that should be asked. Each letter of the word SAMPLE represents a specific question or series of questions:

S — Signs/symptoms?
A — Allergies?
M — Medications?
P — Pertinent past medical history?
L — Last oral intake?
E — Events leading to the illness or injury?

SAMPLE history ■ a system of information gathering that allows the rescuer to ask questions about past or present medical or injury problems. Letters stand for *signs/symptoms, allergies, medications, pertinent past medical history, last oral intake,* and *events leading to the illness or injury.*

3–1.19 Explain the components of the SAMPLE history.

When taking a history, maintain eye contact with the patient. This will improve personal communication and build the patient's confidence in you. If you look away while asking questions or while listening to answers, it may indicate to your patient that you are not as concerned as you should be or not giving him your full attention. A simple touch can also improve communications. You touch the patient's forehead to note relative skin temperature and moisture, and, by touching the patient, you are also showing caring and concern. However, respect a patient's wish not to be touched. Patients are often fearful and anxious. Your calm, caring, and professional attitude often can do as much for the patient as any medical care you provide.

Bystander Interview

You may encounter a patient who is unresponsive or unable to answer your questions regarding his history. If this is the case, you must depend on family or bystanders for information. Ask specific, directed questions to shorten the time required to obtain the information. Questions to bystanders include:

3–1.18 Explain what additional questions may be asked during the physical exam.

1. *What is the patient's name?* If the patient is a minor, ask if the parents are there or if they have been contacted.
2. *What happened?* You can receive valuable information when asking this question. If the patient fell from a ladder, did he appear to faint or pass out first? Was he hit on the head by something? Clues from the answers to this question are limitless.
3. *Did you see anything else?* For example, was the patient holding his chest before he fell? This gives the bystander a chance to think again and add anything he remembers.
4. *Did the patient complain of anything before this happened?* You may learn of chest pain, nausea, shortness of breath, a funny odor where the patient was working, and other clues.

5. *Did the patient have any known illness or problems?* Family or friends who know the patient may know his medical history, such as heart problems, diabetes, allergies, or other problems that may cause a change in his condition.

6. *Does the patient take any medication?* Again, family or friends who know the patient may be aware of the medications he takes. When talking with the patient, family, friends, or bystanders, remember to use the word *medication* or *medicine* instead of *drugs*. Medicines or medications are considered prescriptions for legitimate medical purposes. The public views drugs as illegal substances. Remember to ask the patient if he is taking over-the-counter medications.

Geriatric Focus

Many elderly patients take prescription medications for various medical conditions. A good trick to help disclose pertinent medical history is to ask to see all medications the patient is currently taking. Even if you do not know the purpose of each medication, having them handy when the EMTs arrive will help them begin to understand the patient's history sooner.

Most of the questions in the preceding list are questions you would normally ask about someone who is hurt or ill. You would usually introduce yourself and ask for a name, just as you would ask what was wrong and how it happened. Much of your Emergency Medical Responder training is simply formalized common sense.

Medical Identification Jewelry

Medical identification jewelry can provide important information if the patient is unresponsive and a history cannot be obtained from family or bystanders. A common one is the MedicAlert medallion worn on a necklace or a wrist or ankle bracelet. One side of the device has a Star-of-Life emblem. Information on the patient's medical problem is engraved on the reverse side, along with a phone number for additional information.

If you must move the patient or any of his extremities, take care to check for medical identification jewelry. Be sure to alert the EMTs who take over care that the patient is wearing one, and tell them what is on it, such as diabetes, heart condition, or penicillin allergy.

VITAL SIGNS

FIRST ➤ Vital signs can alert you to problems that require immediate attention. Taken at regular intervals, they can help you determine if the patient's condition is getting better, worse, or staying the same. For most Emergency Medical Responders, vital signs include pulse, respirations, and skin signs. Some Emergency Medical Responders include pupils and blood pressure. (Taking blood pressure is described in Appendix 1.) ▪

The first set of vital signs is called *baseline vital signs*. Compare all other vital sign readings to the baseline vital signs. This comparison helps determine if the patient is stable or unstable, improving or growing worse, and benefiting or not benefiting from care procedures. For example, comparing baseline vital signs before and after administering oxygen to the patient can tell the EMTs who take over patient care objective information about how that intervention may be affecting the patient. Certain combinations of vital signs point to possible serious medical or traumatic conditions. For example, cool, clammy skin, a rapid but weak pulse, and increased breathing rate can indicate possible shock in the presence of a significant MOI. Hot, dry skin with a rapid pulse may indicate a serious heat-related emergency. You can determine which patients are a high priority for immediate transport by taking vital signs.

For an adult, a continuous pulse rate of less than 60 beats per minute or more than 100 beats per minute is considered abnormal. Likewise, a respiratory rate more than 28 breaths per minute or less than 8 breaths per minute is considered serious. You should be concerned about these vital signs because they indicate unstable situations that could become life threatening, and the patient could worsen quickly. Stay alert and monitor the patient closely. Keeping the patient quiet or at rest, caring for shock, and reassuring the responsive patient can make a difference in the outcome.

Geriatric Focus

Obtaining accurate vital signs can be challenging with the elderly patient. Small, frail arms can make it painful for them when you try to get a blood pressure. The bones of the chest have become more rigid, making it more difficult to see chest rise and fall. You may have to use other techniques, such as listening for breath sounds or watching the movement of the abdomen, when counting respirations.

Pulse

When taking a patient's pulse, you must assess for three characteristics: rate, strength, and rhythm (Figure 7.5). Pulse rate is a count of the number of heartbeats per minute and is used to determine if the patient's pulse is normal, rapid, or slow. Strength is the force of the pulse. It will be either strong or weak. Rhythm is the steadiness of the pulse, which will be either regular or irregular.

Is It Safe?

If you cannot feel a radial pulse, check for the presence of a carotid pulse in the neck. Often when there is no radial pulse, the patient does have a carotid pulse. Never begin CPR without first checking the carotid pulse.

During the initial assessment of a responsive patient, you can check the radial pulse in the patient's wrist. For an unresponsive patient, the carotid pulse in the neck should be used. The term *radial pulse* refers to the radial artery found in the

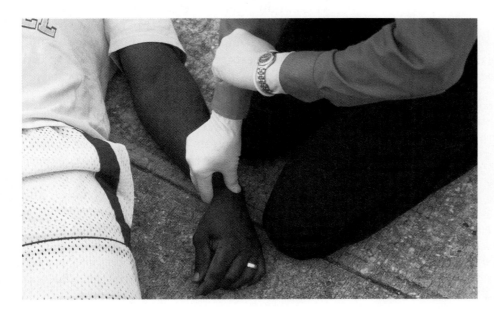

FIGURE 7.5 Rate, strength, and rhythm are characteristics of a pulse.

lateral portion of the forearm, on the thumb side of the wrist. If for any reason you are unable to feel the radial pulse, assess the carotid pulse. The absence of a radial pulse when there is a carotid pulse indicates possible shock. A radial pulse may not be detectable if the patient's blood pressure is too low or if there is an extremity injury that is interrupting blood flow to the distal arm. Do not start CPR based only on the absence of a radial pulse.

FIRST ➤ To measure a radial pulse rate:

1. Use the three middle fingers of your gloved hand. Do not use your thumb because it has its own pulse, which could be mistaken for the patient's.
2. Place your fingertips on the lateral side of the patient's anterior wrist, just above the crease between hand and wrist. Slide your fingers from this position toward the thumb side of the wrist (lateral side). Keeping the fingertip of the middle finger on the crease between wrist and hand will ensure you are placing the fingertip over the site of the radial pulse.
3. Apply moderate pressure to feel the pulse beats. If the pulse is weak, you may have to apply more pressure. Too much pressure can cause the pulse to fade. By having all three fingers in contact with the patient's wrist and hand, you should be able to judge how much pressure you are applying.
4. Once you feel the pulse, make a quick judgment as to the rate. Does the pulse feel normal, rapid, or slow?
5. Count the beats for either 15 or 30 seconds, depending on local practice or protocols.
6. While counting, assess strength and rhythm.
7. Multiply your 30-second count by 2 or your 15-second count by 4 to determine the number of beats per minute. ∎

The normal pulse rate for adults at rest is between 60 and 100 beats per minute. Any rate more than 100 is considered rapid (tachycardia), and any rate less than 60 is considered slow (bradycardia). In emergency situations, because of anxiety or excitement, it is not unusual for the pulse to be about 100 beats per minute. You should consider a pulse rate more than 100 or less than 60 to be an indication of a serious problem. One exception to this is a well-conditioned athlete whose normal resting pulse may be about 50 beats per minute or less.

Newborn infants can have pulse rates around 120 to 160 beats per minute. Children up to 5 years old will show ranges from 80 to 140 beats per minute, depending on their age. The normal range of the pulse of children from 5 to 12 years of age is 70 to 110 beats per minute. Adolescents typically have a pulse rate ranging from 60 to 105 beats per minute.

Measuring pulse rates efficiently takes experience. Practice taking both "at rest" rates and rates after mild exercise of both males and females, adults and children. Practice often. It will help you develop an ability to judge normal and rapid rates quickly and accurately.

See Table 7–2 for the relationship between pulse and certain emergency problems you may see as an Emergency Medical Responder.

FIRST ON SCENE

"Are you having trouble breathing, Craig?" Jared watched the driver's chest and counted his shallow, rapid breaths at 20 per minute.

"A little," the man said. "That's not a big deal though, right? I mean I was just unloading boxes and all."

"Honestly, Craig, it could be a big deal. I'm not really trained to make that determination." Jared turned to Ray and said, "Why don't you go ahead and call 9-1-1."

"Oh! Hold on a minute," the driver protested as he stood up. "I'm ... I'm ... I think...." He grew pale again and Jared helped him sit back on the pallet of boxes.

"Just relax, Craig," Jared said and placed a nonrebreather mask on the driver's face. He could hear Ray talking to the 9-1-1 operator through the thin, plywood walls of the dock manager's office.

TABLE 7-2	Assessment Sign—Pulse
OBSERVATION	**POSSIBLE PROBLEM**
Rapid, strong pulse	Internal bleeding (early stages), fear, heat emergency, overexertion, high blood pressure, fever
Rapid, weak pulse	Shock, blood loss, heat emergency, diabetic emergency, failing circulatory system
Slow, strong pulse	Stroke, skull fracture, brain injury
No pulse	Cardiac arrest

Respiration

As with pulses, there are several characteristics you will want to evaluate when assessing a patient's respirations (breathing) (Figure 7.6): rate, depth, sound, and ease of breathing. A single respiration is one entire cycle of breathing in and out.

The respiratory rate is a count of the patient's breaths and is classified as normal, rapid, or slow. While you are counting respirations, note if the depth is normal, shallow or deep. Notice if the breathing is easy or whether it appears labored, difficult. Listen for any abnormal sounds during breathing, such as snoring, gurgling, gasping, wheezing, or crowing. If the patient is responsive, ask if he is having any problems or pain while he breathes. A patient who has to work at breathing is in serious condition.

Table 7–3 shows some of the problems that are associated with variations in respirations.

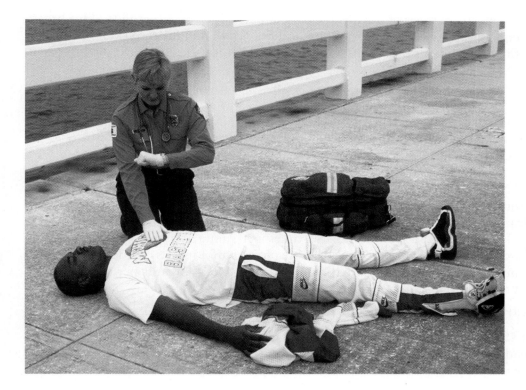

FIGURE 7.6 Rate, depth, sound, and ease are characteristics of breathing.

TABLE 7–3 | Assessment Sign—Respirations

OBSERVATION	POSSIBLE PROBLEM
Rapid, shallow breaths	Shock, heart problems, heat emergency, diabetic emergency, heart failure, pneumonia
Deep, gasping, labored breaths	Airway obstruction, heart failure, heart attack, lung disease, chest injury, diabetic emergency
Slowed breathing	Head injury, stroke, chest injury, certain drugs
Snoring	Stroke, fractured skull, drug or alcohol abuse, partial airway obstruction
Crowing	Airway obstruction, airway injury due to heat
Gurgling	Airway obstruction, lung disease, lung injury due to heat
Wheezing	Asthma, emphysema, airway obstruction, heart failure
Coughing blood	Chest wound, chest infection, fractured rib, punctured lung, internal injuries

FIRST ➤ To assess respirations, follow these steps:

1. After completing the pulse count, leave your hand in the same position at the patient's wrist, as if you were still counting the pulse rate. Do this because many patients will unknowingly alter their respiratory rate when someone is watching them breathe.

2. Observe the patient's chest move and listen for sounds.

3. Count the number of breaths the patient takes in 15 or 30 seconds. (One breath equals one inspiration plus one expiration.) To obtain the respiratory rate, multiply the number of breaths in 15 seconds by 4, or the number of breaths in 30 seconds by 2.

4. While counting respirations, note depth and ease of breathing. ◾

If you cannot visually count the patient's respiratory rate from watching chest movement, gently place your hand on the patient's chest near the notch in the lower sternum. Let the patient know you are going to touch his chest and why. This will allow you to feel each inspiration and expiration.

Normal respiratory rates for adults at rest are from 12 to 20 breaths per minute. Older adults breathe more slowly than younger adults. For adults, a respiratory rate of more than 28 or less than 8 breaths per minute is serious.

Infants breathe from 25 to 50 times per minute. If the patient is a child between one and five years of age, a rate more than 30 or less than 20 breaths per minute is serious. A rate more than 30 or less than 15 breaths per minute is serious for children six to ten years old.

Skin Color, Temperature, and Moisture

FIRST ➤ Skin color, temperature, and moisture are assessed at the patient's forehead (Figure 7.7), unless this is not possible. The patient's abdomen may also be used as a site for this assessment. Some jurisdictions may have you check the

FIGURE 7.7 Color, temperature, and moisture are characteristics of the skin.

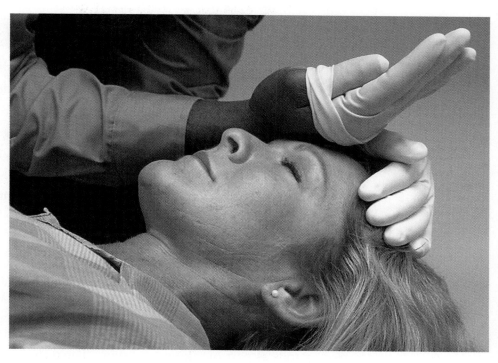

extremities. Use the back of your hand to determine if the skin is normal, hot, or cool. At the same time, notice if the skin is dry or moist. Look for "goose bumps," which are associated with chills. Observe skin color. Does it appear normal, or is the color abnormal in any way? ▪

Tables 7–4 and Table 7–5 list some of the problems associated with skin color, relative skin temperature, and moisture.

Blood Pressure

Although patient assessment is more reliable when the patient's blood pressure is taken and monitored, some Emergency Medical Responders do not carry the

TABLE 7–4	Assessment Sign—Skin Color
OBSERVATION	**SIGNIFICANCE/POSSIBLE CAUSES**
Pink	Normal in light-skinned patients; normal in inner eyelids, lips, and nail beds of dark-skinned patients
Pale	Constricted blood vessels possibly resulting from blood loss, shock, decreased blood pressure, emotional distress
Blue (cyanotic)	Lack of oxygen in blood cells and tissues resulting from inadequate breathing or heart function
Red (flushed)	Heat exposure, high blood pressure, emotional excitement; cherry red indicates late stages of carbon monoxide poisoning
Yellow (jaundiced)	Liver abnormalities
Blotchiness (mottling)	Occasionally in patients in shock

TABLE 7–5	Assessment Sign—Skin Signs
SKIN SIGNS	**SIGNIFICANCE/POSSIBLE CAUSES**
Cool, moist (clammy)	Shock, heart attack, anxiety
Cold, dry	Exposure to cold, diabetic emergency
Hot, dry	High fever, heat emergency, spine injury
Hot, moist	High fever, heat emergency, diabetic emergency
Goose bumps accompanied by shivering, chattering teeth, blue lips, and pale skin	Chills, communicable disease, exposure to cold, pain, or fear

necessary equipment to measure this vital sign (Figure 7.8). If your EMS system requires that you determine blood pressure, see Appendix 1.

Pupils

Many EMS systems have the Emergency Medical Responder assess the patient's pupils as part of taking vital signs. The technique used and information gathered are described on pages 192–193 as part of the head-to-toe examination. Table 7–6 provides observations you may make when assessing a patient's pupils and lists possible causes.

PHYSICAL EXAM

If your trauma patient has no significant MOI and appears to have an isolated minor injury (supported by the MOI and what the patient tells you), perform a focused trauma assessment on the injury site and the area close to it. If the patient

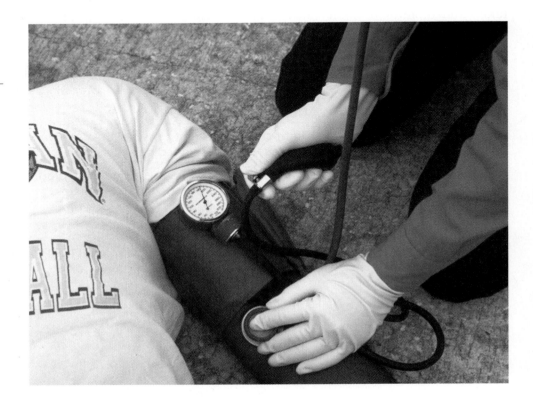

FIGURE 7.8 Blood pressure is a vital sign that some Emergency Medical Responders may be required to measure.

TABLE 7–6	Assessment Sign—Pupils

OBSERVATION	POSSIBLE PROBLEM
Dilated, nonreactive pupils	Shock, cardiac arrest, bleeding, certain medications, head injury
Constricted, nonreactive pupils	Central nervous system damage, certain medications
Unequal pupils	Stroke, head injury

has a significant MOI, a serious injury, or is unresponsive, perform a rapid trauma assessment of the entire body.

The physical exam of a medical patient may be brief. If the patient is responsive, perform a focused physical exam based on the patient's chief complaint. If the patient is unresponsive, conduct a rapid physical exam of the entire body.

When assessing a trauma patient, you may use a memory aid, such as **BP-DOC** or **DCAP-BTLS,** to help you remember what to look for during any physical exam. The letters stand for:

BP-DOC

B — Bleeding.

P — Pain.

D — Deformities.

O — Open wounds.

C — **Crepitus** (a grating noise or sensation).

DCAP-BTLS

D — Deformities.

C — Contusions.

A — Abrasions.

P — Punctures and penetrations.

B — Burns.

T — Tenderness.

L — Lacerations.

S — Swelling.

BP-DOC ▪ a memory aid used to recall what to look for in a physical exam. The letters stand for *bleeding, pain, deformities, open wounds,* and *crepitus.*

DCAP-BTLS ▪ a memory aid used to recall what to look for in a physical exam. The letters stand for *deformities, contusions, abrasions, punctures and penetrations, burns, tenderness, lacerations,* and *swelling.*

crepitus (KREP-i-tus) ▪ a grating noise or the sensation felt when broken bone ends rub together.

NOTE

It is not necessary to learn each and every memory tool for assessment. The important thing is to find one that you understand and are comfortable with and then use it consistently.

Rapid Trauma Assessment—Trauma Patient with Significant MOI

The rapid trauma assessment is a head-to-toe physical exam of the patient that should take no more than 90 seconds to two minutes. It is performed on patients who have a significant MOI. These patients will most likely have a high priority for transport. Take great care not to move the patient unless absolutely necessary. Neck and spine injuries may be present. To save time, another Emergency Medical Responder may take vital signs while you perform the exam.

It is usually not necessary for the Emergency Medical Responder to remove the patient's clothing during a head-to-toe exam. Of course, you may remove or readjust clothing that interferes with your ability to examine the patient. Cut away, lift, slide, or unbutton clothing covering a suspected injury site, especially the chest, back, and abdomen, so you can fully inspect the area. Also, check the patient's clothing for evidence of bleeding.

REMEMBER

No matter what other injuries a patient has or does not have, a patient who is unresponsive or who has an altered mental status is a high priority for immediate transport.

Suspect internal injuries if your responsive patient indicates pain in the area or pain when you touch the area during your exam. If the patient is unresponsive, you may want to remove or rearrange clothing covering the chest, abdomen, and back to examine those areas of the body completely. If you must remove or rearrange the clothing of a responsive patient, tell him what you are doing and why. Take great care to respect the modesty of the patient. Also protect him from harsh weather conditions and temperatures.

Geriatric Focus

There are many factors that contribute to the high incidence of trauma in the elderly, including arthritis, slower reflexes, poor vision, and hearing loss. Their ability to heal efficiently from injury is also diminished and therefore can lead to much longer recovery times.

Many EMS systems recommend or require having another woman present when a male Emergency Medical Responder examines a female patient. However, do not delay examining any patient. As a trained Emergency Medical Responder in an emergency situation, your intentions should be respected.

Is It Safe?

Often there is no way to know for sure if an unresponsive patient experienced spinal trauma. Therefore, when assessing and caring for an unresponsive patient, maintain a high degree of suspicion for spine injuries. Maintain manual stabilization of the head and spine until you can positively rule out injury or until you can immobilize the patient on a long spine board.

While performing a rapid trauma assessment, avoid contaminating your patient's wounds and aggravating his injuries. Be sure to take the appropriate BSI precautions.

FIRST ▶ To perform your assessment:

1. Check the scalp for cuts and bruises (Figure 7.9). Take care not to move the patient's head. Run your fingers through the patient's hair to look for blood. Gently feel for cuts, swelling, or any other injuries. Do not part the hair over a suspected scalp injury. This could cause more bleeding. Gently slide your gloved fingers under the back of the patient's neck and upward to the back of the head. Check your glove for blood.

2. Check the skull for deformities and depressions and check the face (Figure 7.10). Note any depressions or bony projections that would indicate an injury to the skull. Check the facial bones for any signs or symptoms of a possible fracture or crushing, swelling, heavy discoloration, or depressions of the bones. Have the patient smile and notice if the muscles of the face move evenly. The smile should be even on both sides.

3. Examine the patient's eyes (Figure 7.11). Note any cuts, impaled objects, or signs of damage. Have the patient open his eyes, or gently open the eyes of an unresponsive patient. Check the pupils for size, equality, and reaction to light. A penlight would be helpful for this. If you are outside in bright sunlight, cover the patient's eye with your hand. Remove your hand quickly and watch for reaction of the pupil to the light. Pupils that are dilated or constricted may indicate possible drug usage, shock, or cardiac arrest. Unequal

3–1.17 State the areas of the body that are evaluated during the physical exam.

REMEMBER

In a rapid trauma assessment, each area of the body is checked for DCAP-BTLS, plus other problems specific to the area.

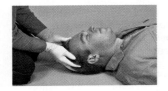

FIGURE 7.9 Examine the scalp. (Step 1)

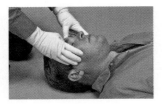

FIGURE 7.10 Check the skull and face. (Step 2)

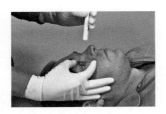

FIGURE 7.11 Examine the eyelids, eyes, and pupils. (Steps 3 and 4)

pupils may indicate a brain or spine injury. Pupils that react sluggishly may indicate shock.

4. Look at the inner surface of the eyelids (conjunctiva). The tissue should be pink and moist. A pale color may indicate poor perfusion.

5. Inspect the ears and nose for drainage, either clear or bloody (Figure 7.12). Use a penlight or other light source for this. Blood in the nose may be caused by a simple nasal tissue injury. But it could also mean a skull fracture. Blood in the ears or clear or bloody fluids in the ears or nose are strong indications of a skull fracture. Also inspect the nose for singed nostrils, which may indicate the inhalation of toxic smoke. Flaring nostrils may be a sign of respiratory distress.

6. Inspect the mouth for foreign material, bleeding, and tissue damage (Figure 7.13). If your patient is unresponsive, you will have to open his mouth. Consider all unresponsive trauma patients to have neck and spine injuries, so open the mouth gently, without moving the head. Look for broken teeth, bridges, dentures, and crowns. Check for chewing gum, food, vomit, and foreign objects. In children, take extra care in looking for toys, balls, and other objects in the mouth and the back of the throat. If you find any objects, follow the directions given in Chapter 6. Inspect the mouth for blood and note any odd breath odors.

7. Check the cervical spine for tenderness and deformity (Figure 7.14). Any tenderness or deformity should be considered an indication of a possible spine injury. If you have already immobilized the patient's head and neck, continue with the exam. If not, stop the exam and immobilize the head and neck now, before continuing. Next, gently check the patient's chin for tenderness and deformity, steadying the patient's chin with one hand. Look for any medical identification jewelry. If one is found, make note of what it says but do not remove it.

8. Check the front of the neck for injury and deformity (Figure 7.15). Also notice if the patient has a stoma, a surgical opening in the front or side of his neck. Observe and palpate for evidence of **tracheal deviation** (any shift of the trachea to one side or the other). Observe for bulging neck veins also known as **jugular vein distention (JVD)** and **accessory muscle use**, which may be a sign of respiratory distress.

9. Inspect the chest for cuts, bruises, penetrations, and impaled objects (Figure 7.16). If necessary, bare the chest and upper abdomen. Leave impaled objects in place. Also check for medical identification jewelry.

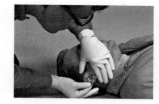

FIGURE 7.12 Check the ears and nose for blood and fluids. (Step 5)

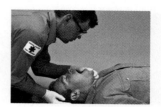

FIGURE 7.13 Examine the mouth for obstructions, bleeding, and tissue damage. (Step 6)

tracheal deviation ■ a shifting of the trachea to either side of the midline of the neck caused by the buildup of pressure inside the chest.

jugular vein distention (JVD) ■ an abnormal bulging of the veins of the neck indicating possible injury to the chest or heart.

accessory muscle use ■ the use of the muscles of the neck, chest, and abdomen to assist with breathing effort.

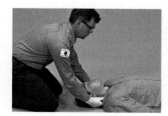

FIGURE 7.14 Check the cervical spine for tenderness and deformity. (Step 7)

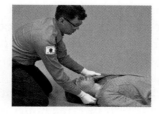

FIGURE 7.15 Check the front of the neck for injuries and openings. Also look for medical identification jewelry. (Step 8)

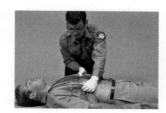

FIGURE 7.16 Inspect the chest for injuries. (Step 9)

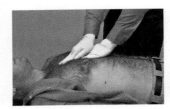

FIGURE 7.17 Check the clavicles and sternum for tenderness and deformity. (Step 10)

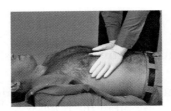

FIGURE 7.18 Check for rib fractures. Then observe for equal expansion of the chest. (Steps 11 and 12)

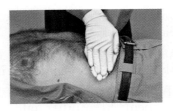

FIGURE 7.19 Inspect the abdomen for injuries. (Steps 13 and 14)

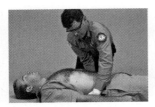

FIGURE 7.20 Check the lower back for point tenderness and deformity. (Step 15)

paradoxical movement ■ movement of an area of the chest wall in opposition to the rest of the chest during respiration.

guarding ■ the protection of an area of injury or pain by the patient; the spasming of muscles to minimize movement that might cause pain.

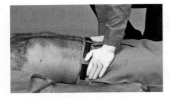

FIGURE 7.21 Check for pelvic injuries. Then inspect the genital region. (Steps 16 and 17)

incontinence ■ loss of bladder and/or bowel control.

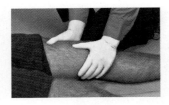

FIGURE 7.22 Examine the legs and feet. *Do not lift or move them.* (Step 18)

10. Examine the chest for possible collarbone (clavicle) and breastbone (sternum) injury (Figure 7.17). Feel for tenderness and deformity.

11. Examine for possible rib fractures (Figure 7.18). Gently apply pressure to the sides of the chest with your hands. Warn the patient of possible pain. Pain here indicates possible rib fractures.

12. Observe and feel for equal expansion of both sides of the chest. Note any portion that appears to be floating or moving in opposite directions to the rest of the chest; this is called **paradoxical movement**. It could indicate an injury called a *flail chest* in which two or more ribs are fractured in two or more places, causing them to float in the chest. When baring the chest of female patients, provide them with as much privacy as possible.

13. Inspect the abdomen for cuts, bruises, penetrations, distention, rigidity, and **guarding**.

14. Feel the abdomen for tenderness (Figure 7.19). Prepare the patient for the possibility of pain. If the patient tells you his abdomen already hurts, leave the area alone, but ask him to describe the pain and where exactly it is located. Gently press on the abdomen with the palm side of the fingers, noting any areas that are rigid, swollen, or painful. As you press on the area, ask the patient if it hurts. Note if the pain is local (just one spot) or general (spread over a wide area). Check each abdominal quadrant, and note any problems in that specific quadrant.

15. Feel the lower back for tenderness and look for deformity (Figure 7.20). Take care not to move the patient. Gently slide your gloved hands into the area of the lower back that is formed by the curve of the spine. Check your gloves for blood.

16. Feel the pelvis for injuries and possible fractures (Figure 7.21). After checking the lower back, gently slide your hands from the small of the back to the lateral wings of the pelvis. Warn the patient of possible pain and gently compress the pelvis. Press in and down at the same time, noting any pain or deformity.

17. Note any obvious injury to the genital region. Look for wetness caused by **incontinence** or bleeding and impaled objects. Do not expose the area unless you suspect there is an injury. In male patients, check for *priapism* (PRI-ah-pizm), the persistent erection of the penis. If there is any reason to suspect spine injury and clothing prevents you from noting the presence of an erect penis, gently brush the genital region with the back of your hand. Priapism is an important indication of spine injury and should be noted during the head-to-toe exam.

18. Examine the legs and feet (Figure 7.22). Examine each leg and foot individually. Compare one limb to the other in terms of length, shape, and any apparent

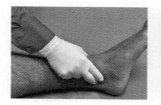
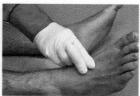

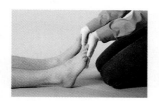

FIGURE 7.23 When possible and without risk to the patient, check for distal pulses. (Step 19)

swelling or deformity. Do not move or lift the legs. Do not change the position of the legs or feet. Note any discoloration, bleeding, bone protrusions, and obvious deformity.

19. Check for distal pulse (Figure 7.23), which would confirm the circulation of blood through the leg and foot. The most useful is the **posterior tibial pulse**, felt behind the medial ankle. If the patient is wearing boots, do not remove them if the patient has indications of crush injury to the leg or foot, objects impaled in the leg or foot, severe leg or foot fractures, or any indications or possibilities of spine injury, unless you must to stop obvious bleeding.

    Another distal pulse is the **dorsalis pedis pulse**, which is located lateral to the large tendon of the big toe. This pulse can be important in assessment because some patients do not have a posterior tibial pulse. Some EMS systems do not have Emergency Medical Responders use the dorsalis pedis pulse in the exam because they would have to unlace or remove the patient's shoe to feel this pulse.

    What you can do about a problem of circulation is minimal. Do not cause additional injury to the patient for the sake of taking a distal pulse. When possible, check both feet for a distal pulse. You may also check capillary refill in pediatric patients (infants and children) at this time.

20. Check the feet for motor function and sensation (Figure 7.24 and 7.25). Touch each toe, and have the patient tell you if he can feel it. You may grasp the toes through the patient's shoe if you believe there are no injuries to the toes. Have the patient gently press the sole of each foot against the palm of your hand and, with your hand on the top of his foot, have him pull up, or flex his foot, lifting your hand. Then pinch the top of the foot. Do these tests on both feet. If the patient does not respond to any one of these tests, assume spine injury. Look for signs of **track marks** and medical identification jewelry.

21. Examine the upper extremities from the shoulders to the fingertips (Figures 7.26 to 7.28). Examine each limb separately. The procedures are similar to those of the lower extremities.

    — Note any cuts, bruises, impaled objects, bleeding, deformities, swelling, discoloration, or obvious fractures. Check for tenderness at any suspected site of fracture. Do not touch open fracture sites.

posterior tibial (TIB-e-al) pulse ■ the pulse felt behind the medial ankle.

dorsalis pedis (dor-SAL-is PEED-is) pulse ■ the pulse located lateral to the large tendon of the big toe.

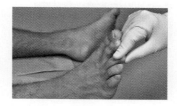

FIGURE 7.24 Check for motor function and sensation. (Step 20)

track marks ■ small dots of infection that form a track along a vein; may be an indication of IV drug abuse.

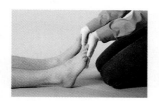

FIGURE 7.25 Can the patient push his foot against the palm of your hand? (Step 20)

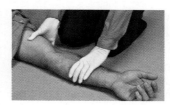

FIGURE 7.26 Check the arms and hands for injuries. (Step 21)

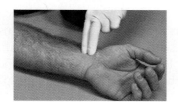

FIGURE 7.27 Take a radial pulse. Remember, you did this for one arm when finding vital signs. (Step 21)

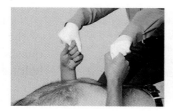

FIGURE 7.28 Can the patient grip your hands with his? (Step 21)

Suspect spine injury if the patient fails to respond properly on any test of the leg or arm. Also, an alert patient who cannot move his hands or arms may suddenly stop breathing due to a spine injury. The patient may also show signs and symptoms of shock. Continually monitor the patient.

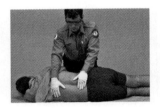

FIGURE 7.29 If there are no injuries to the head, neck, spine, or extremities, inspect the back surface. (Step 22)

— Confirm a radial (wrist) pulse in both arms. Do not measure pulse rate. Simply confirm circulation. You may also check capillary refill in pediatric patients.

— Check for motor function and sensation. If alert, have the patient identify the finger you touch and grip your hand. When checking grip, test both hands at once to determine equality of strength. Have the patient grip your thumbs, one in each hand; having the patient squeeze your whole hand may be painful for you. If the patient is unresponsive, pinch the back of his hand.

— Look for evidence of track marks and medical identification jewelry.

22. Inspect the back surfaces of the patient for bleeding and obvious injury (Figure 7.29). Do not lift or roll the patient if there is any indication of skull, neck, spine, or serious extremity injury. Consider any unresponsive trauma patient as having a neck injury. ◾

Focused Trauma Assessment—Trauma Patient with No Significant MOI

When your trauma patient has no significant MOI, the steps of the focused trauma assessment are appropriately simplified. Instead of examining the patient from head to toe, focus your assessment on just the areas that the patient tells you are painful or that you suspect may be injured because of the MOI. The assessment includes a physical exam, vital signs, and a patient history.

Your decision on which areas of the patient's body to assess will depend partly on what you see and partly on the patient's chief complaint. Be sure to consider potential injuries based on the MOI. For example, if the patient's chief complaint is pain in his leg after falling down several stairs, consider possible back or neck injuries and care for the patient accordingly. Use the memory aid DCAP-BTLS to help you properly perform your assessment.

Rapid Physical Exam—Unresponsive Medical Patient

The rapid physical exam of an unresponsive medical patient is almost the same as the rapid trauma assessment of a trauma patient with a significant MOI. You will rapidly assess the patient's head, neck, chest, abdomen, pelvis, extremities, and posterior. As you assess each area of the body, look for signs of illness. Be sure to assess for:

- *Neck.* Look for neck vein distention and medical identification jewelry.
- *Chest.* Check presence and equality of breath sounds.
- *Abdomen.* Assess for distention, firmness, or rigidity.
- *Pelvis.* Check for incontinence of urine or feces.
- *Extremities.* Check circulation, sensation, and motor function, and for presence of medical identification jewelry.

Focused Physical Exam—Responsive Medical Patient

The focused physical exam of a responsive medical patient is usually brief. The most important assessment information is obtained through the patient history and the taking of vital signs. Focus the exam on the body part that the patient has a complaint about. For example, if the patient complains of abdominal pain, focus your exam on that area of the body. Another memory aid used to help assess the responsive medical patient is known as the **OPQRST** assessment. Just as with the acronym SAMPLE, each of the letters represents a word, and each of the words is designed to trigger specific questions that the Emergency Medical Responder should ask. OPQRST is especially helpful when the chief complaint is related to pain or shortness of breath:

OPQRST ◾ a memory device used for assessing the responsive medical patient. It stands for *onset, provocation, quality, region/radiate, severity,* and *time.*

O — *Onset.* This letter is designed to trigger questions pertaining to what the patient was doing at the onset of pain (when the pain or symptoms began). For example, "What were you doing when the pain began?" or "What were you doing when you first began to feel short of breath?"

P — *Provocation.* Ask questions pertaining to what provokes or affects the pain. For example, "Does anything you do make the pain better or worse?" or "Does it hurt to take a deep breath or when I push here?"

Q — *Quality.* Ask about the quality of the pain; that is, find out what the pain or symptom actually feels like. For example, ask, "Can you describe how your pain feels?" or "Is the pain sharp, or is it dull?" or "Is it steady, or does it come and go?"

R — *Region and radiate.* Ask where the pain is originating and to where it may be moving or radiating. For example, "Can you point with one finger to where your pain is the worst?" or "Does your pain move or radiate to any other part of your body?" or "Do you feel pain anywhere else besides your chest?"

S — *Severity.* Ask about the severity of the pain or discomfort. A standard 1-to-10 scale is typically presented like this: "On a scale of 1 to 10, with 10 being the worst pain you have ever felt, how would you rate your pain right now?" Using the same scale, also ask the patient to describe the severity of his pain when it first began. Once you have been with the patient a while and provided care, you will want to ask the severity question again to see if his pain is getting better or worse.

T — *Time.* Ask the patient how long he may have been experiencing the pain or discomfort. A simple question such as, "When did you first begin having pain today?" or "How long have you had this pain?" will usually suffice.

Geriatric Focus

Many elderly patients have a much higher tolerance for pain and may not always feel the result of a significant injury or illness. A thorough and methodical assessment may reveal areas of involvement that were not initially seen or part of the chief complaint.

Be careful not to put words in the patient's mouth. Instead, provide the patient with choices and then allow him to choose. It is also important to use the patient's own words when documenting the call or when transferring care of the patient to more highly trained personnel. For example, if the patient tells you he feels as though an anvil is sitting on his chest, quote his words to describe the pain. Do not paraphrase or attempt to translate what he said into medical terminology.

Completing the Exam

On completing the physical exam of the patient, you must consider all the signs and symptoms found that could indicate an illness or injury. Certain combinations of signs and symptoms can point to one specific problem. A finding as simple as pain in a certain region of the body may be significant. The lack of certain findings may also lead you to a conclusion. For example, if a patient has an obvious injury but feels no pain at the site, you must consider problems such as spine injury, brain damage, shock, or drug abuse.

FIRST ON SCENE

"Okay, Craig," Jared said and knelt in front of the driver. "While we wait for the ambulance, let's talk about your chest pain." The driver, now frightened by his symptoms, nodded with wide eyes. "I already know that you were unloading the truck when the pain started, right?"

"Yes," Craig said, his voice somewhat muffled by the plastic oxygen mask.

"Does anything make it better or worse? You know, like if you move a certain way or push on it?"

The driver moved his upper body back and forth and pressed harder on his chest. "No," he answered.

The sound of sirens quickly approached the parking lot next door to the loading dock. "Okay," Jared was now writing in a small notebook. "What does the pain feel like?"

The driver thought for a moment and pulled the mask up to speak. "Like a pressure. Like a heavy weight or something right on my chest."

TABLE 7–7	**Rules for Patient Assessment**
1.	Do no further harm.
2.	If anything about the patient's awareness or behavior does not seem "right," consider that something is seriously wrong.
3.	Patients who appear stable may worsen rapidly. You must be alert to all changes in a patient's condition.
4.	Watch the patient's skin for color changes.
5.	Look over the entire patient, and note anything that appears to be wrong.
6.	Unless you are certain that the patient is free of spine injury, assume every trauma patient has a spine injury.
7.	Tell the patient that you are going to examine him, what you will be doing, and why you are doing it. Stress the importance of the exam.
8.	Take vital signs.
9.	Conduct a head-to-toe exam. If anything looks, sounds, feels, smells, or "seems" wrong to you or the patient, assume that there is something seriously wrong with the patient.
10.	Failure of the patient to respond properly on any test for sensation or motor function in the leg or arm must be considered a sign of spine injury.

During your assessment of the patient and throughout the time you are caring for him, remember the first rule of emergency care: *Do no further harm*. Be sure to do only what you have been trained to do. Avoid adding injury and aggravating existing injuries and problems. (See a summary of Rules for Patient Examination in Table 7–7.) Later in your training, you will learn what you can do to help the patient based on the findings in your physical exam.

Detailed Physical Exam

Usually, a full detailed physical exam is performed on the patient while en route to the hospital or medical facility. If the response time of the EMTs is lengthy, you may perform this exam if time permits. Sometimes, the Emergency Medical Responder is part of the crew or may accompany the ambulance crew to assist in continuing care of the patient. During that time, a detailed physical exam is done by repeating the rapid trauma assessment in much more detail and by taking more time. Detailed physical exams are performed on trauma patients with a significant MOI. You also may perform a detailed physical exam on responsive medical patients, but you may be too involved in necessary patient care to do one on unresponsive medical patients.

Ongoing Assessment

3–1.20 Discuss the components of the ongoing assessment.

When performing the ongoing assessment either at the scene or en route to the hospital, repeat the initial assessment, reassess vital signs, and check any interventions to ensure they are still effective. Reassess the patient, watching closely for any changes in his condition. Repeating assessments and noting any changes in patient condition are ways of **trending** a patient's condition. Remember that patients will get better, get worse, or stay the same. Seriously ill or injured patients should be reassessed every five minutes. A good rule to follow is that by the time you finish the ongoing assessment from start to finish, it is time to start over with the beginning of the next ongoing assessment. Patients who are not seriously ill or injured should be reassessed every 15 minutes.

trending ■ monitoring the patient's signs and symptoms and documenting any changes, both good and bad.

Hand-off to EMTS

When additional EMS providers arrive at the scene, it is important to communicate with them well. Give the responding EMTs a verbal report, including:

3–1.21 Describe the information included in the hand-off report.

- Name and age.
- Chief complaint.
- Mental status.
- Airway, breathing, and circulatory status.
- Physical findings.
- Patient history.
- Interventions applied and the patient's response to them.

Some EMS systems also require the Emergency Medical Responder to provide a written report to the EMT crew. It usually includes the same information as the verbal report. The written report and the information in it will become part of the EMT crew's patient care report. Accuracy is vital in any verbal or written report because care given by the responding EMTs and the hospital emergency department staff may be based, in part, on your evaluation of the patient.

 FIRST ON SCENE WRAP-UP

Before Jared could ask the next question, Ray, his partner in this incident, led a group of firefighters to the loading dock. They were carrying several bags and a bright green AED. "Okay," the firefighter in the lead said, pulling on a pair of purple exam gloves. "Who do we have here?"

Jared introduced Craig and explained the situation. Just as he finished, an ambulance crew arrived, noisily rolling a wheeled stretcher across the metal grating of the loading dock floor. In one fluid motion, the ambulance crew had obtained a set of vitals, loaded the patient onto the wheeled stretcher, switched the nonrebreather mask onto their own oxygen tank, and rolled him out to the waiting ambulance. Jared and Ray stood and watched the firefighters and ambulance crew load up into their vehicles and disappear from the parking lot.

"Boy," Ray said as the men turned and returned to the building. "That went just like clockwork."

"Yes it did." Jared held the door open for Ray and patted him on the shoulder as they walked back into the darkness of the loading dock. "And next time you get to do patient care."

Summary

Patient assessment is one of the most important skills you will learn as an Emergency Medical Responder. Even though it may seem time consuming, it is necessary to properly and completely examine the patient if you are to determine what care the patient requires. You must detect life-threatening problems and correct them as quickly as possible. Then you must detect problems that may become life threatening if left without care. Always keep the following in mind:

- *Arrival.* Perform a scene size-up. Make sure the scene is safe to enter. Gain information quickly from the scene, the patient, and bystanders. If possible, determine the patient's NOI or MOI.

- *Initial assessment.* Determine if the patient is responsive. If you suspect a spine injury, maintain manual stabilization of the head and neck. Make certain that the patient has an open airway, adequate breathing, and a pulse. Control all serious bleeding.

- *Focused history and physical exam.* Look over the patient. Look for medical identification jewelry. Begin gathering information by asking questions and listening. The more organized your interview and physical exam are, the better your chances of gaining the needed information. Use the SAMPLE, DCAP-BTLS, and OPQRST assessment tools as appropriate.

  As part of your examination of the patient, take vital signs. Remember that baseline vital signs—plus repeated vital signs over time—are valuable to the personnel who take over patient care. Determine the pulse and respiratory rate and character. Assess skin for color, temperature, and moisture. In some areas, Emergency Medical Responders also assess pupils and measure blood pressure.

The physical exam of a patient varies somewhat, depending on whether the patient is a medical or trauma patient. A head-to-toe exam consists of the following:

- *Head.* Check the scalp for cuts, bruises, swellings, and the skull and facial bones for deformities, depressions, and other signs of injury. Inspect the eyelids and the eyes for injury and check pupil size, equality, and reactions to light. Note the color of the inner surface of the eyelids. Look for blood, clear fluids, or bloody fluids in the nose and ears. Examine the mouth for airway obstructions, blood, and any odd odors.

- *Neck.* Examine the cervical spine for tenderness and deformity. Recheck to see if the patient has a stoma. Note obvious injuries and look for medical identification jewelry.

- *Chest.* Examine the chest for cuts, bruises, penetrations, and impaled objects. Check for possible bone fractures. Look for equal expansion and note chest movements.

- *Abdomen.* Examine the abdomen for cuts, bruises, penetrations, and impaled objects. Check for local and general pain as you examine the abdomen for tenderness.

- *Lower back.* Feel for point tenderness, deformity, and other signs of injury. Check the rest of the back last and only if it is safe to roll the patient (no suspected spine injuries).

- *Pelvis.* Press in and down to check for possible fractures and note any signs of injuries.

- *Genital region.* Note any obvious injuries. Look for wetness. Note the presence of priapism when examining male patients.

- *Extremities.* Examine for deformities, swelling, bleeding, discoloration, bone protrusions, and obvious fractures. Check for point tenderness on all suspected closed fracture sites. Check for distal pulse. In pediatric patients, check for capillary refill. Determine motor function and sensation as appropriate. Remember to look for medical identification jewelry.

  Although EMTs usually complete the detailed physical exam en route to the hospital, in some systems Emergency Medical Responders may assist by repeating the initial assessment and vital signs. If you also assist with the ongoing assessment, note any changes in patient condition or the need for additional interventions.

Remember and Consider

It is extremely important that you constantly review the systematic approach to patient assessment.

➤ Take time now to review the rules for patient exam in Table 7–7. You might consider copying each rule onto a three-by-five card and keeping them as quick reminders.

Consider the importance of vital signs and what they can tell you about a patient's condition. Keep in mind:

➤ In an adult, a pulse rate of less than 60 beats per minute or more than 100 beats per minute is considered serious.

➤ In an adult, a respiratory rate more than 28 breaths per minute or less than 8 breaths per minute is considered serious.

➤ Skin signs can signal serious problems such as shock, heart attack, decreased blood pressure, and heat and cold emergencies.

➤ Also remember the memory aids DCAP-BTLS, SAMPLE history, and OPQRST assessment. Work with a partner and practice using them in various scenarios.

Investigate

Additional vital signs that some Emergency Medical Responders may be required to take include determining blood pressure and examining the patient's pupils.

➤ Find out if your service or company requires you to know how to take a patient's blood pressure. If so, review Appendix 1. Are you required to examine the patient's pupils? If so, review Table 7–6.

Quick Quiz

1. For most patients, an Emergency Medical Responder's assessment begins with performing a scene size-up followed by:
   a. conducting a focused history.
   b. performing an initial assessment.
   c. obtaining vital signs.
   d. determining the nature of illness.

2. After arriving on scene, but before making patient contact, you should:
   a. perform an initial assessment.
   b. contact medical direction.
   c. perform a patient assessment.
   d. take appropriate BSI precautions.

3. There are six components to the initial assessment, beginning with:
   a. assessing the patient's mental status.
   b. assessing the patient's airway.
   c. forming a general impression of the patient.
   d. evaluating patient's circulation.

4. The assessment of a patient's mental status or responsiveness includes using the_____scale.
   a. AVPU
   b. ABC
   c. QRS
   d. TUV

5. In a SAMPLE history, "E" represents:
   a. EKG results.
   b. evaluation of the neck and spine.
   c. events leading to illness or injury.
   d. evidence of airway obstruction.

6. When assessing circulation for a responsive adult patient, you should assess:
   a. the carotid pulse.
   b. radial pulses on both sides of the body.
   c. the radial pulse on one side.
   d. a distal pulse.

7. When assessing a trauma patient with NO significant mechanism of injury, perform a focused trauma assessment, followed by:
   a. rapid physical exam.
   b. a SAMPLE history.
   c. a rapid trauma assessment.
   d. vital signs.

8. The adequate flow of oxygenated blood to all cells of the body is called:
   a. circulation.
   b. perfusion.
   c. compensation.
   d. systole.

9. When assessing a patient's respirations, you need to determine both rate, depth, and:
   a. regularity.
   b. count of expirations.
   c. ease.
   d. count of inspirations.

10. There are 10 rules for a patient examination, the first of which is always:
    a. if patient behavior does not seem "right," consider that something is seriously wrong.
    b. do no further harm.
    c. take vital signs.
    d. watch for skin color changes.

11. Following is a list of steps carried out during a rapid trauma assessment. The steps are not listed in the correct order. On separate sheet of paper, write the numerals 1 to 22 in a column. Then copy these steps in the correct order.

a. Inspect chest for penetrations, cuts, bruises, and impaled objects.

b. Feel pelvis for possible fractures.

c. Inspect scalp for cuts and bruises.

d. Check each upper extremity for injury and paralysis.

e. Inspect the back surfaces.

f. Examine the eyes (including the pupils).

g. Inspect the mouth for possible airway obstructions.

h. Inspect genital region (groin) for obvious injury.

i. Examine chest for possible rib fracture.

j. Feel lower back for point tenderness and look for deformity.

k. Inspect ears and nose for blood, clear fluids, or bloody fluid.

l. Check the lower extremities for sensation and motor function.

m. Observe and feel for equal expansion of both sides of chest.

n. Inspect abdomen for cuts, bruises, penetrations.

o. Check for distal pulses in the feet.

p. Look at inner surface of eyelids (conjunctiva).

q. Feel abdomen for tenderness.

r. Check the cervical spine for point tenderness and deformity.

s. Examine the legs and feet.

t. Check the front of neck for injury and deformity.

u. Check the face and skull for deformity and depressions.

v. Examine the chest for possible collarbone or breastbone fractures.

8 Resuscitation and Use of the AED

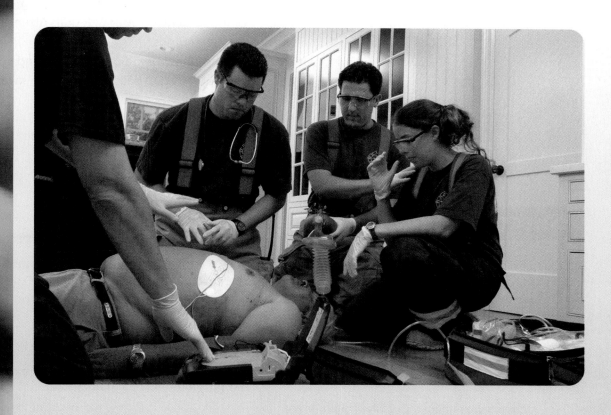

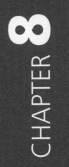

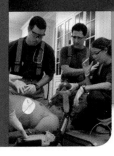

Resuscitation and Use of the AED

Research and statistics from the American Heart Association (AHA) show that there are approximately 900,000 deaths each year due to cardiovascular disease. Approximately one-third of those people die suddenly from cardiac arrest. Over the years, researchers have studied and refined CPR so that emergency care providers can learn it easily and provide it effectively when a patient needs it. Emergency Medical Responders are often the closest and quickest sources of assistance for those experiencing cardiac arrest. It is important to make a point of practicing your CPR skills often and keeping up to date with the latest research findings.

This chapter presents the latest guidelines for CPR and for the use of the automated external defibrillator (AED), skills that can help save lives.

OBJECTIVES

This chapter is based on the objectives of the U.S. DOT's First Responder National Standard Curriculum. Note that cognitive objectives are listed below and beside corresponding text throughout the chapter. You will also notice as you read each objective that the term Emergency Medical Responder is used. This is simply a name change and reflects the new name for the First Responder.

By the end of this chapter, you should be able to (from cognitive or knowledge information):

4–1.1 List the reasons for the heart to stop beating. (p. 207)

4–1.2 Define the components of cardiopulmonary resuscitation. (p. 208)

4–1.3 Describe each link in the chain of survival and how it relates to the EMS system. (pp. 206–207)

4–1.4 List the steps of one-rescuer adult CPR. (pp. 216–219)

4–1.5 Describe the technique of external chest compressions on an adult patient. (pp. 213–214)

4–1.6 Describe the technique of external chest compressions on an infant. (p. 225)

4–1.7 Describe the technique of external chest compressions on a child. (pp. 213–214)

4–1.8 Explain when an Emergency Medical Responder is able to stop CPR. (pp. 230–232)

4–1.9 List the steps of two-rescuer adult CPR. (pp. 220–223)

4–1.10 List the steps of infant CPR. (pp. 223–226)

4–1.11 List the steps of child CPR. (pp. 216–219)

CHAPTER 8

By the end of this chapter, you should be able to feel comfortable enough to (by changing attitudes, values, and beliefs):

4–1.12 Respond to the feelings that the family of a patient may be having during a cardiac event. (pp. 230–231)

4–1.13 Demonstrate a caring attitude toward patients with cardiac events who request emergency medical services. (pp. 230–231)

4–1.14 Place the interests of the patient with a cardiac event as the foremost consideration when making any and all patient-care decisions. (pp. 230–231)

4–1.15 Communicate with empathy with family members and friends of the patient with a cardiac event. (pp. 230–231)

By the end of this chapter, you should be able to show how to (through psychomotor skills):

4–1.16 Demonstrate the proper technique of chest compressions on an adult manikin. (pp. 213–214)

4–1.17 Demonstrate the proper technique of chest compressions on a child manikin. (pp. 213–214)

4–1.18 Demonstrate the proper technique of chest compressions on an infant manikin. (p. 225)

4–1.19 Demonstrate the steps of adult one-rescuer CPR on a manikin. (pp. 216–219)

4–1.20 Demonstrate the steps of adult two-rescuer CPR. (pp. 220–223)

4–1.21 Demonstrate child CPR on a manikin. (pp. 216–219)

4–1.22 Demonstrate infant CPR on a manikin. (pp. 223–226)

ADDITIONAL LEARNING TASKS

This chapter explains the functions of the heart and lungs as they work together to circulate life-giving, oxygen-rich blood to the brain and other vital organs. It also will help you apply that knowledge during your study of CPR. As you work through this chapter, you will be able to:

➤ Recognize the signs of cardiac arrest.
➤ Explain how CPR works to keep the brain and other vital organs supplied with oxygen-rich blood.

It is important that you learn the latest steps for performing CPR so that you can perform them in an emergency without hesitation. One way to develop proficiency is to work with your classmates and coach one another as you use manikins to:

➤ Locate the proper compression site on an infant, child, and adult.
➤ State the compression/ventilation ratios for infant, child, and adult CPR.
➤ Practice performing infant, child, and adult CPR.

It can be difficult and tiring to maintain one-rescuer CPR for any length of time. Two-rescuer CPR has some distinct advantages, but it takes a little more training and practice. After this chapter, you will be able to:

➤ State the advantages of two-rescuer CPR over one-rescuer CPR.

When you become tired during two-rescuer CPR, you may switch or change positions with your partner. This switch takes practice so that CPR remains effective. With practice, you should be able to:

➤ List the steps for changing positions during two-rescuer CPR.

When you apply new knowledge, you must be able to determine if you are applying it correctly. Watch one another as you practice and be able to:

➤ State how you can determine that CPR is being performed correctly.
➤ Discuss some of the complications that can occur while performing CPR.

A heart attack is only one of the many causes of cardiac arrest. You must be able to:

> ➤ List other causes of cardiac arrest.
> ➤ Discuss some of the unique considerations when performing CPR on victims of trauma and hypothermia.

When you approach any emergency scene, be sure to perform all patient assessment steps. Remember and be able to:

> ➤ Demonstrate the steps of the initial assessment to determine if a patient is in cardiac arrest.

Your jurisdiction may allow Emergency Medical Responders to use an automated external defibrillator (AED) and have them ready for use on your unit or where you work. You must complete appropriate training before using an AED, and in your training, you will:

> ➤ List the criteria for the use of an AED.
> ➤ Demonstrate the proper use of an AED for a patient in cardiac arrest.

 FIRST ON SCENE

"What do you think, Paul?" Laryn Axton, security manager for Western Legends Hotel and Casino, was examining a CCTV video screen closely. "Paul?" She turned to see why the hotel's lead security agent hadn't answered her.

Paul sat several feet from her, both hands on his chest and face ghostly pale. "What's wrong, Paul? Paul?"

She stood quickly, sending her chair crashing into a metal rack of DVD cases. Paul looked up at her, his bulging eyes reflecting the wall of video monitors next to him. He tried to speak several times and then collapsed into a heap onto the floor.

"Paul!" Laryn screamed and dropped to her knees next to him, shaking his shoulders. "Are you okay?" There was no response and his eyes, partially hidden behind half-closed lids, stared vacantly at her.

"Okay," Laryn said to herself. "Okay, calm down. First thing's first." Laryn searched her memory for the procedures that she had learned in last spring's Emergency Medical Responder course. She took a deep breath, rolled Paul onto his back and, after opening his airway, checked for signs of breathing.

---

chain of survival ■ the idea that the survival of the patient in cardiac arrest depends on the linkage of early access, early CPR, early defibrillation, and early advanced life support.

4-1.3 Describe each link in the chain of survival and how it relates to the EMS system.

cardiac arrest ■ when the heart stops beating. Also, the ineffective circulation caused by erratic muscle activity in the lower chambers of the heart (ventricular fibrillation).

Cardiopulmonary Resuscitation

CHAIN OF SURVIVAL

Chapter 1 describes the chain of human resources and services in the EMS system. If each link in the chain works quickly and efficiently, the EMS system can provide effective prehospital emergency care. The **chain of survival** is another linked system of patient-care events. For a patient to have the best chance of survival following **cardiac arrest**, each link in this chain must be strong. The links are:

■ *Early access to EMS.* Early access refers to recognizing a possible cardiac emergency and having a quick way to call for the help the patient needs. It usually begins with a family member or bystander calling 9-1-1 (or the emergency phone number for the area). The dispatcher can then activate an appropriate EMS response.

- *Early CPR.* The sooner that **cardiopulmonary resuscitation (CPR)** can be initiated, the sooner circulation can be restored to the patient's brain and vital organs. Pre-arrival instructions provided by an Emergency Medical Dispatcher to the 9-1-1 caller can help sustain life until more advanced assistance arrives on scene.
- *Early defibrillation.* **Defibrillation** is the application of an electric shock to a patient's heart in an attempt to convert a lethal rhythm into a normal one. The time from cardiac arrest to defibrillation is an essential factor in the survival rate of out-of-hospital cardiac arrest patients. The shorter the time is between collapse and defibrillation, the better.
- *Early advanced life support.* **Advanced life support (ALS)** is the care provided by more highly trained personnel such as Advanced Emergency Medical Technicians (AEMTs) and Paramedics. ALS providers have many hours of training in the recognition and care of cardiac emergencies. In addition to defibrillators, they provide other interventions, such as oxygen to support ventilation, intravenous access for fluids, and medications that control heart rate and rhythm, relieve pain, and help to stabilize the patient.

Each link in the chain of survival is essential to improving patient survival. However, research has shown that of all the links, early defibrillation has the most effect on positive patient outcomes. In recent years, defibrillator technology has improved to the point that an **automated external defibrillator (AED)** can be operated with minimal training. Today, AEDs are found in many public areas such as airports, shopping malls, stadiums, and other gathering places.

If Emergency Medical Responders in your jurisdiction are permitted to use AEDs, your instructor or Medical Director will provide the appropriate training. Do not attempt to use one without training.

CIRCULATION AND CPR

At the center of the circulatory system is the heart. When the heart beats, it acts as a pump. Blood from the body flows into the heart and is sent to the lungs. In the lungs, the blood releases carbon dioxide gathered while circulating through the body and exchanges it for oxygen. This oxygen-rich blood is then sent back to the heart, where it is pumped back out to the body.

Many things can affect the proper function of the heart, including injury due to trauma and heart attack. When everything is working properly, the circulatory system keeps oxygenated blood moving to all parts of the body. As blood flows through the body, it also gathers nutrients from the small intestines, picks up secretions from special glands, and gives up wastes to the kidneys. This constant exchange is important for proper functioning of the vital organs—and for life.

There is a strong relationship between the brain and the activities of circulation and breathing (Figure 8.1). That relationship includes the following:

- When breathing stops, blood circulating to the brain will contain little or no oxygen.
- Without an adequate supply of oxygen, the brain cannot direct the work of all other body functions. The heartbeat slows, then becomes irregular, and finally stops beating altogether.
- When the heart stops beating, the oxygen supply remaining in the brain is then used up in about four to six minutes.

cardiopulmonary resuscitation (KAR-de-o-PUL-mo-ner-e re-SUS-ci-TA-shun) (CPR) ▪ combined compression and breathing techniques that maintain circulation and breathing.

defibrillation ▪ the application of an electric shock to a patient's heart in an attempt to convert a lethal rhythm into a normal one.

advanced life support (ALS) ▪ prehospital emergency care that involves the use of intravenous fluids, drug infusions, cardiac monitoring, defibrillation, intubation, and other advanced procedures.

automated external defibrillator (AED) ▪ an electrical device that can detect certain abnormal heart rhythms and deliver a shock through the patient's chest. This shock may allow the heart to resume a normal pattern of beating.

4–1.1 List the reasons for the heart to stop beating.

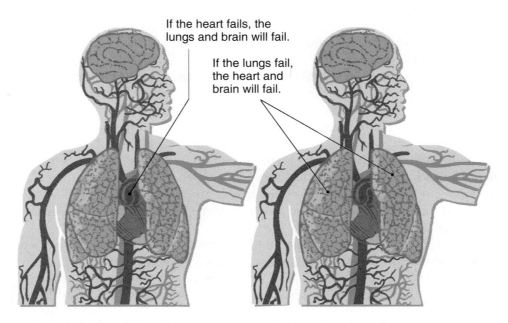

If the heart fails, the lungs and brain will fail.

If the lungs fail, the heart and brain will fail.

FIGURE 8.1 The activities of the heart, lungs, and brain are interdependent.

REMEMBER

In some areas, the ABCs of emergency care have one more letter—the letter "D," which stands for defibrillation.

4-1.2 Define the components of cardiopulmonary resuscitation.

chest compressions ▪ putting pressure on the chest to artificially circulate blood to the brain, lungs, and the rest of the patient's body.

FIRST ➤ When the heart stops beating, a person is said to be in cardiac arrest. The signs of cardiac arrest are (in the order in which you would check them during your initial assessment):

▪ Unresponsive.
▪ No breathing.
▪ No pulse. ▪

CPR—What It Is

Cardiopulmonary resuscitation, or CPR, is an emergency procedure that involves the application of both external chest compressions and ventilations when heart and lung actions stop. (*Cardio-* refers to the heart, and *pulmonary* refers to the lungs. *Resuscitation* means to revive.) You studied pulmonary resuscitation in Chapter 6. When performing CPR, you will perform that skill in addition to **chest compressions**.

FIRST ➤ During CPR, you must:

▪ Ensure and maintain an open airway.
▪ Breathe (ventilate) for the patient.
▪ Perform chest compressions to circulate the patient's blood. ▪

CPR—How It Works

During the period between clinical death and biological death, irreversible brain damage begins. Approximately 10 minutes after breathing and pulse have stopped, it is unlikely that the patient will ever regain normal responsiveness. By performing CPR early, you can circulate oxygenated blood to the brain and help delay the onset of biological death and irreversible brain damage.

However, the time frame for beginning CPR is not always within 10 minutes after the onset of cardiac arrest. In a cold-water near-drowning, for example, people have been successfully resuscitated after being submerged 20 minutes or more. Usually, you will not know exactly when a patient's breathing and pulse actually stopped, even if a bystander reported the person to be unresponsive for what

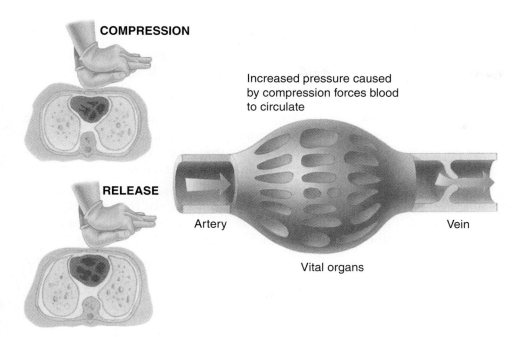

COMPRESSION

Increased pressure caused
by compression forces blood
to circulate

RELEASE

Artery

Vein

Vital organs

FIGURE 8.2 During CPR, pressure in the chest cavity increases with compression, which forces blood into circulation.

seemed to them a long time. Such estimates are generally unreliable. So, in general, you will almost always start CPR in cases of cardiac arrest.

CPR is a series of specific steps that must be performed in a certain manner. (Note that for adults, children, and infants the steps vary slightly to accommodate size and anatomical differences.) Generally, CPR begins with the patient lying on his back on a firm surface. You will compress the patient's chest straight down along its midline at a point over the lower half of the breastbone (sternum). This squeezing of the heart plus the increase of pressure in the chest (thoracic) cavity forces blood out of the heart and into the arteries to circulate to all parts of the body. When compression is relaxed and pressure is released, blood flows back to the heart. One-way valves in the patient's heart and veins keep the blood moving in the proper direction (Figure 8.2).

FIRST ➤ During CPR, your breaths provide oxygen to the patient's blood, which is then circulated to the brain and other vital organs with each compression. ▪

Is It Safe ?

The American Heart Association strongly suggests the use of appropriate barrier devices when performing CPR on any patient. If you do not have an appropriate barrier device, it is important to attempt compression-only CPR. The act of compressing the chest moves some air in and out of the lungs and is more beneficial than not doing CPR at all. ▪

There may be times when no appropriate barrier device is available and the rescuer does not want to take the risk of being exposed to the patient's bodily fluids. According to the American Heart Association, providing compressions only is significantly better than providing no assistance at all, and it minimizes the risk of the rescuer coming in contact with bodily fluids. Studies have shown that there is some air movement in and out of the lungs with each chest compression, provided the patient has an open airway.

When to Begin CPR

FIRST ➤ As an Emergency Medical Responder, you must always perform an initial assessment on your patient. Your actions leading to CPR should include the following:

1. Form a general impression of the patient as you approach. Notice what the patient looks like. Form an immediate opinion and react based on that opinion. Does the patient look sick, appear to be having trouble breathing, or seem unresponsive? Also note the patient's sex, approximate age, and level of distress.

2. Assess responsiveness, using the AVPU scale. Start with a gentle tap on the shoulder and shout, "Are you okay?" If the adult patient does not respond, shake her gently and confirm that she is unresponsive. If she is unresponsive, a serious condition exists and you should make sure that an ambulance has been requested.

3. Position the patient on her back on a firm surface and begin CPR. If you are alone and the patient is a child or an infant, begin CPR immediately and perform rescue support for two minutes. Then, if not already done, call 9-1-1. ALS personnel with defibrillators and ventilation devices can be dispatched to the scene while you perform CPR.

4. Open the airway, using the head-tilt, chin-lift or jaw-thrust maneuver, as appropriate.

5. Assess breathing. Look, listen, and feel for at least five seconds, but no more than 10 seconds. If the patient is not breathing, attempt to deliver two slow breaths. If you do not see the chest rise, the airway may be obstructed, so reposition the head and try again. If you still do not see the chest rise, assess circulation.

6. Assess circulation. Feel for a pulse for at least five seconds, but no more than 10 seconds. If there is no pulse, proceed to chest compressions. To assess for a pulse in an adult or child (age one year and older), check the carotid pulse in the neck (Figure 8.3). To assess the pulse of an infant (younger than one year), check the brachial pulse in the upper arm (Figure 8.4). ■

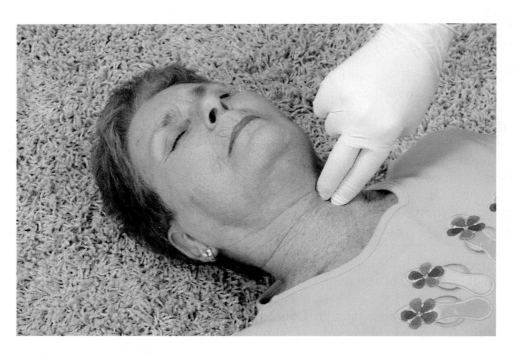

FIGURE 8.3 Use the carotid (neck) pulse for both an adult and a child.

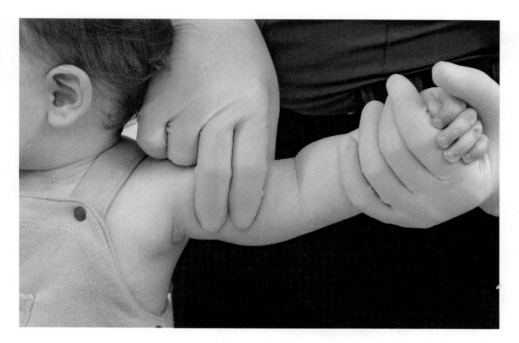

FIGURE 8.4 Feel for a brachial (medial upper arm) pulse for an infant.

Geriatric Focus

One of the consequences of aging is that the bowels become less efficient, making constipation a common problem among the elderly. This can be dangerous to those patients who have heart conditions as they bear down during a difficult bowel movement. The pressure changes inside the chest and abdominal cavity can cause a slowing of the heart and dangerous changes in the heart rhythm. This is one of the reasons why so many elderly are found unresponsive in the bathroom.

NOTE

From here on, discussion centers on adult and child CPR, unless noted otherwise. Infant CPR is addressed later in this chapter.

Locating the CPR Compression Site

External chest compressions are not effective unless they are delivered to a specific site on the patient's chest (Scan 8–1). If you apply compressions to the wrong site, you may injure the patient or provide ineffective CPR. Steps for locating the compression site on an adult patient are listed as follows.

FIRST ➤ After determining that the patient needs CPR, you will:

1. Place the patient face up on a firm surface, such as the ground or the floor. This is necessary for CPR to be effective. If the patient is in bed, move him to the floor or place a board under his back. Do not delay CPR to find a board.
2. Kneel at the patient's side near his shoulder.
3. Quickly move or remove clothing that may be covering the patient's chest.
4. Place the heel of one hand on the center of the patient's bare chest, right between the nipples.
5. Put your other hand on top of the first. Either extend or interlace your fingers to keep them off the patient's chest. ■

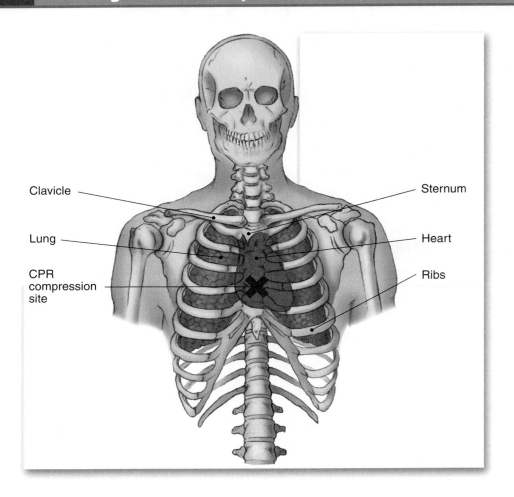

Clavicle

Sternum

Lung

Heart

CPR compression site

Ribs

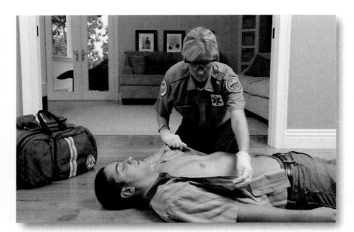

1 ■ Quickly move or remove clothing that may be covering the patient's chest.

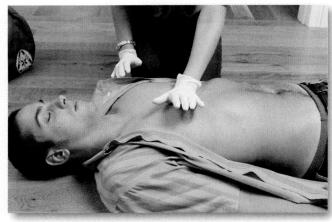

2 ■ Then place the heel of one hand on the center of the patient's bare chest, right between the nipples, along the axis of the sternum.

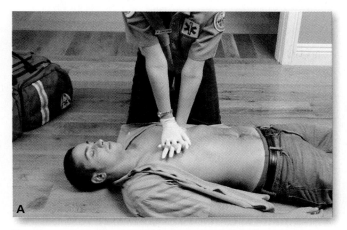

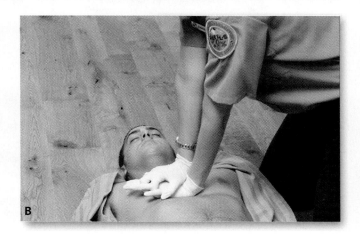

3 ▪ Put your other hand on top of the first hand. Either extend or interlace your fingers to keep them off the patient's chest. (A) side view and (B) front view.

External Chest Compressions

FIRST ➤ The correct technique for external chest compressions is as follows:

1. Keep the heels of both hands parallel to each other, one on top of the other, with the fingers of both hands pointing away from you.

2. Keep your fingers off the chest, either extended or interlaced (Figure 8.5). For some, it may be easier to do compressions by grasping the wrist of the hand placed at the compression site. Practice different positions until you find one that is comfortable for you.

3. Keep your elbows straight and locked. Do not bend your elbows when delivering or releasing compressions.

4. Position your shoulders over your hands (Figure 8.6). Keep both of your knees on the ground about shoulder width apart.

5. Deliver compressions straight down and apply enough force to the adult patient to depress the sternum 1.5 to 2 inches. For a child, compress the chest one-third to one-half of the depth of the chest with one or two hands (Figure 8.7). CPR will be effective for the patient and less tiring for you if you bend from the

4–1.5 Describe the technique of external chest compressions on an adult patient.

4–1.7 Describe the technique of external chest compressions on a child.

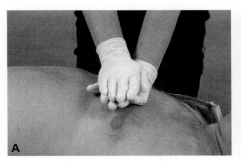

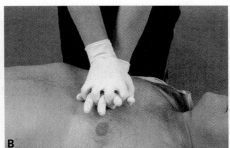

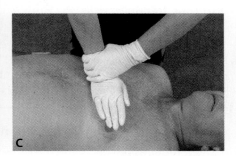

FIGURE 8.5 Hand positions at the CPR compression site: **A.** extending fingers, **B.** intertwining fingers, and **C.** second hand at wrist.

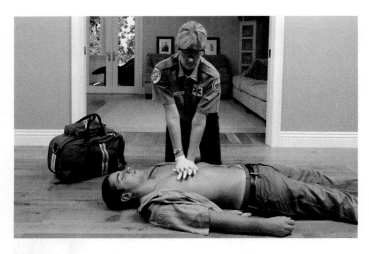

FIGURE 8.6 Position your shoulders directly over the compression site.

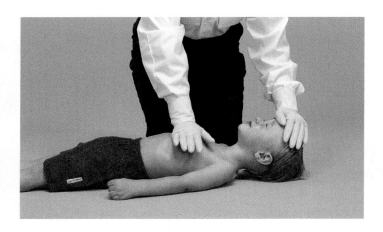

FIGURE 8.7 For child chest compression, use the heel of one hand.

hips in a smooth up-and-down motion. Perform chest compressions at a rate of approximately 100 per minute.

6. Release pressure on the chest completely to allow the patient's heart to refill. Do not bend your elbows in order to release pressure. Do not lift your hands off the patient's chest. Lift up from your hips to return your shoulders to their original position. The release of pressure should take the same amount of time as compression (50% compression and 50% release). ■

Geriatric Focus

A youthful skeleton has lots of flexibility and strength not seen in the geriatric skeleton. For this reason, providing proper chest compressions to the elderly can be a challenge. Significantly more effort may be required to achieve the desired two inches of compression during the first several compressions. In addition, the dry bones of the elderly will be much more brittle, and you will likely hear the sound of breaking bones during your first several compressions. This is rarely the actual sound of bones breaking but instead the sound of cartilage breaking. This is an expected and necessary outcome of good chest compressions. When you hear the sound, double-check your hand position and adjust if necessary. Then continue with chest compressions.

Providing Ventilations During CPR

Along with chest compressions (artificial circulation), you must provide artificial ventilation when performing CPR. Breaths are provided between each set of compressions, using a pocket face mask, face shield, or bag-valve mask. Open the patient's airway using the head-tilt, chin-lift or, if you suspect spine injury, attempt the jaw-thrust maneuver. Place and seal the mask or barrier device over the patient's face and ventilate until you see the chest rise and fall.

Follow these guidelines when providing ventilations during CPR:

■ Deliver each breath slowly over one second.
■ Provide two breaths, one right after the other, after every 30 compressions.

Is It Safe ?

Remember to provide ventilations slowly over one second. Providing slow steady breaths minimizes the chance that your breath will push air into the patient's stomach. ■

■ Do not overventilate the patient. If you force too much air into the patient's lungs, the excess air will begin to fill the stomach and may eventually cause gastric distention. To prevent this, feel for resistance as you ventilate and watch for the patient's chest to rise.

To provide effective mouth-to-mask ventilations, you may position yourself either in the **cephalic position** (at the patient's head) or in the **lateral position** (at the patient's side) (Figure 8.8). The cephalic position is preferred for patients with a pulse but no respirations and for two-rescuer CPR. The lateral position is preferred for one-rescuer CPR. Practice both positions on a manikin. Determine which one enables you to provide the most effective CPR to a patient. Remember that good CPR delays the onset of biological death and increases the patient's chances for survival.

cephalic (seh-FAL-ik) position
■ at the top of the supine patient's head.

lateral position ■ at the supine patient's side.

▬▬▬ Geriatric Focus

Due to the drying out of the bones in the elderly, the ribs can become much less flexible and therefore allow far less chest wall movement during breathing. As you check for breathing or provide ventilations, you might not see as much chest rise and fall as on a younger patient. Observe the abdomen for signs of movement, when you assess breathing or provide ventilations. You should see a steady rise and fall of the abdomen much like you normally would of the chest. Of course, a lack of movement is never good, and you must consider the possibility of a total airway obstruction and provide care accordingly.

Rates and Ratios of Compressions and Ventilations

FIRST ➤ Effective CPR depends on the correct rate and ratio of compressions and ventilations. For effective CPR, you must:

- Deliver compressions at a rate of approximately 100 per minute.
- Provide ventilations at a ratio of two breaths for every 30 compressions. Deliver each breath over one second.
- Once you have begun CPR, avoid interrupting compressions for longer than 10 seconds. Interrupt compressions only for ventilations, for changing rescuer positions, or for moving the patient. ▪

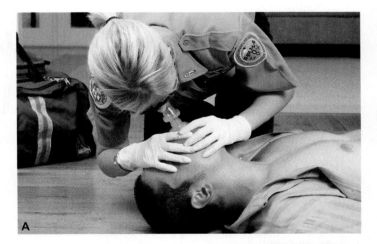

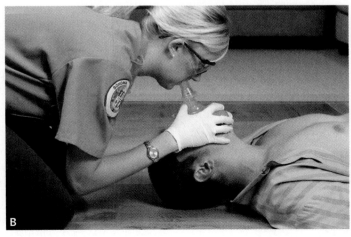

FIGURE 8.8 Deliver ventilations using **A.** the lateral position or **B.** the cephalic position.

NOTE

The rate for chest compressions refers to the speed rather than the number of compressions the rescuer delivers in one minute. Because a single rescuer must interrupt chest compressions to deliver breaths, the actual number of compressions will be less than 100 per minute. To be sure that you provide compressions at the proper rate of 100 per minute, count out loud as you deliver compressions: "One-and, two-and, three-and, four-and . . ." until you reach 30. Then, deliver two ventilations, each over a period of one second, quickly relocate the CPR compression site, and continue the next set of compressions.

REMEMBER

Oxygen must reach the air-exchange levels of the patient's lungs if CPR is to be effective.

FIRST ➤ You can be certain that you are performing CPR correctly if:

- Another trained provider feels and confirms the carotid pulse as you compress the patient's chest. Do not apply constant pressure to the carotid artery, since this could impair blood flow to the brain. Also, do not try to deliver compressions with one hand and check for a pulse with the other.
- You see the chest rise and fall during ventilations. ▪

If you are performing CPR correctly, you may notice the patient's skin color improve, but this does not always occur. Sometimes the patient may try to swallow, gasp, or move his limbs. These actions do not necessarily mean that he is recovering. However, such movements are signs of life and do mean that you should stop CPR and check for the return of breathing and pulse.

FIRST ➤ If the patient regains a pulse but is not breathing, stop compressions and continue with ventilations only. If there is no pulse, continue CPR. Patients will usually require defibrillation and possibly other special medical procedures before they regain heart function. CPR only delays the onset of biological death until special medical procedures can be provided. ▪

Adult and Child CPR

The following is a step-by-step procedure for performing one- and two-rescuer CPR. These procedures follow the American Heart Association recommendations. The extensive research done by the AHA has found these procedures to be most efficient in saving the lives of patients in cardiac arrest. Also, remember that the following steps are a part of the initial assessment. (See Table 8–1 for a summary of CPR techniques.)

ONE-RESCUER CPR

4–1.4 List the steps of one-rescuer adult CPR.

4–1.11 List the steps of child CPR.

FIRST ➤ To perform one-rescuer CPR on an adult or child (Scan 8–2):

1. Check for responsiveness (Figure 8.9). Gently tap the patient's shoulder and ask, "Are you okay?" If the patient is not responsive, call out for help. If you are alone with an unresponsive adult patient, call 9-1-1 immediately and get a defibrillator if available (Figure 8.10). If you are alone with an unresponsive child, provide five cycles of compressions and ventilations (for approximately two minutes), and then call 9-1-1.
2. Position the patient face up on a hard surface. Then kneel beside the patient's chest (Figure 8.11).
3. Open the airway by using the head-tilt, chin-lift maneuver or, if you suspect a spine injury, by using the jaw-thrust maneuver (Figure 8.12).
4. Check for breathing. Place your ear next to the patient's nose and mouth and look, listen, and feel for air exchange. Assess for at least five seconds, but no more than 10 seconds (Figure 8.13).
5. Provide two slow breaths, one right after the other. Watch for chest rise and feel for resistance (Figure 8.14). Follow the steps for mouth-to-

REMEMBER

Each rescuer should use his own barrier device with one-way valve and HEPA filter insert in order to perform two-rescuer CPR safely.

TABLE 8–1 | Summary of CPR Techniques

PROCEDURE	ADULT	CHILD	INFANT
Compressions			
Method	Heels of two hands	Heel of one or two hands	Two fingers or two thumbs with hands encircling chest
Depth	1.5 to 2 inches	One-third to one-half depth of chest	
Rate	100/minute		
Ventilations			
Method	Mouth-to barrier device		
Rate	One breath every 5 to 6 seconds	One breath every 3 to 5 seconds	One breath every 3 to 5 seconds
Ratio of Compressions to Breaths			
One Rescuer	30:2	30:2	30:2
Two Rescuers	30:2	15:2	15:2
Counts	1 and 2 and 3 and 4 and 5 … 30 and breathe, breathe		

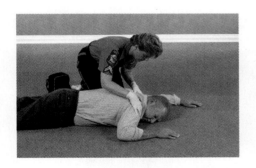

FIGURE 8.9 Determine unresponsiveness.

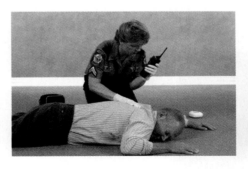

FIGURE 8.10 Activate EMS immediately if the patient is unresponsive.

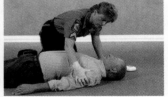

FIGURE 8.11 Properly position yourself and the patient.

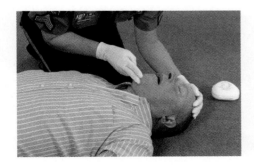

FIGURE 8.12 Open the airway.

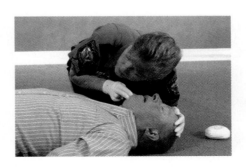

FIGURE 8.13 Check for breathing.

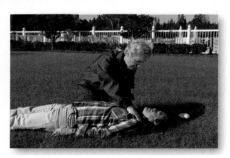

1 ■ Establish unresponsiveness and activate EMS. Position the patient and yourself.

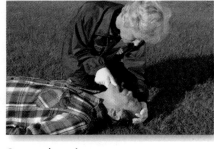

2 ■ Open the airway.

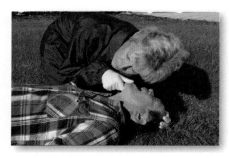

3 ■ Look, listen, and feel for breathing for at least five seconds, but no more than 10 seconds.

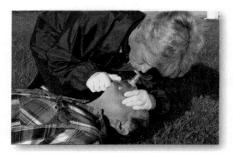

4 ■ Give two slow breaths over one second each.

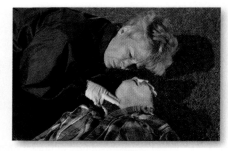

5 ■ Check for a carotid pulse for at least five seconds, but no more than 10 seconds.

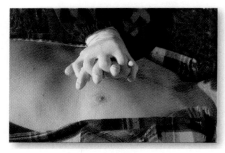

6 ■ Locate the compression site and position your hands.

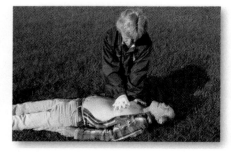

7 ■ Begin compressions. Compression rate is 100 per minute.

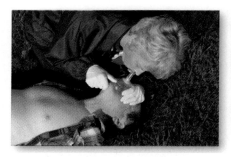

8 ■ Give two ventilations. One cycle consists of two ventilations every 30 compressions.

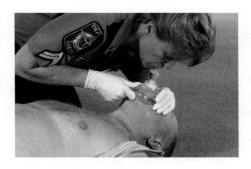

FIGURE 8.14 Use a barrier device to provide two slow breaths.

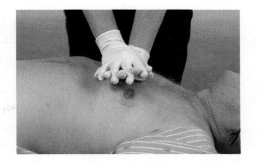

FIGURE 8.15 Position your hands between the nipples over the lower half of the sternum.

mask or mouth-to-face shield ventilation or for using a bag-valve mask (see Appendix 2).

6. Check for a carotid pulse for at least five seconds, but no more than 10 seconds.

7. If the patient has a carotid pulse, but no respirations, provide one breath every five to six seconds for an adult and one breath every three to five seconds for a child. If there is no pulse . . .

8. Locate the CPR compression site (Figure 8.15). Place both hands on the center of the chest, keeping your fingers off the surface.

9. Deliver 30 chest compressions. Keep your arms straight, elbows locked, and shoulders directly over the compression site. Bend at the hips to use your upper body weight when performing compressions.
   — Deliver compressions directly over the CPR compression site.
   — Compress the adult patient's breastbone 1.5 to 2 inches. Compressions on a child should be one-third to one-half the depth of the chest.
   — Deliver compressions at a rate of 100 per minute, counting "one-and, two-and, three-and . . ." until you reach 30.
   — Release pressure completely to allow the heart to refill. Each release should take the same amount of time as a compression. Do not take your hands off the patient's chest while delivering chest compressions.
   — Deliver 30 compressions, then . . .

10. Provide two slow breaths, one right after the other. Provide ventilations at a rate of two breaths after every 30 compressions and watch for chest rise.

11. Continue CPR. Deliver 30 compressions at the rate of 100 per minute followed by two ventilations.

12. Do not interrupt CPR for any longer than is absolutely necessary. If the patient regains a pulse and/or breathing, stop CPR. If there is a pulse but no breathing, continue ventilations at the rate of one breath every five to six seconds. Confirm the continued presence of a pulse frequently.

13. Continue CPR until another trained person can take over, the patient regains a pulse and breathing, or you are too tired to continue. ▪

NOTE

Health-care providers, such as Emergency Medical Responders, who have a duty to perform CPR, should also be trained, equipped, and authorized to use an AED.

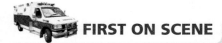

FIRST ON SCENE

"Joey, do you copy?" Laryn grabbed the portable radio after confirming that Paul was not breathing and didn't have a pulse.

"Yeah, go ahead," came a reply with a strong Australian accent.

"I need you to get an ambulance here and bring an AED to the CCTV office right now! Paul is in cardiac arrest!" She then dropped the radio onto the floor next to her, watched Paul's chest rise and fall as she gave him two slow breaths, and began chest compressions.

As Laryn counted out loud, she focused on the hallway monitor to see when Joey was coming with the AED. Also, because the compressions were making Paul's head bob slowly from side to side, and she didn't like how his unseeing eyes kept meeting hers.

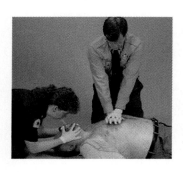

FIGURE 8.16 Two-rescuer CPR.

4–1.9 List the steps of two-rescuer adult CPR.

Is It Safe ?

Doing CPR as a single rescuer can be very tiring. The more tired you become, the less effective you will be. It is recommended that you change places with another rescuer after every five cycles of 30 compressions and two ventilations. This will minimize the chances of becoming overly tired during the resuscitation effort. It also will provide the best possible CPR for the patient. ▪

TWO-RESCUER CPR

All EMS personnel should learn and remain proficient in both one- and two-rescuer CPR techniques. CPR that is performed by two rescuers who have trained together is more efficient and less tiring for both rescuers (Figure 8.16). Two-rescuer CPR minimizes the transition time between ventilations and compressions and, therefore, maximizes the effectiveness of both.

Use of an AED is also more efficient with two rescuers. One rescuer can begin to set up the AED and attach the electrodes to the patient, while the other rescuer begins an initial assessment of the patient. If you arrive on scene and find that an AED is being used, ensure that the individuals are performing the steps properly and taking the necessary safety precautions. Offer to assist them and support their actions. You may also need to relieve or guide someone who is unsure of the procedures.

Changing from One- to Two-Rescuer CPR

When you assess a patient who has collapsed, your first action is to assess for unresponsiveness. Tap the patient and shout, "Are you okay?" If there is no response, direct someone to activate the EMS system (or phone the appropriate emergency number). If you are alone, leave the patient long enough to call for help. Then return and continue your assessment. If the patient is a child or infant, provide two minutes of rescue support before calling 9-1-1.

In many situations, a bystander may start one-rescuer CPR before Emergency Medical Responders arrive. On arrival, assess the patient's breathing and pulse before taking over and performing two-rescuer CPR with your partner.

If you arrive as a lone Emergency Medical Responder and determine that a bystander's CPR techniques are inadequate or incorrect, take over one-rescuer CPR. If the bystander is CPR-trained but has no barrier device and is reluctant to ventilate a stranger, perform the ventilations yourself with your own pocket face mask. Have the bystander take over chest compressions and monitor his effectiveness.

FIRST ➤ If a member of the EMS system is performing CPR when you arrive, begin two-rescuer CPR. To help make a smooth transition from one-rescuer to two-rescuer CPR, follow these steps:

1. If on arriving on scene, you see a rescuer performing CPR, identify yourself. Then, if not already done, activate the EMS system.
2. While the first rescuer is delivering two breaths, get in position next to the patient's chest.

3. After the two slow breaths, resume chest compressions. The first rescuer should then resume ventilations, providing two ventilations after every set of compressions.

4. Provide compressions at the rate of 100 per minute with a pause after every set of compressions to allow for two ventilations.

5. After two minutes of CPR, both you and the other rescuer may change positions. ▪

> **NOTE**
>
> The compression-ventilation ratio for two-rescuer adult CPR is 30:2. The compression-ventilation ratio for a child is 15:2.

If the Emergency Medical Responder who arrives on scene to see CPR being performed is equipped with an AED, he should immediately set it up, turn it on, and attach electrodes in preparation for early defibrillation.

Compressions and Ventilations

During two-rescuer CPR, deliver 30 compressions at a rate of 100 compressions per minute. After every 30 compressions, deliver two ventilations. The compressor (the rescuer providing compressions) will count aloud so that both rescuers will be able to establish and maintain the correct rate. By hearing the count, the ventilator (the rescuer providing ventilations) will be prepared to provide a breath after every 30 compressions while the compressor pauses to allow for adequate ventilation.

CPR Procedure

FIRST ➤ The complete sequence for two-rescuer CPR is illustrated in Scan 8–3. In that scan, both rescuers are shown on the same side of the patient for teaching purposes only. In actual two-rescuer CPR, the ventilator is usually in a cephalic position. Your instructor will demonstrate how to ventilate a patient in both positions—cephalic and lateral—using the barrier devices and oxygen delivery equipment that your jurisdiction requires. ▪

As the ventilator, check frequently for a carotid pulse, which should be felt with each compression. If a carotid pulse cannot be found, have the compressor recheck his hand position, his body position (arms straight, shoulders over sternum, bend at hips), and the depth of his compressions. Make sure the compressor does not rest his weight on the patient's chest, but instead allows the chest wall to completely recoil after each compression. If you notice that the compressor is getting tired, start the process for changing positions.

Changing Positions

Is It Safe ?

Changing positions during two-rescuer CPR can maximize the effectiveness of CPR. This change should only take approximately five seconds to complete. Remember to interrupt CPR only when absolutely necessary and only for as little time as possible. ▪

FIRST ➤ Either rescuer may request a change in position if he becomes tired. However, it is usually the compressor who needs the break. Unless the ventilator finds

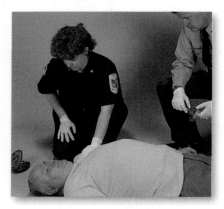

1 ■ The first rescuer determines unresponsiveness, sends someone to activate EMS, and positions the patient.

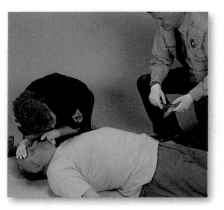

2 ■ Open the airway. Look, listen, and feel for breathing for at least five seconds, but no more than 10 seconds.

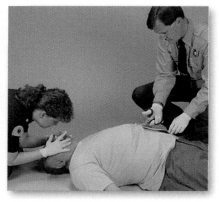

3 ■ Give two slow breaths over one second each.

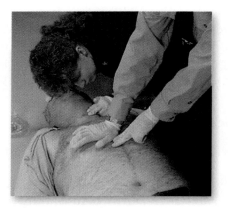

4 ■ Assess for a carotid pulse for at least five seconds, but no more than 10 seconds.

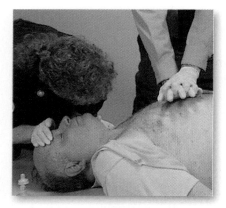

5 ■ If no pulse, the second rescuer locates the compression site and begins compressions at a rate of 100 per minute.

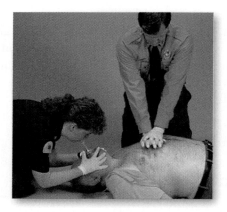

6 ■ The first rescuer provides two slow breaths after each set of compressions. The second rescuer should pause compressions to allow for adequate ventilations. Continue with two ventilations every 30 compressions for an adult and two ventilations every 15 compressions for a child.

that the compressor cannot generate a pulse during compression, the compressor will decide when to change positions. At the beginning of a cycle, the compressor will give a clear signal to the ventilator to switch places, but will complete a set of 30 compressions before any moves are made. At the end of 30 compressions, the ventilator will provide two ventilations. Then the rescuers will quickly change positions. Your instructor will teach you the preferred switching signals to use. ▪

Infant CPR

For purposes of field resuscitation, infant and child patients are defined as follows:

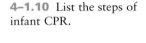

4–1.10 List the steps of infant CPR.

- *Child.* A child is one year old to the onset of puberty, which is typically determined by the presence of chest or underarm hair in boys and the development of breasts in girls.
- *Infant.* A baby from birth through one year of age is considered an infant.

In general, use adult CPR techniques on any child who has reached the age of puberty. However, because children develop at different rates, you may find that many infants and children are large for their age. Some adolescents are small enough to be mistaken for children. Thus, the previous age categories are guidelines, not absolutes. It is more important to begin CPR and check for effective ventilations and compressions than to spend time determining a patient's exact age. For example, if you think the patient is younger than one year and find that you cannot adequately compress the chest with just two fingers, then begin one-handed compressions as you would if the patient was older than one year.

PREPARING FOR INFANT CPR

Positioning the Infant
Just as you do for adults and children, place the infant patient face up on a hard, flat surface. Be aware that when an infant is on his back, his large head can cause the neck to flex forward, potentially closing the airway. To help ensure an open airway, maintain the head in a neutral position. It may be necessary to provide support under the shoulders with a folded blanket or towel (Figure 8.17).

Opening the Airway

Is It Safe?

It takes little effort to open an infant's airway. Extending the neck of an infant too far can cause the airway to close off and thus keep air from entering the lungs. For best results, place the infant's head in a neutral position with nose pointing straight up (sniffing position). ▪

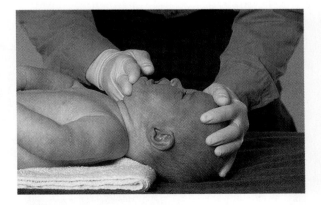

FIGURE 8.17 To help keep the head and neck in a neutral position, place a folded blanket or towel under the shoulders to fill the void.

FIRST ➤ For the infant with no spine injury, use the head-tilt, chin-lift maneuver. Tilt the head gently back to a neutral or slightly extended position with one hand. A slight head-tilt is often all that is needed. Place your fingers under the bony part of the chin and lift to finish the technique of opening the airway. Be careful not to compress the soft tissues of

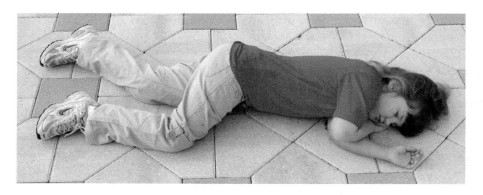

FIGURE 8.18 If the patient begins to breathe and regains a pulse, place her in the recovery position.

the neck because this may obstruct the airway. In cases of suspected spine injury, use the jaw-thrust maneuver. Airway obstructions should be cared for as described in Chapter 6. ■

Assessing Breathing

To assess for breathing, place your ear next to the patient's nose and mouth. Then look, listen, and feel for air exchange for no less than five seconds, but no more than 10 seconds. Look for the rise and fall of the chest and abdomen. Listen and feel for exhaled air. If there is breathing, maintain an open airway. Place the patient in the recovery position, if you do not suspect spine injury (Figure 8.18). If there is no breathing, use an appropriate barrier device and give two slow breaths, each breath over one second while watching for the chest to rise.

Checking for a Pulse

FIRST ➤ Follow these steps when assessing for a pulse in an infant:

1. With your ear next to the patient's nose and mouth, look, listen, and feel for breathing.
2. Feel for a pulse at the brachial artery for no less than five seconds, but no more than 10 seconds. The brachial pulse point is located on the medial side of the arm between the elbow and armpit (Figure 8.19). ■

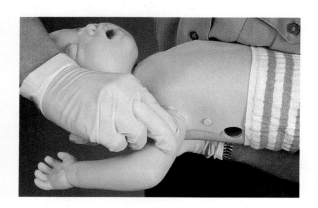

FIGURE 8.19 For infants, feel for a brachial pulse.

INFANT CPR TECHNIQUES

Ventilations

If your assessment finds that the infant patient has a good pulse but is not breathing adequately or at all, provide rescue breaths (ventilations). With the airway open and using an appropriate barrier device, provide slow ventilations at a ratio of one breath every three to five seconds. The correct volume for each ventilation is the volume that causes the chest to rise. Be careful not to overinflate the lungs, which can cause air to enter the stomach (gastric distention) and, eventually, vomiting.

The following ventilation steps are optional if barrier devices are not available. It is unusual for infants to have contagious diseases, so it is generally considered comparatively safer to give mouth-to-nose or mouth-to-mouth ventilations to them.

FIRST ➤ Provide one breath every three to five seconds using an appropriate barrier device or mouth-to-mouth or mouth-to-nose technique if a barrier device is not available. Watch carefully for the rise and fall of the patient's chest. ◼

You may find it easier to seal your mouth over the infant's mouth and nose. If the patient is a very large infant, seal your mouth over the patient's mouth and pinch the nostrils closed. If you do not see the chest rise after repositioning the airway, begin chest compressions.

External Chest Compressions

For infant CPR, external chest compressions and artificial ventilation can easily be performed by a single rescuer or shared between two trained rescuers, depending on available resources.

4–1.6 Describe the technique of external chest compressions on an infant.

FIRST ➤ In infant CPR, apply compressions to the lower half of the breastbone (sternum). Place two fingers on the sternum, one finger-width below the imaginary nipple line (Figure 8.20). Compress the infant's sternum one-third to one-half the depth of the chest, at a rate of at least 100 per minute.

If possible, maintain an open airway with one hand while compressing the chest with two fingers of the other hand. Provide two rescue breaths after each set of 30 compressions. Watch carefully for the rise and fall of the infant's chest. ◼

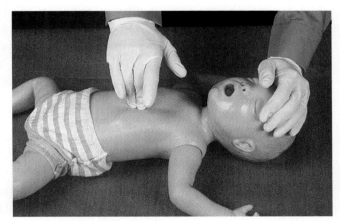

When there are two rescuers, the preferred method for chest compressions for the infant is the two-thumbs, encircling-hands technique. One rescuer (the compressor) places both thumbs side by side over the lower half of the infant's sternum or about one finger width below the nipple line (Figure 8.21). For very small infants or newborns, you may place one thumb on top of the other. The other rescuer provides ventilations.

FIGURE 8.20 For infant chest compression, use the tips of two fingers.

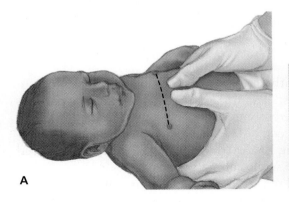
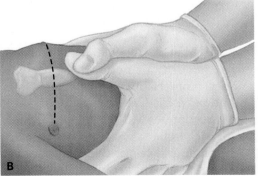

FIGURE 8.21 A. For the infant, place two thumbs side by side on the center of the chest on the imaginary nipple line. **B.** For newborns, place one thumb on top of the other.

Infant CPR Rates and Ratios

FIRST ➤ For infant CPR, deliver compressions at the rate of at least 100 per minute. For a single rescuer, perform compressions and ventilations at a ratio of 30:2. For two rescuers, perform compressions and ventilations at a ratio of 15:2. ∎

> **NOTE**
>
> Because the most common cause of cardiac arrest in infants and children is respiratory arrest, the number of breaths per minute provided by two rescuers is double that for an adult. However, one rescuer is unable to perform this ratio effectively and should therefore use the adult ratio of 30:2.

The following steps outline key points for infant CPR:

1. Determine unresponsiveness by gently tapping the bottom of the infant's feet and shout, "Are you all right?" If no response . . .

2. Direct someone to call EMS. If you are alone, provide two minutes of CPR before calling EMS. (There are exceptions to this rule, such as in the case of near-drowning, congenital heart disease, or respiratory failure.)

3. Position the infant. Place him in a supine (face up) position on a flat, hard surface. You may support small infants on your forearm.

4. Open the airway. Place the infant's head in a neutral position. If you suspect spine injury, use the jaw-thrust maneuver.

5. Check for breathing. Place your ear next to the patient's nose and mouth and look, listen, and feel for breathing. If the patient is not breathing, maintain the airway and . . .

6. Using an appropriate barrier device, provide two slow breaths, each being one second in duration, while watching for adequate chest rise. Look for and clear any airway obstruction as necessary. Use your gloved finger to sweep the mouth only if you see the obstruction.

7. Determine the presence of a brachial pulse. If there is a pulse but no respirations, provide ventilations at a rate of one breath every three to five seconds. If there is no pulse, or the patient is an infant with a heart rate of less than 60 per minute with signs of poor perfusion . . .

8. Provide chest compressions. Place two fingers in the center of the chest, one finger width below the nipple line. Compress at a rate of at least 100 per minute and provide ventilations at a 30:2 ratio.

Activating the EMS System

pediatric patients ∎ refers to infants and children. For the purposes of CPR, patients from birth to one year of age are considered infants. Patients from one year old to the onset of puberty are considered children.

The majority of **pediatric patients** with cardiac arrest result from some type of respiratory failure or respiratory arrest. For this reason, most pediatric patients who need CPR are treated a little differently than adults. With pediatric patients, it is recommended that the lone Emergency Medical Responder provide two minutes of rescue support before activating EMS. You may be able to carry the child or infant and continue emergency care while calling EMS.

 If the patient begins to breathe and regains a pulse, place him on his side in the recovery position. Do not place anyone in the recovery position if you suspect a spine injury. Monitor the breathing infant patient or continue CPR on the pulseless, nonbreathing infant patient until help arrives.

Ensuring Effective CPR for All Patients

Unless the proper techniques are performed (Scan 8–4), CPR will not be as effective and the patient has a greater chance of dying. For effective CPR for all patients, be sure to remember these important points:

- Place the patient face up (supine) on a hard surface.
- Maintain an open airway using the most appropriate technique.
- Use an appropriate barrier device, place it securely over the face, and ensure a good seal.
- During ventilations, watch the chest for adequate rise and fall.
- Compress smoothly and to the proper depth. Relax pressure completely between compressions to allow the heart to refill.
- Use the correct rates and ratios.
- Limit necessary interruptions such as pulse and breathing checks to no more than 10 seconds.

FIRST ➤ Emergency Medical Responders must be aware of the complications that may be caused by the use of both proper and improper CPR techniques.

Certain complications occur because the rescuer places his hands improperly during compressions. Emergency Medical Responders must be aware of such complications:

- If you place your hands too high on the patient's chest, you can cause damage to the collarbones (clavicles) and not provide adequate compression of the heart.
- If your hands are too low, there is a risk of damaging internal organs.
- If you place your hands too far to either side, you may fracture the ribs and possibly damage internal organs. ▪

Is It Safe ?

Providing proper chest compressions on an adult will likely result in the separation of the cartilage where the ribs meet the sternum. During the first few compressions, you are likely to feel and hear a popping sound, much like the popping of knuckles. Do not stop CPR. Instead, reconfirm proper hand position and continue to provide good compressions. This is a normal side effect of good chest compressions. ▪

In some cases, rib fractures occur even when you are performing CPR properly. In adult patients, the ribs may actually break during correct compressions. Children's chests are more pliable; their ribs are not likely to break. However, on any patient, you may hear a cracking sound while performing compressions, which may be a separation of the cartilage that connects the ribs to the sternum. If you think you have heard ribs crack, do not stop CPR. Check the position of your hands, reposition them properly, and resume CPR. A fractured rib will heal; stopping CPR will result in death.

Another problem occurs when too much air is forced into the patient's lungs. The excess air overflows out of the lungs and enters the stomach by way of the esophagus. This can result in gastric distention. Do not try to force excess air out of the stomach. To do so might cause the patient to vomit, which could lead to an airway obstruction. In some cases, the patient may *aspirate* (inhale) stomach contents and, if you try to provide breaths, you will force the vomit into the lungs.

ONE RESCUER	FUNCTIONS		TWO RESCUERS
	• Establish unresponsiveness • If no response, call 911 • Position patient • Open airway • Look, listen, and feel (no more than 10 seconds)		
	• Deliver two breaths (1½–2 sec each). If unsuccessful, reposition head and try again. Clear airway if necessary.		
	• Check carotid pulse . . . (5–10 seconds) If no pulse . . . • Begin chest compressions		
	DELIVER COMPRESSIONS		
	1½–2 inches 100/min	1½–2 inches 100/min	
	DELIVER VENTILATIONS **10–12 breaths/min**		
	30:2	15:2–child 30:2–adult	
	• Do five cycles • Ventilator checks pulse for effective CPR		
	CONTINUE PERIODIC ASSESSMENT		

Changing Positions

• Compressor—signal to change; finsh compression cycle • Ventilator—two ventilations	New ventilator checks pulse. If no pulse, says "No pulse, continue."	Continue CPR sequence

NOTE: Wear latex or vinyl gloves. Rescuers should have their own pocket face masks with one-way valves and HEPA filter inserts.

To avoid or reduce the amount of air forced into the stomach, always look for the patient's chest to rise as you deliver ventilations. Adjust the size of your breaths so that you see the chest rise, and then allow the patient to passively exhale. If you see the stomach begin to bulge, reposition the patient's head and adjust your ventilations.

If the patient vomits, stop CPR. Take time to clear the patient's airway as best as you can by repositioning the patient for drainage and by using your gloved fingers to sweep the mouth. After clearing the airway, resume CPR. ■

Special CPR Situations

MOVING THE PATIENT

Usually, there are only two reasons for an Emergency Medical Responder to move a patient who is receiving CPR: transport and immediate danger at the scene. Most of the time, the patient is moved after the EMTs assume responsibility for care. In preparation for transport when the EMTs arrive, place the cardiac arrest patient on a long spine board. This will allow for easy transfer to the stretcher and provide a firm surface when doing compressions.

TRAUMA

Many factors complicate CPR when dealing with a victim of trauma. Severe injuries to the patient's face may interfere with your attempts to provide ventilations. Crushing injuries to the patient's chest may lessen the effectiveness of chest compressions. Head, neck, and spine injuries may require that you handle the patient in a special manner.

Many rescuers are unsure about starting CPR on trauma patients. When rescuers find obvious indications of spine injuries, they may feel it is more important to immobilize the spine before they start CPR. If rescuers find a patient with a crushed chest, they may be afraid of causing internal injuries if they perform chest compressions. Patient injuries should not prevent you from starting CPR. If you delay or do not start CPR, the patient will die.

Moving the trauma patient into proper position is a major problem. One concern is spine injury, but CPR is not effective if the patient is in a seated position. Nor is CPR likely to be effective if the patient is on a soft surface, such as a car seat. Patients must be moved to hard surfaces and placed on their backs. While doing so, take into account the possibility of neck and spine injury, and use your hands and arms to initially control and stabilize the head and neck whenever you have to move a patient.

When moving an adult, cradle the head and shoulders in your forearms and attempt to move the patient so that his head stays in line with his body. When moving an infant or a child, always use one hand to support the head and neck of the patient. Again, for CPR to be effective, the patient must be lying face up on a hard surface.

If you must move the patient after starting CPR because of the dangers at the scene, then do so. Try not to interrupt CPR for more than 15 to 30 seconds during a move. The total move may have to be done in several stages if conditions allow. Even if your patient has possible neck and spine injuries, start CPR as soon as possible. Do not delay CPR in order to fully stabilize the neck and spine with a collar and immobilization devices. Use the jaw-thrust maneuver for ventilations in order to reduce the chances of causing greater injury to the patient.

NEAR-DROWNING

Rescuer safety and emergency care procedures at the scene of a drowning or near-drowning incident require special training in water rescue (see Appendix 6). If CPR is needed, begin as soon as possible, but remember your personal safety comes first. You may begin ventilations while the patient is still in the water. Be aware that mouth-to-mask methods may be difficult to perform under these conditions.

In a diving incident, suspect neck injury and use the jaw-thrust maneuver to open the airway. Very little water is ever aspirated, and any water in the lungs will be absorbed into the circulation when you ventilate the patient. Chest compressions are not effective when the patient is in the water. Attempts to begin compressions while the patient is in the water will delay removal of the patient from the water and the start of effective CPR.

ELECTRIC SHOCK

Some of the special problems of emergencies involving electricity are covered in Chapter 10. Your first priority is to avoid placing yourself in danger. Assess the patient and start artificial ventilation as soon as possible after you are sure the power is turned off. CPR, when needed, is performed in the same way for a victim of electric shock as it is for any other patient in cardiac arrest.

HYPOTHERMIA

Patients who are victims of hypothermia may have vital signs that are very difficult to assess. You should take extra time, at least a full minute, when assessing both pulse and breathing. Resuscitation attempts should continue until the patient can be rewarmed by the receiving facility. In most cases, a patient is not considered dead until his core temperature has been raised and he remains unresponsive to resuscitation efforts.

CPR—Responsibilities of the Emergency Medical Responder

4–1.8 Explain when an Emergency Medical Responder is able to stop CPR.

When caring for a patient in cardiac arrest, your duties are twofold: to have someone activate EMS and to start CPR immediately. Only a physician at the scene who has accepted responsibility for the patient may order you not to begin CPR. You may also choose not to begin CPR if there are obvious signs of prolonged death, such as the presence of muscle rigidity (rigor mortis) and pooling of blood (lividity). Bystanders and members of the patient's family may tell you that the patient would not want to be resuscitated. You are not to obey such requests.

Even though the patient may have a terminal illness or may be very old, you will still need to provide CPR unless there is an advance directive such as an official do not resuscitate (DNR) order. Quickly let the family know that you understand their concerns, but your duty as an Emergency Medical Responder is to begin CPR. Suggest that they try to contact the patient's doctor to get further directions. Without an advance directive such as a DNR, you have no way of knowing that this is what the patient would have you do. (Be sure you are familiar with prehospital DNR orders in your region.) If in doubt, contact medical direction for assistance and, when EMTs arrive, you or one of them should talk with the family to comfort and reassure them. Offer to call friends or other family members for them, and make sure they know where their family member is being transported.

The longer a patient is in cardiac arrest before CPR is started, the less likely CPR will be effective. However, there are documented cases of adults in cardiac arrest for more than 10 minutes who have been resuscitated with no major brain damage. Children and infants usually can survive longer periods of time in cardiac arrest than adults. Do not refuse to begin CPR because someone has been in cardiac arrest for 10 minutes, although, in most cases, CPR will probably not be effective. However, the moment the patient was seen to collapse and the moment of cardiac arrest are usually not the same. A patient may be unresponsive with minimum lung and heart function for quite some time before cardiac arrest occurs. Always start CPR immediately.

Cold-water drowning victims can be successfully resuscitated after long periods of submersion. There are documented cases of arrest that have lasted more than 45 minutes before successful resuscitation. The same is true of people whose body temperatures are lowered by cold (hypothermia). You must provide resuscitation. The emergency department staff will continue resuscitation while they rewarm the patient's body. They will not declare biological death until the patient is rewarmed adequately and all efforts to revive him have failed.

FIRST ➤ Once you have started CPR, continue to provide CPR until:

- The patient regains a pulse. Then provide ventilations only.
- Spontaneous pulse and breathing begin.
- Equally or more highly trained members of the EMS system or someone certified in CPR can continue in your place.
- You turn over responsibility for patient care to a physician.
- You are exhausted and no longer able to continue. ◼

Rescuers are often concerned that they may have to stop CPR when they become exhausted, but you must be realistic. If you reach that point, realize that you have done all you could. CPR has its physical limitations on the rescuer. It also has its physical limitations on the patient. If you are becoming exhausted and know that you will not be able to continue, look for help from bystanders. Even if they are not trained in CPR, you may be able to tell them what they should do.

If you want to reduce the chances that you will have to stop CPR because of fatigue, then you should:

- Keep yourself in good physical condition. Exercise to improve your heart and lung functions.
- Become a CPR instructor. Help the American Heart Association, American Red Cross, National Safety Counsel, American Safety and Health Institute, Medic First Aid, or similar organizations in their efforts to train all citizens in basic cardiac life support. Your efforts to train others will help increase the number of bystanders who are able to assist you in providing CPR.
- Support your local EMS system by participating in educational events and fundraisers so that it may have the personnel and equipment needed to reach all victims in your area.
- Practice what you have learned about CPR. Your instructor can tell you how to review CPR, keep yourself up to date. Depending on who trained you, you may need to be retrained every year or two to remain certified.

WARNING

Do not practice CPR on anyone. It can cause serious problems when applied to someone with a normal heartbeat. Practice only on manikins. Finding the CPR compression site may be practiced on both people and manikins.

Automated External Defibrillation

There have been two early problems with recognizing and caring for cardiac arrest patients. The first problem—delay in starting CPR—has been dramatically reduced through the training of more people who can administer CPR before EMS personnel arrive. The second problem stems from the fact that many heart attacks are fatal no matter how soon CPR is started. These deaths are often caused by certain abnormal heart rhythms, or *dysrrhythmias,* that must be corrected as soon as possible if patients are to survive.

In response, EMS personnel and laypeople are now being trained in the use of an amazing device called an *automated external defibrillator (AED)*. AEDs can assess a heart's rhythm, determine if defibrillation is necessary, and deliver an electrical shock to convert a lethal (deadly) rhythm to a normal one. Almost all jurisdictions have approved and adopted the use of AEDs. Your organization or service may already have purchased one or more AEDs and may include AED training in emergency care programs.

> **NOTE**
>
> American Heart Association guidelines suggest that all health-care providers are trained and equipped to provide defibrillation at the earliest possible moment for victims of sudden cardiac arrest.

EXTERNAL DEFIBRILLATION

Defibrillators are designed to deliver an electrical shock that will stimulate the heart to begin beating normally. The shock does not start a heart that has stopped or is in arrest, but it will give the heart a chance to spontaneously re-establish an effective rhythm on its own. The entire process is called *defibrillation*.

There are many kinds of defibrillators available today. The two basic kinds are manual defibrillators and AEDs. Manual defibrillators are carried by most ALS providers. They require the rescuer to interpret the patient's heart rhythm and then decide whether or not the patient should receive a shock. The skills needed to accomplish those tasks require significant training beyond the level of most Emergency Medical Responders and EMTs.

The other type of defibrillator, the AED (Figure 8.22), can be fully automated or semi-automated. The fully automated AED assesses the patient's heart rhythm, advises that a shock is necessary, and delivers the shock without any input from the rescuer. Semi-automated defibrillators analyze the patient's rhythm and simply advise the rescuer if a shock is needed. It is then up to the rescuer to push a button to deliver the shock. For safety reasons, the semi-automated AED is the recommended choice for Emergency Medical Responders.

AEDs are capable of recognizing two very specific abnormal heart rhythms: ventricular fibrillation and ventricular tachycardia. The term **fibrillation** refers to a disorganized electrical activity within the heart that renders the heart incapable of pumping blood. The most common cause of fibrillation is a heart attack. Fibrillation results in a disorganized quivering of the heart muscle much like a spasm or seizure (Figure 8.23). The most common type of fibrillation affects the lower half (ventricles) of the heart and is called **ventricular fibrillation** (ven-TRIK-u-ler fib-ri-LAY-shun), VF or V-fib for short. When a person's heart goes into VF, the brain and other vital organs no longer receive an adequate supply of oxygenated blood, and the patient becomes unresponsive. VF does not produce a pulse, so the patient will be found unresponsive

fibrillation ■ a disorganized electrical activity within the heart that renders the heart incapable of pumping blood.

ventricular fibrillation (ven-TRIK-u-ler fib-ri-LAY-shun) (VF) ■ uncoordinated electrical activity, causing rapid ineffective contractions of the lower heart chambers and the absence of a pulse. See *defibrillation*.

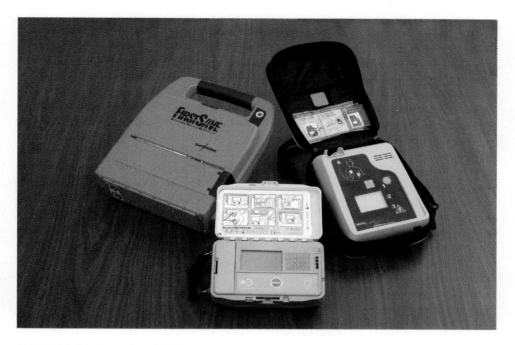

FIGURE 8.22 Examples of AEDs.

with no pulse and no breathing. It is believed that a high percentage of all adult cardiac arrest patients are in VF in the first few minutes following cardiac arrest. The sooner that VF can be defibrillated, the better the patient's chances are for survival.

AEDs also can recognize the abnormal heart rhythm called **ventricular tachycardia,** or *V-tach* for short. V-tach is a rapid rhythm that originates in the ventricles and rarely produces a pulse. It does not pump blood very efficiently. Less than 10% of the prehospital cardiac arrest cases have this problem. Defibrillation may help some of these patients.

In situations where there is no electrical activity within the heart—a condition called **asystole** (ah-SIS-to-le) or sometimes "flatline"—AEDs will not be effective.

ventricular tachycardia (ven-TRIK-u-ler tak-e-KAR-de-ah) ■ the abnormally rapid contraction of the heart's lower chambers, resulting in very poor circulation. Also called *V-tach.*

asystole (ah-SIS-to-le) ■ no electrical activity in the heart; cardiac arrest. Also called *flatline.*

NOTE

Some patients with specific heart conditions may have a small automated defibrillator surgically implanted inside their chest or abdomen. These devices are like external AEDs, only much smaller. You might not know that such a device is in place unless the patient or a family member tells you it is there. Your care of a patient in cardiac arrest will not change with the presence of an internal defibrillator.

EMS AND DEFIBRILLATION

Time is one of the most critical elements in the effort to save the life of a victim of cardiac arrest. Minimizing the time between collapse and the initiation of CPR, between CPR and the delivery of the first AED shock, and between defibrillation and the arrival of more advanced care is the goal of a strong chain of survival. The time between collapse and defibrillation can be divided into four segments:

■ *EMS access time.* This is the time from patient collapse until the EMS system is alerted.

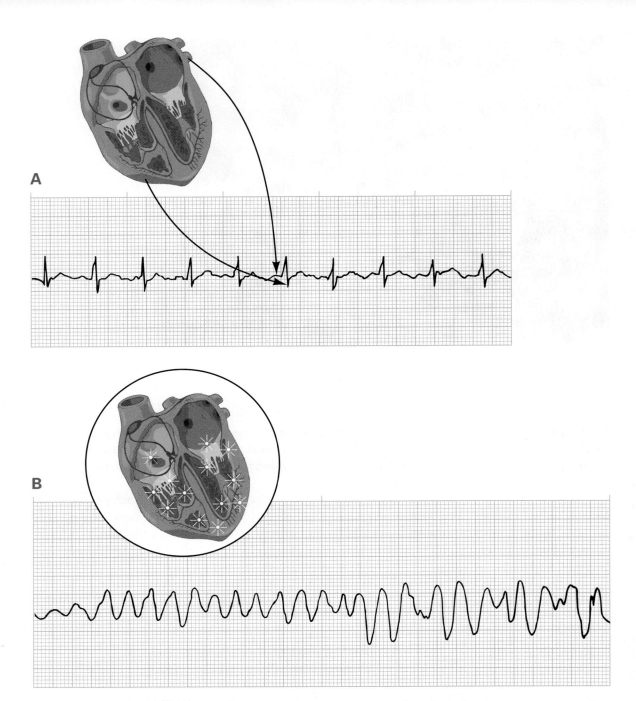

FIGURE 8.23 A. Normal heart rhythm, or normal sinus rhythm, and **B.** ventricular fibrillation.

- *Dispatch time.* This is the time from the call to the EMS dispatcher to the alert of the personnel who will respond and defibrillate.
- *Response time.* This is the time it takes for the rescuer or crew to reach the patient.
- *Shock time.* This is the time it takes from reaching the patient until the first shock is delivered.

The goal of every EMS system is to reduce the time of each of those four segments. In particular, having rescuers with defibrillators available 24 hours a day shortens the time from dispatch to the arrival of the defibrillator. If the patient can receive the first shock within three to five minutes of collapse, survival is more likely.

USING AEDs

A defibrillator must be ready for use at any given moment. Make certain that you follow manufacturer guidelines to ensure that the defibrillators you use are in working order and prepared for use. Always carry fully charged spare batteries.

Basic Warnings

Emergency Medical Responders may be trained to use either fully automated or semi-automated defibrillators. The Medical Director for your EMS system may have approved one or both of these devices. Whichever your system uses, you are responsible for noting certain warnings when working with AEDs:

- Follow the same precautions that you would for operating any electrical device.
- Only place the AED on a patient who is over the age of one year, unresponsive, pulseless, and not breathing.
- Do not place defibrillator patches over a patient's medication patch or implanted pacemaker. With gloved hands, remove the medication patch and wipe the chest dry.
- Make certain that no one is touching the patient during the analyze or shock phases.
- Do not attempt to assess or shock a patient who is moving or when the defibrillator or its leads are being moved.
- Do not attempt to defibrillate a patient in a moving ambulance or other moving vehicle.
- Do not attempt to defibrillate a patient who has an obstructed airway. The patient who is in respiratory arrest but not in cardiac arrest (assess pulse) does not need defibrillation.
- Do not attempt to defibrillate a patient who is lying in a puddle of water.
- Do not attempt to defibrillate a child younger than one year. Your Medical Director may have specific guidelines for defibrillating children from 12 months to eight years old with a special pediatric AED. Follow your local protocols.

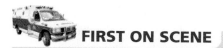

FIRST ON SCENE

Laryn's arms and lower back were just beginning to ache when Joey turned the corner at the end of the hall and sprinted to the locked office door. The sound of his footfalls grew louder until they slid to a halt just outside and she heard him fumbling with a set of keys, find the right one, and push the door open.

Fluorescent light flooded the small office, making Laryn squint and causing Paul to look hideously pale. "Quick!" Laryn shouted. "Get the AED on him!"

Joey popped the black nylon cover open, glancing at the large, cartoon-like directions as he turned the unit on and pulled the electrode pads out. "Okay, stop," Joey said to Laryn as he grabbed Paul's shirt and tore it open, sending small plastic buttons skittering in all directions.

Laryn stretched her back, panting, as Joey yanked the paper backing from the electrodes and placed them on Paul's lifeless body.

Is It Safe ?

The American Heart Association does not recommend for or against the use of AEDs on patients who are younger than one year of age. It is important to always learn and follow your own local protocols. ▪

Is It Safe ?

The American Heart Association has indicated that it is safe and appropriate to use an AED on a patient who is laying on a wet surface. It is, however, important to ensure that he is *not* lying in a puddle of standing water. If this is the case, simply drag the patient out of the puddle and continue your care. Also, it is important that the surface of the patient's chest where the pads are to be placed is dry.

American Heart Association guidelines also indicate that metal surfaces pose no shock hazard to either the patient or the rescuer. ▪

It is not uncommon for an elderly patient to have an implanted pacemaker/defibrillator. This will be seen as a small round or rectangular object beneath the skin, just below the clavicle or high in the abdomen. You should never alter your care due to the presence of one of these devices. You must perform an appropriate initial assessment, and if the patient is pulseless and nonbreathing, then you must begin CPR and apply an AED as if the patient did not have such a device. One of the reasons why the patient is having an emergency may be that the device has failed. Although this is rare, it does happen.

Protocols for the use of AEDs for trauma patients vary by state and jurisdiction. Follow your EMS system's protocols and carefully assess the patient and mechanism of injury or the nature of the illness. If you are not certain as to what you are to do, phone or radio medical direction.

Emergency Medical Responder Care

The use of a defibrillator must follow specific procedures of care and assessment. You must determine if the patient is indeed a candidate for the placement of an AED. The patient must:

- Be unresponsive.
- Be older than one year.
- Have no carotid pulse.
- Have no respirations.

These criteria must be met before you can place an AED on a patient in suspected cardiac arrest.

Perform an initial assessment to confirm that the patient is indeed in cardiac arrest. If you are first on the scene and have confirmed that the patient meets all of the criteria, perform two minutes of CPR before placing the AED. After two minutes of CPR, activate the AED.

If you arrive on scene with a defibrillator and someone else is providing CPR, your job will be to prepare and attach the defibrillator. Make certain that both of you are clear of the patient before delivering a shock.

Attaching the Defibrillator

The procedure for attaching the defibrillator to a patient is the same for both semi-automated and fully automated AEDs. While the first rescuer performs CPR, the rescuer operating the AED should perform the following steps:

1. Bare the patient's chest. If the patient's chest is wet, quickly wipe it dry. Make certain the patient is not lying in a puddle of standing water. Ground that is wet with no standing water is safe for defibrillation.

2. Place electrodes on the patient's bare, dry chest, one at a time. It may be necessary to shave the chest because hair can prevent the electrodes from sticking properly. Place one pad on the patient's upper right chest below the collarbone (clavicle) and next to the breastbone (sternum). Place the second pad on the patient's left side well below the armpit. Most pads and devices have illustrations on them showing the correct placement of the pads (Figure 8.24).

3. Finally, ensure that the electrodes are firmly plugged into the device. Some electrodes come already connected and others need to be plugged in after the pads have been placed. Follow the specific directions for your device.

AEDs will not function properly unless the pads fully adhere to the patient's chest and the cables are tightly inserted into the device. If either of these prob-

---

REMEMBER

Make certain that dispatch is informed of the emergency.

REMEMBER

On the basis of the published evidence to date, the Pediatric Advanced Life Support Task Force of the International Liaison Committee on Resuscitation (ILCOR) has made the following recommendation as of July 2003: "AEDs may be used for children one to eight years of age who have no signs of circulation. Ideally, the device should deliver a pediatric dose."

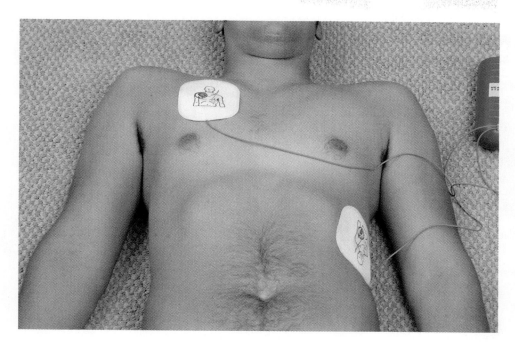

FIGURE 8.24 Correct placement of defibrillator pads.

lems exist, the "no contact" or "check electrodes" prompt will sound or appear on the AED.

Operating the Fully Automated Defibrillator

The following describes the operational procedures for a typical fully automated defibrillator. There are many models available. You must be familiar with the one that you will use. Follow the manufacturer's operating instructions for the specific AED you will be using.

Is It Safe ?

The fully automated AED is not recommended for use by Emergency Medical Responders because it will deliver a shock without any input from the operator. If you find yourself on the scene where a fully automated AED is in use, listen carefully to the device for voice prompts prior to the delivery of a shock. Be certain that no one is touching the patient when the device delivers a shock. ■

Once turned on and attached to the patient, the latest models of fully automated defibrillators will assess the patient's heart rhythm, determine if a shock is indicated, charge to the preset energy level, and deliver the shock to the patient, all without further input from the rescuer. Many of these defibrillators have voice and text prompts that advise the rescuer with messages, such as "Shock advised. Do not touch the patient," "Charging. Stand clear," and "Stop CPR. Check breathing and pulse." If this voice system fails, the rescuer is expected to know what to do and how to ensure personal safety.

To operate a fully automated external defibrillator, you should (Scan 8–5):

1. Assess the patient to confirm that he is in cardiac arrest.

2. Have your partner or someone trained in CPR begin CPR while you set up the AED. If you are alone, do not start CPR. Instead make sure that EMS has been called and immediately attach the AED.

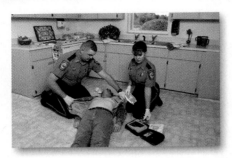

1 ▪ Turn on the AED and bare the patient's chest.

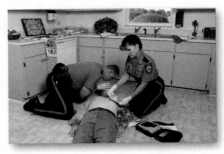

2 ▪ Place the pads and connect the cable to the device (if not already connected).

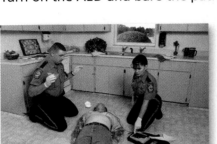

3 ▪ Press the "analyze" button to begin analyzing the patient's rhythm and then follow the prompts.

3. Turn on the AED and attach the electrodes. Once the electrodes are in place, the AED will begin to analyze the patient's rhythm.

4. Depending on the patient's rhythm, the AED will deliver one shock.

5. Following the shock, the AED will advise you to begin CPR. (The most current AEDs are programmed to pause for two minutes after each shock to allow for CPR.)

6. After two minutes, the AED will advise you to stop CPR. It will then re-analyze the heart rhythm and, if indicated, deliver another shock. This sequence of one shock and two minutes of CPR should continue until more advanced care providers arrive.

If at any time the patient goes into a rhythm that is not shockable, the AED will advise you to begin CPR. If the patient does have a pulse, leave the defibrillator attached to him in order to monitor the patient. Maintain an open airway and continue life support procedures until more advanced EMS personnel arrive and take over patient care. The patient would benefit from oxygen therapy and, if necessary, assisted ventilations.

NOTE

The AED sequence presented here is a typical protocol that is programmed into many AEDs from the factory. Each EMS system has its own protocols for the use of AEDs and may differ from what is presented here. Some jurisdictions may require Emergency Medical Responders to give a different number of shocks before transporting or continuing CPR, while others may require rescuers to perform CPR for two full minutes or perform some other step before preparing and attaching the defibrillator. Always know and follow local protocols before attempting to use an AED.

Operating the Semi-Automated Defibrillator

The following is an example of the operational procedure for a semi-automated defibrillator. There are several semi-automated models currently available. Follow the instructions given in the manufacturer's manual for your specific model and always follow your EMS system's protocols for the defibrillator you use.

Once turned on and applied to the patient, semi-automatic defibrillators will analyze the rhythm and advise if a shock is necessary. Some models require the rescuer to push a button to begin the analysis sequence. In either case, the AED will automatically charge to a preset energy level. At this point, it is necessary for the rescuer to push a button to deliver the shock (Figure 8.25).

The same assessment and safety procedures that apply to the fully automated defibrillator also apply to the operation of the semi-automated defibrillator. Some older models may not have a voice synthesizer. Regardless of the model, they all require the rescuer to push a button to deliver the shock.

To operate a semi-automated defibrillator, you should:

1. Assess the patient to confirm that he is in cardiac arrest.

2. Have your partner or someone else trained in CPR begin CPR while you set up the AED. If you are alone, perform two minutes of CPR before attaching the AED.

3. Turn on the AED and attach the electrodes. Once the electrodes are in place, the AED will begin to analyze the patient's rhythm. If necessary, push the analyze button.

4. If a shockable rhythm is detected, the AED will advise so and charge to the appropriate energy level. When needed, the AED will prompt you to push the shock button.

5. After you push the shock button, the AED will deliver one shock.

6. Following the shock, the AED will advise you to begin CPR. (The most current AEDs are programmed to pause for two minutes after each shock to allow you to perform CPR.)

7. After two minutes, the AED will advise you to stop CPR. It will then re-analyze the heart rhythm and, if indicated, advise the rescuer to deliver another shock. This sequence of one shock and two minutes of CPR should continue until more highly trained providers arrive.

The maximum number of shocks that any AED will deliver is typically preset at the factory, as is the energy level of each shock, and follows local protocols. If you are in doubt as to what to do, contact medical direction.

Potential Problems

Most of the problems with defibrillator operations can be easily corrected. Most problems involve the poor attachment of the pads and/or cables. Making certain that the pads are in full contact with the patient's chest and that the cables are tightly connected to the device usually is all that is needed.

Make sure the patient's chest is dry and free of anything that can prevent the pad from adhering well, such as hair or medication patches that occupy the pad placement sites. With gloved hands, remove

REMEMBER

Always follow the manufacturer's manual and your EMS system's guidelines for the defibrillator you use.

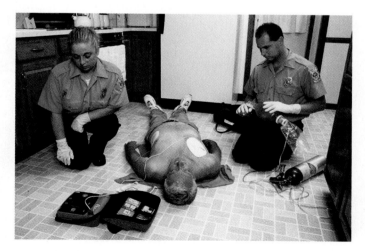

FIGURE 8.25 Operating a semi-automated defibrillator. Do not apply shock until everyone, including you, is clear of the patient.

any medication patches and wipe off any medication remaining on the patient's chest. If you have to shave the pad placement areas of the patient's chest, use a disposable safety razor provided in the AED kit for this purpose.

Most AEDs are programmed to run self-diagnostic checks every 24 hours. If one of these self-checks detects a failure of any of the AED's internal systems, an error message and/or audible alarm will sound alerting the rescuer to the failure. It is important to know the error messages that can be displayed by your specific device. Some errors are only advisory in nature and allow continued use of the device, while others indicate a failure of a major system, rendering the AED inoperable. Be sure to read the manufacturer's operating manual for the device you use and become familiar with all error messages and alarms.

Assessment and Quality Assurance

To be effective, a prehospital defibrillation program requires ongoing evaluation in order to identify and correct any problems. This process of assessment and quality assurance should focus on specific situations that involve standard operating procedures, physician-directed standing orders, care delivered by the rescuers, performance of the equipment, routine maintenance, and effectiveness of training programs. Changes in any aspect of the program must be the result of physician evaluation and orders.

Some AEDs have a voice-recording device built in that will provide an audible record of the resuscitation and defibrillation incident. All AEDs have an internal recording device that can capture a digital recording of the patient's heart rhythm, including shocks delivered. This information can be downloaded onto a computer so that a physician can evaluate the event to determine how the various aspects of the defibrillation program performed. Evaluation is an important part of any AED program and serves to improve and ensure quality patient care.

Be certain to carefully document all incidents involving the use of an AED. Your notes should include the time you arrived on scene, your assessment findings, how many shocks you delivered, and the patient's response following each shock.

Part of your equipment inspection and assessment should include the operation of your defibrillator recording devices. Follow the manufacturer's instructions and your EMS system's recommendations to correct any problems before the unit is put into service. In addition, it is important to ensure that the AED kit includes the necessary supplies at all times, such as an extra battery, an extra set of electrode pads (adult and pediatric), razors, and towels. You may find it helpful to carry duplicate supplies with the unit.

 FIRST ON SCENE WRAP-UP

The afternoon crowd in the casino was sparse (mostly retirees whose RVs were parked haphazardly in the adjoining lot), so not many people noticed as the ambulance crew pulled their gurney through the main doors and walked quickly to the bank of elevators. Once on the third floor, they met a man with an Australian accent who directed them down a long, doorless hallway to the facility's CCTV room. A woman, in a disheveled business suit, was sitting cross-legged on the floor next to an older man in the recovery position.

"It worked," she said with a huge, tired smile. The patient was breathing steadily and slowly running his fingers over the foam pads stuck to his chest.

"You're a very lucky man," one of the EMTs said as she placed an oxygen mask on the patient's face. "It looks like this young lady over here saved your life."

Paul looked over at Laryn, who was now blushing, and smiled weakly as he patted her hand. "Thank you," he mouthed, the hissing oxygen louder than his quiet words.

Summary

Like the chain of EMS resources, the chain of survival is also a linked system of patient-care events. These events include early access, early CPR, early defibrillation, and early advanced life support (ALS). Remember that the chain of survival is different for adults and children.

There is a strong relationship between the brain and the activities of breathing and circulation. When the heart stops beating, a patient is in cardiac arrest and cannot circulate oxygenated blood to the brain. The major signs of cardiac arrest are unresponsiveness, no breathing, and no pulse.

Check for breathing by placing your ear next to the patient's nose and mouth and looking, listening, and feeling for air exchange. Check the carotid pulse in the neck for any patient older than one year of age; check the brachial pulse on an infant (younger than one year of age).

If a patient is unresponsive, check airway, breathing, and circulation (ABCs). After determining that the adult patient is unresponsive, alert the EMS system. If you are alone and caring for a pediatric patient, provide two minutes of CPR before activating EMS. To provide proper CPR, you will:

1. Place the patient in a supine position on a hard surface and then open his airway. Be careful not to overextend the neck of an infant or child.
2. Check for breathing for at least five seconds, but no more than 10 seconds. If the patient is not breathing . . .
3. Provide two slow breaths. (Clear the airway if necessary.)
4. Check for signs of circulation, including a pulse. If there are none . . .
5. Find the appropriate compression site.
   — For an adult and child, the site is on the center of the chest between the nipples.
   — For an infant, the site is on the center of the chest, one finger width below an imaginary line drawn between the nipples.
6. Position your hands for compressions.
   — For an adult, place the heel of one hand on the center of the patient's bare chest, right between the nipples. Put your other hand on top of the first. Either extend or interlace your fingers to keep them off the patient's chest.
   — For a child (age one to onset of puberty), place the heel of one hand on the center of the patient's bare chest, right between the nipples, being sure to keep the fingers off the chest. If necessary, you may use two hands for compressions on a child.

   — For an infant (up to one year of age), place two fingers on the sternum one finger width below the nipple line.
7. Provide external chest compressions.
   — For an adult (older than eight years), provide compressions at a rate of 100 per minute and a depth of 1.5 to 2 inches.
   — For a child (age one to onset of puberty), provide compressions at a rate of 100 per minute at one-third to one-half the depth of the chest.
   — For an infant (up to one year of age), provide compressions at a rate of at least 100 per minute at one-third to one-half the depth of the infant's chest.
8. Compression/ventilation ratios are two breaths every 30 compressions for an adult, child, or infant.
9. Check for pulse.
   — In an adult or child, check the carotid pulse.
   — In an infant, check the brachial pulse.
10. If the circulation check shows:
    — No pulse and no breathing, then begin CPR.
    — Pulse but no breathing, provide artificial ventilation. Continue to monitor pulse every few minutes.
    — Heart rate less than 60 for a child or infant, start CPR. If the heart rate is above 60 beats per minute, continue to assist ventilations and monitor the heart rate to ensure that it increases.

Do not stop CPR for more than 10 seconds other than to move the patient because of danger on scene. If you have to move the patient, do not stop CPR for more than 15 to 30 seconds. Continue CPR until the patient regains a pulse and/or breathing, or until you are relieved by an equally or more highly trained person, care for the patient is accepted by a physician, or until you can no longer continue because of exhaustion.

Start CPR immediately on a patient in cardiac arrest, even if you may worsen existing injuries. Without CPR, the patient will go from clinical death to biological death within 10 minutes. If the patient has a DNR order, do not start resuscitation. Check with your jurisdiction about advance directives.

Emergency Medical Responders use automated external defibrillators (AEDs) in many jurisdictions. These lifesaving units are placed in many public areas, and Emergency Medical Responders should be able to assist the public in using them and in performing CPR. AEDs can convert certain lethal heart rhythms to a normal cardiac rhythm. AEDs are electrical devices and must be used with caution and according to specific protocols. The general steps for the use of a typical AED are:

- Confirm that the patient is unresponsive and has no breathing or pulse.

- Turn on the AED, expose the patient's chest, and securely attach the pads. Wipe dry or shave hair if necessary.
- Follow the AED's prompts to defibrillate and check breathing and pulse.
- Follow AED prompts for a pulse or start CPR if no pulse.

Remember and Consider

As long as the heart pumps, the blood circulates. If the heart stops pumping, the blood stops circulating and CPR is needed to restart and maintain circulation. You will practice CPR in class and may have done so already. Think about what you have read in the text and what you will do during practice.

➤ What equipment do you need to perform CPR?

➤ How many people do you need to perform CPR?

Were the answers to the previous questions easy? Or did you say, "It depends"? Does it depend on the age or size of the patient, on the number of rescuers available to help, or on whether you have a barrier device, gloves, or oxygen? Can you do CPR without these things? Is it safe to do so? What are your obligations for performing CPR on someone in cardiac arrest? Do you think you need to carry your own barrier device and gloves with you at all times? What if you do not have a barrier device and someone in a restaurant has a heart attack and goes into cardiac arrest before the ambulance gets there? Is there anything handy that you can use as an improvised barrier device?

➤ If you start CPR on a cardiac arrest patient in a public place, how would you work with someone who wants to help but is doing CPR incorrectly? Do you feel that you could coach someone or give directions while you are performing CPR? Would you ventilate and tell the person how to do chest compressions, or would you do chest compressions and tell the person how to ventilate? Would it be better to send the person for help or to ask him or her to control the crowd while you perform one-rescuer CPR?

Practice chest compressions while you coach a classmate or station member on artificial ventilation. Switch your position and practice ventilations while you coach someone on chest compressions. Do you think this is effective? Can it work? Or do you think it is easier to just do it yourself? How long can you last?

➤ Have someone time you while you do CPR until you get tired. How long were you able to perform CPR before you felt you were no longer effective?

Investigate

Whether you are on or off duty when you are in a public place, you may need to assist in the care of a patient before an ambulance arrives. Plan ahead.

➤ Which public places and stores in your area keep emergency care supplies handy for public use? When you go to the library, the grocery store, the mall, the theater, or restaurants, do you see signs that tell you they have first aid kits with barrier devices or AEDs available? If you do not see signs, ask if these items are kept for public use in the event of an emergency. Can they be retrieved quickly? Or are they locked away, causing someone to wait while the key is found?

Many malls are beginning to keep emergency care supplies at special locations or at a first aid center.

➤ Do the security guards know where these supplies are kept? Do they have access to these supplies? How hard is it to locate and retrieve these supplies? What supplies are kept? Are there barrier devices and gloves, different sizes of airways and bag-valve masks, an AED? What

training do mall, airport, or other large public place personnel have for using these items?

Part of the learning experience—and an effective quality assurance step—is wanting to know if your emergency care delivery was appropriate and effective. How do you find out if the CPR that you performed on a patient was effective?

➤ Does your department get follow-up information on patients that you cared for in the prehospital setting? Are you able to check the records for patient outcomes? If the new patient privacy laws will not let you, how can you find out what you must do to get that information from the hospital?

You may find that your procedures were performed correctly, but the patient could not be resuscitated because of other medical or trauma conditions or circumstances. Knowing that you performed correctly is a positive reinforcement for your efforts. Finding out what you need to do to correct your performance is a learning experience.

Quick Quiz

1. The appropriate rate of compressions during adult CPR is _____ per minute.
   a. 80 to 100
   b. no faster than 80
   c. about 100
   d. no faster than 120

2. You are caring for an adult patient who was found unresponsive. After opening the airway and checking for breathing, you discover the patient has very slow shallow respirations. You give two successful breaths and then find him to be pulseless. What is the most appropriate next step?
   a. Reposition the airway and try again.
   b. Recheck for a pulse.
   c. Begin chest compressions.
   d. Provide rescue breaths only.

3. The recommended location for assessing for the presence of a pulse on a child is at the _____ artery.
   a. brachial
   b. carotid
   c. radial
   d. femoral

4. What is the recommended rate of compressions for infant CPR?
   a. at least 100 per minute
   b. as fast as possible
   c. 80 to 100 per minute
   d. 60 to 80 per minute

5. What is the recommended ratio of chest compressions to ventilations for an adult patient in cardiac arrest?
   a. 30 to 2
   b. 15 to 2
   c. 5 to 1
   d. 3 to 1

6. You are caring for an adult victim of sudden cardiac arrest. To give this patient the best chance for survival, you should provide immediate:
   a. CPR and no defibrillation.
   b. defibrillation without CPR.
   c. CPR with defibrillation within 10 minutes.
   d. CPR with defibrillation within 5 minutes.

7. Which one of the following is the best reason to provide rescue breathing to a nonbreathing patient?
   a. It is an effective way to provide oxygen to the patient.
   b. It can clear a blocked airway with little effort.
   c. It can defibrillate the heart if done quickly enough.
   d. It helps to circulate blood to the brain and lungs.

8. You are caring for a child who has a good pulse but is not breathing on his own. You should provide rescue breaths for this patient once every _____ seconds.
   a. three to five
   b. five to six
   c. six to seven
   d. 10 seconds

9. Which one of the following statements best describes the appropriate ventilation volume for a nonbreathing child patient?
   a. twice that of an infant
   b. the weight minus the age
   c. enough to cause the chest to rise
   d. exactly half the volume of an adult

10. Before providing rescue breaths, you must check for the presence of adequate breathing. Do this by listening for air flow from the patient's nose and mouth and by:
    a. shaking the patient.
    b. looking for chest rise.
    c. observing pupil response.
    d. sweeping the mouth for obstructions.

11. You are caring for a responsive five-year-old patient who is showing signs of a complete airway obstruction. Care for this patient by providing:
    a. finger sweeps.
    b. abdominal thrusts.
    c. five back blows and chest thrusts.
    d. rescue breaths every three to five seconds.

12. You are alone when you discover and remove a four-year-old child from a public pool. When should you call 9-1-1?
    a. after providing two minutes of CPR
    b. immediately after removing him from the pool
    c. after 10 minutes of CPR with no response
    d. after rescue breaths but before compressions

13. Which one of the following represents the most appropriate hand location for chest compressions on an adult?

    a. at the nipple line
    b. at the top of the sternum
    c. over the left side of the chest
    d. on the very bottom of the sternum

14. You are caring for an infant who is unresponsive and not breathing. Your initial attempt at rescue breathing is not successful. Which one of the following is most likely the cause?

    a. The child has asthma and cannot breathe.
    b. The airway is likely blocked by an airway spasm.
    c. The child is choking on a foreign object.
    d. You probably did not open the airway properly.

15. You are at a local Little League baseball game and see a parent collapse onto the ground. You are the first person to reach the man. What is the first thing you should do?

    a. Place him in the recovery position.
    b. Send someone to call 9-1-1.
    c. Check for responsiveness.
    d. Give two slow breaths.

MODULE **5** Illness and Injury

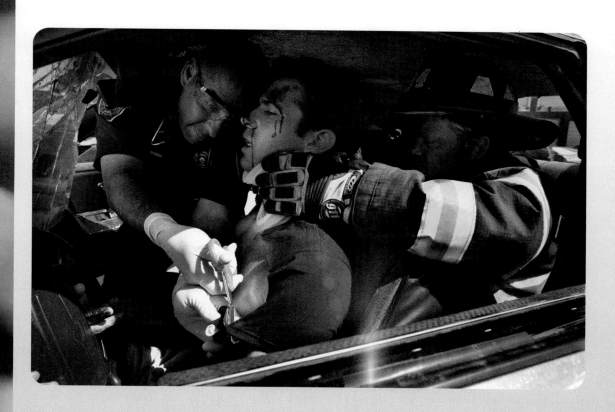

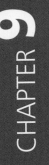

CHAPTER 9

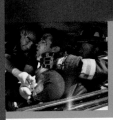

Caring for Medical Emergencies

All patient emergencies can be categorized in one of two ways—either as medical or as trauma. Emergencies that result in injury, such as from a fall or a vehicle crash, are categorized as trauma. Illnesses and conditions that can affect the body are known as *medical emergencies*. You must be prepared to provide appropriate emergency care to the various medical patients you encounter. Although some situations will require you to intervene with specific skills, others will be referred to as *common medical complaints*.

This chapter provides an overview of medical emergencies and emergency care for specific complaints, including chest pain, congestive heart failure (CHF), respiratory emergencies, stroke, seizures, diabetes, and abdominal pain. It also provides emergency care information on poisons, bites, and stings; heat and cold exposure; behavioral change; and alcohol and drug abuse.

OBJECTIVES

This chapter is based on the objectives of the U.S. DOT's First Responder National Standard Curriculum. Note that cognitive objectives are listed below and beside corresponding text throughout the chapter. You will also notice as you read each objective that the term Emergency Medical Responder is used. This is simply a name change and reflects the new name for the First Responder.

By the end of this chapter, you should be able to (from cognitive or knowledge information):

5–1.1 Identify the patient who presents with a general medical complaint. (p. 249)

5–1.2 Explain the steps in providing emergency medical care to a patient with a general medical complaint. (p. 249)

5–1.3 Identify the patient who presents with a specific medical complaint of altered mental status. (pp. 263–271)

5–1.4 Explain the steps in providing emergency medical care to a patient with an altered mental status. (pp. 265–271)

5–1.5 Identify the patient who presents with a specific medical complaint of seizures. (pp. 267–268)

5–1.6 Explain the steps in providing emergency medical care to a patient with seizures. (p. 268)

5-1.7 Identify the patient who presents with a specific medical complaint of exposure to cold. (pp. 287, 289)

5-1.8 Explain the steps in providing emergency medical care to a patient with an exposure to cold. (pp. 287, 289)

5-1.9 Identify the patient who presents with a specific medical complaint of exposure to heat. (pp. 285, 286)

5-1.10 Explain the steps in providing emergency medical care to a patient with an exposure to heat. (pp. 285, 286)

5-1.11 Identify the patient who presents with a specific medical complaint of behavioral change. (pp. 289–290)

5-1.12 Explain the steps in providing emergency medical care to a patient with a behavioral change. (p. 291)

5-1.13 Identify the patient who presents with a specific medical complaint of psychological crisis. (pp. 289–290)

5-1.14 Explain the steps in providing emergency medical care to a patient with a psychological crisis. (p. 291)

By the end of this chapter, you should be able to feel comfortable enough to (by changing attitudes, values, and beliefs):

5-1.15 Attend to the feelings of the patient and/or family when dealing with the patient with a general medical complaint. (p. 249)

5-1.16 Attend to the feelings of the patient and/or family when dealing with the patient with a specific medical complaint. (pp. 253, 255–256, 258, 262, 265, 267, 268, 285, 286, 289)

5-1.17 Explain the rationale for modifying your behavior toward the patient with a behavioral emergency. (pp. 289–293)

5-1.18 Demonstrate a caring attitude toward patients with a general medical complaint who request emergency medical services. (p. 249)

5-1.19 Place the interests of the patient with a general medical complaint as the foremost consideration when making any and all patient-care decisions. (p. 249)

5-1.20 Communicate with empathy to patients with a general medical complaint, as well as with family members and friends of the patient. (p. 249)

5-1.21 Demonstrate a caring attitude toward patients with a specific medical complaint who request emergency medical services. (pp. 253, 255–256, 258, 262, 265, 267, 268, 285, 286, 289)

5-1.22 Place the interests of the patient with a specific medical complaint as the foremost consideration when making any and all patient-care decisions. (pp. 258, 259, 261, 263–264, 271, 272, 273, 293, 296)

5-1.23 Communicate with empathy to patients with a specific medical complaint, as well as with family members and friends of the patient. (pp. 253, 255–256, 258, 262, 265, 267, 268, 285, 286, 289)

5-1.24 Demonstrate a caring attitude toward patients with a behavior problem who request emergency medical services. (pp. 289–293)

5-1.25 Place the interests of the patient with a behavioral problem as the foremost consideration when making any and all patient-care decisions. (pp. 289–293)

5-1.26 Communicate with empathy to patients with a behavioral problem, as well as with family members and friends of the patient. (pp. 289–293)

By the end of this chapter, you should be able to show how to (through psychomotor skills):

5-1.27 Demonstrate the steps in providing emergency medical care to a patient with a general medical complaint. (p. 249)

5-1.28 Demonstrate the steps in providing emergency medical care to a patient with an altered mental status. (pp. 265–271)

5-1.29 Demonstrate the steps in providing emergency medical care to a patient with seizures. (p. 268)

5-1.30 Demonstrate the steps in providing emergency medical care to a patient with an exposure to cold. (pp. 287, 289)

5-1.31 Demonstrate the steps in providing emergency medical care to a patient with an exposure to heat. (pp. 285, 286)

5-1.32 Demonstrate the steps in providing emergency medical care to a patient with a behavioral change. (p. 291)

5-1.33 Demonstrate the steps in providing emergency medical care to a patient with a psychological crisis. (p. 291)

In addition to the National Standard Objectives, you will need to understand the importance of performing an initial assessment on medical patients and identifying any life-threatening conditions. As you work through this chapter, you will also need to know:

➤ Signs and symptoms of cardiac compromise, including heart attack and congestive heart failure.

➤ Signs and symptoms of respiratory difficulty and the care for those patients, including patients who appear to be hyperventilating.

➤ Conditions associated with abdominal pain, including signs and symptoms, causes, and emergency care.

➤ Signs and symptoms of poisonings, bites, and stings, including types and emergency care.

➤ Signs and symptoms and emergency care for patients suffering from an overdose of alcohol and/or drugs.

FIRST ON SCENE

"Micah!" There was a shout from somewhere. "Micah, will you wake up!" Micah Garibaldi shot up in his bed and quickly looked around the dorm room. Nothing seemed out of place. His vacationing roommate's movie posters still hung at odd angles from multicolored pushpins, clothing and books were still scattered around in piles, and the filter on the little octagon-shaped goldfish tank was still humming away, even though the fish were long gone. Just as he was starting to lie back down, someone pounded on the door, rattling it with each booming impact.

"Micah! Are you in there?" Micah slid out of bed and stomped across the room to the door.

"What?" he shouted as he pulled the door open. The look on that new freshman Frank Kline's face told him immediately that something really was wrong.

"There's this girl down in our room," Frank was wide-eyed and whispering hoarsely. "And she's like, like having some sort of, I think she's dying or something!" Micah, the dorm "doctor" ever since completing an Emergency Medical Responder course, quickly threw on a robe as he ran down the hall.

"Airway, breathing, circulation," he repeated in a running whisper, his nerves tightening his stomach and making his hands shake. "Remember the ABCs. Remember the ABCs."

Medical Emergencies

Patients may request EMS for a variety of medical complaints. Medical emergencies may be caused by infections, poisons, or the failure of one or more of the body's organs and systems. You must assess each patient and determine the chief complaint, as well as any signs and symptoms that might be present. The patient or a bystander may be able to tell you of an existing disease or condition. However, in most cases, what you observe and what the patient describes will be your main clues to the patient's problems.

A patient's medical emergency may be hidden because of an injury. For example, a diabetic patient may collapse because of very low blood sugar or may be involved in a vehicle crash and become injured. As an Emergency Medical Responder, your primary job will be to provide care for the patient's most obvious problem; in the case of a car crash, it would be his injuries. The medical problem, however, should not go unnoticed. During your assessment of a trauma patient, keep in mind that there may also be an underlying medical problem.

SIGNS AND SYMPTOMS

To detect a medical emergency, you have to be aware of common signs and symptoms, such as:

5-1.1 Identify the patient who presents with a general medical complaint.

- Altered mental status.
- Abnormal pulse rate and rhythm.
- Abnormal breathing rate and depth.
- Abnormal skin signs.
- Abnormal pupil size and/or response.
- Unusual breath odors.
- Tenderness or rigidity in the abdomen.
- Abnormal muscular activity such as spasms or paralysis.
- Bleeding or discharges from the body.

A patient may complain of some of the following symptoms:

- Pain.
- Numbness, tingling, or weakness.
- Shortness of breath.
- Fever or chills.
- Upset stomach and/or vomiting.
- Dizziness or feeling faint.
- Chest or abdominal pain.
- Unusual bowel or bladder activity.
- Itching or burning skin.
- Thirst, hunger, or odd tastes in the mouth.

ASSESSMENT

Emergency care for medical emergencies is based on the patient's signs and symptoms. That is why it is so important to complete an appropriate patient assessment. For general medical complaints, you should:

5-1.2 Explain the steps in providing emergency medical care to a patient with a general medical complaint.

1. Complete a scene size-up before you begin emergency medical care.
2. Perform an initial assessment.
3. Perform a patient history.
4. Perform a physical exam, as appropriate.
5. Complete ongoing assessments, as appropriate.
6. Comfort and reassure the patient while awaiting additional EMS resources.

FIRST ➤ When assessing the patient, keep in mind the following:

- If the patient appears or feels unusual in any way, suspect that there is a medical emergency.
- If the patient has abnormal vital signs, conclude that there is a medical emergency. ■

Patient assessment and care for medical emergencies are summarized in Figure 9.1.

Geriatric Focus

Assessment of the elderly must consider that due to the process of aging and to complications from and treatment of various diseases, signs and symptoms may not be as significant as you would expect them to be in a younger or healthier patient.

Care for Medical Emergencies

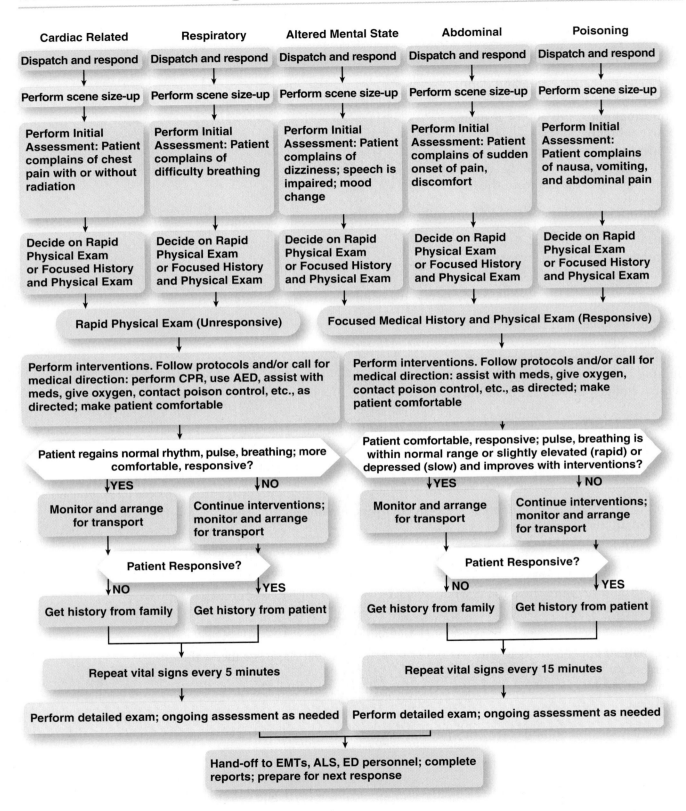

FIGURE 9.1 Algorithm for the emergency care of medical patients.

Specific Medical Emergencies

CARDIAC COMPROMISE

The term **cardiac compromise** is used to describe patients who present with specific signs and symptoms that indicate some type of emergency relating to the heart. Medical conditions such as myocardial infarction (MI) (heart attack), angina pectoris, and congestive heart failure (CHF) are some of the most common causes of the cardiac compromise. The following is a list of the more common signs and symptoms of the cardiac compromise:

- Chest discomfort. Typically described as pain or a dull pressure, tightness, or a squeezing sensation in the chest, the discomfort may also radiate to the arms, shoulders, back, neck, or jaw.
- Sudden onset of sweating (**diaphoresis**).
- Shortness of breath (**dyspnea**).
- Nausea/vomiting.
- Anxiety, irritability.
- Feeling of impending doom.
- Abnormal pulse rate (may be rapid, slow, and/or irregular).
- Abnormal blood pressure (may be high or low).
- Indigestion.

Cardiac compromise has many causes and can present with any one or all of the above signs and symptoms. As an Emergency Medical Responder, you must use your assessment skills to quickly gather a patient history and perform a physical exam to identify the potential for cardiac involvement. When in doubt, provide care for the worst possible scenario and call for an ALS ambulance, if available (Figure 9.2).

Myocardial Infarction

The medical term for what we commonly know as a heart attack is **myocardial infarction (MI)**. *Myo-* meaning muscle, *cardial-* meaning heart, and *infarction* meaning a deadening of tissue due to a loss of adequate blood supply. The heart must have an adequate supply of well-oxygenated blood to continue to function

cardiac compromise ■ a term used to describe specific signs and symptoms that indicate some type of emergency relating to the heart.

diaphoresis ■ perspiration, especially when it is heavy and caused by a medical condition.

dyspnea ■ difficulty breathing.

REMEMBER

A systolic pressure greater than 140 mmHg or a diastolic pressure above 90 mmHg may be an indication of high blood pressure. If you detect a low or a falling blood pressure, consider that the patient may be developing shock.

myocardial infarction (MI) ■ a condition in which the heart has suffered tissue damage due to a lack of adequate circulation to the heart muscle.

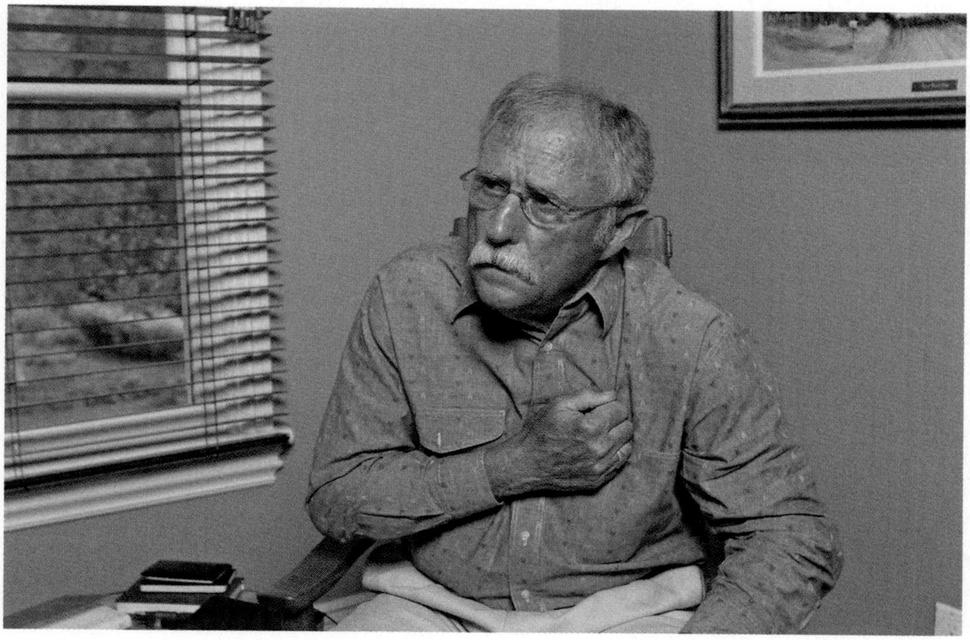

FIGURE 9.2 Chest pain is the primary symptom of a heart attack.

properly. The heart receives its blood supply through vessels known as *coronary arteries*. When these arteries become excessively narrow or blocked from disease and can no longer supply the heart with enough oxygenated blood, the tissue of the heart begins to die. A heart attack may be the result.

It is important to understand that a heart attack, or MI, and cardiac arrest are not the same thing. Patients suffering a cardiac arrest are unresponsive, not breathing, and have no pulse. These patients should receive immediate CPR and the application of an AED. Although it is true that most cardiac arrests are the result of an MI, most MIs do not result in a cardiac arrest.

There are many factors that will ultimately determine whether or not a heart attack will result in a cardiac arrest, but the most common are where the damage occurs on the heart and how much of an area actually dies. Damage that occurs over an important electrical pathway or to the left ventricle is more likely to cause a cardiac arrest than a heart attack.

FIRST ➤ When you suspect that a patient is having or is about to have a heart attack, activate EMS. Report the signs and symptoms. It may be possible for dispatch to send an ALS unit. ▪

The following are common signs and symptoms of an MI, or a heart attack (Scan 9–1):

- Chest or upper abdominal sensations of pressure, tightness, or heaviness. Some patients describe a burning sensation that can easily be mistaken for indigestion.
- The pain or discomfort may be described as behind the sternum (substernal) and radiate to either of the arms or shoulders. In some cases, the pain may extend to the hand, neck, jaw, and teeth, back, or upper abdomen.

FIRST ➤ Many times, chest pain is associated with other signs and symptoms suggestive of a heart attack in progress. They include shortness of breath, nausea, sweating, and weakness. ▪

Patients most likely to have symptoms other than those noted above are women, diabetics, and the elderly. Although they often do present with common signs and symptoms, it is important to remain suspicious even if they do not. During a heart attack, these populations may experience nausea and vomiting; indigestion; or back, neck, or jaw pain. The only symptom that these patients may tell you is, "I don't feel right," or "Something is wrong with me, but I don't know what it is," or "My teeth hurt."

As an Emergency Medical Responder, you must be very aware of all possible presentations of cardiac compromise and not just the typical "Hollywood" presentation of the man who suddenly grasps his chest and falls to the ground. You must be very suspicious of the elderly, female, or diabetic patient who may be insisting that they just have the flu. Provide care as if they are suffering cardiac compromise.

Angina Pectoris

angina pectoris (an-JI-nah PEK-to-ris) ▪ chest pain caused by an insufficient blood supply to the heart muscle.

Another cause of cardiac compromise is known as **angina pectoris**, or as it is more commonly called, *angina*. Literally translated, *angina pectoris* means pain in the chest. Angina occurs when one or more of the coronary arteries are unable to provide an adequate supply of oxygenated blood to the heart muscle. Although this may sound like what happens in a heart attack, the similarity ends there. With angina, there is no actual damage to the heart muscle. The supply of oxygenated blood is never cut off entirely, and the pain is caused by the muscles starving for more blood and oxygen.

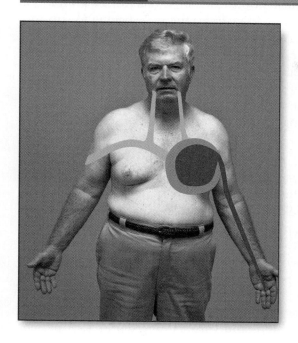

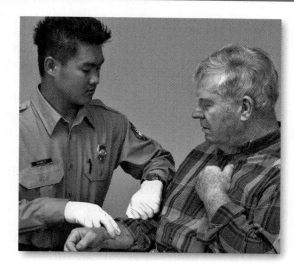

Signs and Symptoms

- Early symptoms generally include chest or upper abdominal discomfort often described as pressure, tightness, heaviness, or burning.
- As an attack worsens, pain may localize behind sternum and radiate to either arm or shoulder (usually the left). Pain may extend to:
  - Hand.
  - Neck, jaw, and teeth.
  - Upper back.
  - Upper, middle abdomen.

  Some patients have pain only in the jaw, neck, or arm.

- Chest pain may be accompanied by other symptoms that suggest a heart attack, including:
  - Shortness of breath.
  - Nausea.
  - Sweating.
  - Weakness.

  Pain may diminish when physical exertion or emotional stress ends or when the patient takes nitroglycerin. Blood pressure may be high or low.

- Additional signs may include:
  - Increased pulse rate; irregular pulse.
  - Low blood pressure (usually a result of repeated doses of nitroglycerin, which dilates blood vessels).

Emergency Care

- Make certain EMS has been activated.
- Obtain a patient history.
- Provide oxygen as to local protocols.
- Provide emotional support. Reassure and calm the patient.
- Keep the patient at rest. Do not allow the patient to move himself.
- Place the patient in a comfortable position.
- Ensure an open airway and adequate breathing.
- Ask if patient took nitroglycerin, when, how much, and over what period of time (see Appendix 3).
- Contact medical facility and let them know:
  - You have a patient with chest pain.
  - Patient's history.
  - If and when the patient took nitroglycerin.
- If local protocols permit, assist patient with prescribed dose of medication. Consult medical direction.
- Do not leave the patient unattended.
- Monitor vital signs.

Angina is often triggered by exertion. Exertion such as physical activity creates a demand on the heart muscle that the coronary arteries are unable to meet. The pain increases until the patient must stop the activity and rest. Within a few minutes, the demand on the heart returns to normal, the pain begins to subside, and eventually it goes away. Some patients are prone to angina attacks and must take medication such as nitroglycerin to help increase circulation to the heart. (Nitroglycerin is discussed in more detail later in this chapter.)

The signs and symptoms of angina are nearly identical to those of a heart attack. For that reason, it is important to care for all suspected cardiac-related pain as though the patient is having a heart attack and to seek immediate advanced medical care.

Congestive Heart Failure

congestive heart failure (CHF) ■ the condition in which the heart cannot properly circulate the blood. This causes a backup of fluids in the lungs and other organs.

Congestive heart failure (CHF) is a term used to describe a backup of fluid when the heart is unable to pump adequately. Because the heart is unable to manage the normal amount of volume, fluid backs up within the circulatory system. This backup of fluids, if left untreated, can cause fluid to be pushed into the alveoli within the lungs resulting in difficulty breathing. The backup can also result in swelling in the lower extremities (pedal edema). Although some patients with CHF have a chief complaint of chest pain, many more have a chief complaint of difficulty breathing.

CHF can be both chronic and acute. Some of the causes of chronic CHF include diseased heart valves, hypertension, and various lung diseases. A patient can experience an acute episode of CHF secondary to a heart attack.

Much like angina and heart attack, the acute CHF patient may complain of chest pain, difficulty breathing, or both. These patients typically have a history of cardiac problems and for that reason will likely have a long list of prescribed medications. Many patients with this condition have difficulty breathing while lying down. The patient will tell you that he cannot lie down and needs to sit upright, or he will tell you that he has to sleep in a recliner in order to breathe. The diabetic patient with CHF may only complain of fatigue.

Geriatric Focus

Just as with chest pain, the elderly patient suffering from congestive heart failure may have vague complaints, with fatigue being one of the most common.

If the patient is in a seated position, you are likely to see obvious swelling of the feet and ankles (pedal edema) because gravity pulls the excess fluids to these areas. If the patient is confined to a bed, you may see edema in the sacral area (sacral edema) because this is typically the lowest part of the body, and once again, gravity pulls the excess fluid downward. Depending on the amount of fluid in the lungs, the patient may experience increased shortness of breath while lying down. Be alert for this and be prepared to place the patient in a position of comfort. You may also see some jugular vein distention (JVD) as a result of the increased pressure inside the circulatory system.

FIRST ➤ The signs and symptoms of congestive heart failure (CHF) include (Figure 9.3):

- Shortness of breath.
- Chest discomfort.
- Rapid pulse rate.
- Pedal and/or sacral edema.

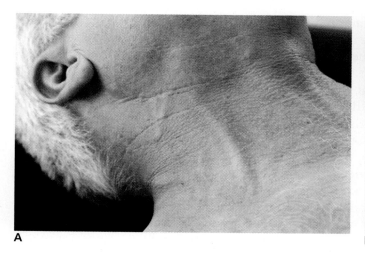
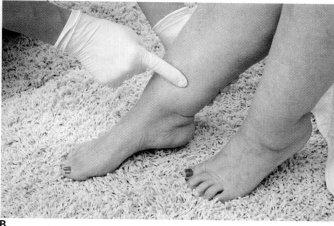

FIGURE 9.3 Signs of congestive heart failure include **A** bulging neck veins and **B** swollen ankles.

- Jugular vein distention (JVD). The veins of the neck may be distended or engorged due to a backup of fluids caused by a weakened heart.
- Pale skin color.
- Altered mental status due to a decrease in perfusion to the brain. ▪

When your patient's chief complaint is chest pain, gather a patient history first, focusing your questions on the chief complaint. The mnemonic OPQRST is a common tool used to assess chest pain. Be sure to look the patient in the eyes as you ask questions to be certain he understands and is not distracted by what is happening to him. Remember that the patient is likely to be frightened. Be very clear with each question and allow plenty of time for him to respond. Following is a review of OPQRST and some sample questions for each component:

O — *Onset.* What were you doing when the pain/discomfort began? With this question you are trying to determine if the patient was at rest or may have been involved in some physical activity when the pain began. Although it may not change how you treat the patient, this information will be valuable to the physician who will be treating the patient at the hospital.

P — *Provocation.* Does anything you do make the pain/discomfort better or worse? This question helps determine if anything the patient does in terms of movement or positioning makes the pain get better or worse. Cardiac-related chest pain is typically a constant pain that will not change with palpation or position. Although the patient may feel as though he can breathe easier in one position or another, the pain/discomfort will not usually change.

Q — *Quality.* Can you describe how your pain/discomfort feels? Try to get the patient to describe his pain/discomfort in his own words. Be careful, because it is easy to accidentally lead the patient. That is, if the patient is having difficulty finding words to describe what he is experiencing, he may agree with the first suggestion you offer him. Instead, a better way to explore what he is feeling is to offer contrasting choices and allow him to select the most appropriate word. For example, you might ask, "Is your pain/discomfort sharp or dull?" or "Is your pain/discomfort steady, or does it come and go?" You must remember that he may be distracted by what is happening to him, so be patient and allow the patient enough time to process the question and provide an appropriate response. Pay attention and notice any use or mention of a clenched fist to describe his pain.

R — *Region and radiate.* Can you point with one finger to where the pain/discomfort is the most intense? Does your pain/discomfort move or radiate anywhere else? The focus of these questions is to determine where the pain/discomfort is located. Watch the patient carefully after you ask this question. See if he is able to pinpoint the pain, or if he motions with an open hand over his chest or other area, suggesting the pain is spread out and perhaps radiating.

S — *Severity.* On a scale of 1 to 10, how would you rate your pain/discomfort? This question will help you determine just how much pain/discomfort the patient is experiencing from the event. It will be important to ask this question three different times. The first time you ask, you are trying to determine the level of discomfort at that moment. You must then ask, "What level was the pain when it first began?" This will provide insight into whether or not the pain has gotten better, worse, or stayed the same. You will then want to ask the question again after you have provided some care and comfort to the patient.

T — *Time.* When did you first begin feeling this pain/discomfort? In many cases of cardiac compromise, time plays an important factor. Although it will not and should not affect the way you care for your patient, it will be an important part of the history you obtain. Ask when the pain/discomfort first began, but you should also find out if the patient felt bad or had any other symptoms prior to its onset. As mentioned previously in this chapter, many patients begin with nausea, lightheadedness, shortness of breath, and fatigue long before the pain or discomfort begin.

FIRST ➤ The emergency care for a patient in CHF is the same as for most patients with a respiratory emergency (see next section). That is, maintain an open airway. Make certain that someone activates the EMS system and requests ALS services, if available. Position the patient to provide the greatest ease when breathing, which is usually an upright position. If the patient is alert, he should be assisted into a sitting position. Administer high-flow oxygen by nonrebreather mask, if allowed to do so (refer to Appendix 2). Keep the patient covered to conserve body heat, but do not overheat. Reassure the patient and calm him if possible. ■

If the patient is in cardiac arrest (no pulse and not breathing), have someone activate EMS and then begin CPR. Otherwise, complete the assessment as required, carefully noting the patient's vital signs (Figure 9.4). If the patient is unresponsive when you arrive, gain what information you can from bystanders. If no one saw the patient prior to the loss of responsiveness, suspect that the patient may have had a heart attack.

FIRST ➤ On gathering signs and symptoms indicating cardiac compromise or the possibility of a heart attack, you should (Figure 9.5):

1. Perform a scene size-up, including taking BSI precautions.
2. Make certain that the EMS system has been alerted. Stay with the patient and monitor his condition. Make certain that if an AED is available it is kept nearby.

Assessment of Chest Pain

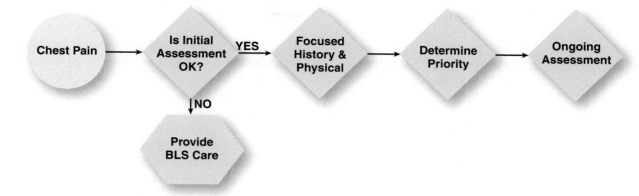

FIGURE 9.4 Algorithm for assessment of patients with chest pain.

3. Obtain a patient history.

4. If possible, provide oxygen per local protocols.

5. Keep the patient at rest. Provide emotional support and reassure the patient.

6. Place the patient into a comfortable position. Do all the work of moving for the patient. This position should be one that allows for easiest breathing. Many patients with the signs and symptoms of a heart attack are most comfortable in a semisitting position.

7. Loosen any restrictive clothing as needed for taking vital signs.

Care for Chest Pain

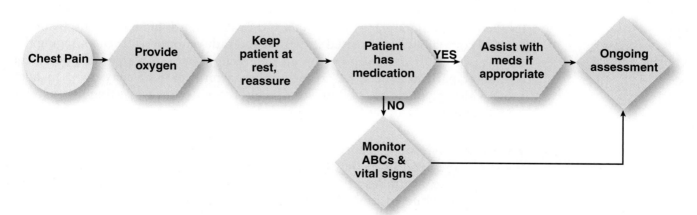

FIGURE 9.5 Algorithm for emergency care of patients with chest pain.

8. Assist the patient with the prescribed dose of medication (nitroglycerin), if your protocols permit. Consult medical direction.

9. Do not leave the patient unattended.

10. Continue to monitor vital signs. ▪

Remember to conduct yourself in a calm, professional manner when caring for any type of patient. It is of particular importance in caring for patients with chest pain who can be anxious, restless, or in denial. Their chances for survival may be increased if they can be calmed and kept at rest.

A patient may ask if he is having a heart attack. It is best to respond by saying, "Your pain could be a lot of things, but let's not take chances." Do all you can to keep the patient calm and still. Remain calm yourself and talk to your patient. Let the patient know that resting is an important part of his care.

Continue to comfort the patient as long as he is in your care. Assure the patient that more highly trained help is on the way. Tell him that you are a trained Emergency Medical Responder and that you will stay with him until further help arrives.

Medications

Usually, Emergency Medical Responders do not administer medications. However, some patients with a history of heart problems have been prescribed medications by their physicians to take when having chest pain. Always ask if a physician has given the patient any medications for the current problem. If medications have been prescribed, then assist the patient in taking them if your local protocols allow (see Appendix 3).

Patients who suffer from angina pectoris usually have nitroglycerin tablets or spray to take when having chest pain. This chest pain may indicate that the heart muscle needs more oxygen. Placing a nitroglycerin tablet or giving one spray under the patient's tongue will allow the drug to rapidly enter the bloodstream. Nitroglycerin dilates (enlarges) blood vessels, allowing an increase in blood flow to the heart muscle. It also reduces the workload of the heart. In doing so, the patient's blood pressure may be lowered. This can cause the patient to become dizzy or lightheaded. Patients receiving nitroglycerin should be sitting or lying down to avoid fainting.

In the form *transdermal patches*, nitroglycerin can pass through the skin and be picked up by the circulatory system. However, the patches are too slow to be of use in a cardiac emergency. The manufacturers state specifically that the patches are prescribed for use to help "prevent angina, not for the treatment of an acute angina attack."

In recent years, the use of aspirin for the treatment of suspected heart attack has become commonplace in hospitals and EMS systems. In fact, several pharmaceutical companies have created television and radio commercials encouraging the use of aspirin for this purpose. As an Emergency Medical Responder, you may encounter patients who have recently taken aspirin or who may want to take some while in your care. Follow your local protocols when assisting any patient with the administration of medication.

FIRST ➤ Help all patients with signs and symptoms of a heart attack take their own medications if they have been prescribed by a physician and you are allowed to do so (unless they have taken the prescribed limit prior to your arrival). Continue to monitor the patient and provide care, even if the pain stops. Do not cancel your request for an EMT or more advanced EMS response. ▪

RESPIRATORY EMERGENCIES

Many conditions cause people to experience difficulty in breathing, or shortness of breath (Scan 9–2). A patient may be unable to stop breathing too rapidly (hyperventilation). Muscle spasms may cause narrowing of the airways (asthma). Or there may be an underlying disease or condition such as emphysema, bronchitis, or pneumonia. Difficulty in breathing may also stem from being exposed to a poison or something to which the patient is allergic. Regardless of the cause, a patient's breathing can be considered adequate or inadequate.

Adequate breathing is breathing that is sufficient to support life. It is easy and effortless. Patients should not have to work hard to breathe. Patients should be able to speak full sentences without having to catch their breath. Adequate breathing is characterized by a normal respiratory rate, depth, and ease of the work of breathing.

Characteristics of adequate breathing include:

- *Normal rate* (number of breaths per minute), which is 12 to 20 for an adult, 15 to 30 for a child, and 25 to 50 for an infant.
- *Normal depth* (the size of each breath), which is also described as *tidal volume*. Normal breaths are not too shallow and not too deep. Your best indicator is good rise and fall of the chest with each breath.
- *Ease of breathing*. Ease of respirations has to do with how much work it takes for the patient to move each breath in and out. Normal respirations are effortless and unlabored as the diaphragm muscle moves up and down with each breath.

Along with rate, depth, and ease of breathing, you must also assess the rhythm of a patient's breathing. Respiratory rhythm should be regular. Breaths should be taken at regular intervals and last the same amount of time. Exhaling (breathing out) should take about twice as long as inhaling (breathing in).

Inadequate breathing is breathing that is not sufficient to support life. Left untreated, such a condition will eventually result in death. In these patients, you may see the following:

- A respiratory rate that is faster or slower than normal.
- Depth of respirations that is either too deep or too shallow.
- Increased work of breathing.
- Irregular breathing rhythm or pattern.
- Audible breath sounds, such as gurgling or wheezing.

When breathing becomes difficult, the patient may have to work extra hard to move air in and out of his lungs. Labored breathing is usually obvious as the patient will be sitting upright, mouth open, and struggling to breathe. Other muscles such as the ones between the ribs and those in the neck and abdomen begin to assist the diaphragm. These are called *accessory muscles* because they assist only when the diaphragm alone is not able to move enough air.

Geriatric Focus

The elderly patient may not appear to be short of breath on initial assessment because he may have only gotten short of breath with exertion. It is important to use the OPQRST approach to this complaint as well.

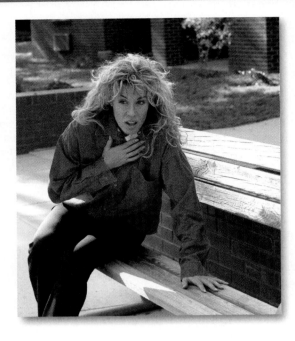

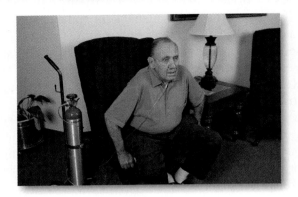

Chronic Obstructive Pulmonary Disease

Signs and Symptoms

- History of respiratory problems or allergies.
- Cough.
- Shortness of breath.
- Tightness in chest.
- Swelling in lower extremities (advanced cases).
- Rapid pulse (some cases).
- Barrel chest (some cases).
- Dizziness (some cases).
- Pale or blue (cyanotic) skin.
- Desire to sit upright at all times.

Emergency Care

Provide the same care as you would for respiratory distress. Be certain not to overheat the patient. Do what you can to reduce stress. If appropriate, encourage coughing.

NOTE

If you are allowed to provide oxygen, follow local guidelines for the COPD patient.

Respiratory Difficulty

Signs and Symptoms

- Difficulty breathing.
- Shortness of breath.
- Temporary cessation of breathing.
- Rapid deep breathing.
- Noisy breathing.
- Dizziness, faintness, or unresponsiveness.
- Restlessness, anxiety, or confusion.
- Strained muscles: face, neck, chest, abdomen.
- Pursed lips or mouth open wide to aid breathing.
- Pale or blue (cyanotic) skin color.
- Sharp chest pains.
- Numbness or tingling in the hands or feet.
- Spasm of the fingers and toes (possible hyperventilation).

Emergency Care

1. Stay with the patient. Have someone call EMS.
2. Ensure an open airway. Check for an airway obstruction.
3. Obtain a patient history.
4. Administer oxygen per local protocols.
5. Check to see if the patient is allergic to anything at the scene. (Remove substance or move patient.)
6. Keep patient at rest.
7. Cover patient to conserve body heat.
8. Monitor patient and provide emotional support.
9. Assist with inhaler per local protocols and medical direction (see Appendix 3).

Respiratory difficulty may be caused by a variety of conditions, ranging from ongoing medical problems such as asthma to sudden illnesses such as a blood clot. Always listen to what a patient tells you about how he perceives the problem before attempting to make a determination of a patient's condition.

The patient may have special medication that needs to be inhaled. He will want to take the medication but may be too upset or frightened to use the inhaler properly. Some jurisdictions allow Emergency Medical Responders to help such patients use an inhaler. Check local protocols, and always call for medical direction before assisting a patient with medications.

Signs and Symptoms

FIRST ➤ For most cases of respiratory difficulty or respiratory distress, any or all of the following signs and symptoms may be noticed (Figure 9.6):

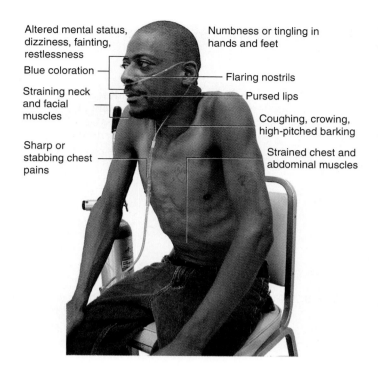

Altered mental status, dizziness, fainting, restlessness

Blue coloration

Straining neck and facial muscles

Sharp or stabbing chest pains

Numbness or tingling in hands and feet

Flaring nostrils

Pursed lips

Coughing, crowing, high-pitched barking

Strained chest and abdominal muscles

FIGURE 9.6 Signs and symptoms of respiratory distress. *(© Ray Kemp/911 Imaging)*

- Labored or difficult breathing; a feeling of suffocation.
- Audible breathing sounds.
- Rapid or slow rate of breathing.
- Abnormal pulse rate (too fast or too slow).
- Changes in skin color, particularly of the lips and nail beds. Usually, the color will change to pale or a bluish color indicating cyanosis.
- Altered mental status.

There are cases in which the patient may not have any signs and reports only symptoms. Provide care as described in the next section, being certain to maintain an open airway. Administer oxygen, if allowed to do so. ■

Emergency Care

FIRST ➤ When caring for most cases of respiratory difficulty (Figure 9.7):

1. Perform scene size-up, including taking BSI precautions.
2. Have someone activate the EMS system. Arrange for ALS response if available.
3. Maintain an open airway. Administer oxygen as per local protocols.
4. Make certain that the problem is not caused by an airway obstruction.
5. Keep the patient at rest.
6. Place the responsive patient in a sitting position. Allow for drainage from the mouth. It often helps if the patient can support himself by the forearms when sitting. This eases the patient's efforts in expanding the chest.
7. Assist with prescribed medication per local protocols and medical direction (see Appendix 3). Obtain vital signs.
8. Continue to monitor the patient and provide emotional support. ■

REMEMBER

Do not withhold oxygen from a patient with inadequate breathing or respiratory distress, including COPD patients.

Care for Respiratory Distress

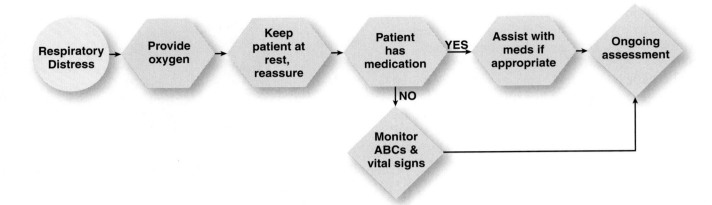

FIGURE 9.7 Algorithm for emergency care of patients in respiratory distress.

REMEMBER

Hyperventilation can be a sign of possible respiratory distress, impending heart attack, or a more serious medical condition. Activate the EMS system and provide care for respiratory distress.

WARNING

Do not use a paper bag in an attempt to treat hyperventilation. These patients can often be cared for with low-flow oxygen and lots of reassurance.

chronic obstructive pulmonary disease (COPD) ■ a variety of lung problems related to diseases of the airway passages or exchange levels, including emphysema complicated by chronic bronchitis.

Hyperventilation

Breathing that is too rapid and too deep is known as **hyperventilation**. Most of the time, it stems from fear or stress, which may cause the patient to appear anxious and frightened. Patients experiencing hyperventilation are receiving too much oxygen and are not retaining enough carbon dioxide. In advanced cases, this could lead to numbness and tingling of the lips, toes, and fingers.

FIRST ➤ Because most cases of hyperventilation are related to conditions of anxiety, your priority in the care of these patients is to reduce anxiety by reassuring and comforting them. Encourage patients to take slow, deep breaths to decrease their breathing rate. Check with medical direction. ■

It will be difficult to determine if the condition is related merely to anxiety or to a more serious condition. Hyperventilation can be a sign of possible respiratory distress, impending heart attack, or a more serious medical condition. Activate the EMS system and provide care for respiratory distress. Be alert for cyanosis (blue discoloration of the skin, lips, and nail beds) or other signs and symptoms of inadequate breathing. Monitor the patient for changes in vital signs, which may indicate serious medical problems. Suspect the worst, and be prepared to respond appropriately.

Chronic Obstructive Pulmonary Disease

A variety of respiratory conditions can be classified as **chronic obstructive pulmonary disease (COPD)**. Such conditions include emphysema and chronic bronchitis. Usually, the COPD patient is middle age or older.

FIRST ➤ The signs and symptoms of COPD may include:

- History of heavy cigarette smoking, respiratory problems, or allergies.
- Persistent cough.

- Shortness of breath. Sometimes the patient breathes through pursed lips and tries to ease breathing effort by sitting a **tripod position** (sitting forward and leaning on hands or elbows).
- Weakness or fatigue.
- Tightness in the chest.
- Wheezing.

tripod position ■ sitting forward, leaning on hands or elbows.

In advanced cases, there may be:

- Irritability and agitation or lethargy and sleepiness.
- Rapid pulse, sometimes irregular.
- Barrel-chest appearance.
- Strong desire to remain sitting, even when asleep.
- Pale or blue discoloration of the skin, lips, and nail beds. ■

COPD can be difficult to distinguish from CHF. However, you do not have to make that distinction. For Emergency Medical Responders, emergency care is the same.

FIRST ➤ When caring for COPD patients, you should:

1. Perform scene size-up, including taking BSI precautions.
2. Ensure an open airway, making certain that the problem is not because of obstruction by the tongue or some form of mechanical obstruction.
3. Have someone activate the EMS system and report the problem as respiratory difficulty with a history of COPD.
4. Help the patient into a position of comfort and provide emotional support.
5. Administer oxygen as per local protocols.
6. Monitor vital signs.
7. Assist with medications if permitted to do so.
8. Cover the patient to conserve body heat, but do not overheat the patient. ■

REMEMBER

Monitor COPD patients carefully. The amount of oxygen you administer may have to be adjusted by medical direction.

ALTERED MENTAL STATUS

An **altered mental status (AMS)** is characterized by a decrease in the patient's alertness and responsiveness to his surroundings. Several conditions may cause a patient to experience an altered mental status, including seizures, strokes, diabetic emergencies, poisonings, breathing problems, and cardiac events (Figure 9.8). Regardless of the underlying cause, you will need to determine the appropriate care procedures by observing and questioning. To start this process, you will need to know and understand the patient's normal mental status.

As you may recall from Chapter 7, the AVPU scale (alert, verbal, painful, unresponsive) is used to categorize a patient's mental status (Table 9–1).

5–1.3 Identify the patient who presents with a specific medical complaint of altered mental status.

altered mental status (AMS) ■ a medical condition characterized by a decrease in the patient's alertness and responsiveness to his surroundings. Also called *altered level of responsiveness*.

▄▄▄ ▟ ◢ ▄▄▄ **Geriatric Focus**

An elderly patient with dementia may not fully comprehend the seriousness of his situation and may not want you to provide care. In other words, the elderly patient with dementia may not be competent to make decisions regarding his own medical care. When presented with an elderly patient who is showing signs of disorientation, a short attention span, confusion, or hallucinations, obtain a detailed history from

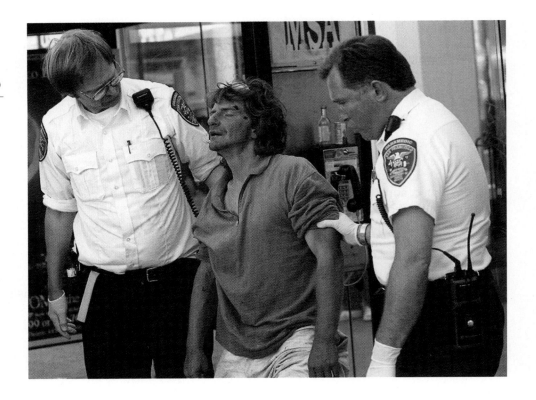

family members or caregivers. It will be important to determine if his mental status is normal for him or if it has gotten worse. Do not allow a patient who is showing signs of dementia to refuse care without further investigation into his normal state of mind. In most cases, you will want to wait for the EMTs to arrive and take over care before you leave the scene.

Stroke

stroke ■ the blocking or bursting of a vessel that supplies blood to the brain. A portion of the brain is damaged or destroyed by this event. Also known as *cerebrovascular (SER-e-bro-VAS-cu-ler) accident (CVA)* or "brain attack."

One potentially serious cause of altered mental status is a **stroke**, or cerebrovascular accident (CVA), also known as "brain attack." Such a condition occurs

TABLE 9–1	The AVPU Scale
A—Alert	Patient is awake and aware of his surroundings. Often, it is stated that a patient is alert and oriented times four (A & O × 4), which means the patient is: A & O × 1 to person. He can tell you his name. A & O × 2 to place. He also can tell you where he is. A & O × 3 to time. He also can tell you exactly or approximately what time it is. A & O × 4 to event. He also can tell you about the event.
V—Verbal	Patient responds only to verbal stimuli (yelling or raised voice).
P—Painful	Patient responds only to painful stimuli (sternal rub).
U—Unresponsive	Patient is not responsive to any stimuli.

when blood to the brain is obstructed or when a vessel ruptures. During a stroke, a portion of the brain does not receive an adequate supply of oxygenated blood and damage occurs. In some cases, this damage is so great that it may lead to death (Scan 9–3).

FIRST ➤ There are many signs and symptoms of stroke, including:

- Headache. This may be the only symptom at first.
- **Syncope** (collapse or fainting).
- Altered mental status.
- Numbness or paralysis, usually to the extremities and/or to the face.
- Difficulty with speech or vision.
- Confusion, dizziness.
- Seizures.
- Altered breathing patterns.
- Unequal pupils.
- Loss of strength, typically to one side of the body.
- Loss of bowel and bladder control.
- Hypertension (patient may report history of high blood pressure). ■

syncope (SIN-ko-pe) ■ collapse or fainting.

There are several assessment tools that can be helpful when assessing a responsive patient suspected of having a stroke. One of the most common of these tools is the Cincinnati Prehospital Stroke Scale (CPSS). The CPSS uses three assessment characteristics to evaluate for the likelihood of a stroke:

- *Facial droop.* Have the patient look directly at you and smile or show his teeth. Observe if the facial muscles do not move symmetrically or if there is facial droop on one side or the other.
- *Arm drift.* Have the patient hold both arms straight out in front of him and close his eyes. Observe for arm drift, one arm that drops down while the other remains up. It is also significant if the patient cannot bring both arms up together.
- *Abnormal speech.* Observe for slurred speech, inappropriate words, or an inability to respond verbally.

Presence of an abnormality in any one of the three areas of the CPSS indicates a strong likelihood of a stroke.

FIRST ➤ When providing emergency care for a possible stroke patient, you should:

1. Perform scene size-up, including taking BSI precautions.
2. Maintain an open airway. Be prepared to provide ventilations or CPR if needed.
3. Administer oxygen as per local protocols.
4. Make sure someone activates the EMS system.
5. Keep the patient at rest, and protect all paralyzed parts.
6. Provide emotional support. Be certain to make an effort to understand everything that the patient says. Remember, the speech centers of the brain may be affected.
7. Position the patient to allow for drainage from the mouth. This is best done by placing him into the recovery position.
8. Do not administer anything by mouth.
9. Continue to monitor the patient. Shock, respiratory arrest, and cardiac arrest are possible. ■

5–1.4 Explain the steps in providing emergency medical care to a patient with an altered mental status.

CAUSES OF CEREBROVASCULAR ACCIDENTS: STROKE

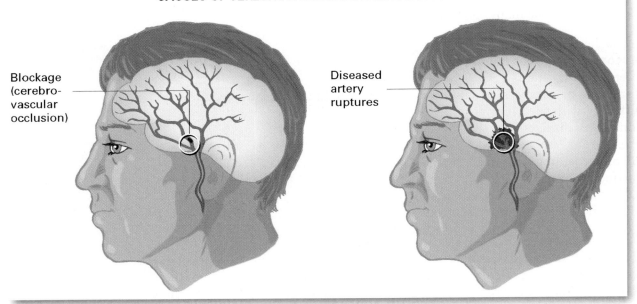

Blockage (cerebro-vascular occlusion)

Diseased artery ruptures

Cerebral Thrombosis (Clot)

Blockage in arteries supplying oxygenated blood will result in damage to affected parts of the brain.

Cerebral Hemorrhage (Rupture)

An aneurysm or other weakened area of an artery ruptures. This has two effects:

- Area of the brain is deprived of oxygenated blood.
- Pooling blood puts increased pressure on the brain, displacing tissue and interfering with function. Cerebral hemorrhage is often associated with arteriosclerosis and hypertension.

Signs and Symptoms of Stroke

- Headache.
- Confusion and/or dizziness.
- Loss of function or paralysis of extremities (usually on one side of the body).
- Numbness (usually limited to one side of the body).
- Collapse.
- Facial paralysis and loss of expression (often to one side of the face).
- Impaired speech.
- Unequal pupil size.
- Impaired vision.

- Rapid or slow pulse.
- Abnormal respirations.
- Nausea, vomiting.
- Convulsions.
- Loss of bladder and bowel control.
- High blood pressure (may have history of hypertension).

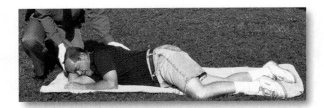

Emergency Care of Stroke Patients

- Ensure an open airway.
- Administer oxygen per local protocols.
- Keep the patient calm.
- Monitor vital signs.
- Give nothing by mouth.
- Provide care for shock.
- Place the patient into the recovery position on affected side to protect extremities.

Prompt recognition is important when dealing with patients exhibiting the signs and symptoms of stroke. There are specific medications that can be given to stroke patients that, if given soon enough, can greatly decrease the long-term effects of the stroke. These medications are called "thrombolytics" and are most commonly given in the hospital setting. Because of the importance of prompt delivery of these medications, some EMS systems are allowing these medications to be delivered by Paramedics in the field setting.

Seizures

Irregular electrical activity in the brain that can cause a sudden change in behavior or movement is called a **seizure**. Seizures can cause uncontrolled muscular movements known as **convulsions**. When a seizure causes the entire body to convulse, it is referred to as a **generalized seizure**. Other seizures characterized by a temporary loss of concentration with no dramatic body movements are known as **partial complex seizures**. Older terms, still in use but becoming rare, are *grand mal* for the generalized seizure and *petit mal* for the partial complex seizure.

Seizures can be frightening for a patient's family, friends, and others to witness. Even though most seizures do not last longer than a minute, it can seem like a much longer period to witnesses. Talk to them to determine what the patient was doing prior to the seizure and if this has happened in the past. Although some people have seizures on a regular basis, the patient should still be evaluated by someone with advanced medical training.

A seizure is not a disease, but a sign of an underlying condition. Some of the causes of seizures are:

- Epilepsy.
- Ingestion of drugs, alcohol, or poisons.
- Brain tumors.
- Infections, high fever.
- Diabetic problems.
- Trauma.
- Stroke.
- Heat stroke.
- Head injury.

FIRST ➤ In cases of generalized seizure, any or all of the following may be present:

- Sudden loss of responsiveness.
- Patient may report bright light, bright colors, or the sensation of a strong odor prior to losing responsiveness.
- Convulsions.
- Loss of bladder and/or bowel control. This is called *incontinence*.
- Breathing may be labored, and there may be frothing at the mouth.

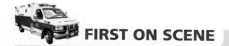

FIRST ON SCENE

The girl, a teen too young to be a student at the college, was convulsing on the dorm room's dirty carpet. Her arms and legs were pulling and pushing slowly in all directions, her back arched severely, and her head snapped rhythmically from side to side, sending foamy splatters of saliva back and forth on the carpet.

"What did you guys give her?" Micah demanded of the small group of terrified young men.

"Nothing!" Frank shouted, holding his palms out in an unconscious effort to show that his hands were empty. "We were just drinking some beer and playing video games! We didn't do anything!"

Micah looked down at the girl and saw that her lips were now bluish and her breathing was coming in hitches and gasps as she convulsed. "How long has she been like this?" he asked.

"Since just before I knocked on your door." Frank kept looking from the girl to his friends and then back to Micah. "Just a couple of minutes."

Micah suddenly felt useless. The freshmen had the sense to pull furniture away so the girl wouldn't crash into anything, and one of them had put a sweatshirt under her head, but as long as she was seizing, there was nothing he could do.

"Frank," Micah said, pointing to the cowering young man. "Bring me a phone right now. She needs an ambulance, and I have to let campus security know what's going on."

seizure ■ irregular electrical activity in the brain that can cause a sudden change in behavior or movement.

convulsions ■ uncontrolled muscular contractions.

5–1.5 Identify the patient who presents with a specific medical complaint of seizures.

generalized seizure ■ a seizure characterized by unresponsiveness and full body convulsions.

partial complex seizure ■ a seizure characterized by a temporary loss of concentration with no dramatic body movements.

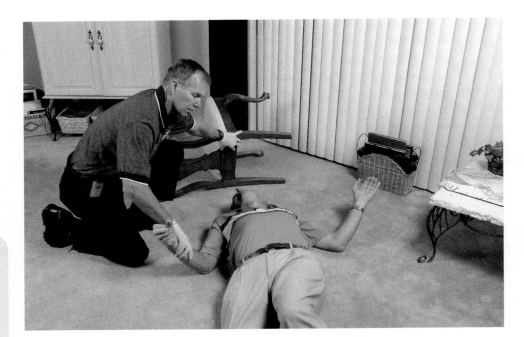

FIGURE 9.9 During a seizure, protect the patient from injury.

REMEMBER

Generalized, or grand mal, seizures usually last only a few minutes and consist of dramatic body movements. Partial complex, or petit mal, seizures last only 10 to 30 seconds with no dramatic body movements.

5–1.6 Explain the steps in providing emergency medical care to a patient with seizures.

WARNING

Do not place any object between the teeth of a convulsing patient. Many objects, such as a pencil, can break and obstruct the patient's airway.

- After the seizure, the patient's body completely relaxes.
- Patient may complain of a headache prior to or following a seizure. ■

FIRST ➤ Basic care for a generalized seizure includes:

1. Perform scene size-up, including taking BSI precautions.
2. Protect the patient from injury (Figure 9.9). If necessary, gently restrain the patient and pad him. Do not attempt to force anything into his mouth to protect the tongue; this can injure the teeth or compromise the airway.
3. Loosen restrictive clothing.
4. After convulsions have stopped, keep the patient at rest, with the head positioned to allow for drainage in case of vomiting (recovery position).
5. Administer oxygen as per local protocols.
6. Protect the patient from embarrassment by asking onlookers to give the patient some privacy. ■

If the patient says that this is the first attack, activate the EMS system. If the patient has a history of seizures and has had other episodes, ask if you may phone the patient's doctor. It is possible that the doctor may want to see the patient or have the patient transported to a medical facility. Remember that the patient has the option to refuse additional care.

After a seizure, the patient will generally feel tired and weak and may not be fully alert. Do not let him wander away. It is best to keep him at rest. Provide emotional support to the patient and family members until additional medical help arrives.

Diabetes

glucose (GLU-kohs) ■ a simple sugar that is the primary source of energy for the body's tissues.

insulin (IN-su-lin) ■ a hormone produced in the pancreas that is needed to move sugar (glucose) from the blood into the cells.

Glucose, a form of simple sugar, is the main source of energy for the body's cells. It is carried to the cells by way of the bloodstream. However, to enter the cells, **insulin**, a hormone secreted by the pancreas, must be present. Insulin allows sugar to enter the blood cells so it can be used effectively. In normal healthy adults, this process works to balance the glucose levels within the body.

Diabetes is a disease that prevents individuals from producing enough insulin or from using insulin effectively. Although some patients can manage their condition with a balanced diet, others require the administration of oral medications, or in severe cases, the patient must inject himself with insulin (Scan 9–4).

Hyperglycemia   High blood sugar, or **hyperglycemia**, is usually a gradual event, taking many hours to several days to develop. If the individual does not take enough insulin or eats too much for the amount of insulin being taken, or if the diabetes has not been diagnosed, hyperglycemia may occur.

Most of the carbohydrates we consume are broken down into glucose to provide energy to the body and to become part of many of the body's own structural carbohydrates. It is very important that diabetics keep track of their intake of carbohydrates and relate this amount to the exercise they get and, if on insulin, the amount of insulin they take. Carbohydrates include sucrose (table sugar), as well as starches such as those found in breads, pastas, rice, potatoes, and dairy products.

FIRST ➤ The signs and symptoms of hyperglycemia include:

- Difficult or abnormal breathing. Typically, the patient will take deep, rapid breaths, often heaving or sighing. This rapid breathing may appear to be hyperventilation.
- Extreme thirst.
- Abdominal pain.
- Dry, warm skin. Sometimes the skin may become reddened.
- Rapid, weak pulse.
- Sweet or fruity odor on the patient's breath, which is called *ketone breath*. Ketones smell like acetone, the same compound found in fingernail polish remover.
- Dry mouth.
- Restlessness and/or stupor.
- Unresponsiveness. ▪

FIRST ➤ Emergency care for hyperglycemia consists of the following:

1. Perform scene size-up, including taking BSI precautions.
2. Have someone activate the EMS system. This patient will have to be transferred to a medical facility.
3. Administer oxygen per local protocols.
4. Keep the patient at rest. If the patient is alert, try to gain additional information through a focused history and physical exam. Ask if the patient is diabetic. Find out if the patient has taken insulin and has eaten recently.
5. If the patient is alert and you are not certain if the problem is too much sugar (hyperglycemia) or too little sugar (hypoglycemia), give the patient sugar, candy, orange juice, or a soft drink. Make certain that the substance contains real sugar, not an artificial sweetener. Some jurisdictions may allow Emergency Medical Responders to give oral glucose. Check local protocols and always call for medical direction before assisting a patient with medications (see Appendix 3) ▪

diabetes ▪ usually refers to diabetes mellitus, a disease that prevents individuals from producing enough insulin or from using insulin effectively.

hyperglycemia ▪ a condition in which the sugar (glucose) level increases in the blood and decreases in the tissue cells. The problem can be serious enough to produce a coma.

REMEMBER

Some patients who are hyperglycemic may appear to be drunk at first. Do not conclude someone is drunk unless there is obvious alcohol abuse and you have ruled out hyperglycemia. Keep in mind that an alcoholic may also be diabetic.

REMEMBER

When in doubt about a patient being hyperglycemic or hypoglycemic, follow the "sugar for everyone" rule. (See Scan 9–4.)

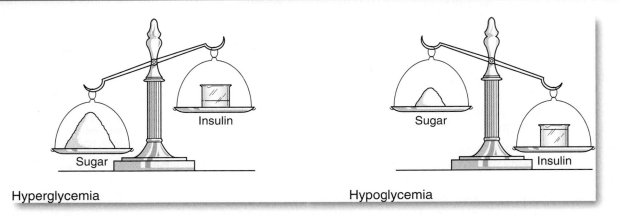

Hyperglycemia

Hypoglycemia

Hyperglycemia (Diabetic Coma)

Causes

- Diabetic's condition has not been diagnosed or treated.
- Diabetic has not taken his insulin.
- Diabetic has overeaten, flooding the body with a sudden excess of carbohydrates.
- Diabetic suffers an infection or other stress that disrupts his glucose/insulin balance.

Signs and Symptoms

- Gradual onset of signs and symptoms over hours or days.
- Patient complains of dry mouth and intense thirst.
- Abdominal pain and vomiting common.
- Gradually increasing restlessness and confusion, followed by stupor.
- Unresponsiveness with these signs:
  Air hunger, or deep, sighing respirations.
  Weak, rapid pulse.
  Dry, red, warm skin.
  Eyes that appear sunken.
- Breath smells of acetone-sickly sweet, like nail polish remover.

Emergency Care

- Monitor ABCs.
- Provide oxygen per local protocols.

Hypoglycemia (Insulin Shock)

Causes

- Diabetic has taken too much insulin.
- Diabetic has not eaten enough to provide her normal sugar intake.
- Diabetic has overexercised or overexerted herself, thus reducing her blood glucose level.
- Diabetic has vomited a meal.

Signs and Symptoms

- Rapid onset of signs and symptoms in minutes.
- Dizziness and headache.
- Abnormal, hostile, or aggressive behavior, which may appear to be alcohol intoxication.
- Fainting, convulsions, and occasionally coma.
- Full rapid pulse or a weak rapid pulse.
- Patient intensely hungry; drooling.
- Skin pale, cold, clammy; profuse perspiration.

Emergency Care

- For a responsive patient with a gag reflex, administer oral glucose or a substitute such as honey, candy, soft drink, or orange juice.
- For an unresponsive patient, give oral glucose per local protocols and medical direction.
- Place patient in the recovery position.
- Administer oxygen per local protocols.

When faced with a patient who may be suffering from either hyperglycemia or hypoglycemia:

- Determine if the patient is diabetic. Look for a medical identification device or information cards. Interview patient and family members.
- If the patient is a known or suspected diabetic, and hypoglycemia (insulin shock) cannot be ruled out, conclude that it is possible hypoglycemia and administer glucose.

Often, a patient suffering from these conditions may appear drunk. Always check for underlying conditions—such as diabetic complications—when caring for someone who appears to be intoxicated.

Hypoglycemia The diabetic who has taken too much insulin, has eaten too little sugar, or is overexerted may develop **hypoglycemia** (low blood sugar), which usually comes on suddenly over a period of several minutes to a few hours.

hypoglycemia ▪ too little sugar in the blood.

FIRST ➤ Signs and symptoms of hypoglycemia and developing **insulin shock** include:

insulin shock ▪ severe hypoglycemia. A form of shock usually caused by too high a level of insulin in the blood, producing a sudden drop in blood sugar.

- Altered mental status.
- Pale, cool, and often moist skin.
- Rapid, strong pulse.
- Dizziness.
- Headache.
- Normal or shallow breathing.
- Very hungry.
- Some patients will develop seizures if they do not receive early care. ▪

Geriatric Focus

The elderly patient with diabetes is usually taking pills to control his blood sugar and may also be taking insulin. While you may administer glucose, his blood sugar may drop again, sometimes many hours later because the pills he takes are long lasting. For this reason, it is generally advised that all elderly hypoglycemia events result in transport to the hospital.

FIRST ➤ Emergency care for hypoglycemia and developing insulin shock consists of the following:

1. Perform a scene size-up, including taking BSI precautions.
2. Perform an initial assessment and ensure adequate ABCs.
3. If the patient is alert, provide oral glucose or a suitable substitute. Do not give liquids or foods to the patient who is unresponsive.
4. Have someone activate the EMS system.
5. Keep the patient comfortable and administer oxygen per local protocols. ▪

FIRST ON SCENE

As Micah hung up the cordless phone and tossed it onto the dorm's old brown couch, he turned to Frank. "Go down to the grass common in front of the building and wait for the ambulance."

As the young man jogged from the room, obviously happy to get out, the girl's seizure tapered off and then stopped altogether. She was still unconscious but was now snoring loudly. Micah squatted next to her, not wanting to kneel in the pools of saliva, and gently opened her airway by placing one hand on her cool, moist forehead and the other under her jaw. The girl's snoring immediately stopped and her lips faded from blue to the same paleness as the rest of her face.

With the help of two of the remaining freshmen, Micah was able to roll the girl into the recovery position. It was then that he noticed something glimmering inside the collar of her denim jacket. He reached into it and pulled out a MedicAlert necklace indicating that the girl is an insulin-dependent diabetic.

ABDOMINAL PAIN

FIRST > The sudden onset of severe abdominal pain is sometimes called an **acute abdomen** or *acute abdominal distress*. The presence of pain alone is enough to indicate that the patient must be seen as soon as possible by someone with more advanced training. ■

The cause of the pain may be anything from simple indigestion to a very serious medical problem. Your role is to assess the patient and provide the needed care, making certain that the EMS system has been activated. Do not attempt to diagnose the patient's problem. If the pain is severe enough for the patient to seek emergency care, then his problem must be considered serious.

Many medical problems are associated with severe abdominal pain. Some examples include appendicitis, ulcers, inflamed abdominal membranes, aortic aneurysm, pancreatitis, obstruction of the intestine, liver disease, gallstones, and kidney stones. Female patients, who do not know they are pregnant, may have severe abdominal pain related to problems with the pregnancy. Identifying the exact nature of the pain is not possible at the Emergency Medical Responder level of care.

Do not assume that pain over the top of a specific organ means that this organ is the location of the patient's problem. Abdominal pain is usually **referred pain**, or pain spread out over one or more areas (Figure 9.10).

acute abdomen ■ the sudden onset of severe abdominal pain; abdominal pain related to one of many medical conditions or a specific injury to the abdomen. Also called *acute abdominal distress*.

REMEMBER

The location of abdominal pain may not be the actual site of the patient's problem.

referred pain ■ pain spread out over one or more areas.

REFERRED AND ACTUAL PAIN AREAS

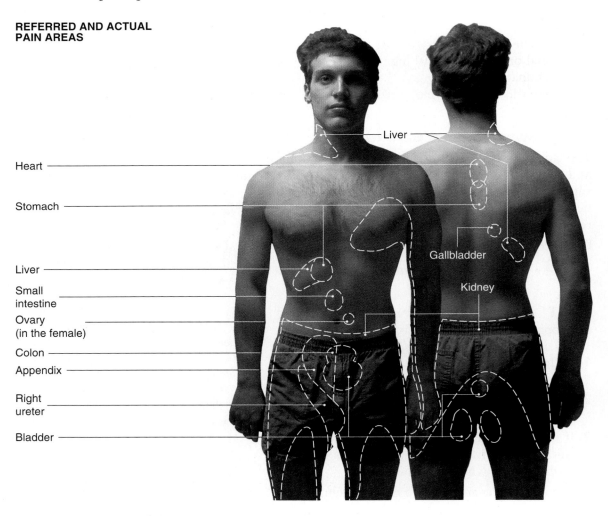

Heart

Stomach

Liver

Small intestine

Ovary (in the female)

Colon

Appendix

Right ureter

Bladder

Liver

Gallbladder

Kidney

FIGURE 9.10 Patterns of abdominal pain.

FIRST ➤ Signs and symptoms associated with an acute abdomen may include:

- Abdominal pain.
- Back pain.
- Nausea and vomiting.
- Rapid pulse.
- Rapid and shallow breathing.
- Fever.
- Signs of developing shock.
- Guarding the abdomen. That is, the patient may fold his arms across his abdomen and draw up his knees. Usually, the patient tries not to move.
- Distention.
- Tenderness.
- Rigidity.
- Pulsating mass, which can be an indication of an abdominal aortic aneurysm.
- Rectal bleeding; dark, tarry stools or changes in stools; blood in the urine; or nonmenstrual vaginal bleeding. ■

As you gather signs and symptoms, carefully watch the patient. Does he appear ill? Does he continue to guard the abdomen? Is he reluctant to move?

Geriatric Focus

The elderly patient will complain of pain when you palpate his abdomen even in the absence of a serious condition. This may be due to his increased frequency of constipation. Be gentle when palpating the abdomen and ask him if his abdomen appears "bloated" or different than usual.

FIRST ➤ Basic care for patients with abdominal complaints requires you to (Figure 9.11):

1. Perform scene size-up, including taking BSI precautions.

2. Maintain an open airway. Stay alert for vomiting.

3. Provide care for shock, including oxygen per local protocols.

4. Make certain that EMS is activated.

WARNING

Do not give the patient with abdominal pain anything by mouth. To do so may cause the patient to vomit.

Care for Abdominal Pain

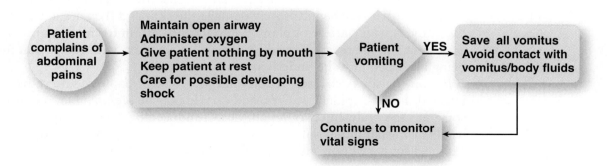

FIGURE 9.11 Algorithm for emergency care of patients with abdominal pain.

5. Keep the patient at rest. Sometimes the patient's pain may be reduced if he is positioned on his back with knees flexed. Do not force the patient to assume this position.

6. Save all vomit for later analysis by the EMTs. Avoid contact with the vomit, discharges, mucous membranes, and body fluids.

7. Reassure the patient and continue to gather information. Use the OPQRST assessment tool as appropriate. Ask if the pain came on suddenly or did it build over time, the nature or quality of the pain (sharp, dull, stabbing), if there were any fevers or chills, any unusual bowel movements (dark, light, tarry, bloody, loose, or hard), or any problems with urination (inability to urinate, frequent urination, or blood in the urine). Ask the patient when he last ate and what was consumed. Make sure you document his answers. Ask the female patient about her menstrual and pregnancy/birth history. ■

Poisonings, Bites, Stings

poison ■ any substance that can be harmful to the body.

Any substance that can be harmful to the body is known as a **poison**. There are more than 2 million incidents of poisoning reported annually in the United States. Although some cases might be related to murder or suicide attempts, most are accidental and often involve children.

Routes of Exposure

ingestion ■ taking into the body by swallowing.

inhalation ■ taking into the body by breathing in.

absorption ■ taking into the body through the skin and body tissues.

injection ■ taking into the body by puncturing the skin.

We usually think of a poison as a liquid or solid chemical that has been ingested (swallowed), but there are actually four routes of exposure, or ways that a poison can enter the body. They are **ingestion, inhalation, absorption,** and **injection.** The following is a description of each:

- *Ingestion.* Poisons taken into the body by way of the mouth are said to be ingested. Ingested poisons include various household and industrial chemicals, certain foods and improperly prepared foods, plant materials, petroleum products, medications (particularly if taken in improper doses), and poisons made specifically to control rodents, insects, and crop diseases.
- *Inhalation.* Poisons taken in by breathing are said to be inhaled. Inhaled poisons take the form of gases, vapors, and sprays, including carbon monoxide (from car exhaust, kerosene heaters, and wood-burning stoves), ammonia, chlorine, volatile liquid chemicals (including many industrial solvents), and insect sprays.
- *Absorption.* Poisons taken into the body through the skin and body tissues are said to be absorbed. Many such poisons damage the skin and then are slowly absorbed into the bloodstream. Some insecticides, agricultural chemicals, and corrosive chemicals may damage the skin and then are absorbed by the body. A wide variety of plant materials and certain forms of marine life can cause allergic reactions and/or damage to the skin, with the poison (toxin) being absorbed into the underlying tissues.
- *Injection.* Poisons delivered directly into the bloodstream are said to be injected. Insects, spiders, snakes, and certain marine life are able to inject poisons into the body. Injection might be self-induced by way of a hypodermic needle. Unusual industrial accidents producing cuts or puncture wounds also can be a source of poisons being injected into the body.

Table 9–2 lists some of the types of poisons that could require emergency care. This information is provided so that you may learn more about various poisons as

TABLE 9–2 | Common Poisons

POISON	SIGNS AND SYMPTOMS
Acetaminophen (Tylenol, Comtrex, Bancap, Datril, Excedrin PM)	Nausea, vomiting, altered mental status (late).
Acids	Burns on or around the lips. Burning in the mouth, throat, and stomach, often followed by heavy vomiting.
Alkalis (ammonia, bleaches, detergents, lye, washing soda, certain fertilizers)	Check mouth to see if the membranes appear white and swollen. There may be a soapy appearance in the mouth. Abdominal pain is usually present. Vomiting may occur, often full of blood and mucus.
Arsenic (most rat poisons and now warfarin)	"Garlic breath," with burning in the mouth, throat, and stomach. Abdominal pain can be severe. Vomiting is common.
Aspirin	Delayed reactions, including ringing in the ears, rapid and deep breathing, dry skin, and restlessness.
Chloroform	Slow, shallow breathing with chloroform odor on breath. Pupils are dilated and fixed.
Corrosive agents (disinfectants, drain cleaners, household acids, iodine, pine oil, turpentine, toilet bowl cleaners, styptic pencil, water softeners, strong acids)	(See Acids.)
Food poisoning	Difficult to detect because signs and symptoms vary greatly. Usually, you will note abdominal pain, nausea and vomiting, gas and bowel sounds, and diarrhea.
Iodine	Upset stomach and vomiting. If a starchy meal has been eaten, the vomit may appear blue.
Metals (copper, lead, mercury, and zinc)	Metallic taste in mouth, with nausea and abdominal pains. Vomiting may occur. Stools may be bloody and dark.
Petroleum products (some deodorizers, heating fuel, diesel fuels, gasoline, kerosene, lighter fluid, lubricating oil, naphtha, rust remover, transmission fluid)	Cough, altered mental status. Note characteristic odors on patient's breath and clothing or in vomit.
Phosphorus	Abdominal pain and vomiting.
Plants: Contact (poison ivy, poison oak, poison sumac)	Swollen, itchy areas on the skin, with quickly forming blister-like structures.
Plants: Ingested (azalea, castor bean, poison, elder, foxglove, lily of the valley, mountain laurel, mushrooms, nightshade, oleander, mistletoe and holly berries, rhododendron, rhubarb leaves, rubber plant, some wild cherries)	Difficult to detect ranging from nausea to coma. Always question in cases of apparent child poisoning.
Strychnine	Face, jaw, and neck will stiffen. Strong convulsions occur quickly after ingesting.

part of your continued training. It is not meant to be memorized as part of your basic course.

POISON CONTROL CENTERS

There are more than 60 regional poison control centers in the United States, most of which are staffed 24 hours a day. The staff at each center is trained to advise you on what should be done for most cases of poisoning. There are several ways the Emergency Medical Responder can access one of these poison control centers. The first is by calling the local poison control center directly. Your instructor can provide you with the location and phone number of the regional poison control center serving your area. Another way is by contacting the EMS dispatcher who, in most cases, can put the Emergency Medical Responder in direct contact with the local center. Finally, there is a nationwide poison control number, which when called will automatically redirect the caller to the closest or most appropriate poison control center (Figure 9.12).

In some EMS systems, rescuers must receive directions for the care of poisoning patients from a physician. This is not always the case for every poison control center. If directions must come from a physician, the Emergency Medical Responder should phone or radio the emergency department or EMS dispatch. You are to follow the method used by your EMS system. Remember, a nurse or the dispatcher may relay the physician's directions. You may not have a chance to speak directly to a physician.

To aid the poison control center or medical direction, note and report any containers at the scene of the poisoning. Let them know if the patient has vomited and describe the vomit (check for pill fragments). When possible, and if it can be done quickly, gather information from the patient or from bystanders before you call the center.

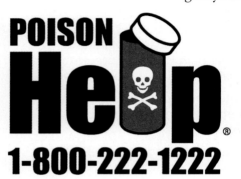

FIGURE 9.12 The phone number of the American Association of Poison Control Centers redirects the caller to the closest or most appropriate poison control center.

> **NOTE**
>
> In your jurisdiction, Emergency Medical Responder care for ingested poisons may include giving the patient syrup of ipecac or activated charcoal. Check local protocols and always call for medical direction before assisting a patient with these medications. (See Appendix 3.)

ASSESSMENT AND EMERGENCY CARE

Ingested Poisons

In cases of possible ingested poisoning, you must gather information quickly. If at all possible, do so while you are conducting your patient assessment. Note any containers that may hold poisonous substances (Figure 9.13). See if there is any vomit. Check for any substances on the patient's clothes or if the patient is wearing clothing that indicates the nature of work (farmer, miner, and so on). Can the scene be associated with certain types of poisonings? Question the patient and any bystanders.

FIRST ➤ The signs and symptoms of ingested poisons can be gathered during the scene size-up and patient assessment. They may include any one or all of the following:

- Burns or stains around the patient's mouth.
- Unusual breath odors, body odors, or odors on the patient's clothing or at the scene.
- Abnormal breathing.
- Abnormal pulse rate and rhythm.

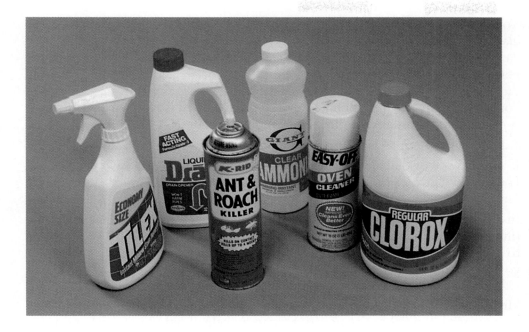

FIGURE 9.13 Common household poisons.

- Sweating.
- Dilated (enlarged) or constricted pupils.
- Excessive saliva formation or foaming at the mouth.
- Burning in the mouth or throat, or painful swallowing.
- Abdominal pain.
- Upset stomach or nausea, vomiting, and diarrhea.
- Convulsions.
- Altered mental status, including unresponsiveness. ▪

   Contact your local poison control center to obtain advice on appropriate care for specific poisons. But do not provide any care, other than for the ABCs to ensure control of life-threatening situations, until you have contacted medical direction.

   Emergency care directions from a poison control center may consist of diluting the poison or using activated charcoal to absorb the poison. Never attempt to dilute the poison or give activated charcoal (see Appendix 3) if the patient is not fully alert. The patient who is unresponsive may not have an intact gag reflex. Follow your local guidelines and the instructions given by the poison control center.

FIRST ➤ Providing liquids by mouth to patients who have ingested poison may be dangerous. This is especially true if the patient has been convulsing, or if the source of the poison is a strong acid, alkali, or petroleum product such as gasoline or diesel fuel. Included in these groups of substances are oven cleaners, drain cleaners, toilet bowl cleaners, lye, ammonia, bleach, and kerosene. Always check for burns around the patient's mouth and for the presence of unusual odors on the patient's breath. Follow the poison control center's instructions. ▪

FIRST ➤ For responsive patients, emergency care typically includes the following:

1. Perform scene size-up, including scene safety and BSI precautions.

2. Ensure an open airway and adequate breathing.

3. Call the poison control center or medical direction for instructions.

WARNING

Always follow the poison control center's instructions before giving liquids by mouth to ingested poisoning patients.

4. You may be directed to dilute the poison by having the patient drink one or two glasses of water or milk, or you may be directed to give syrup of ipecac or activated charcoal. Check local protocols, and always call for medical direction before assisting a patient with medications. The poison control center or medical direction may tell you to have the patient consume the fluids in sips to prevent vomiting. Do not give anything by mouth if the patient is having convulsions or is gagging, unless otherwise directed by a physician or the poison control center.

5. Administer oxygen as per local protocols. Assist ventilations as necessary.

6. If supplies are available and you are directed to do so, give activated charcoal. For an adult, give 25 to 50 grams. For a child, give 12.5 to 25 grams. (See Appendix 3.)

7. In case of vomiting, position the patient so that no vomit will be aspirated (inhaled). Put him on one side or in a semisitting position with the head turned to the side.

8. Save all vomit for later analysis by hospital staff. ■

In cases of ingested poisons, be realistic about the limits of emergency care. Some poisons kill quickly. Some patients can be helped only by special antidotes, and there are no antidotes at all for some poisons. Understand that even when you have done all that can be done, the patient may still die from an ingested poison.

> **NOTE**
>
> In addition to the usual risks, if the patient has ingested a highly concentrated dose of certain poisons, such as arsenic or cyanide, and if deposits remain on the patient's lips, there is a chance the rescuer may be harmed. The current recommendation is to use a pocket face mask with HEPA filter, a bag-valve mask, or your EMS system's approved protective barrier device on all poisoning patients who need rescue breathing. Keep in mind that patients receiving a high dose of these poisons may die within minutes.

Inhaled Poisons

Gather information from the patient and bystanders as quickly as possible. Look for indications of inhaled poisons. Possible sources include automobile exhaust systems, stoves, charcoal grills, industrial solvents, and spray cans.

FIRST ➤ Signs and symptoms of inhaled poisons vary depending on the source of the poison. Shortness of breath and coughing are common indicators. Pulse rate is usually fast or slow. Often, the patient's eyes will appear irritated. ■

FIRST ➤ Emergency care consists of safely removing the patient from the source of the inhaled poison, maintaining an open airway, administering oxygen, providing needed life support measures, contacting the poison control center or medical direction, and making certain that the EMS system has been activated. Remember to gather information from the patient and bystanders (substance inhaled, length of time exposed, early care measures, patient's initial reactions and appearance).

Is It Safe ?

Be especially cautious when caring for patients who may have suffered an inhalation poisoning. Due to the nature of the poisoning, you may be at risk for exposure. If in doubt about the safety of the scene, wait a safe distance away and call for a specialty hazmat team.

WARNING

Do not attempt to rescue the victim of an inhaled poisoning unless you are absolutely certain that the scene is safe. This is true even when the incident occurs outside or in a well-ventilated area. Unless you are trained to enter such a scene and have the proper equipment, do not try to provide care for a patient in a poisonous atmosphere. Do only what you have been trained to do.

It may be necessary to remove contaminated clothing from the patient. Avoid touching this clothing because it may cause skin burns. Wear latex or vinyl gloves to protect yourself. ■

Fire presents problems other than thermal burns. One such problem is smoke inhalation. The smoke from any fire source contains poisonous substances. Modern building materials and furnishings often contain plastics and other synthetics that release toxic fumes when they burn or overheat. It is possible for the substances found in smoke to burn the skin, irritate the eyes, injure the airway, cause respiratory arrest, and, in some cases, cause cardiac arrest. Do not attempt a rescue unless you have been trained to do so and have all the required personnel and equipment.

As an Emergency Medical Responder, you will probably see irritation to the eyes and airway associated with smoke. Irritations to the skin and eyes may be cared for by flushing with water. But your first priority will be the patient's airway. In cases of smoke inhalation, you should:

1. Move the patient to a safe, smoke-free area.
2. Perform an initial assessment and supply life support measures as needed.
3. Administer oxygen, if you have been trained and your jurisdiction permits Emergency Medical Responders to do so.
4. If the patient is responsive and without signs of neck or spine injury, place him in a sitting or semisitting position. The patient may find it easier to breathe in a different position, so let him assume a position of comfort. Always provide support for the back, and be prepared if the patient becomes unresponsive.

Carbon monoxide poisoning is often present at fire scenes. This gas enters the patient's bloodstream, where it is picked up by red blood cells that should be carrying oxygen. The patient will complain of headache and dizziness, and may experience confusion, seizures, and coma. Proper care requires moving the patient away from the source and the same basic procedures as would be provided for any smoke inhalation or victim of an inhaled poison. EMT-level care and transport are required in all cases of carbon monoxide poisoning. Look for soot around the nose and/or mouth. This may be a sign of smoke inhalation, along with inhalation of the superheated gases from the combustion process of fire.

Absorbed Poisons

As mentioned previously in this chapter, absorbed poisons usually irritate or damage the skin or eyes. However, there are cases in which a poison can be absorbed with little or no damage to the skin. The patient, bystanders, and other clues at the scene will help you determine if you are dealing with such rare cases. In Emergency Medical Responder care, most cases of absorbed poisoning will be detected because of skin reactions related to chemicals or plants at the scene.

FIRST ➤ Signs and symptoms of absorbed poisoning include any or all of the following:

■ Skin reactions, ranging from mild irritations to severe burns.
■ Itching.
■ Eye irritation.
■ Headache.
■ Increased skin temperature.
■ Anaphylactic (allergy) shock. ■

The body's reaction to toxic gases and foreign matter in the airway often can be delayed. It is good Emergency Medical Responder practice to alert 9-1-1 for all cases of smoke inhalation.

REMEMBER

Carbon monoxide poisoning may also occur under circumstances other than a fire. Malfunctioning furnaces and other heating devices are common sources.

REMEMBER

You are responsible for all clothing, jewelry, documents, and money removed from the patient. Obtain an official receipt for these items when you turn them over to the proper authorities and include it in the patient's medical records. Your instructor will inform you of the forms used in your state.

FIRST ➤ Emergency care for absorbed poisons includes moving the patient from the source of the poison (when safe to do so) and immediately flooding with water all the areas of the patient's body (including the eyes) that have been exposed to the poison. After flushing with water, remove all contaminated clothing (including shoes and jewelry), and wash the affected areas of the patient's skin with soap and water. If no soap is available, continue to flush the exposed areas of the patient's skin. Be certain to have someone contact the poison control center or medical direction and activate the EMS system.

If the poison is in the form of a powder, you may have to brush it from the patient's clothing, skin, and hair. It is best done with you wearing gloves and eye protection. If available, protect the patient's eyes as well. Take precautions so that no one—you, the patient, or onlookers—do not inhale the powder. Some inhaled powders can set off asthmatic events or anaphylactic (allergy) shock. More specific directions for chemical burns appear in Chapter 10. ∎

Injected Poisons

Insect stings, spider bites, stings from marine life, and snakebites can all be sources of injected poisons. Some of these poisons cause serious emergencies in all patients, though others cause problems only for those patients sensitive to the poison. In all cases of injected poisons, be alert for anaphylactic (allergy) shock (see page 282).

Poisons can also be injected into the body by a hypodermic needle. Drug overdose and drug contamination can produce serious medical emergencies.

FIRST ➤ Gather information from the patient, bystanders, and the scene. Signs and symptoms of injected poisoning may include:

- Noticeable stings or bites to the skin.
- Puncture marks to the skin. Pay careful attention to the fingers and hands, forearms, toes and feet, and lower legs.
- Pain at or around the wound site.
- Itching.
- Weakness, dizziness, or collapse.
- Difficulty breathing and abnormal pulse rate.
- Headache.
- Nausea.
- Anaphylactic (allergy) shock. ∎

FIRST ➤ Because a patient may go into anaphylactic (allergy) shock, alert the poison control center and the EMS system or medical direction as soon as possible for all cases of injected poisoning. Emergency care for injected poisons (except snakebite) includes:

1. Perform scene size-up, including taking BSI precautions.
2. Administer oxygen as per local protocols.
3. Scrape away bee and wasp stingers and venom sacs. Do not pull out stingers. Always scrape them from the patient's skin. A plastic credit card works well as a scraper.
4. Place an ice bag or cold pack over the bitten or stung area. ∎

REMEMBER

Part of the patient assessment is to look for medical identification devices.

Some patients sensitive to stings or bites carry medication to help prevent anaphylactic shock. Help all such patients to take their medications (see Appendix 3). Your Emergency Medical Responder course may include training in how to administer medications by injection when the patient cannot inject himself. Do only what you have been trained to do. Remember to look for medical identification devices.

SNAKEBITES

Between 7,000 and 8,000 people in the United States are bitten by poisonous snakes each year, with fewer than 20 deaths being reported annually. (In the United States, more people die each year from bee and wasp stings than from snakebites.) Signs and symptoms of poisoning may take several hours to develop. Death from snakebite is usually not a rapidly occurring event unless anaphylactic shock also occurs. Staying calm, as well as keeping the patient calm, is critical. There is usually time to activate the EMS system and provide care for the patient.

Consider all snakebites to be from poisonous snakes. The patient or bystanders may indicate that the snake was not poisonous. They could be mistaken. If you see the live snake, do not approach it to determine its species. Only if safe to do so from a distance, note its size and coloration. Unless you are an expert in capturing snakes, do not try to catch it. However, if possible, do contact animal control authorities.

FIRST ➤ Signs and symptoms of snakebite may include:

- Noticeable bite to the skin. This may appear as nothing more than a discoloration.
- Pain and swelling in the area of the bite. This may be slow to develop, taking 30 minutes to several hours.
- Rapid pulse and labored breathing.
- Weakness.
- Vision problems.
- Nausea and vomiting. ▪

FIRST ➤ Emergency care for snakebite includes:

1. Perform a scene size-up, including taking BSI precautions.
2. Keep the patient calm and lying down.
3. Have someone activate the EMS system.
4. Locate the fang marks, and gently clean this site with soap and water.
5. Remove from the bitten extremity any rings, bracelets, and other constricting items.
6. Keep any bitten extremities immobilized. Try to keep the bitten area at the level of the heart, or when possible, below the level of the heart.
7. Provide care for shock, conserve body heat, and monitor vital signs. ▪

If you know that the patient will not reach a medical facility within 30 minutes after having been bitten, or if the signs and symptoms of the patient begin to worsen, apply a constricting band two to four inches above the fang marks. The band should be about 1.5 to 2 inches wide, placed about two inches from the wound, or above the swelling. (Never place a band directly on a joint.)

The constricting band should be placed so that you can slide your finger underneath it. Do not place it so tight that it cuts off arterial flow. Monitor for a distal pulse at the wrist or ankle, depending on the extremity involved. Many EMS systems recommend constricting bands for all cases of snakebite. Check with your instructor.

Do not place an ice bag or cold pack on the bite unless you are directed to do so by a physician or the poison control center. Do not cut into the bite and/or apply suction unless you are directed to do so by a physician. Never suck the venom from the wound using your mouth.

REMEMBER

The coral snake has a small mouth. Usually, its bites are limited to the patient's finger or toe. When the bite is known to be from a coral snake, apply one constricting band above the wound site.

ANAPHYLACTIC SHOCK

anaphylactic (AN-ah-fi-LAK-tik)
shock ■ a severe allergic reaction in which a person goes into shock. Also called *allergy shock*.

Anaphylactic shock, or allergy shock, occurs when people come into contact with a substance to which they are allergic. The body considers the substance an invader and reacts to counteract it. This is a life-threatening emergency. There is no way of knowing if patients will stabilize, grow worse slowly or rapidly, or overcome the reaction on their own. Many patients become worse rapidly. For some, death is a certain outcome unless special care is provided quickly.

There are many different causes of anaphylactic shock, such as insect bites and stings, including bee stings; foods (nuts, spices, shellfish); inhaled substances, including dust and pollens; chemicals, inhaled or when in contact with the skin; and medications, injected or taken by mouth, including penicillin.

FIRST ➤ Signs and symptoms of anaphylactic shock are:

■ Burning, itching, or breaking out of the skin, such as hives or some type of rash.
■ Breathing that is difficult and rapid, with possible chest pains and wheezing.
■ Pulse that is rapid, very weak, or not detected.
■ Lips often turn blue (cyanosis), and the face and tongue may swell.
■ Restlessness.
■ Changes in mental status, such as fainting or unresponsiveness. ■

When you interview patients, ask if they are allergic to anything and if they have been in contact with that substance. Look for a medical identification device, which may indicate that there is an allergy problem. If you are in the patient's residence, look for a "Vial of Life" or similar type sticker on the main entrance, the closest window to the main door, or the refrigerator door. This sticker indicates the presence of patient information and medications in a vial kept in the refrigerator.

FIRST ➤ To provide emergency care to patients in anaphylactic shock, follow the same procedures used for shock (see Chapter 10). Even though the danger to the patient may be immediate, do not attempt to transport him unless you are allowed to do so. It is usually better to wait for the EMTs to respond. In many cases, EMTs can respond to the scene and administer the medications required to stabilize the patient before transport. Some jurisdictions may allow Emergency Medical Responders to give medications to counteract the effects of allergic reaction or anaphylactic shock. Check local protocols, and always call for medical direction before assisting a patient with medications. ■

Some people who are sensitive to bee stings or who have other allergy problems carry prescribed medications to take in case of an emergency. These medications, usually epinephrine and/or antihistamines, can be administered by the patient (see Appendix 3). Your jurisdiction may allow Emergency Medical Responders to help the patient take medications. State laws and protocols will govern if you can assist the patient in administering the medication. Your instructor will inform you of local policies for the care of these patients.

Heat Emergencies

hyperthermia ■ an increase in body core temperature above its normal temperature.

Exposure to hot and humid environments can cause the body to generate too much heat, which can create an abnormally high body core temperature known as **hyperthermia**. Such a condition could result from a patient being outside on a hot, humid afternoon for a prolonged period of time, or from exposure to excessive heat while indoors, such as a boiler room. Left unchecked, this condition could lead to death.

The body generates heat by creating energy during digestion and metabolism. Heat is lost through the lungs and skin. The entire process is controlled by a structure in the brain (the hypothalamus) that acts as the body's thermostat. It is responsible for regulating all processes to maintain a normal body temperature (98.6°F, or 37°C).

Geriatric Focus

The elderly are particularly prone to both extremes of temperature. Sweating may be reduced due to aging of their skin and the effects of their medications. The normal response to a loss of fluids is to increase the heart rate to maintain blood pressure. This reflex is often weaker in the elderly and can easily lead them to passing out before reaching a cooler place.

Sweating is one of the body's ways of ridding itself of excess heat. On a really hot day, you can lose up to one liter (about two pints) of sweat per hour. The sweat, in turn, is evaporated from the motion of the wind or gentle breeze. Heat is then lost at the same time. A problem develops on humid days or days without breezes, which inhibits the evaporative process.

Dry heat (low humidity) can often fool individuals, causing them to continue to work in or be exposed to heat far beyond the point that can be accepted by their bodies. For this reason, the problems caused by dry heat exposure are often far worse than those seen in moist heat exposure.

When dealing with problems created by exposure to excessive heat, you must perform a thorough history and physical exam (Figure 9.14). A previous history

Assessment of a Heat Emergency

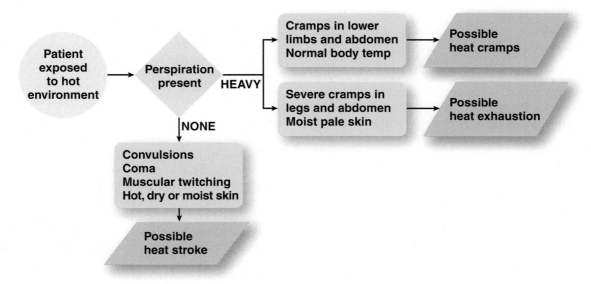

FIGURE 9.14 Algorithm for the assessment of patients with a heat emergency.

of blood pressure or lung problems may quicken the effects of heat exposure. What appears to be a problem related to heat exposure could be a heart attack. Also, remember that certain types of patients are at risk for heat emergencies. Children, the elderly, the chronically ill, and alcoholics are especially susceptible to temperature extremes. Individuals who are taking certain heart or other medications may also be prone to such conditions, along with anyone with a pre-existing illness or condition (Scan 9–5).

SCAN 9–5 | Heat-Related Emergencies

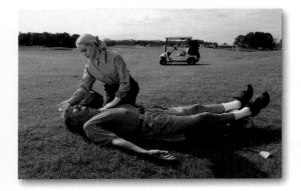

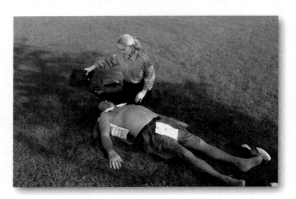

Heat Cramps/Exhaustion

Heat cramps and heat exhaustion are typically early signs of a heat emergency.

Signs and Symptoms

- Mild to severe muscle cramps in legs and abdomen.
- Exhaustion, possible altered mental status (dizziness, faintness, and unresponsiveness).
- Weak pulse and rapid, shallow breathing.
- Heavy perspiration.
- Normal to pale skin color.

Emergency Care

- Move patient to nearby cool place. Loosen or remove clothing. Do not chill. Watch for shivering.
- Provide oxygen at 15 LPM by nonrebreather mask if allowed.
- Give water to the responsive patient.
- Position the responsive patient on his back with legs elevated; unresponsive patient on the left side, monitoring airway and breathing.
- Help ease cramps by applying moist towels over cramped muscles or, if the patient has no history of circulatory problems, apply gentle but firm pressure on the cramped muscle.

Heat Stroke

Heat stroke is a true life-threatening emergency.

Signs and Symptoms

- Altered mental status.
- Skin that is hot to the touch.
- Heavy perspiration.
- Rapid, shallow breathing.
- Strong and rapid pulse.
- Weakness, unresponsiveness.
- Little to no perspiration.
- Dilated pupils.
- Seizures or muscular twitching.

Emergency Care

- Rapidly cool the patient in any manner. Move to a cool place. Remove clothing. Keep skin wet by applying wet towels. Fan the patient.
- Wrap cold packs or ice bags, if available, and place them at the neck, armpits, wrists, and groin (latest protocols often request only positions that touch trunk). Fan the patient to increase heat loss.
- If transport is delayed, find tub or container and immerse patient in cool water. Monitor to prevent drowning.
- Continue to monitor the patient's vital signs.
- Provide oxygen at 15 LPM via nonrebreather mask if allowed.

HEAT EXHAUSTION

The typical heat emergency patient with moist, pale, normal-to-cool skin is a healthy individual who has been exposed to excessive heat while working or exercising. The circulatory system of the patient begins to fail because of fluid and salt loss. During this process, sometimes known as **heat exhaustion**, the individual perspires heavily, and becomes very thirsty.

FIRST ➤ Signs and symptoms of heat exhaustion include:

- Mild to moderate perspiration.
- Skin temperature may feel normal or cool.
- Skin color may be normal to pale.
- Weakness, exhaustion, or dizziness.
- Muscle cramps (usually in legs or abdomen).
- Rapid, shallow breathing.
- Rapid, weak pulse.
- Altered mental status. ▪

FIRST ➤ Emergency care for heat exhaustion includes (Figure 9.15):

1. Complete a scene size-up, including taking BSI precautions.
2. Make sure the EMS system has been activated.
3. Perform an initial assessment. Provide oxygen as per local protocol.
4. Remove the patient from the hot environment and place him in a cool area.
5. Loosen or remove clothing.
6. Cool the patient by fanning. Be careful not to chill the patient.
7. If the patient is not alert, place him in the recovery position.
8. Provide emotional support and reassure the patient. ▪

HEAT CRAMPS

Heat cramps are painful muscle spasms following strenuous activity in a hot environment, usually caused by an electrolyte (such as salt) imbalance. Sometimes,

> **heat exhaustion** ▪ prolonged exposure to heat, which creates moist, pale skin that may feel normal or cool to the touch.

> **5–1.9** Identify the patient who presents with a specific medical complaint of exposure to heat.

> **5–1.10** Explain the steps in providing emergency medical care to a patient with an exposure to heat.

> **heat cramps** ▪ common term for muscle cramps in the lower limbs and abdomen associated with the loss of fluids and salts while active in a hot environment.

Care for a Heat Emergency

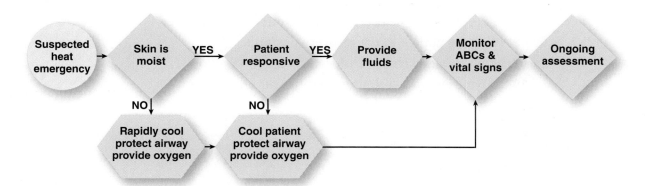

FIGURE 9.15 Algorithm for the emergency care of patients with a heat emergency.

these cramps are accompanied by signs and symptoms of heat exhaustion. In most cases, however, the patient will be mentally alert and sweaty with a normal body temperature. The care for these victims is to simply remove them from the heat and replenish fluids by having them drink water. If symptoms persist, activate the EMS system for an EMT or more advanced response.

HEAT STROKE

Sometimes, the body's temperature-regulating mechanism fails and is unable to rid the body of excess heat. Temperature then rises significantly, causing the patient to become very hot. This condition is known as **heat stroke** and should be considered a life-threatening condition. A patient's body temperature may increase to 105°F (40.5°C) or higher, and the patient may experience a decreased level of responsiveness. The skin will be hot and dry. The patient with heat stroke will almost always present with an altered mental status. If you are caring for a patient with a heat emergency and he has an altered mental status, provide care for heat stroke.

FIRST ➤ Patients suffering from heat stroke may have the following signs and symptoms:

- Altered mental status.
- Skin that is hot to the touch.
- Skin that is slightly moist to dry.
- Rapid, shallow breathing.
- Full and rapid pulse.
- Convulsions.
- Generalized weakness. ▪

FIRST ➤ Emergency care for heat stroke (hot, moist to dry skin) includes the following:

1. Complete a scene size-up, including taking BSI precautions.
2. Make sure EMS has been activated.
3. Perform an initial assessment. Provide oxygen as per local protocol.
4. Remove the patient from the hot environment and place him in a cool area.
5. Loosen or remove clothing. Pour cool water over wet wrappings.
6. Cool patient by fanning. Be sure not to chill the patient.
7. Wrap cold packs or ice bags, if available, and place one under each of the patient's armpits, one on each wrist and ankle, one on the groin, and one on each side of the neck. Note that testing indicates that cold packs at wrists and ankles may not be useful. Follow your local protocol.
8. Place the patient in the recovery position.
9. Monitor vital signs.
10. Provide emotional support and reassure the patient. ▪

Cold Emergencies

HYPOTHERMIA

When body heat is lost faster than it is generated, a condition called **hypothermia**, a generalized cold emergency, may develop. Hypothermia becomes generalized when the temperature at the center of the body—the body's core temperature—

drops too low. To prevent this condition from occurring, the body will attempt to compensate by increasing muscle activity (shivering) to increase metabolism and maintain body heat. But as the core body temperature continues to drop, shivering stops and the body can no longer warm itself.

As with heat exposure, young children and the elderly are more susceptible to cold emergencies. Those with previous medical problems might also be prone to such problems. Many cold exposures are more obvious than others, such as a victim who is working or playing outside in a cold environment during the winter months. Sometimes, however, the exposure can be subtle. For example, elderly patients who do not maintain the home thermostat at a proper level during the winter are often affected by cold exposure. Refrigeration accidents and incidents in mild climates also occur.

The patient experiencing a generalized cold emergency will present with cool or cold abdominal skin temperature. Place the back of your ungloved hand against the patient's abdomen to assess the general temperature of the patient. In healthy adults, the abdomen should be warm, dry, and pink.

REMEMBER

The environmental temperature does not have to be below freezing for hypothermia to occur.

FIRST ➤ Signs and symptoms of a generalized cold emergency may include the following:

- Cool or cold skin temperature.
- Shivering.
- Decreased mental status.
- Initially rapid, then slow pulse.
- Lack of coordination.
- Stiff or rigid posture.
- Muscle rigidity.
- Impaired judgment.
- Complaints of joint/muscle stiffness. ▪

5–1.7 Identify the patient who presents with a specific medical complaint of exposure to cold.

REMEMBER

Do not allow the patient to smoke or drink alcohol or caffeine. These substances may affect blood vessels and worsen the patient's condition.

FIRST ➤ Emergency care for generalized cold emergencies includes:

1. Perform a scene size-up, including taking BSI precautions.
2. Make sure that someone activates the EMS system.
3. Perform an initial assessment. Administer oxygen as per local protocols.
4. Remove the patient from the cold environment, but do not allow the patient to walk or exert himself in any way.
5. Protect the patient from further heat loss.
6. Remove any wet clothing, and place a blanket over the patient. If there are no indications of possible spine injuries, place a blanket under the patient using a log roll. Remember to handle the patient gently.
7. Monitor vital signs.
8. Comfort the patient and reassure him. While awaiting additional EMS resources, do not give the patient anything to eat or drink (including hot coffee, tea, or alcohol). ▪

5–1.8 Explain the steps in providing emergency medical care to a patient with an exposure to cold.

Some cases of generalized cold emergency are extreme. The patient might be unresponsive and show no vital signs, with skin cold to the touch. You cannot assume that this patient is dead. Assess the pulse for 30 to 45 seconds. If there is no pulse, begin CPR immediately. Arrange for transportation to an emergency department. The doctors at the hospital will pronounce a patient biologically dead only after they have rewarmed the tissues and there is still no response.

LOCALIZED COLD INJURY

frostbite ▪ localized cold injury in which the skin is frozen.

Another environmental emergency that is characterized by the freezing or near freezing of a body part is known as **frostbite**, or a localized cold injury. It is caused by a significant exposure to cold temperature (below 0°F or 17°C). It mainly occurs in the extremities and in areas of the fingers, toes, ears, face, and nose (Scan 9–6).

A classic example of a victim of a cold emergency is someone who is outdoors during the winter for a prolonged period of time. Perhaps he is unprotected by scarves,

SCAN **9–6**	Cold-Related Emergencies		
CONDITION	**SKIN SURFACE**	**TISSUE UNDER SKIN**	**SKIN COLOR**
Early, superficial	Soft	Soft	White
Late, deep	Hard	Initially soft, progressing to hard	White and waxy progressing to blotchy white, then to yellow-gray to blue-gray

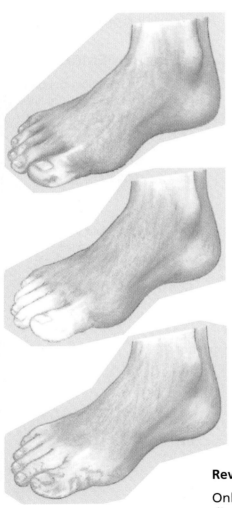

Early, Superficial
Slow onset with numbing of affected part. Have the patient rewarm the part with his own body heat. Tingling and burning sensations are common during rewarming.

Late, Deep
Tissues below the surface initially will have their normal bounce. Protect the entire limb. Handle gently. Keep the patient at rest and provide external warmth to injury site. Untreated, this will progress to where the tissue below the surface will feel hard. Provide the same care you would for early superficial cooling. Immediate EMS transport is recommended.

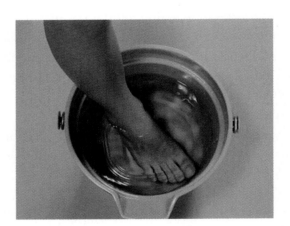

Rewarming
Only if transport is delayed in case of late or deep local cooling and if medical direction allows, rewarm the affected part by immersing it in warm water (100°F to 105°F; 37.7°C to 40.5°C). Do not allow the body part to touch the container bottom or side. After rewarming, gently dry the part and pad between fingers or toes. Dress the affected area, cover and elevate the limb, and keep the patient warm. *Do not rewarm* if there is any chance that the tissue may refreeze, usually due to extended exposure.

gloves, or boots. The core of the body continues to be warmed by metabolism, but the exposed areas are susceptible to the impact of cold and wind. Most patients will describe a localized cold injury as starting with a cold sensation to the extremities that leads to pain, followed by numbness. This is the classic progression of symptoms.

FIRST ➤ Signs and symptoms of a localized cold injury may include the following:

Early
- Blanching of the skin (after palpation of the skin, color does not return).
- Feeling of cold, pain, or loss of feeling and sensation to the injured area.
- Skin remains soft.
- If thawed, tingling sensation is present.

Late
- White, waxy skin (in light-skinned patients).
- Firm to frozen feeling on palpation.
- Swelling may be present.
- Blisters may be present.
- If thawed, may appear flushed with areas of purple and blanching. ■

FIRST ➤ Emergency care for a localized cold injury is as follows:

1. Perform a scene size-up, including taking BSI precautions.
2. Perform an initial assessment.
3. Make sure that someone activates the EMS system.
4. Remove the patient from the cold environment.
5. Protect the patient from further cold exposure.
6. Remove any wet or constrictive clothing.
7. If it is an early injury:
   - Manually stabilize the extremity.
   - Cover the extremity.
   - Do not rub or massage it.
   - Do not re-expose the injured part to cold.
8. If it is a late injury:
   - Remove jewelry from the injured area.
   - Cover the injured part with dry, sterile dressings.
   - Do not break blisters.
   - Do not rub or massage the injured area.
   - Do not apply heat.
   - Do not rewarm. (Some jurisdictions allow rewarming. Check with medical direction.)
   - Do not allow the patient to walk on affected legs.
9. Comfort and reassure the patient. ■

Behavioral Emergencies

Behavior is the manner in which a person acts or performs. This includes any or all of a person's activities, including physical and mental activity. The behavior of most people is considered typical or normal because it is accepted by their families and society. It does not interfere with the daily activities of life. Behavior that is unacceptable or intolerable to others is known as abnormal (atypical) behavior.

5–1.11 Identify the patient who presents with a specific medical complaint of behavioral change.

behavioral emergency ■ a situation in which an individual exhibits abnormal behavior that is unacceptable or intolerable to the patient, family, or community.

5–1.13 Identify the patient who presents with a specific medical complaint of psychological crisis.

WARNING

If the patient creates an unsafe scene and you are not a trained law enforcement officer following standard operating procedures (SOPs), get out and find a safe place until the police arrive.

Although caring for this type of patient might be challenging, it is crucial that you remain professional and provide appropriate care.

A **behavioral emergency** exists in situations where the patient exhibits abnormal behavior that is unacceptable or intolerable to the patient, family, or community. Such behavior may occur because of extremes of emotion or a psychological or medical condition. Other causes of behavioral change include situational stress (patient reacting to events at the scene); mind-altering substances; psychiatric problems; and psychological crises, including panic or paranoia.

ASSESSMENT AND EMERGENCY CARE

FIRST ➤ When performing an assessment on behavioral emergency patients, do the following (Figure 9.16):

- Identify yourself and let the patient know you are there to help.
- Inform the patient of what you are doing.
- Ask questions in a calm, reassuring voice.
- Without being judgmental, allow the patient to tell what happened.
- Show that you are listening by rephrasing or repeating part of what is said.
- Assess the patient's mental status: appearance, activity, speech, and orientation to person, place, time, and event. ■

Is It Safe ?

Responding to a behavioral emergency can present many risks for responders. Although most patients want your care, behavioral emergency patients may not want any part of it. Consider the need for law enforcement early in the call and do not get yourself cornered in a room with the patient.

FIGURE 9.16 Evaluate the scene and maintain a safe distance as you begin to ask questions and reassure the patient.

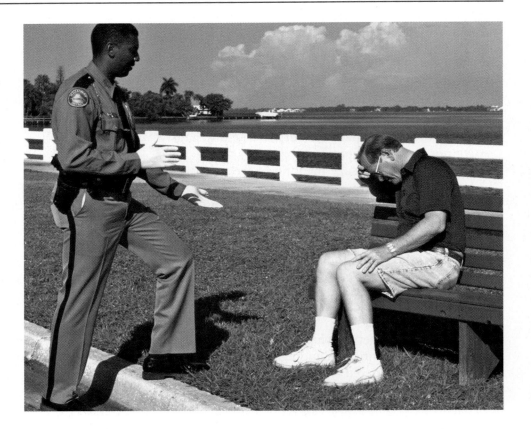

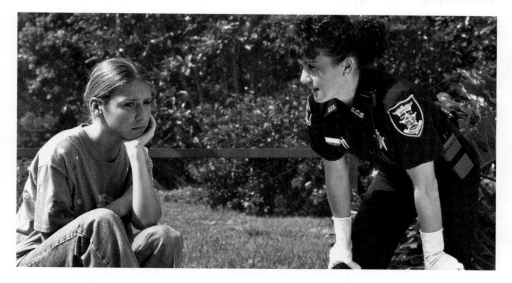

FIGURE 9.17 Encourage the emotionally distraught patient to tell you what is troubling her.

FIRST ➤ Emergency care of a patient with a behavioral emergency includes the following:

- Perform a scene size-up, including taking BSI precautions and considering the need for law enforcement.
- Make sure that someone has activated the EMS system.
- Perform an initial assessment by observing the patient from a safe distance.
- Acknowledge that the patient seems upset and restate that you are there to help.
- Inform the patient of what you are doing.
- Ask questions in a calm, reassuring voice.
- Maintain a comfortable distance.
- Encourage the patient to state what is troubling him (Figure 9.17).
- Do not make quick moves.
- Answer questions honestly.
- Do not threaten, challenge, or argue with disturbed patients.
- Do not "play along" with hallucinations or auditory disturbances.
- Involve trusted family members or friends, if appropriate.
- Be prepared for an extended scene time.
- Avoid unnecessary physical contact.
- Leave yourself a way out. Never let the potentially violent patient come between you and your exit. ▪

5–1.12 Explain the steps in providing emergency medical care to a patient with a behavioral change.

5–1.14 Explain the steps in providing emergency medical care to a patient with a psychological crisis.

ASSESSING THE POTENTIAL FOR VIOLENCE

Sometimes patients experience conditions that cause them to become violent and uncooperative. As an Emergency Medical Responder, your priority is to prevent the patient from harming himself or others, while also protecting yourself. Consider contacting law enforcement (Figure 9.18), and note the following:

- *Scene size-up.* Use caution when approaching a scene. Observe the patient and the surroundings for any indication that he might be a danger to himself or others. Ensure that he has no weapons or anything that may be used as a weapon.
- *History.* Often, patients who have exhibited violent behavior in the past will repeat it. Take such past history into consideration during your assessment.

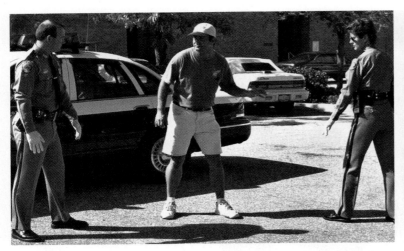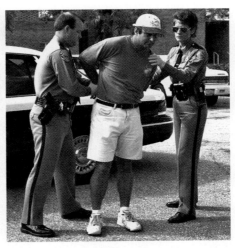

FIGURE 9.18 Law enforcement officers may be needed to approach and control a behavioral patient who may become violent.

- *Posture.* How is the patient standing? Is he in an offensive stance? What does his body language tell you? Are you positioned at a safe distance?
- *Verbal activity.* Often, verbal abuse is a precursor to violence. If a patient continues to use foul language or raise his voice, consider such action as a possible warning sign of violent behavior.
- *Physical activity.* Patients may begin to pace or wave their arms in the air with increased activity. Such movements may escalate into more violent behavior.

Geriatric Focus

Do not let the age of the patient lull you into a false sense of security. A violent elderly patient can be just as dangerous as any other patient given the right circumstances and/or availability of a weapon.

REMEMBER

When there is reasonable cause to restrain a person, a physician or law enforcement officer may order restraint. Ask your instructor to explain your state's laws and EMS guidelines for such a situation.

RESTRAINING PATIENTS

In some cases, behavioral emergency patients might become violent to the point that it is necessary to physically restrain them. Although this task should be avoided, it is often necessary to protect the patient, yourself, and others. In these situations, follow your local guidelines for contacting police and consulting medical direction. Remember the emotional disturbance may be caused by an underlying medical condition that the patient is not aware of, does not understand, or cannot control. Because of this, emotionally disturbed patients may threaten those who are trying to help and will often resist emergency care.

You cannot provide emergency care to a patient without proper consent, so you must have a reasonable belief that the patient will harm himself or others and would want help if he were able to understand and consent to it. Contact medical direction for guidance before attempting to provide care for a patient without consent. In these cases, local protocols may require you to contact law enforcement for assistance.

Do not approach a violent patient alone. While waiting for assistance, try the following:

- Talk and listen to the patient to divert his focus and keep him from harming himself and others.
- Sit or stand passively but remain alert to the patient's actions and responses.
- Avoid any action that may alarm the patient and cause him to react violently.

- Wait for law enforcement assistance to arrive if restraining the patient is necessary, and let police officers take the lead in restraining the patient.
- Use reasonable force only to defend yourself against attack.

Geriatric Focus

Often, it is enough to simply place the elderly patient on the cot and apply the adjustable straps. If you need to restrain his arms or legs, try to use soft restraints to prevent injury to his skin or cause restriction of circulation.

Alcohol and Other Drugs

For all situations involving patients with alcohol or other drug emergencies, perform a thorough scene size-up and remain alert for changes. Once you can approach the patient, let him know who you are and what you are going to do before you start a patient assessment. You may have to modify your approach and communication techniques as you try to determine whether the situation also involves a medical or a trauma problem. It may be difficult to perform the detailed physical exam, the ongoing assessment, or any care procedures until you can calm the patient and gain his confidence.

ALCOHOL ABUSE

Alcohol is a drug, socially acceptable in moderation, but still a drug. Abuse of alcohol, as with any other drug, can lead to illness, poisoning of the body, antisocial behavior, and even death. A patient under the influence of alcohol is not funny. He may have a medical problem or an injury requiring your care. The patient may become injured or could hurt others.

As an Emergency Medical Responder, try to provide care to the patient suffering from alcohol intoxication as you would any other patient. It is often difficult to determine that the problem has been caused by alcohol and if alcohol abuse is the only problem. Even trained mental health professionals can miss making a dual diagnosis. Do not depend on the smell of alcohol on the patient's breath or clothing to be a meaningful sign, especially if the source of alcohol is vodka.

If the patient allows you to do so, conduct a patient assessment that includes a thorough history. In some cases, you will have to depend on bystanders for meaningful information. Also, remember that diabetes, epilepsy, head injuries, high fevers, and other medical problems can make a patient appear drunk.

FIRST ➤ The signs of alcohol abuse in an intoxicated patient may include:

- Odor of alcohol on the patient's breath or clothing. This is not enough by itself unless you are sure that this is not "acetone breath," a sign of the diabetic patient.
- Swaying and unsteady, uncoordinated movements.
- Slurred speech and the inability to carry on a conversation. Do not be fooled into thinking that the situation may not be serious because the patient jokes or clowns around.
- Flushed appearance, often with sweating and complaining of being warm.
- Nausea and vomiting or feeling the need to vomit. ▪

delirium tremens (DTs) ■ temporary state of mental confusion characterized by sweating, anxiety, trembling, and hallucinations.

FIRST ➤ A patient suffering from alcohol abuse may be going through withdrawal from having been without alcohol. **Delirium tremens (DTs)** may result from sudden withdrawal. In such cases, look for:

■ High blood pressure, rapid heart rate.
■ Confusion and restlessness.
■ Atypical behavior, to the point of being "mad" or demonstrating "insane" behavior.
■ Hallucinations.
■ Gross tremor (obvious shaking) of the hands.
■ Convulsions. ■

As you see, some of the signs displayed in alcohol intoxication are similar to those found in some medical emergencies. Be certain that the only problem is alcohol intoxication. Remember, persons who abuse alcohol may also be injured or ill. The effects of the alcohol may mask the typical signs and symptoms observed during assessment. Also, be on the alert for other signs, such as depressed vital signs, because of the patient mixing alcohol and drugs. Never ask if the patient has taken any "drugs." The patient may think that you are gathering evidence of a crime. Ask if any "medications" have been taken while drinking. Most patients, however, will not report recreational drugs or even over-the-counter medications.

FIRST ➤ The basic care for the alcohol abuse patient consists of the following:

■ Perform a scene size-up, and take appropriate BSI precautions.
■ Perform a proper history and physical exam to detect any medical emergencies or injuries. Remember that alcohol may mask pain. Look carefully for mechanisms of injury and the signs of illness.
■ Monitor vital signs, staying alert for respiratory problems.
■ Talk in an effort to keep the patient alert.
■ Help the patient when he is vomiting, so the vomit will not be aspirated (inhaled).
■ Protect the patient from further injury without the illegal use of restraint.
■ Alert dispatch and let them decide if the police must be alerted or if EMTs are to respond on their own. ■

DRUG ABUSE

uppers ■ stimulants that affect the central nervous system to excite the user.

downers ■ depressants that affect the central nervous system to relax the user.

narcotics ■ a class of drugs for the relief of pain. Illicit use is to provide an intense state of relaxation.

hallucinogens ■ mind-altering drugs that act on the central nervous system to excite the user or to distort perception of surroundings.

volatile chemicals ■ vaporizing chemicals that cause excitement or produce a "high" when they are inhaled by the abuser (huffing).

FIRST ➤ Drugs may be classified as uppers, downers, narcotics, hallucinogens (mind-affecting drugs), or volatile chemicals. **Uppers** are stimulants affecting the nervous system to excite the user. **Downers** are depressants meant to affect the central nervous system to relax the user. **Narcotics** affect the nervous system and change many of the normal activities of the body. Often they produce an intense state of relaxation and feelings of well-being. **Hallucinogens**, or mind-altering drugs, act on the nervous system to produce an intense state of excitement or distortion of the user's surroundings. **Volatile chemicals** give an initial rush, but then depress the central nervous system. ■

Some courses that train rescuers and EMS personnel have spent considerable time in the past teaching specific drug names and reactions. As an Emergency Medical Responder, you will not need such knowledge. For you, it is important to be able to detect possible drug abuse at the overdose level and to relate certain signs to certain types of drugs. Your care for the drug abuse patient will be basically the same as for any drug that may have been used. Your care will not change unless you are ordered to do so by medical direction or a poison control center. Figure 9.19 and Table 9–3 list some of the names of common drugs that are abused, but you do not need to memorize them.

The signs and symptoms of drug abuse and drug overdose can vary from patient to patient, even for the same drug. The scene, bystanders, and the patient

REMEMBER

Many drug abusers will abuse more than one drug, often mixing several at one time. It may be impossible through simple physical examination to tell what drugs are causing the patient's problem.

TABLE 9–3	Commonly Abused Substances

UPPERS

Amphetamine (Benzedrine, bennies, pep pills, ups, uppers, cartwheels)	Methamphetamine (speed, meth, crystal, diet pills, Methedrine)
Biphetamine (bam)	Methylphenidate (Ritalin)
Cocaine (coke, snow, crack)	Preludin
Desoxyn (black beauties)	
Dextroamphetamine (dexies, Dexedrine)	

Downers

Amobarbital (blue devils, downers, barbs, Amytal)	Nonbarbiturate sedatives (various tranquilizers and sleeping pills; Valium or Diazepam, Miltown, Equanil, meprobamate, Thorazine, Compazine, Librium or chlordiazepoxide, reserpine, Tranxene or clorazepate, and other benzodiazepines)
Barbiturates (downers, dolls, barbs, rainbows)	
Chloral hydrate (knockout drops, Noctec)	
Ethchlorvynol (Placidyl)	
Glutethimide (Doriden, goofers)	
Methaqualone (Quaalude, ludes, Sopor, sopors)	

Narcotics

Codeine (often in cough syrup)	Heroin (H, horse, junk, smack, stuff)
Meperidine	Paregoric (contains opium)
Demerol	Methadone (dolly)
Morphine	Fentanyl
Dilaudid	Oxycodone (perc), OxyContin
Opium (op, poppy)	

Hallucinogens and Mind-Altering Drugs

Hallucinogenics	Nonhallucinogenics
Psilocybin (magic mushrooms)	Mescaline (peyote, mesc)
DMT	Marijuana (grass, pot, weed, dope)
STP (serenity, tranquility, peace)	Morning glory seeds
LSD (acid, sunshine)	Hash
	PCP (angel dust, hog, peace pills)
	THC

Volatile Chemicals

Amyl nitrate (snappers, poppers)	Nail polish remover
Glue	Furniture polish
Butyl nitrate (locker room, rush)	Paint thinner
Hair spray	Gasoline
Cleaning fluid (carbon tetrachloride)	

REMEMBER: The most commonly abused substance in the United States is alcohol (ethanol). In addition to its direct effects, alcohol is often mixed with other abused substances, worsening effects on the body.

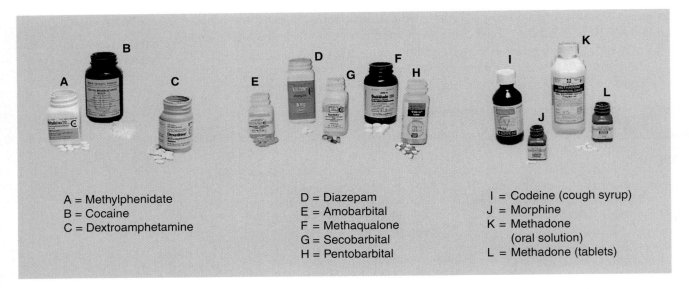

A = Methylphenidate
B = Cocaine
C = Dextroamphetamine

D = Diazepam
E = Amobarbital
F = Methaqualone
G = Secobarbital
H = Pentobarbital

I = Codeine (cough syrup)
J = Morphine
K = Methadone
    (oral solution)
L = Methadone (tablets)

FIGURE 9.19 Commonly abused substances.

may be your only sources of finding out if you are dealing with drug abuse and the substance involved. When questioning the patient and bystanders, you will get better results if you ask if the patient has been taking any medications, rather than using the word "drugs." If you have any doubts, then ask if the patient has taken drugs or is "using anything." Patients may not give information about their drug use.

FIRST ➤ Some significant signs and symptoms related to specific drugs include:

- *Uppers.* Uppers can cause excitement, increased pulse and breathing rates, rapid speech, dry mouth, dilated pupils, sweating, and the complaint of having gone without sleep for long periods.
- *Downers.* The use of downers can cause the patient to be sluggish or sleepy, lack normal coordination of body movements, and have slurred speech. Pulse and breathing rates are low, often to the point of a true emergency.
- *Hallucinogens.* These can cause a fast pulse rate, dilated pupils, and a flushed face. The patient often sees things and hears voices or sounds that do not exist, has little concept of real time, and may not be aware of the true environment. Often, the patient makes no sense when speaking. Many show signs of anxiety and fearfulness. They have been described as paranoid. Some patients become very aggressive. Others tend to withdraw.
- *Narcotics.* Reduced pulse and breathing rates and a lowered skin temperature are often seen in the patient who is abusing narcotics. The pupils are constricted, muscles are relaxed, and sweating is heavy. The patient is very sleepy and does not wish to do anything. In overdoses, coma is a common event. Respiratory arrest may occur.
- *Volatile chemicals.* The user may seem dazed or show temporary loss of contact with reality. This patient may go into a coma. The inside of the nose and mouth may show swollen membranes. The patient may complain of numbness or tingling inside the head or a headache. The face may be flushed and the pulse rate accelerated. There may be a chemical odor to the patient's breath, skin, or clothing. ▪

These signs and symptoms have a lot in common with many medical emergencies. Never assume drug abuse or drug abuse occurring by itself.

REMEMBER

For all cases of possible drug overdose, first contact medical direction. Then contact your local poison control center if protocol directs you to do so.

FIRST ➤ Withdrawal varies from patient to patient and from drug to drug. In most cases of drug withdrawal, you will see shaking, anxiety, nausea, confusion, irritability, sweating, and increased pulse and breathing rates. ■

FIRST ➤ When providing care for drug abuse patients, you should:

1. Provide life support measures, if required.
2. Alert dispatch as soon as possible. They should be informed that the problem may be caused by drugs.
3. Administer oxygen as per local protocols.
4. Monitor vital signs and be alert for respiratory arrest.
5. Talk to the patient to gain his confidence and to maintain his level of responsiveness.
6. Protect the patient from further harm.
7. Continue to reassure the patient throughout all phases of care. ■

Medical direction in your area may require you to induce vomiting if an overdose is suspected within 30 minutes of your arrival at the scene. Your instructor will give you the protocols and exceptions for your area. For all cases of possible drug overdose, it is good practice to contact medical direction and your local poison control center.

Is It Safe ❓

Many drug abusers may appear calm at first and then become violent as time passes. Always be on the alert and be ready to protect yourself. If the patient creates an unsafe scene and you are not a trained law enforcement officer, get out and find a safe place to wait until the police arrive. ■

> **NOTE**
>
> Always consider PCP users dangerous, even when they appear to be calm. PCP usage leads to aggressive behavior. The drug can build up in the body and cause a violent reaction without warning. If PCP is the cause of the problem, wait for police to arrive, unless the patient is unresponsive or in need of life support measures.

 FIRST ON SCENE WRAP-UP

The small room was bustling with firefighters, ambulance personnel, campus security, and two police officers from the city. Micah had described the patient's seizure and pointed out the medical identification necklace to the firefighters who were the first on scene.

"Who took care of this patient before we got here?" the Paramedic from the ambulance asked as he started an IV on the unconscious girl. A firefighter pointed at Micah, who was now self-consciously tightening his green robe.

"You did a great job!" The Paramedic was now administering a clear fluid into the IV line with a huge syringe. "You kept her airway open and got her into the lateral recumbent position. I couldn't have asked you to do better than that."

Micah smiled and felt his face get hot at the compliment. Before he walked from the room, he was happy to see the girl blink her eyes several times and begin to ask questions of the Paramedic.

Summary

Various illnesses and conditions can bring about a medical emergency. Medical emergencies involve illnesses and related conditions, whereas traumatic emergencies involve injuries. All patients will be categorized as either medical or trauma. The signs and symptoms gained from patient assessment and history-taking will help you recognize a medical emergency. Abnormal pulse, breathing, skin color, and temperature are some of the important signs in determining a medical emergency. Lip color, any odors of the breath, abdominal tenderness, nausea, vomiting, and altered mental status are also important signs. Listen to the patient and bystanders for reports of other symptoms, including pain, fever, nausea, dizziness, shortness of breath, problems with bowel and bladder activities, burning sensations, thirst, hunger, and odd tastes in the mouth. Look for medical identification devices and question the patient. There may be medication that should be taken during medical emergencies.

If the patient appears or says he feels unusual or has unusual vital signs and there is no injury present, conclude that there is a medical emergency. An injury can mask a medical emergency or problem. Always check for medical emergencies.

Consider chest pain in any patient as a possible heart attack. Ask if the patient has chest, arm, neck, or jaw pain. Nausea, shortness of breath, sweating, and weakness also may indicate a heart attack. Alert dispatch. Keep the patient at rest and in a position to ease difficult breathing. Loosen restrictive clothing and prevent chill. Monitor vital signs and provide emotional support.

Respiratory difficulties, including those seen in congestive heart failure (CHF), may produce the same signs and symptoms regardless of the cause of the distress. Check for labored breathing, unusual breath sounds, rate, and quality. Make sure there is no airway obstruction. Skin color change is an important sign in serious cases. Check for altered mental status. Look for swelling at the ankles and engorged neck veins, which may indicate CHF.

In all cases of respiratory difficulty, have someone call dispatch. Care for all respiratory difficulty cases by maintaining an open airway and making sure the patient is breathing adequately. Place the patient in a sitting position and conserve body heat. Keep the patient at rest and provide emotional support.

Numerous conditions can cause a patient to experience an altered mental status: seizures, strokes, diabetic emergencies, poisonings, breathing problems, and cardiac events. Signs and symptoms of an altered mental status include dizziness, impaired speech, hearing loss, confusion, or rapid mood changes. To check patient status, use the AVPU scale to categorize a patient's level of responsiveness.

A stroke patient may complain of nothing more than a headache. Consider all headaches to be a serious complaint. In cases of possible stroke, you may notice altered mental status, numbness or paralysis, speech or vision difficulty, confusion, convulsions, breathing difficulty, or unequal pupils. Maintain an open airway, keep the patient at rest, and place in the recovery position. Protect all paralyzed limbs. Provide emotional support and monitor vital signs.

A seizure patient may have a sudden loss of responsiveness and collapse. The body will stiffen, and there may be a loss of bowel and bladder control. Convulsions may occur, followed by body limpness. On regaining responsiveness, the patient is usually confused and tired. Protect the patient from physical harm during the seizure and from embarrassment after the seizure. Keep the patient at rest.

Diabetes patients may have trouble with hyperglycemia or hypoglycemia. In both cases, the patient may become unresponsive and go into a coma. In severe hyperglycemia, expect to find labored breathing with a fruity or sweet odor on the breath, rapid and weak pulse, and dry and warm skin. In severe hypoglycemia, there is no labored breathing and no fruity odor, but the pulse is strong and rapid, and skin is cold and moist. The only indication of a diabetes-related problem may be an altered mental status. Activate EMS and keep the patient at rest. When in doubt as to whether the condition is hyperglycemia or hypoglycemia, give the patient sugar.

In the case of an acute abdomen, keep the patient at rest and as comfortable as possible. Monitor for vomiting, give nothing by mouth, and activate EMS.

Anaphylactic shock, or allergy shock, is a life-threatening emergency. It is brought about when people come into contact with a substance to which they are allergic (bee stings, insect bites, chemicals, foods, dusts, pollens, drugs). Signs may include burning or itching skin, breaking out (hives), rapid and difficult breathing, very weak pulse, swelling of the face and tongue, blue lips, and sudden loss of responsiveness. Care for anaphylactic shock is the same as for other cases of shock. Transport the patient to a hospital as soon as possible and care for the patient according to local protocol. Ask the patient about allergies during the interview. Be certain to look for a medical identification device.

When dealing with a possible poisoning, look for evidence of the nature of the poison. Signs and symptoms associated with ingested poisons include burns or stains around the patient's mouth, unusual breathing and pulse rate, and sweating. Abdominal pain, nausea, and vomiting are common. (Save all vomit.) Emergency care of ingested poisons may include diluting with water or milk, or using activated charcoal to absorb the poison. Be prepared for vomiting. If an unresponsive patient vomits or convulses, assure an open airway and alert the EMTs.

Inhaled poisons can cause shortness of breath or coughing, irritated eyes, rapid or slow pulse rate, and changes in skin color. Emergency care includes removing the patient from the source (when safe to do so), providing life support measures as needed, and removing contaminated clothing.

Absorbed poisons can be severe, irritating, or damaging to the skin and eyes. Emergency care includes removing the patient from the source, flushing with water all areas of the body that came into contact with the poison, and removing contaminated clothing and jewelry.

Injected poisons usually cause pain and swelling at the site, difficulty breathing, and abnormal pulse rate. In cases of poisoning, contact the poison control center and medical direction. (Follow your EMS guidelines.) When providing care for injected poisons other than snakebite, care for shock, scrape away stingers and venom sacs, and place an ice bag or cold pack over the area. For snakebite, keep the patient calm and lying down, clean the site, keep bitten extremities immobilized, alert the dispatcher, and provide care for shock.

A hot and humid environment may cause the body to generate too much heat, which can create an abnormally high body temperature, known as hyperthermia. Early symptoms of hyperthermia include heat cramps and heat exhaustion. Heat cramps are sudden and sometimes severe muscle cramps, most often occurring in the legs. Heat exhaustion results from prolonged exposure to heat, which creates moist, pale skin that may feel normal or cool to the touch. Signs and symptoms include excessive sweating, rapid weak pulse, weakness, and possible altered mental status. Heat stroke results from prolonged exposure to heat and causes hot, dry or moist skin; altered mental status; and rapid breathing. This is a life-threatening emergency. Emergency care for heat emergencies includes removing patients from the hot environment, cooling them with water, and fanning them. Alert dispatch.

In cold environments, body heat may be lost faster than it can be generated. Rapid heat loss creates a state of low body temperature known as hypothermia, or a generalized cold emergency. Patients will have cool skin temperature, shivering, decreased mental status, stiff or rigid posture, and poor judgment. The environmental temperature does not have to be below freezing for hypothermia to occur. Another environmental emergency that is characterized by the freezing or near freezing of a body part is known as a localized cold injury, or frostbite. Frostbite patients will experience a feeling of cold followed by pain and finally numbness or tingling. Emergency care includes removing the patient from the cold environment, removing any wet clothes, keeping the patient calm and warm, and stabilizing any cold extremity.

Emergency Medical Responders might encounter patients whose behavior is unacceptable or intolerable to others. This is known as abnormal (atypical) behavior. There are many causes for a patient to act in this manner, such as stress, mind-altering substances, psychiatric problems, psychological crises, and medical causes. When assessing a patient with abnormal behavior, it is important to use methods of keeping the patient calm.

Patients may experience conditions that cause them to become violent and uncooperative. Exercise caution when approaching these patients. Consider any past history of behavioral difficulties or violence. Remember that a patient's posture and verbal activity may be warning signs of potential violent behavior. Notify law enforcement to assist you in dealing with these patients.

In some cases, patients with a behavioral emergency might become violent to the point that it is necessary to physically restrain them, but the patient must be endangering himself or others in order for Emergency Medical Responders to have the legal right to restrain him.

Patients suffering from alcohol abuse should receive the same professional level of care as any other patient. The problem may be because of alcohol or alcohol withdrawal, but there may be a medical problem or injuries. Try to detect the odor of alcohol, slurred speech, swaying, and unsteadiness of movement. Find out if the patient is nauseated. Be alert for vomiting. In cases of alcohol withdrawal, look for tremors that may indicate the DTs. In all cases of alcohol abuse, monitor vital signs and be alert for respiratory arrest.

Drug abuse can show itself in many ways, depending on the drug, the patient, and whether it is withdrawal or overdose. Withdrawal from most drugs will produce shaking, anxiety, nausea, confusion, irritability, sweating, and increased pulse and breathing rates.

In cases of drug overdose or drug withdrawal, provide life support as needed and alert dispatch. Monitor vital signs and talk to the patient. Protect the patient and provide care for shock. Reassure the patient through the entire process.

Remember and Consider

Medical emergencies are very common. As an Emergency Medical Responder, you will more than likely encounter many patients with medical complaints. In this chapter and in your classes, you have discussed how to assess these patients and manage certain specific conditions. Remember the overview of medical emergencies and how to approach a victim with a generalized medical complaint or a specific illness.

➤ What will you do for a victim of a seizure in a public place?

➤ What are the various causes of an altered mental status?

> How do you feel about providing care to a patient who is experiencing a behavioral emergency?

You should feel comfortable answering these questions. Review what you have learned in this chapter and in class and try applying it to your life. How will these things be useful to you, your coworkers, family, friends, and others?

Investigate

Regardless of where you live or what type of job you have, you should be prepared to handle any medical emergency. Remember, by definition, an emergency happens when and where you least expect it. There are several things you may be able to predict and prepare for ahead of time, based on the area in which you live. For example, many areas in the United States are exposed to extreme heat and humidity conditions.

> What are the major types of medical emergencies you might encounter in your area?
> What can you do to prepare for an emergency in your area or organization?

Quick Quiz

1. Which one of the following patients would be categorized as having a general medical complaint?
   a. 66-year-old fall victim
   b. 8-year-old having an asthma attack
   c. 23-year-old victim of a motorcycle crash
   d. 43-year-old with a severely twisted ankle

2. When assessing a patient with a medical complaint, the best way to determine the problem is to:
   a. identify the medications he is taking.
   b. perform a thorough physical exam.
   c. assess the mechanism of injury.
   d. determine the chief complaint.

3. Altered mental status is best defined as a patient who:
   a. is unresponsive.
   b. cannot speak properly.
   c. cannot tell you what day it is.
   d. is not alert or responsive to surroundings.

4. A patient who is unresponsive and having full body muscle contractions is likely experiencing:
   a. stroke.
   b. seizure.
   c. heart attack.
   d. respiratory distress.

5. Which one of the following is the best example of appropriate care for a seizure patient?
   a. Keep him from injuring himself and place him in the recovery position following the seizure.
   b. Place him in a semisitting position and apply oxygen following the seizure.
   c. Place him in a prone position and provide oxygen by nasal cannula.
   d. Restrain him and assist ventilations with a bag-valve mask.

6. A patient who is experiencing an abnormally low body core temperature is said to be:
   a. hyperthermic.
   b. cyanotic.
   c. hypothermic.
   d. hyperglycemic.

7. An injury characterized by the freezing or near freezing of a body part is known as:
   a. frostbite.
   b. frostnip.
   c. hypothermia.
   d. cold bite.

8. All of the following are appropriate steps in the management of a patient with a generalized cold emergency EXCEPT:
   a. remove the patient from the cold environment.
   b. protect him from further heat loss.
   c. provide warm liquids to drink.
   d. monitor his vital signs.

9. A patient who presents with warm moist skin, weakness, and nausea is likely experiencing:
   a. heat exhaustion.
   b. heat stroke.
   c. heat cramps.
   d. mild heat stroke.

10. A patient who presents with abnormal behavior that is unacceptable to family members and others is said to be experiencing a(n):
    a. psychosis.
    b. mental breakdown.
    c. altered behavioral state.
    d. behavioral emergency.

11. One of the best techniques for dealing with a patient experiencing a behavioral emergency is to:

    a. not let the patient know what you are doing.
    b. not believe a thing the patient says.
    c. speak in a calm and reassuring voice.
    d. acknowledge the "voices" he is hearing.

12. The term _____ is used to describe patients who present with specific signs and symptoms that indicate some type of emergency relating to the heart.

    a. respiratory compromise
    b. myocardial compromise
    c. cardiac compromise
    d. angina pectoris

13. Blockage of a coronary artery resulting in damage to the heart muscle is known as:

    a. cerebrovascular accident.
    b. myocardial infarction.
    c. cardiac compromise.
    d. angina pectoris.

14. During an episode of chest pain caused by _____, the patient does not experience any actual damage to the heart muscle.

    a. congestive heart failure
    b. myocardial infarction
    c. cardiac compromise
    d. angina pectoris

15. A term used to describe an overload of fluid in the body's tissues when the heart is unable to pump an adequate volume of blood is:

    a. congestive heart failure.
    b. myocardial infarction.
    c. angina pectoris.
    d. emphysema.

16. Shortness of breath, swelling of the ankles, and distended neck veins are common signs and symptoms of:

    a. congestive heart failure.
    b. myocardial infarction.
    c. angina pectoris.
    d. heat stroke.

17. "Does anything you do make the pain/discomfort better or worse?" This question is associated with which letter of the OPQRST assessment mnemonic?

    a. O—onset
    b. P—provocation
    c. Q—quality
    d. S—severity

18. Nitroglycerin is a common medication used to treat:

    a. congestive heart failure.
    b. respiratory problems.
    c. cardiac chest pain.
    d. allergic reactions.

19. Breathing that is effortless and at a good rate and volume is described as:

    a. regular.
    b. adequate.
    c. irregular.
    d. inadequate.

20. Emphysema and bronchitis are both examples of:

    a. myocardial infarction.
    b. cerebrovascular accident.
    c. congestive heart failure.
    d. chronic obstructive pulmonary disease.

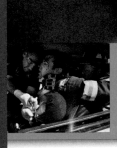

Caring for Bleeding, Shock, and Soft-Tissue Injuries

CHAPTER 10

The leading cause of death in the United States for people under the age of 40 is trauma. As an Emergency Medical Responder, you will be called on to provide emergency care to trauma patients with injuries that range from minor to life threatening. Early assessment and intervention is crucial to the proper care of these patients. As an Emergency Medical Responder, you must know how the body responds to bleeding, how to help keep bleeding under control, and how to manage shock.

This chapter covers bleeding, shock, and various soft-tissue injuries and provides descriptions of the skills you will need to care for such emergencies.

OBJECTIVES

This chapter is based on the objectives of the U.S. DOT's First Responder National Standard Curriculum. Note that cognitive objectives are listed below and beside corresponding text throughout the chapter. You will also notice as you read each objective that the term Emergency Medical Responder is used. This is simply a name change and reflects the new name for the First Responder.

By the end of this chapter, you should be able to (from cognitive or knowledge information):

5-2.1 Differentiate between arterial, venous, and capillary bleeding. (pp. 307–308)

5-2.2 State the emergency medical care for external bleeding. (pp. 309–320)

5-2.3 Establish the relationship between body substance isolation (BSI) and bleeding. (p. 307)

5-2.4 List the signs of internal bleeding. (pp. 322–324)

5-2.5 List the steps in the emergency medical care of the patient with signs and symptoms of internal bleeding. (p. 324)

5-2.6 Establish the relationship between body substance isolation (BSI) and soft-tissue injuries. (p. 307)

5-2.7 State the types of open soft-tissue injuries. (pp. 332–334)

5-2.8 Describe the emergency medical care of the patient with a soft-tissue injury. (pp. 334–336)

5-2.9 Discuss the emergency medical care considerations for a patient with a penetrating chest injury. (pp. 336–338, 350–352)

5-2.10 State the emergency medical care considerations for a patient with an open wound to the abdomen. (pp. 339, 353–354)

5-2.11 Describe the emergency medical care for an impaled object. (p. 352)

5-2.12 State the emergency medical care for an amputation. (pp. 338–339)

5-2.13 Describe the emergency medical care for burns. (pp. 357–361)

5-2.14 List the functions of dressing and bandaging. (p. 317)

By the end of this chapter, you should be able to feel comfortable enough to (by changing attitudes, values, and beliefs):

5–2.15 Explain the rationale for body substance isolation when dealing with bleeding and soft-tissue injuries. (p. 307)

5–2.16 Attend to the feelings of the patient with a soft-tissue injury or bleeding. (pp. 331, 336, 345, 354–355, 361)

5–2.17 Demonstrate a caring attitude toward patients with a soft-tissue injury or bleeding who request emergency medical services. (pp. 331, 336, 345, 354–355, 361)

5–2.18 Place the interests of the patient with a soft-tissue injury or bleeding as the foremost consideration when making any and all patient-care decisions. (pp. 307, 308, 322, 332, 339, 342, 343, 350, 351, 354, 361)

5–2.19 Communicate with empathy to patients with a soft-tissue injury or bleeding, as well as with family members and friends of the patient. (pp. 331, 336, 345, 354–355, 361)

By the end of this chapter, you should be able to show how to (through psychomotor skills):

5–2.20 Demonstrate direct pressure as a method of emergency medical care for external bleeding. (pp. 311–313)

5–2.21 Demonstrate the use of diffuse pressure as a method of emergency medical care for external bleeding. (pp. 311–313)

5–2.22 Demonstrate the use of pressure points as a method of emergency medical care for external bleeding. (pp. 313–315)

5–2.23 Demonstrate the care of the patient exhibiting signs and symptoms of internal bleeding. (p. 324)

5–2.24 Demonstrate the steps in the emergency medical care of open soft-tissue injuries. (pp. 334–336)

5–2.25 Demonstrate the steps in the emergency medical care of a patient with an open chest wound. (pp. 336–338, 350–352)

5–2.26 Demonstrate the steps in the emergency medical care of a patient with open abdominal wounds. (pp. 339, 350–354)

5–2.27 Demonstrate the steps in the emergency medical care of a patient with an impaled object. (p. 352)

5–2.28 Demonstrate the steps in the emergency medical care of a patient with an amputation. (pp. 338–339)

5–2.29 Demonstrate the steps in the emergency medical care of an amputated part. (pp. 338–339)

ADDITIONAL LEARNING TASKS

This chapter explains the functions of blood and the blood vessels, and describes the effects bleeding has on the body. You will need to understand the relationship between bleeding and shock. As you work through this chapter, you will also need to know and recognize:

➤ Differences between internal and external bleeding and what actions should be taken for each.
➤ Methods used to control profuse bleeding versus the methods used to control mild bleeding.

You will learn how to perform the steps of emergency care for:

— Foreign objects in the eye.
— Impaled objects.
— Injuries to the ear.
— Nosebleeds and other soft-tissue injuries to the face.
— Injuries to the mouth.
— Bleeding from the neck.
— Injuries to the genitalia.

It will be important for you to learn about internal bleeding, what causes it, and how it can affect the body. As you gain knowledge, you will also be able to:

➤ Define hemorrhagic shock.
➤ List the signs and symptoms of hemorrhagic shock.

- Describe the step-by-step procedures used to care for hemorrhagic shock.
- Describe how to reduce a patient's chances of fainting.

As you work through this chapter, you will learn about the assessment and care of burns and will be able to:

- Distinguish among superficial, partial-thickness, and full-thickness burns.
- Use the rule of nines for estimating body surface area affected.
- Demonstrate the appropriate care for burn injuries.

 FIRST ON SCENE

"This darn fifth wheel lock is sticking," Randy Mower shouted to his partner, Bobby Churchgood, as he crouched with his left arm under the trailer. "Rock the tractor a little."

Sitting in the driver's seat of the big rig watching his partner in the side mirror, Bobby slipped the transmission into reverse and eased off the clutch. The semi lurched backward, thundering into the empty trailer as Randy pulled on the handle to unlock it. Bobby then pulled the stick down into a low forward gear and eased the clutch again.

The truck bounced forward this time, and the fifth wheel lock snapped free. Bobby pulled the tractor forward about 10 feet, put it in neutral, and set the noisy parking brake. As he climbed down out of the cab he noticed Randy rolling around on the ground, holding his left hand close to his body. It took Bobby a second before he saw the blood. And there was a lot of it.

"What happened, Randy?" He jogged over to his friend, careful not to step in the bright blood.

Randy, his face contorted in pain, just kept cursing under his breath and rolling from side to side in the parking lot.

"Let's see your hand." Bobby bent over and touched the other man's arm. Randy held his left hand up for a moment, long enough for Bobby to see that all of the skin and most of the flesh was gone from the ring finger. From the tip to where it met the hand was now nothing more than a spindly red bone. Randy then buried his hand back close to his body and cursed through clenched teeth.

Heart, Blood, and Blood Vessels

The Heart

The heart is the center of the circulatory system. It pumps blood through the many miles and types of vessels to all the body's tissues, organs, and systems. If the heart stops functioning, as in cardiac arrest, blood does not circulate or carry fuel and oxygen to the body's parts, and they die.

The heart has four separate chambers (Figure 10.1). The top two are called *atria* (plural), or the right and left *atrium* (singular). The right atrium receives deoxygenated blood from the body; the left atrium receives oxygenated blood from the lungs. The bottom two chambers are called *ventricles* (plural), or the right or left *ventricle* (singular). The right ventricle receives the deoxygenated blood from the right atrium and pumps it to the lungs through the *pulmonary artery* (the only artery that carries deoxygenated blood and is named so because arteries carry blood away from the heart). The left ventricle receives oxygenated blood from the left atrium, which received it from the lungs through the *pulmonary veins* (the only veins that carry oxygenated blood but they are still called veins because they return blood to the heart).

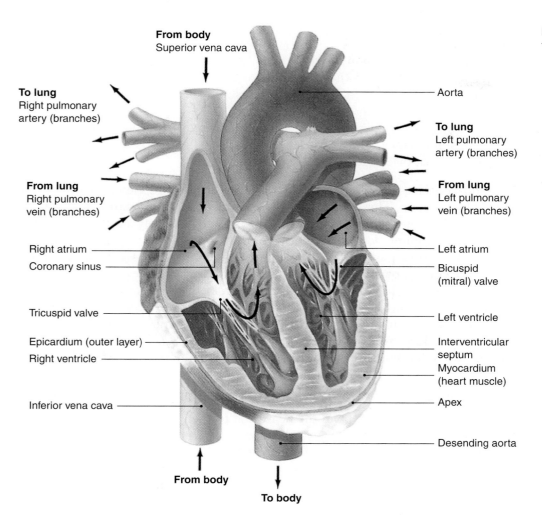

FIGURE 10.1 The heart.

From body
Superior vena cava

To lung
Right pulmonary
artery (branches)

Aorta

To lung
Left pulmonary
artery (branches)

From lung
Right pulmonary
vein (branches)

From lung
Left pulmonary
vein (branches)

Right atrium

Left atrium

Coronary sinus

Bicuspid
(mitral) valve

Tricuspid valve

Left ventricle

Epicardium (outer layer)

Interventricular
septum

Right ventricle

Myocardium
(heart muscle)

Inferior vena cava

Apex

Desending aorta

From body

To body

The ventricles are larger than the atria because they do the more difficult task of pumping blood to the lungs and body. The atria only have to pump blood to the ventricles below them. The left ventricle pumps blood to the body, leaving the heart by way of the aorta. The venous system carries blood from the body back to the heart, entering by way of the superior vena cava and inferior vena cava.

Blood

Blood performs many functions necessary to sustain life. Blood carries oxygen to the body's cells and carries away carbon dioxide (Figure 10.2). It transports nutrients to the cells and carries away certain waste products. The blood contains cells that destroy bacteria and produce substances that help resist infection. There are elements in the blood that act with calcium and chemical factors to combine blood cells, forming sticky clots around cuts to help control bleeding. Compounds carried in the blood called *hormones*, such as insulin, regulate many body activities. Without blood circulating through your body, you would quickly die.

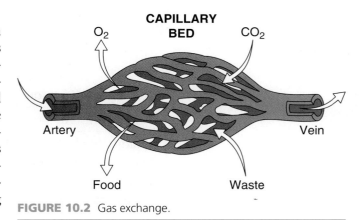

FIGURE 10.2 Gas exchange.

The functions of blood are to:

- Carry oxygen and carbon dioxide.
- Carry food to the tissues (nutrition).
- Carry wastes from the tissues to the organs of excretion—kidneys, lungs, and liver.
- Carry hormones, water, salts, and other compounds needed to keep the body's functions in balance (body regulation).
- Protect against disease-causing organisms (defense).

plasma (PLAZ-mah) ▪ the fluid portion of the blood.

REMEMBER

The typical adult has six liters (about 12 pints) of blood. This volume must be maintained for proper circulatory function.

Blood contains red blood cells, white blood cells, and elements involved in forming blood clots. These are carried by a watery, salty fluid called **plasma**. The volume of blood in the typical adult's body is approximately six liters (about 12 pints). When bleeding occurs, the body not only loses blood cells and clotting elements, it also loses plasma and total fluid volume. This loss can be significant because the volume of blood must be maintained at a certain level in order to have proper heart action, blood flow, and nutrient exchange between the blood and the body's cells. The body has more blood than is needed to produce minimum circulation. During bleeding, once this reserve is gone, the patient experiences circulatory system failure, followed very quickly by death. See Table 10–1 for blood volumes and lethal blood loss volumes for adults, children, and infants.

Blood Vessels

artery ▪ any blood vessel that carries blood away from the heart.

Arteries carry blood away from the heart and to the tissues, organs, and systems of the body. The largest artery is the *aorta*. The smallest artery is called an *arteriole*. All sizes between the aorta and the arteries are referred to as *arteries*. At certain points in the body, where arteries are close to the skin surface, you can feel the blood pumping through the artery. These points are called *pulse points*, places where you can feel the pumping heart at work and assess pulse rate.

vein ▪ any blood vessel that returns blood to the heart.

Veins carry blood from the tissues, organs, and systems of the body back to the heart. The largest veins are the superior and inferior *vena cava*. The smallest vein is called a *venule*. Sizes in between are just referred to as veins. On some parts of the arms (inside the wrist and elbow) and legs (lower leg and ankle), and sometimes the face (temple), you can see the blue of veins showing through skin where they are close to the surface.

capillaries ▪ the microscopic blood vessels that connect arteries to veins; where exchange takes place between the bloodstream and the body tissues.

The oxygen and nutrients carried by arteries are passed off to the body's cells when the blood reaches a small system of vessels called **capillaries**. Capillaries act as an exchange point for nutrients and wastes. Some of our organs act as disposal

TABLE 10–1	Blood Volumes and Serious Blood Loss	
PATIENT	**TOTAL BLOOD VOLUME**	**LETHAL BLOOD LOSS (RAPID)**
Adult male (154 pounds)	6.6 liters	2.2 liters
Adolescent (105 pounds)	3.3 liters	1.3 liters
Child (early to late childhood: depends on size)	1.5 to 2.0 liters	0.5 to 0.7 liters
Infant (newborn, normal weight range)	300+ milliliters	30 to 50 milliliters

and maintenance organs, such as the kidneys and liver, but the heart is the organ that works with the lungs to replenish oxygen. Once the blood has dropped off all its supply of oxygen for the body's cells to use, it travels from the capillary system into the veins and back to the heart, through the lungs to pick up oxygen, and back to the heart again to be pumped through vessels to the body. By the time blood reaches the capillaries, pressure and speed are greatly reduced and the beating action of the heart no longer causes pulsations. Blood moving through the capillaries in a constant flow is called **perfusion**. (A reduction in blood volume can seriously affect perfusion.)

perfusion ■ the adequate supply of well oxygenated blood to body tissues.

FIRST ➤ For now, you should know:

- Arteries carry blood away from the heart.
- Veins return blood to the heart.
- Capillaries are where oxygen, nutrient, and waste exchange takes place.
- Perfusion is the adequate flow of well oxygenated blood through the body. ■

Bleeding

Having an idea of how blood and blood vessels work within the body will assist you in assessing patients with bleeding problems. Keep the following general considerations in mind while you learn how to care for patients:

5–2.3 Establish the relationship between body substance isolation (BSI) and bleeding.

- *Body substance isolation (BSI) precautions.* The risk of infectious disease should always be assessed and minimized when caring for bleeding patients. BSI precautions must be taken routinely to avoid skin contact with mucous membranes and body fluids. Gloves should be worn during every patient encounter. Additional equipment (goggles, gown, mask) should also be used when there is an increased risk of contact with blood or other body fluids (for example, in cases of childbirth or when a patient is spitting or vomiting blood).
- *Severity of blood loss.* The severity of blood loss should be based on the patient's signs and symptoms and an estimation of blood loss. If signs and symptoms of shock are present, bleeding should be considered serious.
- *Body's normal response to bleeding.* The body's automatic response to bleeding is blood vessel constriction and clotting. In cases of major bleeding, however, clotting might not occur because the flow of blood washes the clot away before it can form. The factors affecting the body's response are discussed throughout this chapter.

5–2.6 Establish the relationship between body substance isolation (BSI) and soft-tissue injuries.

Uncontrolled bleeding should be taken seriously. If not stopped, it will lead to shock and death.

External Bleeding

Bleeding can be classified as external or internal. The assessment and care of both kinds of bleeding are presented in this chapter.

FIRST ➤ External bleeding may be classified as (Figure 10.3):

5–2.1 Differentiate between arterial, venous, and capillary bleeding.

- *Arterial bleeding.* Blood spurts from an artery with each beat of the heart. The color of the blood is bright red because it contains oxygen. Depending on the size of the artery, a great deal of blood can be lost in a short amount of time.

FIGURE 10.3 Three types of bleeding.

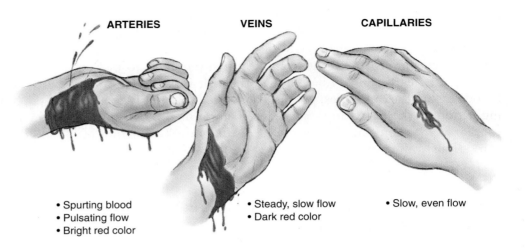

ARTERIES   VEINS   CAPILLARIES

- Spurting blood
- Pulsating flow
- Bright red color

- Steady, slow flow
- Dark red color

- Slow, even flow

- *Venous bleeding.* Blood flows steadily from a vein. The color of the blood is dark red, often appearing deep maroon (because it contains little oxygen). However, it may look or become a brighter red when exposed to the oxygen in the air. Depending on the size of the vein affected, venous bleeding can also be profuse.
- *Capillary bleeding.* Blood oozes from a bed of capillaries. The color of the blood is bright red, but usually less bright than arterial blood. The flow is slow, as seen in minor scrapes and shallow cuts to the skin. ▪

> **NOTE**
>
> Large veins may produce profuse bleeding, but there is no pulsation as is typically seen with arterial bleeding. Rate of flow and pulsation are more significant factors than color in determining if the bleeding is arterial or venous.

Evaluating External Bleeding

Of the three types of external bleeding, arterial bleeding is usually the most serious. The action of the heart and the pressure in the arteries can prevent blood clot formation because of the pressurized flow. Arterial bleeding can take 10 minutes or more to clot. Because arteries are located deep within body structures, capillary and venous bleeding is seen more often than arterial bleeding.

Venous bleeding can range from very minor to very severe, leading to death within minutes. Some veins are located near the surface of the body. Many are large enough to be seen through the skin. Other veins are deep in the body and can be as large as arteries. Bleeding from a deep vein will produce rapid blood loss. Surface bleeding from a vein can be profuse, but blood loss is not as rapid as that seen from arteries and deep veins because of their smaller diameters and lower pressure. Veins have a tendency to collapse as soon as they are cut. This often reduces the severity of venous bleeding.

Is It Safe ?

Do not be fooled by capillary bleeding. Even though it is rarely life threatening, patients can fall prey to severe infection if the wound is not cared for properly. Be sure to always use proper BSI precautions when caring for a patient with open wounds. ▪

Most individuals experience little difficulty with capillary bleeding. The blood oozes slowly, and clotting is very likely to occur within six to eight minutes. However, the larger the area of the wound, the more likely is the chance of infection. Capillary bleeding requires care to stop blood flow and reduce contamination.

In emergency care, arterial and large vein bleeding are given priority over small vein and capillary bleeding. If bleeding is severe and considered an immediate threat to life, bleeding control has to begin while you are observing for signs of breathing during the initial assessment. Even though it may prove awkward, an Emergency Medical Responder may be faced with the task of stopping severe bleeding while also evaluating airway and pulse.

Estimating external blood loss requires some experience (Figure 10.4). It is important in cases where slow bleeding has been occurring for a long time or in cases where both internal and external bleeding are present. To get a good idea of how to estimate blood volume loss, pour a pint of water on the floor next to a fellow student or a manikin. Also, try soaking an article of clothing with a pint of water and then note how much of the article is wet and how wet it feels.

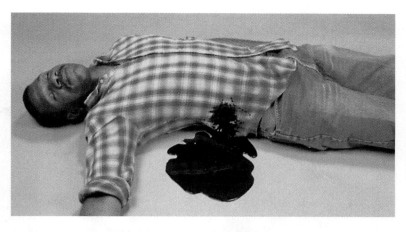

FIGURE 10.4 External blood loss of about one-half liter (approximately one pint).

REMEMBER

Always take appropriate BSI precautions prior to initiating emergency care for bleeding.

REMEMBER

Finding and stopping profuse bleeding is a component of the initial assessment.

5–2.2 State the emergency medical care for external bleeding.

Controlling External Bleeding

FIRST ➤ There are four steps to the procedure used by Emergency Medical Responders to control external bleeding (Figure 10.5 and Scan 10–1):

- Direct pressure, including use of pressure dressing.
- Elevation combined with direct pressure.

Control of External Bleeding

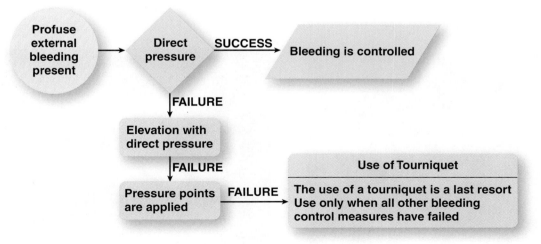

FIGURE 10.5 Algorithm for control of external bleeding.

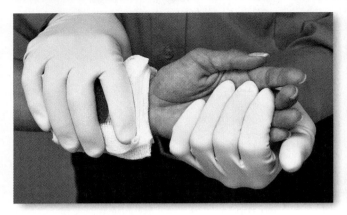

1 ■ Direct pressure

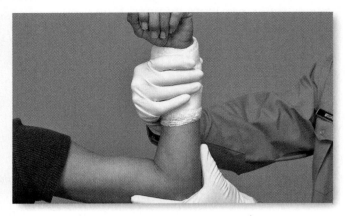

2 ■ Elevation

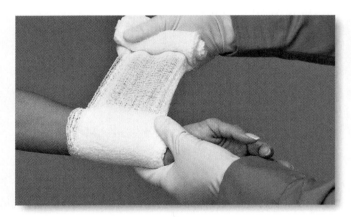

3 ■ Pressure dressing

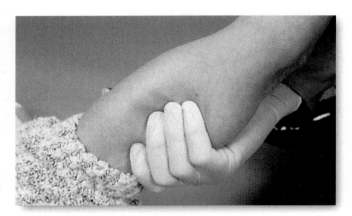

4 ■ Pressure point: arm (brachial artery)

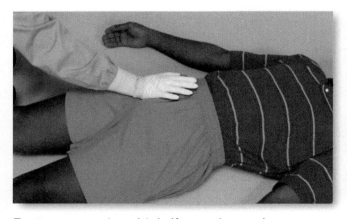

5 ■ Pressure point: thigh (femoral artery)

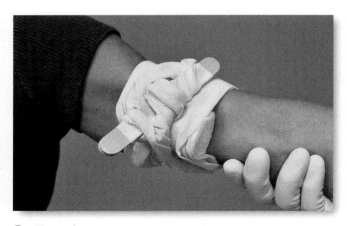

6 ■ Tourniquet

FIGURE 10.6 In cases of profuse bleeding, use your gloved hand. Do not waste time hunting for a dressing.

- Pressure points in the upper arm and groin.
- Tourniquet, which is used only as a last resort when other bleeding control steps fail. ▪

Direct Pressure Most cases of external bleeding can be controlled by applying **direct pressure** to the site of the wound. Ideally, a clean dressing should be used. However, hunting in your pocket for a clean dressing, going back to your car, going to a kit found in the next room, or other such activities may be a waste of precious time. If profuse bleeding is found during the initial assessment and you do not have dressings immediately available (Figure 10.6):

direct pressure ▪ the quickest, most effective way to control most forms of external bleeding. Pressure is applied directly over the wound site.

1. Place your gloved hand directly over the wound and apply pressure.
2. Keep applying steady, firm pressure.

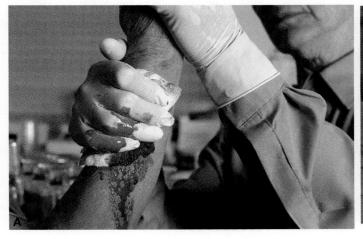
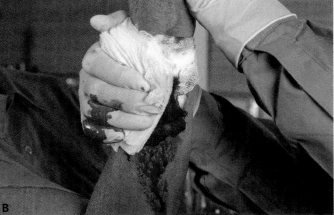

FIGURE 10.7 A. To control bleeding, place several (a small stack) 4 × 4s on the wound and apply direct pressure. **B.** If the wound bleeds through the dressings, apply several more 4 × 4s.

If dressings are immediately available, then (Figure 10.7):

1. Apply firm pressure using clean dressings or a clean cloth.
2. Apply pressure until bleeding is controlled. In some cases, this may take 10 minutes, 30 minutes, or longer. Resist the temptation to remove pressure repeatedly in order to determine if the bleeding has stopped. Assume it has stopped as long as you do not see bleeding through or around the dressing.
3. Secure the dressing in place with a bandage to create a pressure dressing.

Never remove or attempt to replace any dressing that is applied directly to the wound. To do so may interrupt clot formation and restart bleeding, or cause additional injury to the wound site. If an outer dressing becomes soaked with blood, replace it with another dressing. Make sure you do not disturb the dressing that is immediately against the wound.

Most bleeding can be controlled by a pressure dressing (Figure 10.8). To apply a pressure dressing:

roller bandage ▪ a long strip of soft, self-adherent gauze, a few inches wide and some yards long; used to secure dressings in place.

cravat ▪ a piece of cloth that can be used to secure a dressing or splint.

1. Place several clean gauze dressings directly on the wound. Maintain pressure with your gloved hand.
2. Use a **roller bandage** or **cravats** (cloth ties) to hold the entire dressing in place. It should be wrapped snugly over the dressing and above and below the wound.
3. Wrap the bandage to produce enough pressure to control the bleeding.
4. Check for a distal pulse to be certain that the pressure has not restricted blood flow.

A pressure dressing should not be removed once it is in place. If bleeding continues, add more pressure by using the palm of your gloved hand, applying more

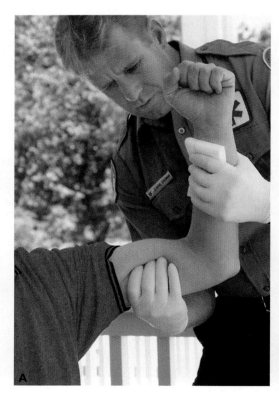
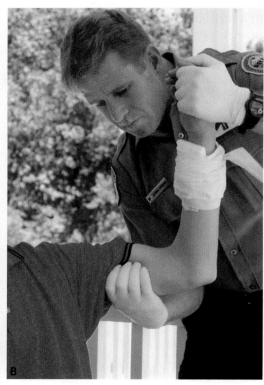

FIGURE 10.8 A. To use a pressure dressing, maintain direct pressure to the wound by applying a bulky pad. **B.** Secure the entire pressure dressing in place with a self-adherent roller bandage or cravat.

dressing pads, and continuing the process of bandaging. (Do not remove the bandage to add more pads.) You also may apply more bandages to increase the pressure. In very few cases (amputations and severe tearing injuries), you will have to create more bulk by using additional dressings.

If you use your gloved hand or a dressing to apply direct pressure, you can apply a pressure dressing once the bleeding is controlled. If you are dealing with bleeding from the chest, abdomen, or neck, attempting to apply a pressure dressing may not be of any real use. Your best approach to such situations is to maintain direct pressure on the wound using your gloved hand and a dressing.

Elevation

FIRST ➤ Elevation may be used in combination with direct pressure when dealing with bleeding from an arm or leg (Figure 10.9). The effects of gravity will help reduce blood pressure and slow the bleeding. This method should not be used, however, with suspected fractures to the extremities, objects impaled in the extremities, or possible spine injury.

To use elevation:

1. Lift the injured extremity. When practical, raise it so that the wound is above the level of the heart. If the forearm is bleeding, you do not have to elevate the entire arm. Simply elevate the forearm.

2. Continue to apply direct pressure to the site of bleeding as explained earlier in this chapter. ▪

Pressure Points

FIRST ➤ Pressure points are sites where an artery that is close to the skin surface lies directly over a bone. The flow of blood through such an artery can be slowed if pressure is applied to the artery. This procedure should be used only after direct pressure or direct pressure with elevation has failed to control the bleeding.

There are 22 pressure point sites that could potentially be used to control bleeding. They occur at 11 sites on each side of the body. Because the combination of direct pressure and elevation is so effective for most areas of the body, only the upper arm and groin pressure points are commonly used to control serious bleeding in the field. These sites are:

▪ **Brachial pressure point** in the upper arm to control bleeding from the arm.
▪ **Femoral pressure point** in the groin to control bleeding from the leg. ▪

Pressure point techniques are to be used only after direct pressure and elevation have failed to control bleeding.

FIRST ➤ For bleeding from the forearm Figure 10.10):

1. Make sure someone activates the EMS system.
2. Take appropriate BSI precautions.
3. Perform scene size-up.
4. Perform an initial assessment, ensuring the patient's ABCs.
5. Apply direct pressure.
6. Elevate the limb.

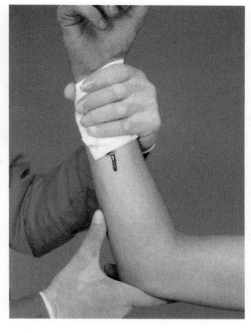

FIGURE 10.9 Combine elevation and direct pressure for bleeding from an arm or leg.

REMEMBER

Use pressure point techniques only after direct pressure and elevation have failed.

brachial (BRAY-ke-al) pressure point ▪ a location in the upper arm, where the brachial artery is close to the skin surface and lies over a bone. It can be used to help control serious external bleeding from the upper limb.

femoral (FEM-o-ral) pressure point ▪ a location at the anterior pelvis in the thigh, which can be used to help control serious external bleeding from the lower limb.

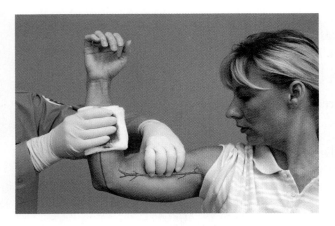

FIGURE 10.10 Apply pressure to the brachial pressure point to control bleeding from the forearm.

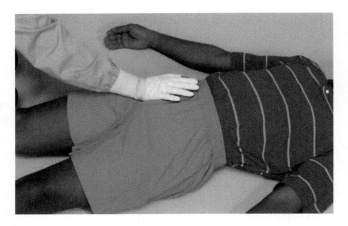

FIGURE 10.11 Apply pressure to the femoral pressure point to control bleeding from the leg.

7. If necessary, use a pressure point. Extend the patient's arm, placing it at a right angle, lateral to the body. This angle will provide the best results, but may be reduced if a 90-degree extension is not possible. Place the palm of the patient's hand in the anatomical position.

8. Press your fingers in the groove found below the biceps muscle.

9. Apply pressure to the brachial artery by pressing your fingers into this groove. Bleeding should slow, and you may no longer be able to feel a radial (wrist) pulse.

10. Provide care for shock. Calm and reassure the patient, maintain normal body temperature, and administer oxygen as soon as possible as per local protocols. ■

FIRST ➤ For bleeding from the leg (Figure 10.11):

1. Make sure someone activates the EMS system.

2. Take appropriate BSI precautions.

3. Perform a scene size-up.

4. Perform an initial assessment, ensuring the patient's ABCs.

5. Apply direct pressure.

6. Elevate the limb.

7. If necessary, use a pressure point. Locate the anterior medial side of the leg where the thigh joins the lower trunk. The femoral artery has a pulse that can be felt at this location.

8. Use the heel of your gloved hand to apply pressure to this site. Keep your arm straight, using your body weight to help apply the pressure. The number of leg muscles, their size, and the fat content of the thigh require that you exert much more pressure than you would use to compress the brachial artery in the arm.

9. Apply the necessary pressure to control bleeding.

10. Reassure the patient and keep him calm.

11. Provide care for shock. ■

Keep in mind that the brachial (upper arm) and femoral (thigh) pressure points are not to be used if there are possible fractures to the bone under the pressure point site. To do so could produce severe pain and cause serious damage to the bone, soft tissues, nerves, and blood vessels in the area. You could cause more bleeding, rather than reduce the bleeding. If there are no indications of spine injury or possible fractures of the extremity (remember to consider the mechanism of injury), elevation and pressure point techniques can be combined to control bleeding. Any patient who has suffered moderate to severe blood loss will benefit from receiving oxygen. If you are an Emergency Medical Responder who carries oxygen, administer it as needed. (See Appendix 2.) Follow local protocols.

Tourniquet

FIRST ➤ A **tourniquet,** is a last resort, used only when the other methods of controlling life-threatening bleeding have failed. In most cases when you think you should use a tourniquet, a pressure dressing would be the better choice. ▪

A partial amputation of the arm or leg may leave you with no other choice than to use a tourniquet. However, many total amputations do not have uncontrollable, profuse bleeding because the ends of the blood vessels tend to collapse. In cases in which there is profuse bleeding from an arm or leg wound, a tourniquet should be applied to stop life-threatening bleeding after direct pressure, elevation, and pressure point techniques have failed. If there is no other way to stop bleeding and save the patient's life, then this is an acceptable action.

FIRST ➤ If all other methods have failed and you must apply a tourniquet, carefully follow these steps (Figure 10.12):

1. Locate the site for the tourniquet. This should be between the wound and the patient's heart, as close to the wound as possible without being on its edge. The most effective and safest location is about two inches from the wound.

2. Place a tourniquet pad on the site you have selected, over the artery. This pad can be a roll of dressing, a folded handkerchief, or a piece of cloth folded to about the same thickness as a folded handkerchief.

3. If you are using a manufactured tourniquet, carefully place it around the limb just above the wound. Pull the free end of the band through the friction catch or buckle and draw it tightly over the pad. Tighten the tourniquet to the point where bleeding is stopped. Do not tighten it beyond this point.

   If you do not have a commercially manufactured tourniquet or you would have to leave the patient to retrieve one, use a flat belt, necktie, stocking, or long dressing material. Flat materials are best. The band should be at least one-inch wide. Do not use any material that could cut into the patient's limb. Carefully slip the tourniquet around the patient's limb and tie a half-knot with the ends of the tourniquet. The knot should be over the pad. A device such as a long stick, wooden dowel, or metal rod should then be placed over the half knot. (Pens and pencils tend to break.) Next, tie a full knot over the stick or rod. Then turn the device until bleeding has been stopped. Do not tighten the tourniquet beyond this point.

4. Once the tourniquet is in place, do not loosen it. Tie it or tape it in place.

5. Attach a tag to the patient. Write on it that a tourniquet has been applied and the time at which it was applied (for example: T/K—5:11 p.m.). If you do not

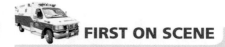

FIRST ON SCENE

Bobby ran across the busy parking lot and crashed through the doors of the truck stop. He was breathing too heavily to say anything, and, as the store's tinny overhead speakers played an upbeat tune, all eyes turned silently toward him. He caught his breath and shouted, "Somebody call an ambulance! A guy just tore his finger off out back."

He then turned, headed back out the door, and stumbled across the parking lot. A woman who had been standing in line at the register set a soft drink down on a candy display and ran out the door after him. They both reached the semi at the same time.

The woman knelt down and put her hand on Randy's shoulder. "Sir," she said. "My name is Stephanie, and I'm an Emergency Medical Responder. I'm trained to care for injuries. May I help you?"

"Oh God." Randy was still squeezing his left hand, trying to make the overwhelming pain go away. "Only if you can knock me out!"

tourniquet ▪ a wide, flat band or belt used to constrict blood vessels to help stop the flow of blood.

REMEMBER

Use a tourniquet only as a last resort.

WARNING

Never practice tightening a tourniquet on anyone.

REMEMBER

As an Emergency Medical Responder, you have the responsibility to advise the EMTs or other more highly trained personnel about the application of a tourniquet and the time it was applied.

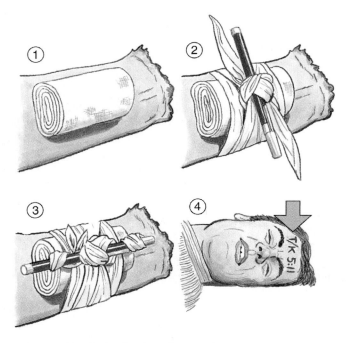

FIGURE 10.12 Application of a tourniquet.

have a tag, write the information in ink on the patient's forehead. If you do not have a pen, write in lipstick, crayon, or whatever is available at the scene. This information must be written so that the tourniquet does not go unnoticed and so that the hospital staff will know how long it has been in place.

6. Provide care for shock, but do not cover the tourniquet. This is an additional safeguard to prevent it from being missed by others who provide care for the patient. ■

NOTE

Over the past several years, the use of a tourniquet fell out of favor for many EMS systems. Recent research by the military suggests that a tourniquet can be an effective tool for controlling severe bleeding and ultimately saving lives. If used properly, a tourniquet can be an excellent tool for the EMS provider.

Splinting   Splinting is not usually considered an Emergency Medical Responder-level method of controlling bleeding. However, some Emergency Medical Responders are trained to use air-inflatable splints. For long wounds on an arm or leg, the application of an air splint can help control bleeding. This is actually a form of direct pressure. Using an air splint requires special training in its application and knowledge of its limitations (see Chapter 11). The air splint can be used even when there is no suspected fracture to the bones of the limb.

Combining the use of an air splint and elevation can work well on long, bleeding wounds. The splint also serves to immobilize the limb, helping reduce the chance of restarting bleeding due to patient movement. Because obtaining and applying air splints consumes time, this procedure is best done in cases of minor bleeding. The skilled rescuer can use air splints to control more serious bleeding if the splint is immediately at hand.

REMEMBER

Always have someone activate EMS for all but the mildest cases of external bleeding.

Special Cases of External Bleeding   There are situations in which a deep cut opens a major artery or vein and then the cut partially closes. Such cuts do not always appear to be major, and the bleeding from these cuts is often mild. Be alert for blood flow from wounds to change quickly from mild to profuse. If there is a wound to the arm or leg and you cannot detect a distal pulse, be prepared for profuse bleeding.

In addition, do not let cuts to the chest and abdomen fool you. Some may appear minor, but they could be very deep and have produced internal injuries that are causing a great deal of internal bleeding. When you find an external wound, you must consider the possibility of internal injuries. Do not open the wound to determine its depth.

Have someone activate EMS for all patients with external bleeding except for the mildest cases (small areas of capillary bleeding) in which there are no other signs of injury.

Bleeding from the eye, ear, nose, mouth, and around impaled objects requires special consideration. Each area is discussed later in this chapter.

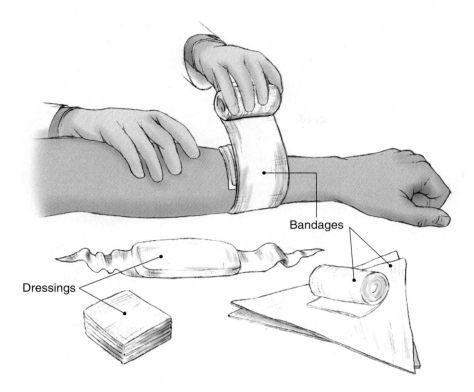

FIGURE 10.13 Dressings cover wounds. Bandages hold dressings in place.

Bandages

Dressings

Dressing and Bandaging

Bandaging is not a difficult skill to learn. In Emergency Medical Responder care, most bandages are simple and easy to apply. If you follow the basic principles of dressing and bandaging wounds, you will provide effective care for the patient.

5–2.14 List the functions of dressing and bandaging.

FIRST ➤ To begin, read the following definitions (Figure 10.13):

- **Dressing.** A dressing is any material (preferably sterile) placed over a wound that will help control bleeding and help prevent additional contamination.
- **Bandage.** A bandage is any material used to hold a dressing in place. ■

dressing ■ any material used to cover a wound; helps control bleeding and reduce contamination.

bandage ■ any material that is used to hold a dressing in place.

Dressings, whenever possible, should be sterile. This means that they have been processed so that all germs and the spores that can grow into active germs are killed. They are nonfibrous so that material particles do not stick to wounds. Commercially prepared dressings are usually sterile. They come in a variety of sizes, with the most common size being four inches square. They are referred to according to size, such as 2 × 2s, 4 × 4s, 5 × 9s, and 10 × 30s.

Throughout this text, you will find reference to **bulky dressings,** or multitrauma dressings. These are thick dressings, often large enough to allow for the complete covering of large wounds. They are used to help control very serious bleeding and to stabilize impaled objects. Sanitary pads can be used in place of these dressings. They are available individually wrapped. Although sanitary pads are not sterile, they are very clean. (Avoid applying any adhesive surface directly to the wound.) Bulky dressings can be formed by applying many layers of simple gauze dressings.

bulky dressing ■ a thick dressing or a buildup of thin dressings used to help control profuse bleeding, stabilize impaled objects, or cover large open wounds.

Another type of special dressing is the **occlusive dressing,** which is used to create an airtight seal to a wound or body cavity. It is used to close an open wound that penetrates a body cavity. Commercially prepared occlusive dressings are available. If these are not on hand, you can use folded plastic wrap or a plastic bag to help seal off an open wound to the chest or abdomen.

occlusive dressing ■ a dressing used to create an airtight seal or to close an open wound of a body cavity.

FIGURE 10.14 Materials used for impro-vised dressings and bandages.

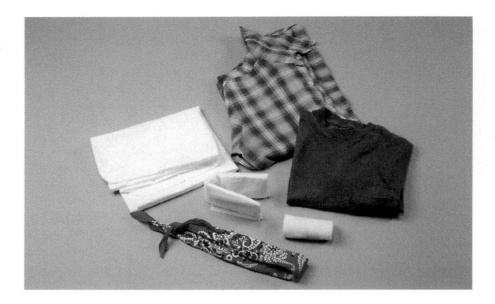

Often, an Emergency Medical Responder will not have any dressing materials at the scene of an emergency. In such cases, you might have to use clean handker-chiefs, towels, sheets, a piece of clothing, or other similar materials (Figure 10.14). When you improvise a dressing, it will not be sterile, but it can be used to help provide proper care for the patient. Because the patient's wound has already been contaminated, your task is to avoid further contamination by using the cleanest material available. The hospital has special wound-cleansing procedures and antibiotics to care for wound contamination and infection. In the field, you must be concerned with controlling bleeding and minimizing contamination.

Dressings are more effective if they are held in place. The adhesive bandage has a sticky backing that will adhere to the patient's skin. If no such bandaging material is on hand, tie a dressing in place by using a gauze roller bandage, a cravat, a hand-kerchief, strips of cloth, or any other material that will not cut into the patient's skin. Do not use elastic bandages. They are often used for injuries to the joints, but they can restrict circulation and apply undesired pressure to injured tissues.

The use of the self-adherent, form-fitting gauze roller bandage eliminates the need for highly specialized bandaging techniques (Figure 10.15). It does not have

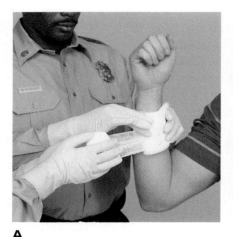
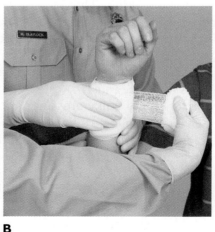
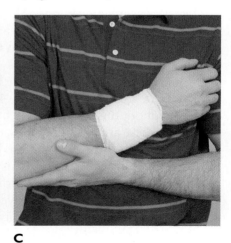

A   **B**   **C**

FIGURE 10.15 A. While maintaining direct pressure to the wound, hold the end of the roller bandage securely in place. **B.** Then begin to circle the limb, applying the bandage firmly. When complete, the bandage should be snug, but not too tight. **C.** Be sure to secure any loose ends.

an adhesive backing, yet clings to itself, making the task of wrapping around a dressing easier, quicker, and more efficient.

Rules for Dressing and Bandaging

FIRST ➤ The following rules apply to dressing wounds:

- A dressing and bandage are of little value if they do not help control bleeding. Continue to apply dressing material and pressure as needed to control bleeding.
- Use sterile or clean materials. Avoid touching dressings in the area that will come into contact with the wound.
- Cover the entire surface of the wound and, if possible, the immediate area surrounding the wound.
- Once a dressing is applied to a wound, it must remain in place. Add new dressings on top of blood-soaked dressings. When a dressing is removed from a wound, bleeding could restart or increase in rate. Removal should be done only in the emergency department. There is an exception to this rule in some EMS systems. (Do only what you have been trained to do.) If a bulky dressing becomes blood soaked, you may have to remove it so that direct pressure can be re-established or a new bulky pad or dressing can be applied. It is best to apply simple gauze pads to wound sites before applying a bulky dressing. This will allow removal of the bulky dressing, if necessary, without directly disturbing the wound. ■

Geriatric Focus

Often, the elderly are taking medications that contain "blood thinners" such as Coumadin. This prevents their blood from clotting. As a result, minor cuts may bleed profusely. Be prepared to aggressively treat any bleeding in the elderly with compression dressings and pressure points.

FIRST ➤ The following rules apply to bandaging (Figure 10.16):

- Do not bandage too tightly. Hold the dressing snugly in place, but do not restrict blood supply to the affected area.
- Do not bandage too loosely. The dressing must not be allowed to slip from the wound or move while on the wound.

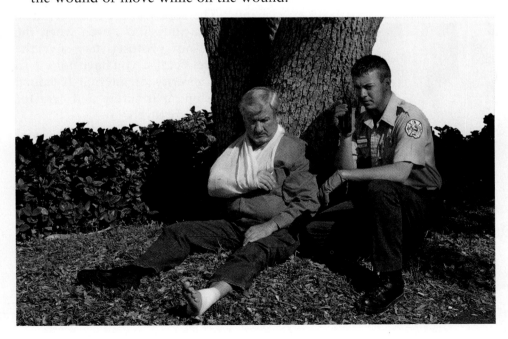

FIGURE 10.16 The rules of bandaging:

- Do not bandage too tightly or loosely.
- Tuck in loose ends.
- Do not cover fingers and toes.
- Bandage from the bottom to the top of a limb.
- Use sterile or clean materials.
- Cover the entire wound.
- Do not remove dressings.

- Do not leave loose ends. Loose ends of tape, dressing, or cloth might get caught on objects when the patient is being moved.
- Do not cover fingers and toes unless they are injured. These areas must be exposed so that you can watch for color changes that indicate a change in circulation. Blue skin; pale skin; and complaints of numbness, pain, and tingling sensations all indicate that the bandage may be too tight.
- Wrap the bandage around the limb starting at its far (distal) end and working toward its origin or near (proximal) end. Taking such action will help reduce the chances of restricting circulation.

Three additional rules for bandaging must be considered when the wound is on a limb:

- Applying the bandage to a narrow area can produce enough pressure to restrict circulation. Instead, wrap a large area of the limb, making certain to maintain uniform pressure as you wrap the bandage.
- Do not bend a joint if it is bandaged. Once the bandage is in place, movement of the joint may restrict circulation or cause the bandage and dressing to loosen.
- Always check distal circulation, sensation, and motor function before and after bandaging. ▪

See Scan 10–2 for examples of general dressing and bandaging techniques.

Internal Bleeding

Internal bleeding can range from a minor bruise to a major life-threatening problem. Most small, simple bruises are examples of minor internal bleeding. Such minor blood loss is not of great significance. Of primary concern to Emergency Medical Responders is internal bleeding that brings about shock, heart and lung failure, and eventual death. Some cases of internal bleeding are so severe that the patient dies in a matter of seconds. Other severe cases of internal bleeding take minutes to hours before death. Emergency Medical Responder-level care might keep these patients alive until the EMTs arrive.

Even when internal bleeding is not profuse, it does not take long for serious reactions to occur in the body. The most important, shock, is covered later in this chapter. The care you provide for internal bleeding and shock, even when the bleeding is not profuse, may save the patient's life. Because you have no way to know the severity of internal bleeding, always assume it is severe and care for the patient aggressively.

Detecting Internal Bleeding

Internal bleeding can occur in many ways (Figure 10.17). It can be caused by wounds that are deep enough to sever major blood vessels or the vessels in organs, such as a deep wound to the chest or abdomen. Open wounds that have cut through major vessels to produce profuse internal bleeding may show only minor external bleeding. Many cases of internal bleeding occur even when there are no cuts in the skin. Internal organs and blood vessels may have

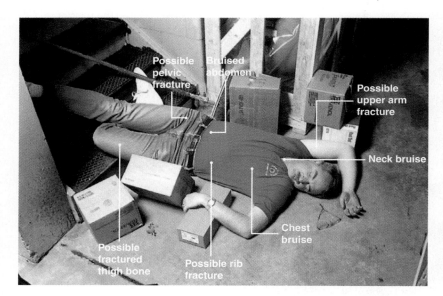

FIGURE 10.17 Certain types of injuries may indicate serious internal bleeding.

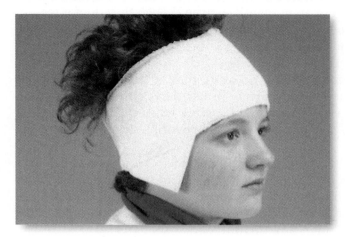

Forehead (no skull injury) or ear. Place dressing and secure with roller bandage.

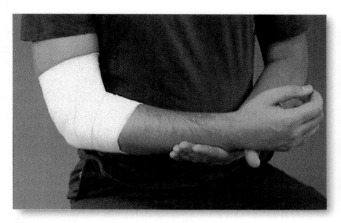

Elbow or knee. Place dressing and secure with cravat or roller bandage. Apply roller bandage in figure-eight pattern.

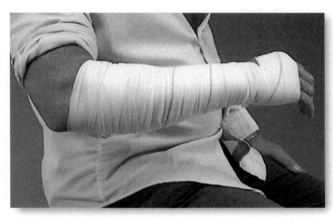

Forearm or leg. Place dressing and secure with roller bandage, distal to proximal. Better protection is provided if palm or sole is wrapped.

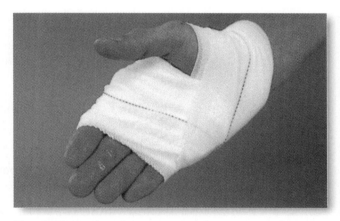

Hand. Place dressing, wrap with cravat, and secure at wrist. Use the same pattern for roller bandage.

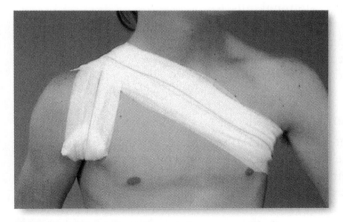

Shoulder. Place dressing and secure with figure-eight bandage made with a cravat or roller bandage. Pad under knot if cravat is used.

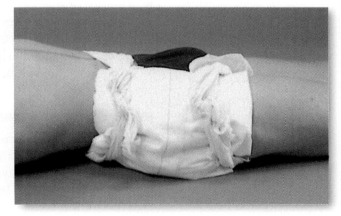

Hip. Place a large dressing to cover hip. Secure with first cravat around waist and second cravat around thigh on injured side.

been ruptured or crushed by a severe blow to the body that did not produce any external wounds. This is an example of **blunt trauma**, an injury caused by an object that was not sharp enough to penetrate the skin. The blunt instrument can be fairly large, such as the steering wheel of an automobile. Even though they do not tend to cause penetrating wounds, blunt instruments can deliver a great deal of force to the body, causing life-threatening internal bleeding.

blunt trauma ■ an injury caused by an object that was not sharp enough to penetrate the skin.

Pay special attention to bruises on the neck, chest, and abdomen. Severe injury with internal bleeding may show no more than a bruise at first, to be followed by the rapid decline of the patient. Bruise detection can be particularly important in assessing possible internal bleeding when the patient is unresponsive and thus unable to complain of pain that would clearly indicate the problem.

To complicate your assessment of the patient, in some cases a blow to one side of the body can cause internal bleeding on the opposite side of the body cavity. In automobile collisions, blunt trauma to the lower right side of the rib cage can cause the spleen, which is on the left side of the body, to rupture and bleed freely, releasing about one liter (two pints) or more of blood.

NOTE

Internal bleeding may be difficult to detect because it can occur in cases where external bleeding is absent or minor and away from the site of noticeable injury, or where there is no obvious external injury. Considering the mechanism of injury (falls, steering wheel injuries, and the like) and conducting a proper patient assessment are of major importance in detecting internal bleeding.

5–2.4 List the signs of internal bleeding.

FIRST ➤ Conclude that there is internal bleeding whenever you detect any of the signs listed below. Notice how the signs follow the order of the head-to-toe physical exam:

- Wounds that have penetrated the skull.
- Blood or clear fluids draining from the ears and/or nose.
- Patient vomits or coughs up blood (coffee-grounds or frothy red appearance).
- Bruises on the neck.
- Bruises on the chest, possible fractured ribs (possible cuts to the lungs and liver), and wounds that have penetrated the chest.
- Bruises or penetrating wounds to the abdomen.
- Rigidity or distention of the abdominal muscles.
- Abdominal tenderness.
- Bleeding from the rectum or vagina.
- Possible fractures (with special emphasis on the pelvis, the long bones of the upper arm and thigh, and the ribs). ■

Geriatric Focus

The signs and symptoms of internal bleeding in the elderly are often different from those in a younger patient. The survival reflexes that the younger body uses, such as increased heart rate, may be blunted due to cardiac disease or the medication the elderly patient is taking. The elderly patient's level of consciousness is the most reliable sign to monitor for shock.

Always suspect that there is internal bleeding if the patient has been injured and the signs and symptoms of shock are present (Figure 10.18). The symptoms of

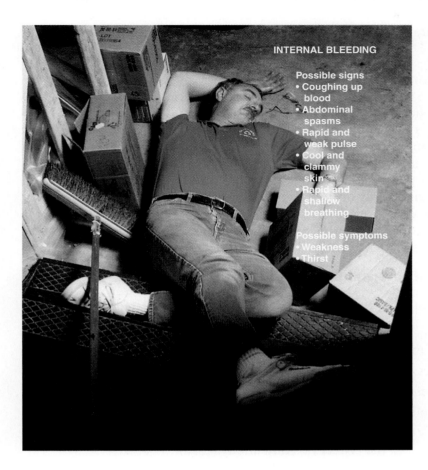

INTERNAL BLEEDING

Possible signs
• Coughing up blood
• Abdominal spasms
• Rapid and weak pulse
• Cool and clammy skin
• Rapid and shallow breathing

Possible symptoms
• Weakness
• Thirst

shock associated with internal bleeding are weakness or dizziness, thirst, feeling cold, anxiety, or restlessness. (More about this later in the chapter.) However, during the early stages of internal bleeding, there may not yet be signs or symptoms. Do not wait for sign and symptoms to develop. Treat the patient based on mechanism of injury and/or history.

FIRST ➤ The signs of shock associated with internal bleeding include:

- Decreasing level of responsiveness.
- Restlessness or combativeness.
- Shaking and trembling.
- Shallow and rapid breathing.
- Rapid and weak pulse.
- Pale, cool, and moist (clammy) skin.
- Dilated (enlarged) pupils, which may respond sluggishly. ▪

Stop now and notice how these signs fit into your assessment of the patient during the physical exam. Remember, none of these signs or symptoms may be present in the early stages of internal bleeding. If the mechanism of injury is severe enough to make you think that there may be internal bleeding, assume that there is such bleeding and provide the necessary care.

FIRST ➤ You can detect internal bleeding by looking for mechanisms of injury that could cause internal bleeding, wounds, and the signs and symptoms of shock. ▪

REMEMBER

Shock can be fatal if action is not taken.

Medical emergencies that can produce internal bleeding are discussed in Chapter 9.

Evaluating Internal Bleeding

It is very difficult to determine the amount of blood lost in cases of internal bleeding. Special hospital procedures and tests are required. However, estimates can be made. Consider blood loss to be severe if there is penetration of the chest cavity over or immediately above the heart, if the spleen or liver may have been injured, or if you suspect the pelvis is fractured. Estimate blood loss of at least one liter (two pints) if there is a suspected major fracture in the upper arm or thigh bone. Where you find badly bruised skin, assume that there is a 10% loss of total blood volume for each bruise the size of the patient's fist. For an adult, this is about a one-pint loss. Such estimates will help you evaluate the chance of the patient going into shock, lung or heart failure, or cardiac arrest.

Management of Internal Bleeding

5–2.5 List the steps in the emergency medical care of the patient with signs and symptoms of internal bleeding.

FIRST ➤ In general, the steps in the care of patients with suspected internal bleeding include:

1. Make certain that someone activates the EMS system.
2. Take appropriate BSI precautions.
3. Perform a scene size-up.
4. Perform an initial assessment. (Maintain the airway and monitor breathing and pulse.)
5. Keep the patient in the proper position and lying still.
6. Loosen restrictive clothing and provide care for shock.
7. Be alert in case the patient starts to vomit.
8. Do not give the patient anything by mouth.
9. Reassure the patient and keep him calm.
10. Report the possibility of internal bleeding as soon as more highly trained EMS personnel arrive at the scene. ■

If you are an Emergency Medical Responder who is allowed to administer oxygen, remember that any patient with possible internal bleeding will benefit from receiving it. Provide oxygen as per local protocols.

Internal bleeding in the abdominal cavity or the chest cavity is a life-threatening situation requiring quick, safe transport to a hospital. Most areas in the United States do not consider transport to be an Emergency Medical Responder's duty. Most EMS medical directors believe it is better if Emergency Medical Responders keep patients at the scene. You must recognize that a patient unattended in the back seat of your car could go into cardiac arrest and die while you are trying to rush to the hospital. Improper movement could also aggravate spine injuries.

Internal bleeding is very serious, often leading to death, even in cases in which the bleeding begins once the patient is at the hospital. You may provide excellent Emergency Medical Responder care for a patient with internal bleeding, only to have him die later. To be a good Emergency Medical Responder, accept the fact that there are limits to emergency care at all levels. Some patients will die no matter what you do. The patient has a better chance to survive, however, if you do as you have been trained to do.

Shock

Development of Shock

When providing patients with emergency care, consider the concept of the "golden hour." This is the first hour after serious injury. Providers must make every effort to provide care and assist in delivering seriously injured patients to the hospital as quickly as possible. The first 60 minutes are critical. If shock can be prevented or if its severity can be reduced during this period, the patient's chances for survival are greatly improved.

FIRST ➤ Any injury or illness must be considered more severe once the patient enters a state of shock. Keeping patients from going into shock and helping stabilize patients who are in shock are two of the most important responsibilities of Emergency Medical Responders. If nothing is done for the patient who is in shock, death will almost always result. ■

Whenever the body is hurt, either by injury or illness, it reacts by trying to correct the effects of the damage. If the damage is severe, one consequence is shock, which often indicates a problem with the circulatory system. The problem can be related to the:

- *Heart.* The heart should be pumping blood and doing so efficiently. If the heart fails to pump an adequate volume of oxygenated blood, shock will develop.
- *Vessels.* Blood circulates throughout the body through a closed system. If there is any opening in this system, such as a cut or rupture, with enough blood loss, shock will develop.
- *Blood volume.* An adequate amount of blood must be present to fill the vessels. If there is loss of blood volume or if the vessels dilate (enlarge) to a size that no longer allows the system to properly fill, shock will develop.

Basically, **shock** is the failure of the body's circulatory system to provide enough oxygenated blood and nutrients (perfusion) to all vital organs. There must be enough blood being pumped efficiently to allow for a steady flow through the capillaries so that exchange can occur (perfusion). Oxygen and carbon dioxide are exchanged, nutrients and waste are exchanged, and fluid and salt balance must be maintained between the blood and the tissues. When this cannot take place, **hypoperfusion** (lack of adequate perfusion), develops and the patient goes into shock.

> **shock** ■ the reaction of the body to the failure of the circulatory system to provide enough blood to the vital organs. Also referred to as *hypoperfusion.*

> **hypoperfusion** ■ the lack of adequate perfusion.

Shock develops or occurs in a step-by-step progression. The development of shock can be rapid or it can come about slowly. Most new rescuers expect shock to develop rapidly; however, this is not always the case. Some patients can go into shock "a little at a time." Experienced rescuers know that you will often have enough warning to slow down the process. They also know that if you do not continue to monitor patients, you can miss some of the subtle, early signs and symptoms. Shock is a dynamic process that can be life threatening.

Care for patients with shock should not be delayed. The problem worsens with time, and early intervention is crucial. Think of shock as a reaction to blood loss. This reaction causes more problems that, in turn, cause more problems. For example, if there is bleeding, the heart rate increases, attempting to circulate blood to all vital parts of the body. By doing this, more blood is lost. The body's immediate response to this problem is to try to circulate more blood by increasing the heart rate even further. This process will continue until death occurs. This cycle of decline must be stopped (Figure 10.19). The initial problem, such as bleeding, must be corrected, and shock must be managed. Emergency Medical Responder-level care should begin to correct problems and stop the decline.

Types of Shock

REMEMBER

The signs and symptoms of shock are not always due to blood loss.

Shock can be classified into several categories, because there is more than one cause of shock. It is not necessary to memorize the following list. It is provided so that you can see the many ways shock develops. A patient in shock may have one or more of the following:

- *Hypovolemic (HI-po-vo-LE-mic) shock* is caused by blood loss or by the loss of plasma (a component of blood) as in cases of burns. (The term *hypovolemic* means low volume.) This term includes all shock caused by fluid loss, such as bleeding, burns, vomiting and diarrhea, and severe dehydration. Shock caused by vomiting and diarrhea is also called *metabolic (MET-ah-BOL-ic) shock*.
- *Hemorrhagic shock* is caused when the body loses a significant amount of blood from the circulatory system. It can be caused by either uncontrolled internal or external bleeding.

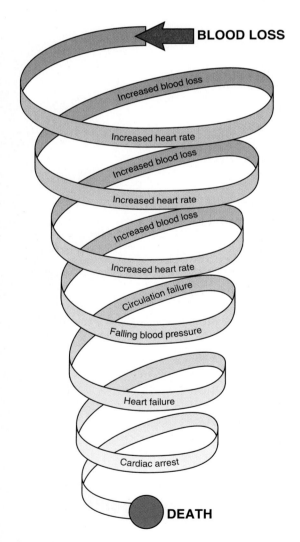

- *Cardiogenic (KAR-di-o-JEN-ic) shock* is heart shock, caused by the heart failing to pump enough blood to all parts of the body. It may be due to the damage of the heart itself as in the case of a heart attack.
- *Neurogenic (NU-ro-JEN-ic) shock* is nerve shock, caused when something goes wrong with the nervous system (such as from an injury to the spinal cord) and there is a failure to control the tone of blood vessels. The vessels become dilated. There is not enough blood in the body to fill this increased space, causing inadequate circulation.
- *Anaphylactic (AN-ah-fi-LAK-tik) shock* is allergy shock, a life-threatening reaction of the body caused by something to which the patient is extremely allergic. This is such a serious problem that it is covered as a special topic in Chapter 9.
- *Psychogenic (SI-ko-JEN-ic) shock* is fainting. It usually occurs when some factor, such as fear, causes the nervous system to react and rapidly dilate the blood vessels. The proper flow of blood to the brain is interrupted. In most cases, fainting is a self-correcting form of shock, with the interruption of proper blood flow being a temporary condition. Fainting is not the same as neurogenic shock.
- *Septic shock* is caused by infection. Poisons are released that cause the blood vessels to dilate. As in other cases of shock, the blood volume is too low to fill the circulatory system. This type of shock is seldom seen by Emergency Medical Responders.

As an Emergency Medical Responder, you do not have to classify shock, with the exception of anaphylactic, or allergy, shock. For all other cases, report that the patient has the signs and symptoms of shock and any factors you notice usually associated with shock, such as bleeding and loss of body fluids.

BLOOD LOSS

Increased blood loss

Increased heart rate

Increased blood loss

Increased heart rate

Increased blood loss

Increased heart rate

Circulation failure

Falling blood pressure

Heart failure

Cardiac arrest

DEATH

FIGURE 10.19 If left untreated, blood loss will lead to death.

Signs and Symptoms of Shock

FIRST ➤ The symptoms of shock are weakness, nausea, thirst, dizziness, anxiety, agitation, and fear (Figure 10.20). The signs of shock are:

- Entire body assessment:
  — Restlessness or combativeness.
  — Profuse external bleeding.
  — Vomiting.
  — Shaking and trembling.
- Altered mental status. The patient may become disoriented, confused, unresponsive (often suddenly), or faint.
- Breathing, shallow and rapid.
- Pulse, rapid and weak.
- Skin, pale, cool, and moist often with blue color (cyanosis) seen at the lips, tongue, and earlobes (may be profuse sweating).
- Eyes, lackluster. Pupils are sluggish and may be dilated. ▪

These signs and symptoms follow the order in which they may be detected during the initial assessment of the patient. However, all signs and symptoms of shock may not be present at once, and they do not necessarily occur in the order listed here. Shock is progressive (becoming worse with time). Look for the following patterns (Scan 10–3):

- *Increased pulse rate.* The body is trying to adjust to the loss of blood and poor perfusion. Unlike the rapid pulse rate associated with the stress of an injury or the fear of needing help during an emergency, this increased rate will not slow down.

FIRST ON SCENE

Stephanie looked at Randy's bloody hand and noticed that it wasn't actively bleeding. She turned to Bobby, who was still trying to catch his breath from the run to and from the convenience store, and asked if there was a first aid kit in the truck. Bobby thought for a moment and brightened, "Oh yeah! We have one next to the emergency triangles in the side box!"

He then turned and hurried to the truck. As he was digging the first aid kit from among the spare bulbs, rags, and jumper cables, he saw the skin of Randy's finger hanging limply from the fifth wheel lock handle. It was dangling from something that flickered like gold, so he stepped closer. It was Randy's wedding ring. It had gotten caught on the lock handle, and when it had finally popped open, the action of the lock handle must have pulled the finger right off the bone.

Bobby turned, feeling queasy, and hurried back over with the dirty first aid kit. Randy was extremely pale now, and Bobby could see that he had thrown up on the pavement.

"Quick," Stephanie said, grabbing the kit from Bobby's shaking hands. "I need you to cover him with your jacket and then go lift both of his feet about a foot or so off of the ground and hold them there."

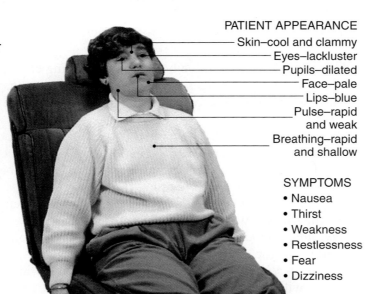

SIGNS
- Restlessness or combativeness
- Becomes unresponsive
- Profuse bleeding
- Vomiting
- Shaking and trembling

PATIENT APPEARANCE
- Skin—cool and clammy
- Eyes—lackluster
- Pupils—dilated
- Face—pale
- Lips—blue
- Pulse—rapid and weak
- Breathing—rapid and shallow

SYMPTOMS
- Nausea
- Thirst
- Weakness
- Restlessness
- Fear
- Dizziness

FIGURE 10.20 Signs and symptoms of shock.

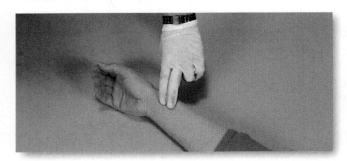

1 ■ Increased pulse: 100+.

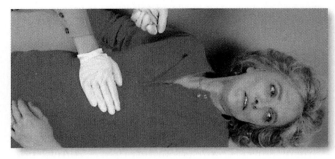

2 ■ Increased breathing rate.

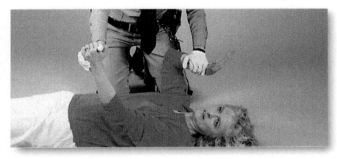

3 ■ Restlessness or combativeness.

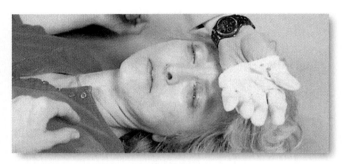

4 ■ Skin changes and sweating.

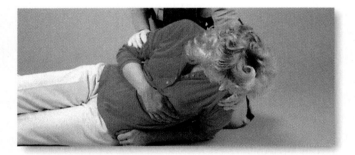

5 ■ Thirst, weakness, and nausea.

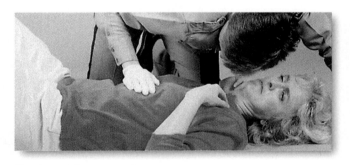

6 ■ Loss of responsiveness.

REMEMBER

Children may compensate for a loss of blood better than adults. This will delay the early indications of developing shock. However, once children and young adults begin to show the first signs of shock, its development may be rapid.

- *Increased breathing rate.* When the body is not receiving enough oxygen and the level of carbon dioxide increases, the body tries to compensate by increasing the breathing rate. This increased rate will not slow down as it usually does after experiencing stress.
- *Restlessness or combativeness.* The patient is reacting to the body's attempt to adjust to the loss of proper circulatory function. The patient feels that something is wrong and may often look afraid. In some cases, this behavioral change may be the first sign of developing shock.
- *Skin appears pale.* Skin, nail bed, and other color changes occur. The skin feels cool to the touch. Sweating may be profuse.
- *Rapid, weak pulse and labored, shallow respirations.* The body is failing in its attempt to adjust to the circulatory system failure.
- *Changes in mental status.* As adequate circulation to the brain continues to fail, the patient will become confused, disoriented, sleepy, or unresponsive.
- *Respiratory and cardiac arrest* can develop.

FIRST ➤ Provide care for all injured patients as if shock will develop. Do the same for all patients with problems involving the heart, breathing, abdominal pain, diabetes, drug abuse, poisoning, and abnormal childbirth. Carefully monitor all patients for the early signs of shock. ■

Preventing and Caring for Shock

FIRST ➤ Help delay the onset of shock by the following (Figure 10.21):

1. Make sure someone activates the EMS system.
2. Perform a scene size-up.
3. Take appropriate BSI precautions.
4. Perform an initial assessment.
5. Control external bleeding. Administer oxygen as per local protocol.
6. Assist the patient in lying down.
7. Provide care for shock. Calm and reassure the patient, and maintain his normal body temperature. Take care not to overheat the patient because overheating can worsen his condition. Place at least one blanket under and one blanket over the patient, covering all body parts except the head. Do not try to place a blanket under a patient who has possible spinal injuries.
8. Properly position the patient. Regardless of the position used, make certain that the patient has an open airway and be alert for vomiting. If there is no indication of spine injury, use one of the following positions (Figure 10.22):
   — *Option 1:* Elevate the lower extremities. This procedure is performed in most cases. Place the patient flat, face up, and elevate the legs 8 to 12 inches. Do not tilt the patient's body. Do not elevate any limbs with possible fractures unless they have been properly splinted. Do not elevate the legs if there are suspected fractures to the pelvis. Remember to consider the mechanism of injury for every patient.
   — *Option 2:* Lay the patient flat, face up. This is the supine position, used for patients with serious injuries to the extremities. If the patient is placed in this position, you must constantly be prepared for vomiting.
   — *Option 3:* Slightly raise the head and shoulders. This position should be used only for responsive patients with no possible neck, spine, chest, or

REMEMBER

Keeping a patient lying down and at rest reduces the risk of developing shock.

Care of Developing Shock

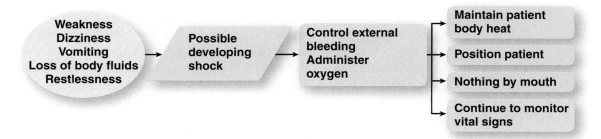

FIGURE 10.21 Algorithm for emergency care of patients with developing shock.

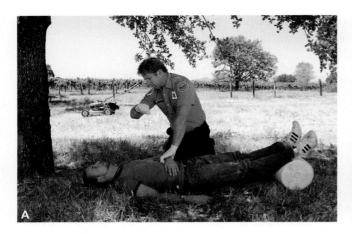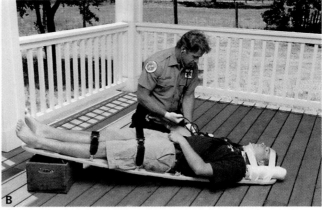

FIGURE 10.22 **A.** In most cases, the patient should lie flat with lower extremities elevated 8 to 12 inches. **B.** The Trendelenberg position is achieved with the patient lying on his back on a backboard or similar device with the foot end elevated.

abdominal injuries, and only for patients having difficulty breathing, but who have an open airway. A semisitting position can also be used for patients with a history of heart problems. It is not recommended for moderate to severe cases of shock. Be certain to keep the patient's head from tilting forward.

9. Do not give the patient anything by mouth. Even if the patient expresses serious thirst, do not give any fluids or food.

10. Monitor the patient's vital signs. This must be done at least every five minutes. Stay alert for vomiting, give nothing to the patient by mouth, and provide emotional support to the responsive patient. ▪

Restlessness may be a sign of someone going into shock. The patient may want to assume a sitting position even when there are no problems with breathing. A patient has less chance of going into shock if kept lying down and at rest.

You will not be able to reverse shock, but you may be able to delay the onset of shock or keep it from worsening by following the previous procedures. The care you provide may reverse the severity of certain aspects of shock and may help the patient avoid immediate danger.

If you are trained to do so and if your state laws allow, oxygen can be significant in helping shock patients. Administer oxygen as per local protocols.

Fainting

Fainting is usually a self-correcting form of mild shock. However, the patient may have been injured in a fall due to fainting. Be certain to examine the patient for injury. Even if no other problems are apparent, keep the patient lying down and at rest for several minutes.

In some cases, fainting is caused by a sudden drop in blood pressure. If you are trained to do so and have the needed equipment, check the patient's blood pressure. Otherwise, have the patient's blood pressure checked by an EMT or a nurse.

Fainting can also be a warning of some serious condition, including brain tumors, heart disease, undetected diabetes, and inner ear problems. Always recommend that the patient see a physician as soon as possible. In a polite but firm manner, tell anyone who has fainted not to drive or operate any machinery until after having been seen by a physician. Make certain that you have witnesses to this warning.

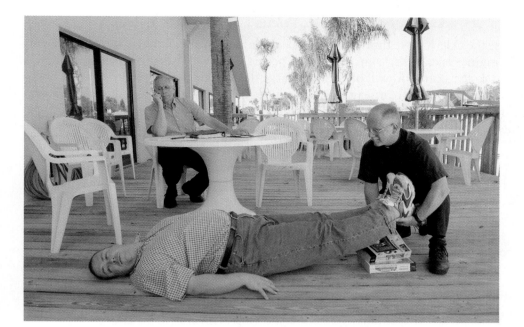

FIGURE 10.23 For some patients, lying down with feet slightly elevated, plus emotional support, can prevent fainting.

Your patient may have fainted because of fear, stress from problems, bad news, or the sight of blood. Be ready to provide emotional support when the patient is alert.

FIRST ➤ You can often prevent a person from fainting by lowering the patient's head. Assist the patient to the floor and have him lie down with his feet slightly elevated. This will increase blood flow to the brain and will often prevent fainting (Figure 10.23). ■

soft tissues ■ the tissues of the body that make up the skin, muscles, nerves, blood vessels, fat, and the cells that line and cover organs and glands.

Soft-Tissue Injuries

This section of the chapter describes injuries to the **soft tissues** of the body—skin, muscles, nerves, blood vessels, fatty tissues, and cells (Figure 10.24). Since childhood, we have learned about soft-tissue injuries such as bruises, scratches, and cuts. The idea of amputations and crush injuries are at least known, if not witnessed, before we enter our teens. Our own experiences and those of the people around us lead to our general understanding of injuries.

This prior knowledge will be useful to you. To be an Emergency Medical Responder, you will have to refine this knowledge, learning how to recognize and provide care for various injuries. However, you should not forget your basic understanding of injuries. Most of your patients will, at best, have the same level of understanding that you had when you started this course. Remembering this will help you with patient interviews and in providing explanations and reassurance. Also, recalling what you knew about injuries as you went through childhood will help when dealing with children who have suffered injuries.

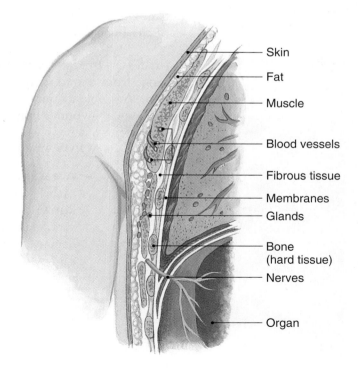

Skin
Fat
Muscle
Blood vessels
Fibrous tissue
Membranes
Glands
Bone (hard tissue)
Nerves
Organ

FIGURE 10.24 Soft tissues and associated underlying structures.

Because the elderly have thin skin that is easily damaged, one of the more common soft-tissue injuries is called a "skin tear." This occurs when a twisting or shearing action is applied to the skin. You will often find a large flap of thin skin similar to a burn hanging from the wound. Treatment for this includes gently laying the flap of skin back into its original position and applying pressure bandages over it to prevent bleeding from the numerous small blood vessels that may be damaged.

Except for cases of spine injury and certain types of internal injury, most adults can look at someone and often tell if there is an injury. Your training will build on this ability so that you will not miss detectable injuries. This is why there has been so much emphasis on patient assessment. As you progress through this course, you will be trained to determine the extent of an injury and the emergency procedures needed to care for it.

Types of Injuries

Soft-tissue injuries can be categorized as either closed wounds or open wounds.

FIRST ➤ A **closed wound** is an injury in which the skin is not broken. Such injuries are usually caused by the impact of a blunt object. Bleeding can range from minor to major, while the extent of injury can range from a simple **bruise** to the rupturing of internal organs. ▪

Most closed wounds detected during Emergency Medical Responder care are bruises (contusions) (Figure 10.25). There is always some internal bleeding associated with a bruise. Because the skin is not broken, the blood leaks between tissues, causing discoloration over time ranging from black and blue to a brownish-yellow. Keep in mind that large bruises can mean serious blood loss and that there may be fractures or extensive tissue damage under the site of the bruise.

FIRST ➤ In cases of **open wounds**, the skin is opened. The extent of injury can range from a mild scrape (abrasion) to a tearing or cutting open of the skin (laceration). A simple scraping of the skin may produce no bleeding, while more severe open wounds may be associated with minor to life-threatening bleeding. ▪

Open wounds may be classified as:

- **Abrasions**. Wounds such as skinned elbows and knees, "road rash," "rug burns," and thorn scratches are minor open wounds known as abrasions (Figure 10.26). Although such scratches and scrapes may be painful, tissue injury is usually not serious because the skin is not fully penetrated and the force causing the injury does not crush or rupture underlying structures. There may be no detectable bleeding or only minor capillary bleeding. Wound contamination tends to be the most serious problem faced when caring for abrasions to the skin.
- **Lacerations**. In cases of lacerations, the skin is fully penetrated, with injury also occurring to tissues lying under the skin. Lacerations may be classified as:
  — Smooth cuts, or **incisions** (Figure 10.27), are produced by very sharp objects, such as razor blades, knives, and broken

closed wound ▪ an internal soft-tissue injury in which the skin is not broken.

bruise ▪ a simple closed wound in which blood leaks between soft tissues, causing a discoloration. Also called a *contusion (kun-TU-zhun)*.

5–2.7 State the types of open soft-tissue injuries.

open wound ▪ an injury to the body in which the skin or its outer layers are opened.

abrasion (ab-RAY-zhun) ▪ the simplest form of open wound that damages the skin surface but does not break all layers of skin; scratches and scrapes.

laceration ▪ a soft-tissue injury in which all layers of skin are opened and the tissues immediately below the skin are damaged.

incision ▪ a laceration with smooth edges, usually caused by very sharp objects such as a razor blade, knife, or broken glass.

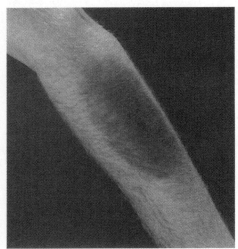

FIGURE 10.25 Bruises are the most common form of closed wounds.

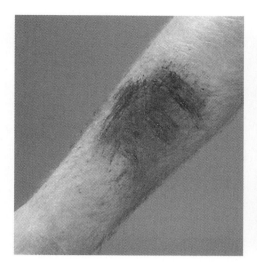

FIGURE 10.26 Abrasions are the least serious form of all open wounds.

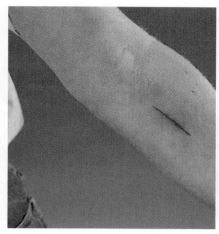

FIGURE 10.27 The edges of a smooth cut (incision) are straight.

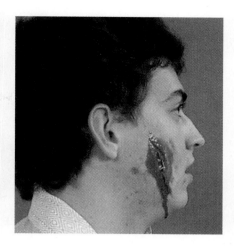

FIGURE 10.28 Tissues along the edges of a jagged cut (laceration) will be torn and rough.

glass. The edges of a smooth cut appear straight, with no apparent tears or jagged areas. Deep incisions can cause severe tissue damage and life-threatening bleeding.

— Jagged cuts are tears with rough edges (Figure 10.28). Sometimes jagged cuts can be produced from the impact of a blunt object. Usually, they occur when the skin is cut by an object that does not have a very sharp edge.

■ **Punctures**. Objects such as knives, nails, and ice picks can produce puncture wounds. An object puncturing the body will tear through the skin and usually proceed in a straight line, damaging all tissues in its path. A puncture wound can range from shallow to deep (Figure 10.29). It may also have both an entrance and an exit wound, as the object, such as a bullet, passes through the body. Often, the exit wound is the larger and more serious of the two (Figure 10.30).

puncture ■ an open wound that tears through the skin and damages tissues in a straight line.

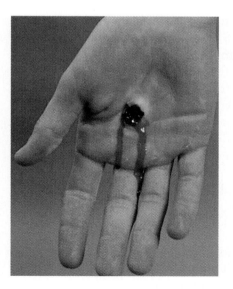

FIGURE 10.29 Puncture wound.

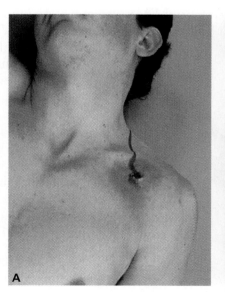

A

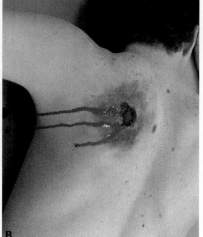

B

FIGURE 10.30 A penetrating wound can have both **A.** an entrance wound and **B.** an exit wound. Often the exit wound is the more serious of the two.

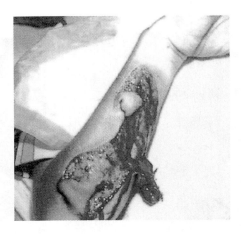

FIGURE 10.31 Avulsions are open wounds.

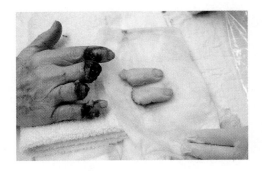

FIGURE 10.32 Amputation. *(© Edward T. Dickinson, MD)*

avulsion (ah-VUL-shun) ▪ a soft-tissue injury in which flaps of skin are torn loose or torn off.

amputation ▪ a soft-tissue injury that involves the cutting or tearing off of a limb or one of its parts. Often, hard tissues are also injured.

crush injury ▪ a soft-tissue injury produced by crushing forces. Soft tissues and internal organs are crushed, and hard tissues are usually damaged.

5–2.8 Describe the emergency medical care of the patient with a soft-tissue injury.

- **Avulsions**. These wounds most frequently involve the tearing loose or the tearing off of large flaps of skin (Figure 10.31). A torn ear, an eyeball removed from its socket, and the loss of a tooth are also examples of avulsions.
- **Amputations**. These wounds involve the cutting or tearing off of the fingers, toes, hands, feet, arms, or legs (Figure 10.32). Because amputation can be done as a surgical procedure, this injury is often called a *traumatic amputation*.
- **Crush injuries**. Most of the time, when people see an incident in which a body part has been crushed, their first thoughts are of fractures. Soft tissues and internal organs are also crushed, often rupturing (Figure 10.33). Both external and internal bleeding can be profuse.

Basic Emergency Care

Bystanders at emergency scenes may begin care before Emergency Medical Responders or other members of the EMS system arrive to provide professional-level assessment and care. Untrained individuals often focus on soft-tissue injuries. Your EMS system may require that you do not attempt to undo what has been done before your arrival until EMTs or other more highly trained personnel arrive. Usually, EMS system protocols state that obviously harmful care must be stopped and corrected. For example, people at the scene may have applied a very tight bandage and stopped circulation in an extremity. In such a situation, you may be required to re-establish distal circulation. Your instructor will alert you to specific protocols for your EMS system.

In situations where care has been rendered by individuals having less training than an Emergency Medical Responder, follow your EMS protocols for assessment and care. If there is any doubt, call or have someone call 9-1-1.

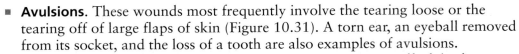

FIGURE 10.33 Both soft tissues and internal organs are damaged in crush injuries.

Care During Assessment

A limited amount of care may be initiated during the patient assessment. Immediately care for injuries involving the ABCs (major bleeding and arrest). As an Emergency Medical Responder, you may begin certain

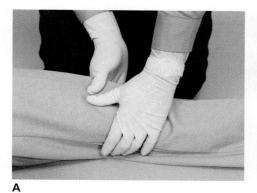

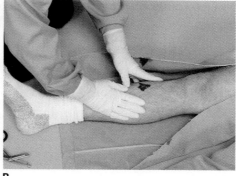

A   B

FIGURE 10.34 A limited amount of care for soft-tissue injury may be started during patient assessment.

types of soft-tissue injury care during assessment (Figure 10.34), but take care to avoid a tunnel-vision approach.

Remember that each patient is different. Follow local protocols and begin care when it is safe to do so. You should care for any life-threatening injuries as you encounter them, but always remember to continue to monitor the ABCs, as they take precedence. Do not be in such a hurry to start patient care that you miss detecting serious injuries.

Care of Closed Wounds

As mentioned previously in this chapter, the most frequently seen closed wound is the bruise or contusion. Generally, bruises do not require emergency care in the field. However, bruises can be a warning sign of possible internal injuries and related bleeding. Look for large bruises or large areas of the body covered with bruises. Remember that a deep bruise the size of the patient's fist equals a blood loss of about 10%. Be certain to look for swelling and deformities that may indicate suspected fractures. Note if the patient's abdomen is rigid, if the patient is coughing up blood, or if there is blood in the mouth, nose, or ears.

Care of Open Wounds

FIRST ➤ To care for open wounds, you should (Figure 10.35):

1. Expose the wound. Clothing over and around an open wound must be cut away. Avoid aggravating the patient's injuries. Do not try to remove clothing by pulling the items over the patient's head or limbs. Simply lift aside, or cut the clothing away from, the site of injury.
2. Remove superficial foreign matter from the surface of the wound with a sterile gauze pad. This method will reduce the chances of contamination from your gloved fingers and will protect your fingertips. Do not try to clean the wound

REMEMBER

Providing care for soft-tissue injuries may place you in contact with blood and body fluids. Take BSI precautions. Also, remember to wash your hands after each patient contact.

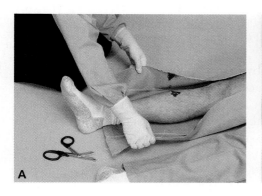

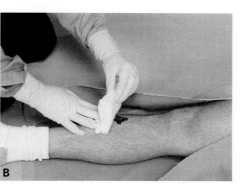

A   B

FIGURE 10.35 Emergency care for open wounds. **A.** Expose the wound. **B.** Control bleeding with direct pressure or direct pressure and elevation.

or pick out any particles or debris. If bleeding from the wound is controlled, take care not to restart or increase the flow of blood.

3. Control bleeding with direct pressure or direct pressure and elevation. If the bleeding continues, try pressure point control. A tourniquet should be used only as a last resort for life-threatening bleeding from a limb. Administer oxygen as per local protocols.

4. Prevent further contamination by using a sterile dressing, clean cloth, or clean handkerchief to cover the wound. After the bleeding has been controlled, bandage the dressing in place.

5. Keep the patient lying still because any activity will increase circulation. Keep the patient lying down, using a blanket or other form of covering to provide protection from the elements.

6. Reassure the patient. This will reduce patient movement and may help lower the patient's blood pressure toward a normal level.

7. Care for shock. This applies to all but the simplest of wounds. Do not elevate a limb if there is the possibility of a fracture, unless the limb is immobilized. ▪

REMEMBER

Do not remove a dressing once it is in place.

If you have to control bleeding from an extremity or if the wound on a limb is long, dress the wound and immobilize the limb with a splint (see Chapter 11). If an air splint is part of your Emergency Medical Responder equipment, use it to help control the bleeding.

Care of Specific Injuries

5–2.9 Discuss the emergency medical care considerations for a patient with a penetrating chest injury.

Care for certain soft-tissue injuries is summarized in Figure 10.36.

Puncture Wounds

FIRST ➤ When dealing with any puncture wound, assume that there is extensive internal injury and internal bleeding. Always check for an exit wound, realizing that exit wounds can be more serious than entrance wounds (in the case of gunshot injury). Care for entrance and exit wounds as you would any open wound.

If a puncture wound contains an impaled object (such as glass, a knife, wood, metal, or plastic), do the following (Figure 10.37):

1. Take appropriate BSI precautions.
2. Do not remove an impaled object.
3. Expose the wound, without disturbing the impaled object. Do not lift clothing over the object.
4. Control bleeding. Administer oxygen as per local protocols.

   NOTE

   Take special care not to cut your gloves or hand on an impaled object. Spread your fingers around the object and apply pressure to the wound site. Do not put any pressure on the object or the tissues that are up against the edge of a sharp impaled object.

5. Attempt to stabilize the impaled object by using bulky dressings. Several layers of dressings, cloths, or handkerchiefs placed on the sides of the object will help stabilize it. An alternative approach is to cut a hole in the center of a bulky dressing, making the cut slightly larger than the impaled object. Gently pass the dressing over the object. Bandaging these dressings in place will improve stability.
6. Provide care for shock.
7. Keep the patient at rest. ▪

Care for Soft-Tissue Injuries

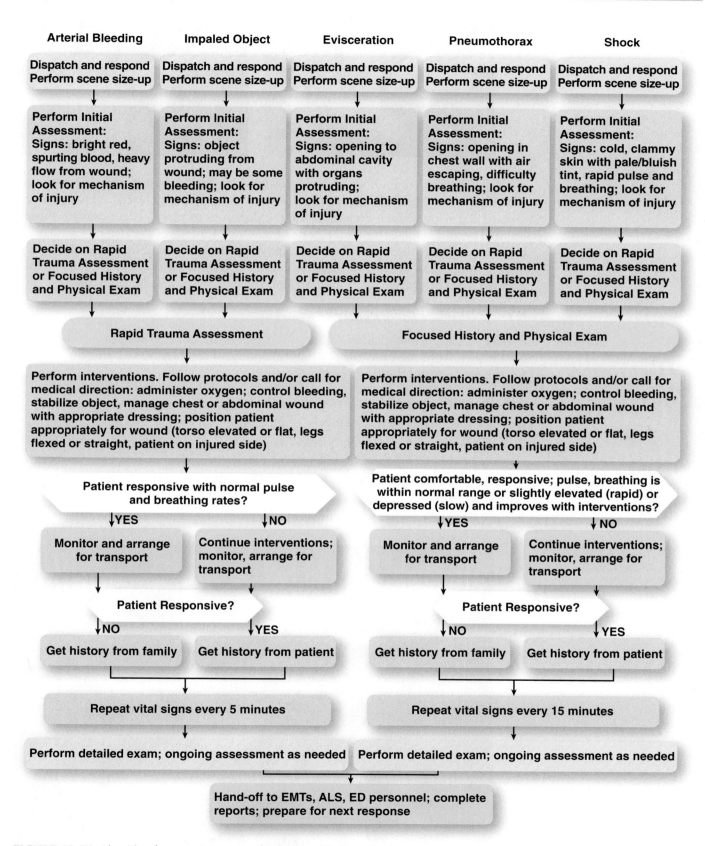

FIGURE 10.36 Algorithm for emergency care of soft-tissue injuries.

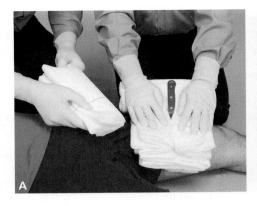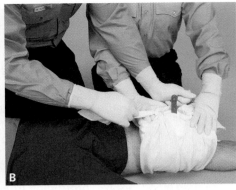

FIGURE 10.37 Emergency care for a wound with an impaled object. **A.** Control bleeding. **B.** Stabilize the object in place.

Adhesive tape often does not stick to the skin around an impaled object wound site. Blood and sweat on the skin, even when the surface is cleared, may cause the tape to slip. Cravats can be used to tie the dressings in place. These cravats should be made from folded triangular bandages. Once folded, the cravats should be at least two inches wide. If the object is impaled in the chest or abdomen, a thin splint or coat hanger can be used to push the cravats under the natural void in the patient's back so that the cravat can be tied around the patient's trunk (Figure 10.38).

Avulsions and Amputations

5–2.12 State the emergency medical care for an amputation.

FIRST ➤ Care for avulsions and amputations is the same. If skin or another body part is torn from the body, or if a flap of skin has been torn loose, you should care for the wound with bulky pressure dressings:

1. Take appropriate BSI precautions.
2. Clear the surface of the wound.
3. If there is an avulsion, gently fold the skin back to its normal position. Follow local protocols for procedures.
4. Control bleeding and care as you would for any open wound, using bulky pressure dressings.
5. Provide care for shock. Administer oxygen as per local protocols. ■

FIGURE 10.38 A thin splint or coat hanger can be used to push the cravat under the natural void in the back, reducing patient movement. Follow local protocol.

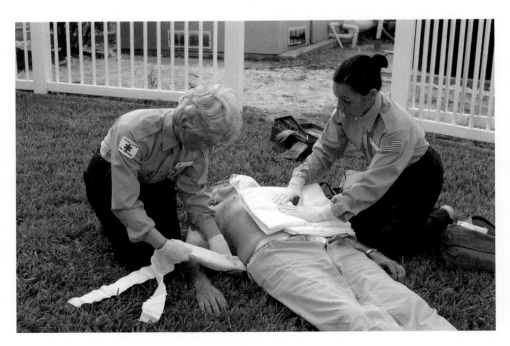

Save and preserve an avulsed or amputated part. This is best done by wrapping the part in a slightly moistened sterile dressing, if available, and placing it into a plastic bag or wrapping it in plastic wrap. If possible, keep the part cool (not cold, avoid freezing). Do not place the avulsed or amputated part in water or in direct contact with ice. Be certain that the bag with the part in it gets transported with the patient. It may be helpful to label the bag with the patient's name.

FIRST ➤ In most cases of avulsion or amputation, bleeding can be controlled by direct pressure, elevation, and a pressure dressing held firmly over the stump or area of avulsion. Use pressure point techniques if the bleeding continues. Should this fail, apply a tourniquet. ∎

Protruding Organs

FIRST ➤ A deep open wound to the abdomen may cause organs to protrude through the wound opening. This is known as an **evisceration.** In such cases:

- Do not try to replace the organ(s).
- Place a plastic covering over the exposed organs. If possible, apply a thick, moist dressing over the top of this covering to help conserve heat.
- Provide care for shock. Do not give the patient anything by mouth. ∎

5–2.10 State the emergency medical care considerations for a patient with an open wound to the abdomen.

evisceration (e-VIS-er-a-shun) ∎ protrusion of the intestines through the abdominal wall.

Scalp Injuries

Injuries to the scalp can be difficult to care for because of the numerous blood vessels found there. Many of these vessels are close to the surface of the skin, producing profuse bleeding even from minor wounds. Additional problems arise if the bones of the skull are involved.

Injuries to the scalp (and face) require an extra effort on the part of the Emergency Medical Responder to provide emotional support for patients. These injuries tend to be very painful, produce bleeding that frightens many patients, and are in a body region where people have concern for their appearance. Talk to patients in a calm, professional manner. Always let them know what you are going to do before you do it. Make certain that they know additional help is on the way.

FIRST ➤ The procedures for the care of soft-tissue injuries covered previously in this chapter apply to the care you should provide for injuries to the soft tissues of the scalp. However, there are three exceptions:

- *Exception 1:* Do not attempt to clear the surface of a scalp wound. This will often cause additional bleeding and may cause great harm if there are fractures to the skull.
- *Exception 2:* Do not apply firm pressure to the wound if there is any chance of skull fracture.

Care of scalp wounds includes the following (Figure 10.39):

- Do not clear foreign matter or dirt from the wound. It will cause more bleeding.
- Control bleeding with a dressing held in place with gentle pressure. Avoid exerting excessive pressure if there are signs of a fractured skull or the injury site feels spongy.
- Adhesive bandages will not work well. A roller bandage or gauze can be wrapped around the patient's head to hold dressings in place once bleeding has been controlled. If there is any indication of neck or spine injuries, do not attempt to wrap the patient's head. Do not wrap the bandage around the patient's lower jaw or neck.

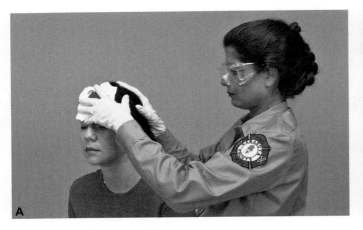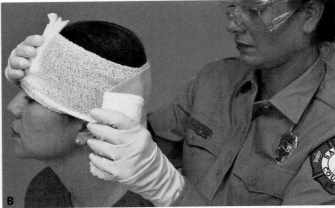

FIGURE 10.39 Emergency care for a scalp wound. **A.** Use a dressing to apply controlled pressure. **B.** When bleeding is controlled, wrap a roller bandage around the patient's head to hold dressings in place.

- If there are no signs of skull fracture or injuries to the spine, neck, or chest, you may position the patient so that the head and shoulders are elevated. ▪

An optional approach to holding a dressing in place over a scalp wound is to use a commercially prepared triangular bandage or one made from gauze or some other cloth. The steps for this procedure are shown in Scan 10–4.

Facial Wounds

The first concern when caring for facial injuries is to make certain that the patient's airway is open and breathing is adequate. Even though bleeding may appear to be the only problem, check the airway and establish the presence of a carotid pulse. Continue to watch the patient to be sure that the airway remains open and clear of fluids and obstructions (tongue, teeth, blood clots).

FIRST ➤ When caring for patients with facial injuries, you should (Figure 10.40):

1. Correct breathing problems, being careful to note and properly care for neck and spine injuries.

FIGURE 10.40 Emergency care of soft-tissue injuries to the face.

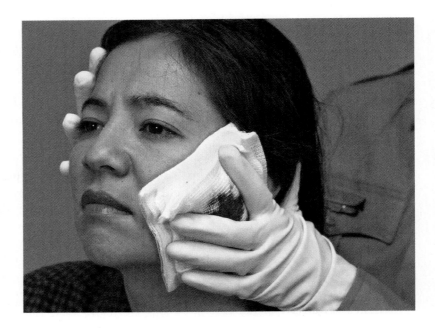

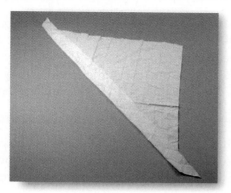

1 ■ Fold the bandage to make a two-inch hem along its base.

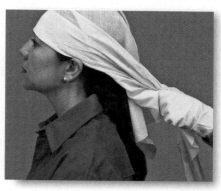

2 ■ Have the folded edge face out when you position the bandage on the patient's forehead, just above the eyes. Make certain that the point of the bandage hangs down behind the patient's head.

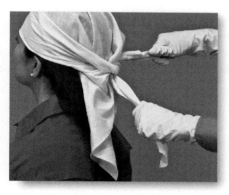

3 ■ Draw the ends of the bandage behind the patient's head.

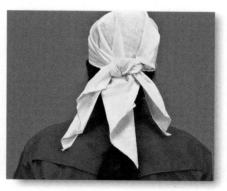

4 ■ Then tie the ends over the point of the bandage.

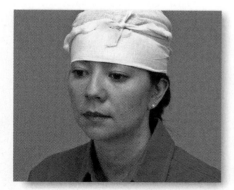

5 ■ Pull the ends to the front of the head and tie them together. Finally, bring the point of the bandage down and tuck it into the crossed fold.

2. Control bleeding by direct pressure, being careful not to press too hard because many facial fractures are not obvious.

3. Apply a dressing and bandage. ▪

Geriatric Focus

Facial injuries generally bleed profusely in any patient, but in the elderly who may be taking "blood thinners" such as Coumadin, warfarin, or aspirin, the bleeding may be life threatening. Be prepared to treat the wounds aggressively with bandages and direct pressure.

If you find the patient has an object that has passed through the cheek wall and is sticking into the mouth, you may have to remove it. This should be done if the object blocks the airway or is loose and may fall into the airway. To remove an impaled object from the cheek (Figure 10.41):

1. Look into the mouth and probe to see if the object has passed through the cheek wall.

2. If you find penetration, pull or safely and carefully push the object out of the cheek wall, back in the direction from which the object entered. Avoid cutting your gloves and yourself. If the object has not penetrated the cheek wall or if you cannot easily remove the object, stabilize it with dressings applied to the outer surface of the cheek.

3. In all cases, except for neck and spine injuries, turn the patient so that blood will drain from the mouth. If there are neck or spine injuries, do not turn the patient. Use dressing material packed against the inside wound to control the flow of blood.

4. If you remove an impaled object, place the dressing material between the wound and the patient's teeth, leaving some of the dressing outside the mouth so that it can be held to prevent swallowing it. Watch closely to be sure that the dressing does not work its way loose and into the airway. Do not assume that the patient's gag reflex will prevent the dressing from becoming an airway obstruction.

5. Dress and bandage the outside of the wound.

6. Provide care for shock.

Eye Injuries

Two rules of soft-tissue injury care apply when caring for an eye injury: do not remove any impaled objects, and do not try to put the eye back into its socket. When caring for a cut eyeball, there is one major exception to the procedures listed for

WARNING

Do not apply direct pressure to an injured eyeball. There are jelly-like fluids inside the eyeball that cannot be replaced.

FIGURE 10.41 Removing an object impaled in the cheek. **A.** Look into the mouth and probe to see if the object has passed through the cheek wall. If it has, remove it. **B.** Use dressing material packed against the inside wound to control the flow of blood.

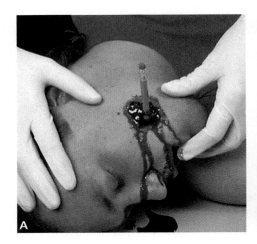
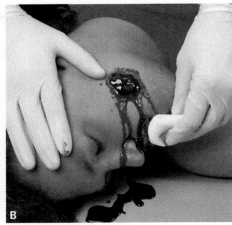

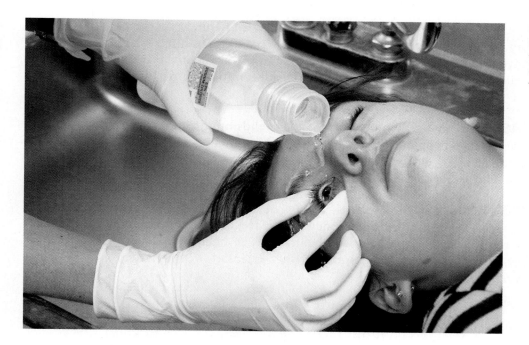

soft-tissue injury care: do not apply direct pressure to an injured eyeball. A loose bulky dressing will help the formation of blood clots to control the bleeding.

Problems resulting from foreign objects in the eyes are common. These problems can range from minor irritations to permanent injury. If the patient's own tears do not wash away a foreign object, use running water to remove it (Figure 10.42). *But do not apply the wash if there are impaled objects or cuts in the eye.* Apply the flow of water at the corner of the eye socket closest to the patient's nose. You may have to help the patient hold open the eyelids. As you pour the water, direct the patient to look from side to side and up and down. Before completing the wash, have the patient blink several times. When possible, continue the wash for at least 20 minutes or for the time recommended by medical direction.

WARNING

Do not apply running water to the eye if there are impaled objects or cuts in the eye.

FIRST ➤ It is critical that you:

- Do not remove impaled objects, including what may appear to be small pieces of glass impaled in the globe of the eye.
- Do not probe into the eye socket.
- Reduce the patient's eye movements. If there are sharp objects in the patient's eye, do not direct the patient to move the eyes during the wash. After the wash, keep the patient's eyes shut. Cover both eyes, bandaging the materials in place. ▪

REMEMBER

After debris is washed from the eye, the patient must be examined by someone with more advanced training. A physician or qualified eye care specialist should see the patient.

Whenever you are caring for a patient with eye injuries, you will have to cover both of the patient's eyes. In most cases, only one eye will actually be injured. However, when one eye moves, the other eye will also move (sympathetic movement). If you cover the injured eye and leave the uninjured eye uncovered, the uninjured eye will continue to react to activities and movement. Each time the uninjured eye moves, so will the injured eye. Having both patient's eyes covered reduces eye movements.

Is It Safe?

In some instances, it may be appropriate to secure the hands of an unresponsive patient who has eye injuries. If the patient becomes responsive, he may attempt to remove the bandages. Do this only if allowed by your local protocols. ▪

Having both eyes covered can cause fear and anxiety in the patient. Tell him why you are covering the uninjured eye. Keep close to him or have someone else stay close. Try to maintain contact with him through conversation and touch. If a friend or loved one of the patient also has been injured, reassure the patient that care is being provided for others.

FIRST ➤ Always remember to close the eyelids of unresponsive patients. Because unresponsive people do not blink, moisture is quickly lost from the eye surface, damaging the eye. If you notice that the patient is wearing contact lenses, be sure to point this out to the EMTs who take over the care of the patient. ■

FIRST ➤ Burns to the eye must always be considered serious, requiring special in-hospital care. As an Emergency Medical Responder, you may have to care for burns to the eyes caused by heat, light, or chemicals (Figure 10.43). Your actions can make the difference as to whether or not the patient's sight can be saved.

- *Thermal (heat) burns.* Do not try to inspect the eyes if there are signs of thermal burns to the eyelids. With the patient's eyelids closed, cover the eyes with loose, moist dressings. If you have no means to moisten the dressings, then apply loose, dry dressings. Do not apply any burn ointment to the eyelids.
- *Light burns.* "Snow blindness" and "welder's blindness" are two examples of light burns. Close the patient's eyelids and apply dark patches over both eyes. If you do not have dark patches, then use thick dressings or dressings followed with a layer of an opaque material such as dark plastic.

FIGURE 10.43 Emergency care for burns to the eye.

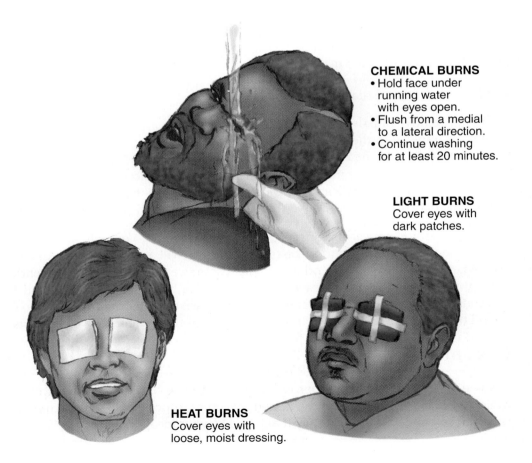

CHEMICAL BURNS
- Hold face under running water with eyes open.
- Flush from a medial to a lateral direction.
- Continue washing for at least 20 minutes.

LIGHT BURNS
Cover eyes with dark patches.

HEAT BURNS
Cover eyes with loose, moist dressing.

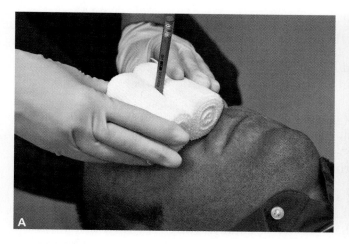
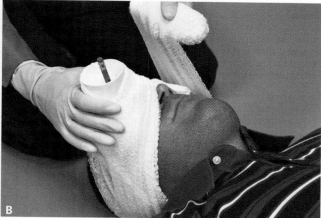

FIGURE 10.44 Emergency care for a patient with an object impaled in the globe of the eye includes **A.** stabilizing the object and **B.** securing it in place.

- *Chemical burns.* Many chemicals cause rapid, severe damage to the eyes. Flush the eyes with water. Do not delay care by trying to locate sterile water. Use any source of clean drinking water. If possible, continue the washing flow for at least 20 minutes. After washing the patient's eyes, close the eyelids and apply loose, moist dressings.

If you find an object impaled in the globe of a patient's eye, you should (Figure 10.44):

1. Use several layers of dressing or small rolls of gauze to make thick pads. Place them on the sides of the object. If you have only enough material for one thick pad, cut a hole, equal to the size of the eye opening, in the center of this pad. Set the pad over the patient's eye, allowing the impaled object to stick out through the opening cut into the pad.

2. Fit a disposable cardboard drinking cup or paper cone over the impaled object. This will serve as a protective shield. Rest the cup or cone onto the thick dressing pad, but do not allow this protective shield to come into contact with the impaled object.

3. Hold the pad and protective shield in place with a self-adherent roller bandage or with a wrapping of gauze or other cloth material.

4. Use dressing material to cover the uninjured eye, and bandage this dressing in place. This will reduce sympathetic eye movements.

5. Provide care for shock.

6. Provide emotional support to the patient. ▪

Wrapping a paper cup or cone with gauze is tricky and cannot be done easily unless you practice. Ideally, you should wrap around the cup and then continue around the patient's head and wrap around the cup again. This procedure is repeated until the cup is stable. Take great care not to push the cup down onto the impaled object or pull the cup out of place.

FIRST ➤ If the eye is pulled out of the socket (avulsed eye), the care provided is the same as for an object impaled in the eye. ▪

REMEMBER

Consider any bleeding from the ear as a sign of a possible head injury.

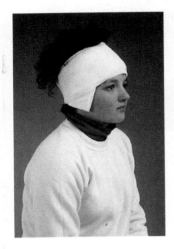

FIGURE 10.45 When caring for injuries to the external ear, apply a dressing and bandage.

REMEMBER

Most nosebleeds are minor, requiring little attention. However, they can be serious. Care for them accordingly.

Ear Injuries

External ear injuries include (Figure 10.45):

- *Cuts.* Apply dressings and bandage in place.
- *Tears.* Apply bulky dressings, beginning with several layers behind the torn tissue.
- *Avulsions.* Use slightly moistened bulky dressings, bandaged into place. Save the avulsed part in a plastic bag or plastic wrap. Keep the part dry and cool. If no plastic is available, then wrap in dressing material. Be certain to label the bag, wrap, or dressing with the patient's name.

Internal ear injuries may appear as bleeding from the ears. Any such bleeding must be considered a sign of serious head injury. Bloody or clear fluids draining from the ear may indicate the presence of skull fracture. For such cases, assume there is serious injury and provide the necessary care. (For more about head injuries, see Chapter 11.)

Do not pack the external ear canal. To do so can cause increased internal injury. If there is bleeding or clear fluid leaking from the ears, apply external dressings, sterile if possible, and hold them in place with bandages. Report this bleeding to the EMTs.

Do not attempt to remove foreign objects from inside the ear. Apply external dressings, if necessary, and provide emotional support to the patient.

If the patient tells you that it feels like his ears are "clogged" or "stopped up," suspect possible damage to the eardrum, fluids in the middle ear, or objects in the ear canal. Many of these problems will clear up quickly after hospital care.

Nose Injuries

FIRST ➤ When dealing with injuries to the nose—when there are no suspected skull fractures or spine injuries—you will have two duties: maintain an open airway and control bleeding. ◾

For a nosebleed in a responsive patient, maintain an open airway. Have the patient assume a seated position, leaning slightly forward. This position will help prevent blood and mucus from obstructing the airway or draining down the throat and into the stomach, which can cause nausea and vomiting. Next, have the patient pinch the nostrils. Bleeding is usually controlled when the nostrils are pinched shut. If the patient cannot pinch them shut, you will have to do so (Figure 10.46). However, if other patients are in need of your help, do not delay their care while you sit pinching someone's nose. Have a bystander put on gloves, pinch

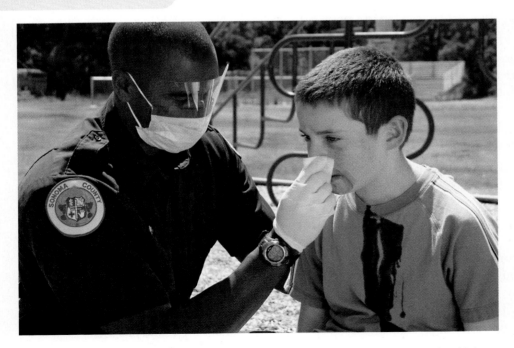

FIGURE 10.46 For a nosebleed, if the patient cannot pinch the nostrils shut, you should do so. Remember to position the patient for drainage.

the patient's nose, and inform you of any problems as you continue to care for the other patients. Do not pack the patient's nostrils. Do not allow the patient to blow his nose if he is bleeding from the nostrils or has recently controlled a nosebleed.

For a nosebleed in an unresponsive patient or in a patient injured in such a way that he cannot be placed in a seated position, place him on one side with the head turned to provide drainage from the nose and mouth. Attempt to control bleeding by pinching the nostrils shut. Do not pack the nose. Do not remove objects or probe into the nose.

For an avulsion of the nose, apply a pressure dressing to the site. Save the avulsed part in plastic or a sterile or clean dressing. Keep the part cool.

(See Scan 10–5 for a summary of care for soft-tissue injury to the head.)

Injury to the Mouth

FIRST ➤ As with all injuries that occur in or around the airway, your first concern will be to ensure an open airway. If there are no suspected skull, neck, or spine injuries, position the patient in a seated position with the head tilted slightly forward to allow for drainage. If the patient cannot be placed in a seated position, position him on one side with the head turned slightly downward to provide some drainage for blood and other fluids. ■

For cut lips, use a rolled or folded dressing. Place the dressing between the patient's lip and gum. Take great care that the patient does not swallow this dressing.

For avulsed lips, apply a pressure bandage to the site of injury. Save the avulsed part in plastic or a sterile or clean dressing. Keep the avulsed part cool.

For cuts to the internal cheek, position a dressing between the patient's cheek and gum. (Do not pack the mouth with dressings.) Hold the dressing in place with a gloved hand. Always leave three to four inches of dressing material outside the patient's mouth to allow for quick removal. This is necessary to prevent the patient from swallowing the dressing. If possible, position the patient's head to allow drainage.

Neck Wounds

FIRST ➤ As an Emergency Medical Responder, be aware of the following signs that indicate soft-tissue wounds to the neck:

- Difficulty speaking, loss of voice.
- Airway obstruction when the mouth and nose are clear and no object can be dislodged from the airway. This is often due to swollen tissues.
- Obvious swelling or bruising of the neck.
- Pain on swallowing or speaking.
- Trachea pushed off to one side (tracheal deviation).
- Depressions in the neck.
- Obvious cuts or puncture wounds.

For all profuse bleeding from the neck, make certain that someone activates EMS and reports the problem and the need for immediate EMS transport. Cut or severed arteries in the neck require the following procedure:

1. Take appropriate BSI precautions.
2. Immediately apply direct pressure over the wound, using the palm of your gloved hand.
3. Try controlling the bleeding with a pressure dressing, taking care not to close the airway and not to apply pressure to both sides of the neck.

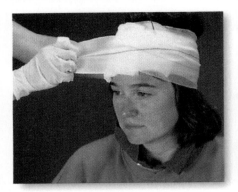

Scalp. Control bleeding, dress, and wrap with roller bandage.

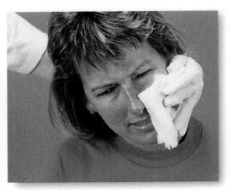

Face. Ensure airway, control bleeding, dress, and wrap with roller bandage.

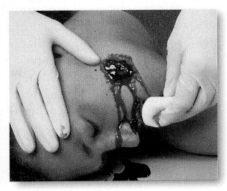

Cheek. Ensure airway, remove impaled object, and control bleeding. Dress and bandage the external wound.

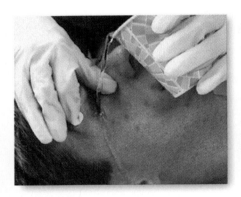

Debris in eye. If eye is not cut, wash objects from surface.

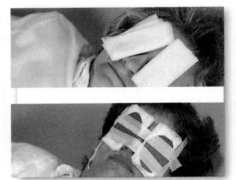

Eye burns. Flush chemical burns (20 minutes). Loosely dress heat burns. Apply dark patches for light burns.

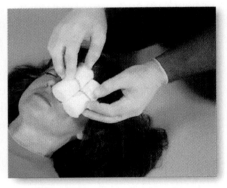

Impaled object in the eye. Stabilize the object and apply rigid protection.

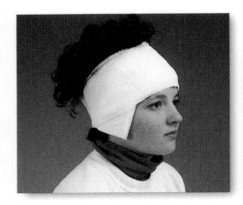

Ear. Do not pack canal. Dress and bandage.

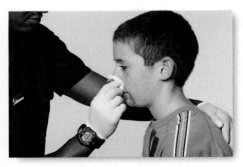

Nosebleed. Pinch nostrils shut.

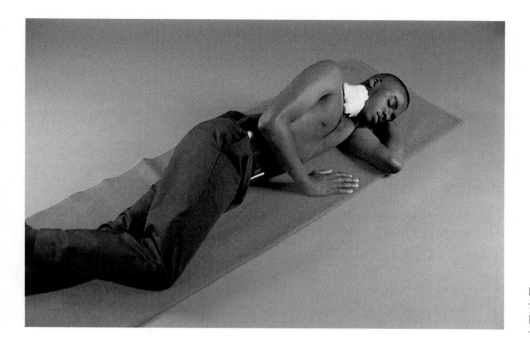

FIGURE 10.47 With open wounds to the neck, place the patient on the left side.

4. Once the bleeding is controlled, place the patient on his left side (Figure 10.47). If possible, lay the patient on a surface that can be slanted (spine board, table, long bench, plywood) so that the entire body can be tilted into a head-down position. The slant should be no more than 15 degrees. This will help trap any air bubbles that may have entered the bloodstream.

5. Provide care for shock. Administer oxygen per local protocols.

Bleeding from a large cut or severed neck veins usually cannot be controlled by pressure dressings. For such emergencies, you should (Figure 10.48):

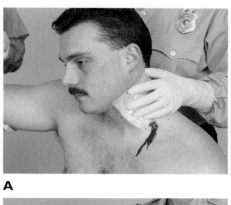

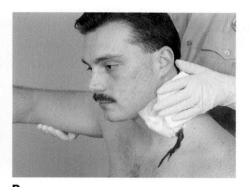

FIGURE 10.48 Use an occlusive dressing to help control bleeding from the neck. **A.** Apply direct pressure. **B.** Apply an occlusive dressing and over that apply a roll of gauze. **C.** Secure all with a figure-eight wrap of self-adherent roller bandage. **D.** Provide care for shock.

A

B

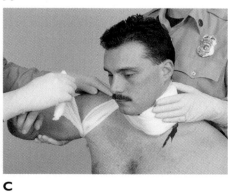

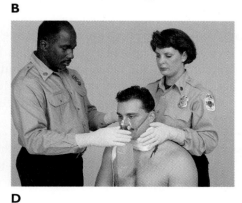

C

D

1. Immediately apply direct pressure to the wound, using the palm of your gloved hand.

2. Apply an occlusive dressing or some type of plastic over the wound. Use tape to seal this dressing on all sides. When complete, the dressing must be air-tight. If you do not have the materials to make an occlusive dressing, use any sterile or clean dressing material and attempt to control bleeding by direct pressure.

3. To help trap any air bubbles that may have entered the bloodstream, place the patient on the left side for transport, with the body slanted as described above.

NOTE

Do not attempt to reposition the patient if there are indications of spine injury.

4. Care for shock by maintaining body warmth and providing oxygen. ■

An alternative method of securing a dressing to the neck is as follows. Your instructor will tell you if the technique is approved for use in your region. This method uses the same procedure for both arterial and venous bleeding of the neck:

1. Immediately apply direct pressure over the wound, using the palm of your gloved hand.

2. Place a plastic occlusive dressing over the wound and continue to apply pressure, using the palm of your hand. Do not use a single layer of plastic wrap. It is too thin and may be sucked into the wound. Ideally, the occlusive dressing should extend one inch beyond the wound on all sides.

3. Place a roll of gauze dressing or dressing materials over the occlusive dressing and continue to apply pressure. Another roll can be placed between the wound and the trachea to help reduce pressure on the trachea.

4. While maintaining pressure, secure the entire dressing with a figure-eight wrap of self-adherent roller bandage. This eliminates the problem of trying to make adhesive tape stick to a bloody surface.

5. Place the patient on his left side for transport, with the body slightly slanted in a head-down position.

6. Care for shock by maintaining body warmth and providing oxygen.

NOTE

These methods take a great deal of practice and review if they are to be done correctly in the field.

Should your attempts to control bleeding from a neck wound fail, a last-resort method would be to place your gloved finger or fingers into the wound and attempt to compress the vessel or pinch shut the ends. This method is to be used only when standard Emergency Medical Responder-level care procedures have failed to control life-threatening profuse bleeding.

Penetrating Chest Wounds

Soft-tissue injuries to the chest receive the same basic type of care as you would give to soft-tissue injuries in other areas of the body. Typically, these injuries are cuts, bruises, and puncture wounds. Serious soft-tissue injuries to the chest include deep puncture wounds, penetrating wounds, and impaled objects.

For puncture and penetrating wounds, apply occlusive dressings. Impaled objects must be stabilized. Wounds from punctures and impaled objects may go through the chest. If this occurs, you will have to care for both an entrance wound and an exit wound. Deep punctures to the chest are generally serious because of the vital organs located there. In addition, as explained in Chapter 6, breathing causes pressure changes in the chest cavity. When the chest wall is punctured, this pressure balance is affected. A lung will collapse because air gets between it and the chest wall, causing extra pressure to build up inside the chest cavity and breathing to be ineffective.

You must seal an open wound to the chest to prevent air from entering the chest space and causing lung collapse. The seal will also allow the lungs to re-expand.

In some cases, the lung itself will be penetrated (Figure 10.49). As the patient inhales, air from this lung will leak out and enter the chest cavity. If the wound has been tightly sealed on the outside, pressure may still build from the inside as air continues to enter the cavity from the punctured lung during each breath. Unless this pressure is released, it may interfere with heart and lung actions.

FIRST ➤ You will be able to tell if a puncture wound has penetrated the lung by noting:

- Open chest wound in which the chest wall is torn or punctured.
- Sucking sound each time the patient breathes. This is why this type of wound is sometimes called a **sucking chest wound**. Bubbling at the injury site may be noted.
- Patient is coughing up bright red, frothy blood. ◾

If you find that a penetrating chest wound has both an entrance and an exit wound, assume that at least one lung has been punctured.

FIRST ➤ The following method is recommended for open chest wounds free of impaled objects. If there is no puncture to the lung, the method will work. If there is a punctured lung, this method will allow release of air trapped in the chest:

1. Have all dressing materials ready. Take appropriate BSI precautions. Then seal the patient's wound with the palm of your gloved hand as the patient exhales.

> **REMEMBER**
>
> Closely monitor the breathing of all patients with open chest wounds.

sucking chest wound ◾ an open chest wound through which air is sucked into the chest cavity each time the patient breathes.

> **REMEMBER**
>
> When the patient has an entrance wound and an exit wound, dress both.

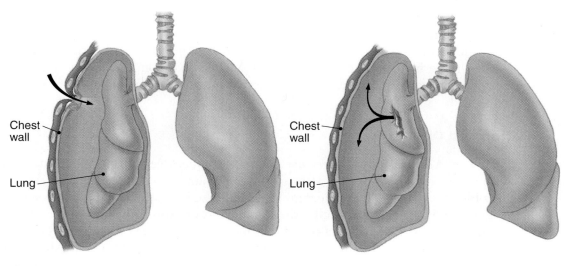

Chest wall

Lung

Chest wall

Lung

FIGURE 10.49 Penetrating chest wounds.

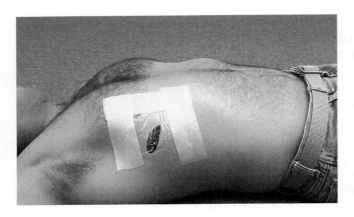

FIGURE 10.50 Apply an occlusive dressing to an open chest wound. If local protocol allows, tape it only on three sides to allow air to escape.

(A forceful exhalation will push trapped air out of the chest cavity.) Do not unseal the wound to prepare dressings. Have others at the scene help prepare the dressings.

2. Place an occlusive dressing under your hand while the patient exhales, and hold it in place.
   — *Taping three sides:* Have someone seal it by placing tape on three sides (Figure 10.50). This will produce a flutter valve effect. That is, when the patient inhales, the free edge will seal against the skin. When the patient exhales, the free edge will break loose from the skin and allow any build up of air in the chest cavity to escape.
   — *Taping four sides:* Some EMS systems prefer that all four sides be taped. The last side is taped as the patient exhales. Your instructor will inform you of local protocol.

With either taping method, the patient must be monitored. If the patient begins to have trouble breathing again, lift up one side of the plastic and have him forcefully exhale. Then quickly reposition the plastic to reseal.

3. Provide oxygen as soon as possible, and care for shock. ▪

A commercial occlusive dressing is the best choice for open chest wounds. Plastic wrap can be used, but it must be folded over several times so that it is thick enough to prevent air from seeping through it and so it will not be sucked into the wound. The occlusive dressing should extend two or more inches beyond the edge of the wound.

If blood or perspiration prevents the tape from sticking to the patient's skin, apply bulky dressings over the occlusive dressing and secure them in place with cravats. You must still monitor the patient and relieve pressure buildup if the patient develops difficulty breathing. In cases when the EMTs will not be delayed in their arrival and tape will not hold the dressing, hold the occlusive dressing in place with the palm of your gloved hand. If the patient's condition declines, periodically release one edge of the seal in order to allow trapped air to escape as described above.

If there is an entrance wound and an exit wound, both wounds will need a dressing. You may have to wait for EMT assistance to roll the patient and apply a dressing to the patient's back.

Penetrating wounds of the chest may also penetrate the heart. When this occurs, there is little that the Emergency Medical Responder can do other than provide care for shock and the open chest wound and provide basic life support as needed.

Impaled Objects

5–2.11 Describe the emergency medical care for an impaled object.

FIRST ➤ An impaled object must be left in place. Even though it created the wound, the impaled object is also sealing the wound. If it is removed, the patient may bleed profusely. The object must be stabilized with bulky dressings or pads (Figure 10.51). Begin by placing these materials on opposite sides of the object, along the vertical line (long axis) of the body. Place the next layer perpendicular (opposite direction) to the first. Use tape or cravats to hold all dressings and pads in place. If tape will not hold, carefully apply cravats according to local protocols. ▪

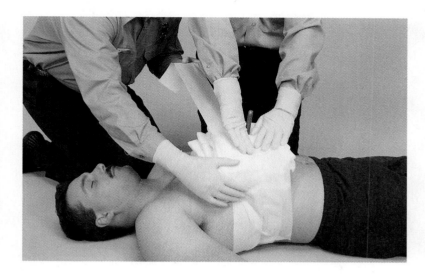

FIGURE 10.51 Never remove an object impaled in the chest. Stabilize it in place.

Abdominal Injuries

(In Chapter 4, the locations of the various body organs were presented. Before continuing with this section, study Scan 4–1, page 70, to review the locations of the major hollow and solid organs of the abdomen and pelvis.)

Internal bleeding can be severe when an internal organ is damaged. In addition, hollow organs can rupture and drain their contents into the abdominal and pelvic cavities, producing a very serious and painful reaction. As an Emergency Medical Responder, you should be aware of the following signs, which indicate injury to organs of the abdomen and pelvis:

- Any deep cut or puncture wound to the abdomen, pelvis, or lower back.
- Indications of blunt trauma to the abdomen or pelvis.
- Pain or cramps in the abdominal or pelvic region.
- Patient is protecting the abdomen (guarding).
- Patient is trying to lie still with legs drawn up.
- Rapid, shallow breathing and a rapid pulse.
- Rigid, distended, and/or tender abdomen.

FIRST ➤ To care for all possible abdominal and pelvic injuries:

1. Take appropriate BSI precautions.

2. Control all obvious external bleeding.

3. Have the patient lie on his back. For open wounds or eviscerations, flex the patient's legs and support them with pillows or a rolled blanket. Do not flex the legs if there are signs of injury to the pelvic bones, lower limbs, or back. For impaled objects, leave the legs in the position found.

4. Care for shock, administer oxygen as per local protocols, and constantly monitor vital signs.

5. Be alert for vomiting.

6. Do not touch exposed internal organs. Cover them with an occlusive dressing. Maintain warmth by placing dressings or a towel over the occlusive dressing (Figure 10.52). (Some EMS systems provide sterile materials to allow the Emergency Medical Responder to apply a moist, sterile dressing in place of the occlusive dressing. Follow local protocols.)

7. Do not remove an impaled object. Stabilize it with bulky dressings. ■

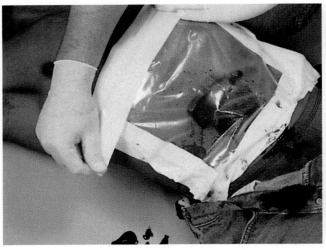
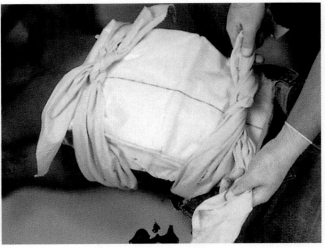

A   B

FIGURE 10.52 Emergency care of an open wound to the abdomen. **A.** Cover the wound with an occlusive dressing. **B.** Help maintain body heat by placing dressings or a towel over the occlusive dressing.

Many patients with abdominal pain find some relief by hugging a bulky, soft object such as a pillow against the abdomen.

Injury to the Genitalia

FIRST ➤ Because of the location, external reproductive organs are not common sites of injury. The pelvis and the thighs usually prevent injury to these organs, which are known as the external **genitalia**. When injury does occur, two types of soft-tissue injury are commonly seen:

- *Blunt trauma.* Such an injury is very painful, but little can be done by the Emergency Medical Responder. An ice pack, if available, can help.
- *Cuts.* Bleeding should be controlled by direct pressure. A sterile dressing or a sanitary pad should be used. If either of these is not available, then use any clean, bulky dressing. Once bleeding is controlled, the dressing can be held in place with a large triangular bandage, applied in the same manner as a diaper.

Other soft-tissue injury care procedures also apply when caring for injuries to the genitalia:

- Do not remove impaled objects.
- Save avulsed parts, wrapping them in plastic, sterile dressings, or any clean dressing. ∎

Emergency Medical Responders are a part of the professional health-care team. As such, you must carry out your role in a manner that will reduce embarrassment for the patient. Tell the patient what you are going to do. Tell him why you must examine and care for the genitalia. Protect him from the sight of onlookers by having them leave the scene. If this is not possible, have them turn their backs to the patient. Then, provide care without any hesitation. Conduct all procedures in the same manner as you would care for an injury to any other part of the body. This is essential if you are to provide proper total patient care.

Genital injury may be the result of rape. Maintain the patient's privacy, and remain professional in your conversation and care. Inform the patient not to wash, urinate, or change clothing. The patient should be transported by EMS to the emergency department. If possible, the caregiver should be of the same gender as the patient in order to lessen any fears that the patient may have.

Many genital injuries are self-inflicted or are the result of abuse. They may also be caused by an attempt to abort an unborn fetus by the mother or other unlicensed person. Whatever the cause, the patient will need emotional support and understanding.

Burns

Emergency Medical Responders should consider burns to be complex soft-tissue injuries that can range from a superficial burn to the skin's surface (epidermis) to a serious deep injury that involves nerves, blood vessels, muscles, and bones. Careful patient assessment is necessary to avoid missing injuries or medical problems that may be far more serious than obvious burns.

Classification of Burns

FIRST ➤ Burns are classified in a number of ways. One way is to categorize burns based on the agent that caused the injury (source of the burn). This information should be gathered and forwarded to more highly trained personnel during transfer of care. Categories of burns based on source include:

- *Heat (thermal) burns,* which may be caused by fire, steam, or hot objects.
- *Chemical burns,* which may be caused by caustics, such as acids and alkalis.
- *Electrical burns,* which originate from outlets, frayed wires, and faulty circuits.
- *Lightning burns,* which occur during electrical storms.
- *Light burns,* which occur with intense light. Light from the arc welder or industrial laser will damage unprotected eyes. Also, ultraviolet light (including sunlight) can burn the eyes and skin.
- *Radiation burns,* which usually result from nuclear sources. ∎

Always investigate the source of a burn carefully. The environment where the patient was burned may be hazardous and may contain hazardous materials. Talk with bystanders and the patient, in addition to performing a patient assessment. This information will assist in finding out exactly what happened to cause the injury.

FIRST ➤ Most often burns are categorized according to the depth of the burn (Figure 10.53):

- **Superficial burns** involve the top layer of skin known as the *epidermis.* Once known as *first-degree burns,* they involve reddening of the skin and pain at the site. A common example is a sunburn.

WARNING

Scenes involving chemical burns may be hazardous to emergency personnel.

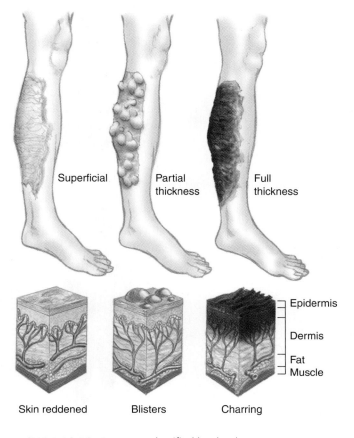

Superficial   Partial thickness   Full thickness

Epidermis
Dermis
Fat
Muscle

Skin reddened   Blisters   Charring

FIGURE 10.53 Burns are classified by depth.

superficial burn ■ a burn involving only the outer layer of skin (epidermis). Also called *first-degree burn*.

partial-thickness burn ■ a burn in which the outer layer of skin is burned through and the second layer (dermis) is damaged. Also called *second-degree burn*.

full-thickness burn ■ a burn involving all layers of skin. Muscles below the skin and bones may also be damaged. Also called *third-degree burn*.

- **Partial-thickness burns** involve both the epidermis and the dermis (the top two layers of skin). Once known as *second-degree burns*, they generally involve intense pain, white to red skin that is moist and mottled (in light-skinned patients), and blisters. A classic example is a steam burn.
- **Full-thickness burns** extend through all dermal layers and may involve subcutaneous layers, muscle, bone, or organs. Once known as *third-degree burns*, they can be dry and leathery and may appear white, dark brown, or charred. Because there is often nerve damage present, there may be little to no sensation of pain present. ■

Severity of Burns

FIRST ➤ An important aspect of care is being able to assess the severity of a burn, or extent of the damage. A superficial or partial-thickness burn that involves less than 9% of the patient's total body surface area is considered a minor burn. The exceptions are if the burn involves the respiratory system, face, hands, feet, groin, buttocks, or major joint.

Any burn to the face (other than a simple sunburn) is an example of a serious burn. Other serious burns include any superficial burns covering a large area of the body, or burns involving the feet, hands, groin, buttocks, or major joints. ■

rule of nines ■ system used to estimate the amount of skin surface burned. The body is divided into 12 regions, 11 of which are estimated as 9% each and one at 1% (the genitals).

One system used for determining the amount of skin surface burned is called the **rule of nines** (Figure 10.54). A quick reference for learning the rule of nines is to keep in mind that a patient's palm is about 1% of his or her body surface area. For example, the front of one leg equals 9% of approximately the same area that nine of the patient's palms would cover.

For adults, the head and neck, chest, abdomen, each arm, the front of each leg, the back of each leg, the upper back, and the lower back and buttocks are each considered equal to 9% of the total body surface area. This gives a total of 99%. The remaining 1% is assigned to the genital area.

For infants and children, a simple approach assigns 18% to the head and neck, 9% to each upper limb, 18% to the chest and abdomen, 18% to the entire back, 14% to each lower limb, and 1% to the genital area. This method adds up to a total of 101% but provides an easy way to make approximate determinations.

FIGURE 10.54 Rule of nines.

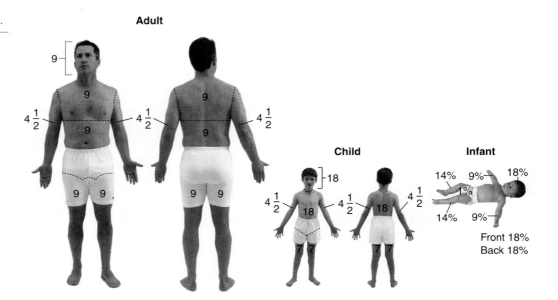

By using the rule of nines, you can add up the areas affected by burns to determine how much of the patient's body has been injured. For example, if an adult patient has full-thickness thermal burns to the chest and front of one leg, this 9% plus 9% means that 18% of the total body surface area has been burned. Note that burns often overlap different body regions. So, when in doubt, always estimate to the higher percentage.

As an Emergency Medical Responder, you may not be required to learn the rule of nines. In most situations, knowing this information will not be necessary to carry out your duties. However, the rule of nines may be useful when communicating patient information to more highly trained EMS personnel.

Rules for Emergency Medical Responders

FIRST ➤ Regardless of the system used to evaluate burns, follow these rules:

- Always perform a scene size-up, initial assessment, and provide basic life support as needed.
- Provide care for all burns, even the most minor or superficial ones.
- Any of the following partial- or full-thickness burns should be considered serious and should be evaluated by someone in the EMS system above the level of Emergency Medical Responder:
  — Burns to the hands, feet, face, groin, buttocks, thighs, and major joints.
  — Any burn that encircles a body part.
  — Burns estimated at greater than 15% of the patient's body.
  — Burns that include respiratory involvement.
- When in doubt, overclassify. For example, consider a serious superficial burn to be partial-thickness burn.
- Always consider the effects of a burn to be more serious if the patient is a child, elderly, the victim of other injuries, or someone with a medical condition (for example, respiratory disease). ▪

WARNING

Do not attempt to rescue people trapped by fire unless you have been trained to do so. The simple act of opening a door or window could cost you your life. Do not endanger yourself and risk creating more patients.

Emergency Care of Burns

FIRST ➤ For Emergency Medical Responder care of a patient with burns, take BSI precautions. Then follow these steps:

5–2.13 Describe the emergency medical care for burns.

1. Stop the burning process immediately after performing a scene size-up. This may require the patient to stop, drop, and roll to extinguish the flames. You might also have to smother the flames and wet down or remove smoldering clothing. If the patient is part of a hazmat response, he may need to be decontaminated before you can treat him. This may mean that you will have to wait until the hazmat technicians remove and decontaminate the patient so you can begin treatment. (Hazardous material responses are discussed in Chapter 15.)

2. Activate EMS and, if a burn involves the mouth, nose, throat, or airway, consider it critical. Request assistance as per local protocol.

3. Flush minor burns with cool or running water (or saline) for several minutes. For serious burns, do not flush burns with cool water unless they involve an area of less than 9% of the total body surface area. Flushing large burn areas may chill the patient and increase the risk of developing shock and infection.

4. Remove smoldering clothing and jewelry. Do not remove any clothing that is melted onto the skin.

5. Continually monitor the airway. Any burns to the face or exposure to smoke may cause airway problems. Administer oxygen as per local protocols.

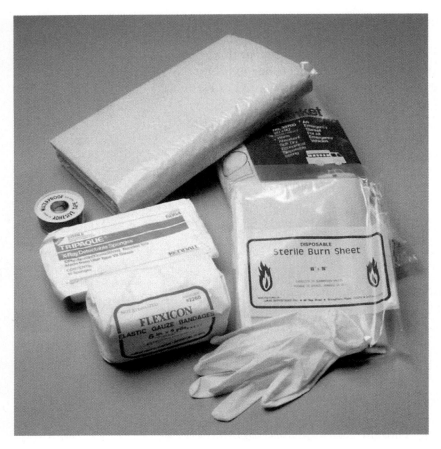

FIGURE 10.55 Emergency Medical Responder supplies for emergency care of burns.

6. Prevent further contamination. Keep the burned area clean by covering it with a dressing. Infection is common with burns.

7. Cover the burn area with dry, clean dressing (Figure 10.55). In some EMS systems, you may be instructed to moisten dressings before placing them on the patient. Otherwise, place dry, sterile dressings onto the burned area. Follow local protocols.

8. Give special care to the eyes. If the eyes or eyelids have been burned, place clean dressings or pads over them. Moisten these pads with sterile water if possible.

9. Give special care to the fingers and toes. If a serious burn involves the hands or feet, always place a clean pad between toes or fingers before completing the dressing.

10. Provide oxygen and care for shock. ▪

Thermal Burns
See Scan 10–6 for a summary of caring for thermal burns.

WARNING

Always make certain the electricity is off before entering the scene of an electrical injury.

Chemical Burns

Many chemicals are harmless if they are used properly or remain contained. However, if those chemicals come in contact with the human body, they can cause harm. Some irritate the skin and create burns very quickly. Others create a slow, painful burning process. In either case, it is crucial to stop the burning process and remove the irritant.

Scenes involving patients with chemical burns can be very dangerous. Thus, completing a scene size-up and ensuring scene safety is important. There may be a pool of dangerous chemicals near the patient. Acids may be spurting from containers. Toxic fumes may be in the air. If you believe there are hazards at the scene that will place you in danger, do not attempt a rescue unless you have been trained to do so and have the necessary equipment.

Remember that taking BSI precautions is required for every patient contact. Wear synthetic gloves and additional equipment if required by local protocol.

The primary method of caring for chemical burns is to wash away the chemical with water. A simple wetting of the burned area is not enough. Flush the area of the patient's body that has been exposed. Continue to flush the area for at least 20 minutes. Be sure to remove all contaminated clothing, shoes, socks, and jewelry from the patient during the wash.

Once you have flushed the area for at least 20 minutes, apply a dry, clean dressing, care for shock, and make sure EMS has been notified. If the patient begins to complain of increased burning or irritation once a dressing is in place, remove the dressing and flush the burned area with water for several minutes more. Then, apply a new dry dressing.

TYPE OF BURN	TISSUE BURNED			COLOR CHANGES	PAIN	BLISTERS
	Outer Layer of Skin	Second Layer of Skin	Tissues Below Skin			
Superficial	Yes	No	No	Red	Yes	No
Partial-thickness	Yes	Yes	No	Deep red	Yes	Yes
Full-thickness	Yes	Yes	Yes	Charred black or white	Yes	Yes

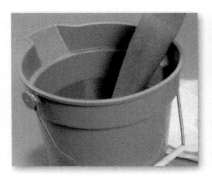
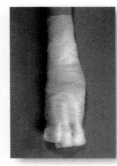

MINOR: Superficial and Partial-thickness

- Have someone alert dispatch.
- Cool the burn if possible.
- Cover entire burn with dry, clean dressing.
- Moisten dressing only if burn is less than 9% of skin surface.

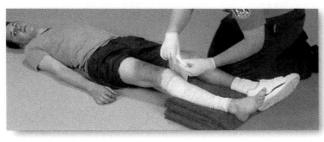

SERIOUS BURNS: Extensive Superficial, Partial-thickness, and any Full-thickness Burns

- Stop burning process.
- Have someone alert dispatch.
- Maintain open airway.
- Wrap area with dry, clean dressing.
- Provide care for shock.
- Moisten dressing only if burn is less than 9% of skin surface.

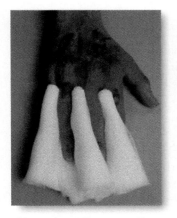
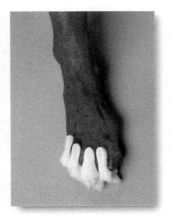

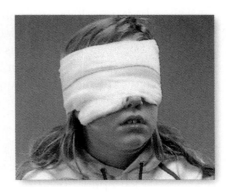

If Hands or Toes are Burned:

- Separate digits with clean gauze pads.
- When appropriate, elevate the extremity.

Burns to the Eyes:

- Do not open eyelids if burned.
- Be certain burn is thermal, not chemical.
- Apply moist, clean gauze pads to both eyes.

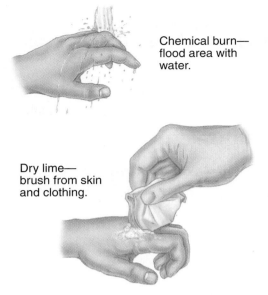

Chemical burn—
flood area with
water.

Dry lime—
brush from skin
and clothing.

FIGURE 10.56 Emergency care of chemical burns.

Activate EMS for all cases of chemical burns.

FIRST > Remember, when providing care for chemical burns:

1. Flush the burned area for at least 20 minutes. If possible and if it can be done quickly, try to identify any chemical powders before applying water. Water could cause a reaction that will produce heat and increase burning of the skin.
2. Apply a dry, clean dressing.
3. If burning continues, remove dressing and flush again. ▪

If dry lime is the agent causing the burn, *do not* begin by flushing with water. Instead, use a *dry* dressing to *brush* the substance off the patient's skin, hair, and clothing. Also have the patient remove any contaminated clothing or jewelry. Once this is done, you may flush the area with water (Figure 10.56).

Chemical burns to the eyes require immediate attention. Assume that both eyes are involved. When caring for chemical burns to the eyes, you should:

1. Perform a scene size-up, including taking appropriate BSI precautions.
2. Perform initial assessment, ensuring the patient's ABCs.
3. Immediately flood the eyes with water.
4. Keep the water flowing from a faucet, bucket, or other source into the eye. You may have to hold the eyelid open to ensure a complete washing.
5. Continue flushing for at least 20 minutes.
6. After flushing the eyes, cover both of them with moistened pads.
7. Remove the pads and flush again if the patient begins to complain about increased burning sensations or irritation.

Electrical Burns

On the scene of an electrical injury, burns are not usually the most serious problem a patient sustains. Cardiac arrest, nervous system damage, fractures, and injury to internal organs may occur with these incidents (Figure 10.57). Activate EMS for all cases involving electrical burns.

The scene of an electrical injury is often very hazardous. Make sure that the source of electricity has been turned off before caring for the victim. If the electricity is still active, do not attempt a rescue unless you have been trained to do so and have the necessary equipment.

To provide care for a patient with an electrical burn, you should:

1. Perform scene size-up, including taking appropriate BSI precautions.
2. Perform an initial assessment. Electricity passing through a patient's body will cause cardiac arrest. Even if the patient appears stable, be prepared for complications involving the airway and heart. Administer oxygen as per local protocols.
3. Evaluate the burn. Look for two burn sites—an entrance and an exit wound. The entrance wound (often the hand) is where the electricity entered the body. The exit wound is where the electricity came into contact with a ground (often a foot). The entrance wound may be small, and you may need to look very carefully for it. The exit wound may be large and obvious.

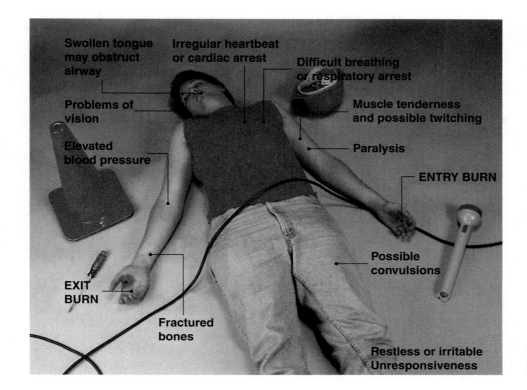

Swollen tongue
may obstruct
airway

Irregular heartbeat
or cardiac arrest

Difficult breathing
or respiratory arrest

Problems of
vision

Muscle tenderness
and possible twitching

Elevated
blood pressure

Paralysis

ENTRY BURN

EXIT
BURN

Possible
convulsions

Fractured
bones

Restless or irritable
Unresponsiveness

FIGURE 10.57 Injuries due to electrical incidents.

4. Apply dry, clean dressings to the burn sites. You may apply moistened dressings if transport is delayed, the burn involves less than 9% of the body, and the patient will not be in a cold environment.

5. Provide oxygen and care for shock.

6. Make certain EMS has been notified.

Infants and Children

The extent of burns to infants and young children can be difficult to assess because the patient may not understand why he hurts, or he may feel the pain is a punishment for something he did wrong. The pediatric patient may be unable to explain how much or exactly where the pain is.

Also, remember that children have a greater skin surface area in relation to total body size. In other words, more areas can be burned. The greater the surface area is, the greater the fluid and heat loss will be. So keep the environment warm whenever possible.

Consider the possibility of child abuse. If the burns are suspicious, do not confront the parents. Report your suspicion to local authorities.

WARNING

External burns do not reflect the true nature of an electrical injury. All such injuries require medical attention.

 FIRST ON SCENE WRAP-UP

Stephanie had just finished dressing and bandaging Randy's finger when an ambulance arrived in the parking lot with sirens blaring. Randy had regained some of his color and said the nausea was pretty much gone, but that the pain was understandably still "10 out of 10."

The EMTs thanked Bobby for activating the EMS system and Stephanie for recognizing and caring for Randy appropriately when he started to go into shock.

As the ambulance pulled out of the parking lot to transport Randy and the rest of his finger to the nearest trauma center, Stephanie took a deep breath, smiled, and walked back into the convenience store with a new bounce in her step.

Summary

Bleeding can be classified as external or internal. Both types of bleeding can range from minor to life threatening. The risk of infectious disease must be considered when caring for bleeding patients. Use the appropriate BSI precautions—including gloves, goggles, gowns, and masks—to protect yourself from infectious bodily fluids.

Bleeding may be classified as arterial, venous, or capillary bleeding. The four major techniques for controlling external bleeding are direct pressure, elevation, pressure points, and a tourniquet.

Dressings cover wounds. To control bleeding, use sterile or clean materials and cover the entire wound. Do not remove any dressing once it is in place. Occlusive dressings are used when an airtight seal is required.

Bandages hold dressings in place. Secure a bandage so that it is not too loose or too tight. It should have no loose ends. Do not cover the patient's fingertips or toes.

Internal bleeding can be very serious. Look for mechanisms of injury that can cause internal bleeding. Look for wounds associated with internal bleeding, and examine the patient for signs and symptoms of shock. Care for internal bleeding the same as you would for shock.

Shock (hypoperfusion) is the lack of perfusion to all vital organs. Unless the process is stopped, the patient will die. The symptoms of shock may include weakness, nausea, thirst, dizziness, and fear. The signs of shock may include restlessness, combativeness, profuse external bleeding, vomiting or loss of body fluids, shaking and trembling (rare), altered mental status, shallow and rapid breathing, rapid and weak pulse, pale skin (with the face often turning blue), cool and moist skin, and dilated pupils.

To care for shock, administer oxygen as per local protocols, calm and reassure the patient, keep the patient at rest, maintain an adequate airway, and maintain normal body temperature. Be sure to control external bleeding and splint injuries you suspect are major fractures. For most cases of shock, elevate the lower extremities.

Both closed and open wounds are soft-tissue injuries. Internal body organs may also be involved. Bruises (contusions) are the most common form of closed wound, while scratches and scrapes (abrasions) and cuts (lacerations and incisions) are the most common forms of open wounds. Puncture wounds are open wounds. If it is a penetrating puncture wound, it may have both an entrance and an exit wound. Avulsions occur when skin or a body part (tip of the nose, fingertip, external ear, tooth, lip) is torn loose or off the body. The cutting or tearing off of fingers, toes, hands, feet, arms, or legs is called an amputation. Crush injuries can have open or closed wounds with severe soft-

tissue damage. Internal and external bleeding is seen with these injuries.

When caring for closed wounds, assume there is internal bleeding. When providing care for open wounds, ensure personal safety, then expose the wound. Control bleeding by dressing the wound. Care for shock (hypoperfusion). Remember to provide emotional support by reassuring the patient.

For puncture wounds, assume that there are internal injuries and bleeding. Remember to look for exit wounds.

Do not remove impaled objects. Control bleeding and stabilize the object. If the object is in the cheek wall, has passed though into the mouth, and causes an airway obstruction, remove the object.

Partially avulsed skin can be placed back in its normal position. If skin is torn loose, preserve the part. Do not try to replace an avulsed eye. Do not try to replace protruding organs. In cases of avulsion, control bleeding and be prepared to care for shock.

Attempt to control bleeding from amputations with direct pressure applied to a dressing held firmly over the stump. Elevate and apply pressure point techniques if needed. Your last resort is a tourniquet.

Specific care procedures require you to remember certain rules and exceptions. For example:

- *Scalp wounds.* Do not try to clean the wound. Do not apply finger pressure if there is any chance of a skull fracture.

- *Facial wounds.* Maintain an open airway, control bleeding, and dress and bandage the wounds. If there are no skull, neck, or spine injuries, position the patient for drainage.

- *Eye wounds.*
  - Do not apply direct pressure to a cut eyeball.
  - Do not remove objects impaled in the eye. Cover with dressing pads and a rigid shield (for example, a paper cup).
  - Do not replace an eyeball pulled from its socket.
  - Do not open the eyes of a patient with burns to the eyelids.
  - Flush foreign objects from the eye.
  - Care for chemical burns by flushing the eyes for at least 20 minutes.
  - Keep the patient's eyelids closed.
  - Always cover both of the patient's eyes.

- *Ear wounds.* Do not probe into the ear. Do not pack the ear canal. For cuts and bleeding from the ear, apply a dressing and bandage. Wrap avulsed parts in plastic.

- *Nose injuries.* Maintain an open airway. Do not pack the nostrils. Control bleeding by pinching nostrils shut. Wrap avulsed parts in plastic.
- *Mouth injuries.* Maintain an open airway and position for drainage. Do not pack the mouth. Use dressings and direct pressure to control bleeding and hold the dressings in place.
- *Neck wounds.* Look for signs of neck wounds. Care for arterial bleeding with pressure dressings and venous bleeding with an occlusive dressing.
- *Open chest wounds.* Place occlusive dressings on open chest wounds. Apply and seal the dressing as per local protocol and monitor the patient for signs of pressure building up in the chest. If you see signs of pressure build up, release the seal and reseal it after the patient has exhaled.
- *Abdominal injuries.* Look for signs of abdominal injury, care for shock, and be alert for vomiting. If there are no injuries to the pelvic bones or lower limbs, flex the patient's legs to reduce pain.

- *Genitalia injuries.* Conduct an examination and provide care in a professional manner. Control bleeding by direct pressure and a pressure dressing. Save avulsed parts.

Burns can be caused by heat, chemicals, electricity, light, or radiation. They may be classified as:

- Superficial (first-degree) burns, which involve the top layer of skin known as the epidermis.
- Partial-thickness (second-degree) burns, which involve both the epidermis and the dermis (the top two layers of skin).
- Full-thickness (third-degree) burns, which extend through all dermal layers and may involve subcutaneous layers, muscle, bone, or organs.

For minor burns, flush the burned area with water (or saline) for several minutes. Do not flush major burns with water unless they involve less than 9% of the total body area. Cover with dry, sterile dressings.

Remember and Consider

Bleeding is a common occurrence. All of us at some point in our lives have suffered a scraped knee, paper cut, or perhaps a laceration to the palm from a broken glass while washing dishes. The good news is that most wounds are relatively minor and bleeding can be controlled easily. Approximately 95% of the time, direct pressure and elevation can effectively control bleeding. The bad news is that even minor bleeding can, in some cases, become serious. Never assume that a condition is minor simply based on the absence of major bleeding.

In your Emergency Medical Responder classes, you will practice bandaging wounds, controlling bleeding, and caring for patients in shock. Bandages do not have to be neat. They simply have to be functional. Think about the types of wounds you may encounter and how you will care for them.

➤ Do you have personal protective equipment readily available for use?

➤ What will you use to control bleeding?

➤ What equipment will you need to care for bleeding/shock victims?

The purpose of the initial assessment is to detect and control life-threatening problems. Go back to Chapter 7 and review the steps involved in performing an initial assessment. Relate the detection of developing shock to all stages of the patient assessment.

➤ What might you find during the initial assessment?

➤ What might you see that would indicate shock when you observe the entire patient?

➤ What will you find when taking vital signs (breathing, pulse, and skin signs)?

➤ What should you notice about a patient's eyes if he is going into shock?

➤ What information related to shock is gathered when you examine the head and face of a patient?

➤ What might have caused this patient to develop shock?

Investigate

➤ Do public places keep emergency care supplies handy for public use?

➤ Does your employer have a first aid kit stocked and ready to use?

➤ How do the contents of the kits relate to the emergency care of problems found during the initial assessment?

First aid kits vary greatly in contents. Search for kits that contain gloves, pocket face masks, barrier shields, gauze pads, and roller bandages.

➤ Did you find any supplies that you would recommend against and why?

Mishaps and injuries can happen anywhere. They often occur when you least expect them.

➤ What would you do if you encountered someone who is bleeding or in shock in a public place or at work?

➤ Are bandages or dressings available that you could use?

➤ What would you do without supplies? What plan could you have in mind in case you run into such a problem?

You might choose to carry a personal first aid kit in your car. This would allow you access to first aid supplies and BSI equipment at any time. Although some malls and shopping centers are beginning to have equipment available at a centralized location, many do not. Know where the equipment is or how to gain access to it. Be prepared to render aid at any time and any place.

Quick Quiz

1. Which one of the following is NOT a typical characteristic of arterial bleeding?
   a. Blood spurts from the wound.
   b. Blood flows steadily from the wound.
   c. The color of the blood is bright red.
   d. Blood loss is often profuse in a short period of time.

2. For each bruise the size of a patient's fist, assume a blood loss of:
   a. 2%.
   b. 4%.
   c. 10%.
   d. 20%.

3. Which one of the following procedures is usually the last resort used to control bleeding?
   a. direct pressure
   b. tourniquet
   c. elevation combined with direct pressure
   d. pressure points

4. Most cases of external bleeding may be controlled by:
   a. applying direct pressure.
   b. using a tourniquet.
   c. securing a pressure dressing.
   d. applying the closest pressure point.

5. The material placed over a wound to help control bleeding is called a(n):
   a. bandage.
   b. elastic bandage.
   c. bulky dressing.
   d. dressing.

6. When the body suffers a significant loss of blood, which type of shock is most likely to occur?
   a. anaphylactic
   b. cardiogenic
   c. hemorrhagic
   d. septic

7. The tearing loose or the tearing off of a large flap of skin is which one of the following types of wound?
   a. abrasion
   b. amputation
   c. laceration
   d. avulsion

8. The first step in caring for an open wound is to expose the wound surface. The next step is to:
   a. control bleeding.
   b. clear the wound surface.
   c. care for shock.
   d. prevent further contamination.

9. When providing care for an open injury to the cheek in which the object has entered through the skin into the mouth, ensure an open airway and:
   a. remove the impaled object.
   b. turn the patient's head to one side.
   c. dress and bandage the outside of the wound.
   d. place dressings into the mouth.

10. When providing care for an open injury to the external ear:
    a. pack the ear canal.
    b. use a cotton swab to clear the ear canal.
    c. wash out the ear canal.
    d. apply dressings and bandage in place.

11. In the case of an open chest wound, place an occlusive dressing over the open wound and then:
    a. cover it loosely with a cloth bandage.
    b. tape it on three or four sides.
    c. hold it in place with a gloved hand.
    d. pack the opening with clean gauze.

12. When caring for a patient with severe burns, you must take BSI precautions and then:
    a. stop the burning process.
    b. prevent further contamination.
    c. flush only large burn areas.
    d. remove jewelry.

13. All of the following are signs or symptoms of internal bleeding EXCEPT:

 a. increased pulse rate.
 b. decreasing blood pressure.
 c. decreasing pulse rate.
 d. pale skin color.

14. Which one of the following is the MOST appropriate care for an open abdominal injury?

 a. Pack the inside of the wound with clean dressings.
 b. Pour sterile saline over the wound.
 c. Cover the wound with a dry clean dressing.
 d. Cover the wound with an occlusive dressing.

15. Which one of the following BEST describes the appropriate care for an amputated body part?

 a. Wrap with clean gauze and place on ice.
 b. Apply a tourniquet to the exposed end of the part.
 c. Bandage the part back onto the body.
 d. Place the part in sterile water.

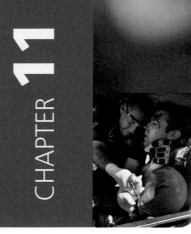

CHAPTER 11

Caring for Muscle and Bone Injuries

Bones are the foundation of the body. Like the steel girders that provide the strength and structure for buildings, bones provide the tough, internal structure and support for the demanding activities we put our bodies through on a daily basis. But unlike steel girders, bones are made of living tissue. Bones are able to move and bend by the actions of muscles and other tissues and by the messages received from a system of nerves controlled by the brain.

In your career as an Emergency Medical Responder, you will manage many patients with muscle and bone injuries. Such injuries are fairly common. To help you learn to evaluate and care for them, this chapter covers the general causes, types, and signs and symptoms of muscle and bone injuries, as well as Emergency Medical Responder care.

OBJECTIVES

This chapter is based on the objectives of the U.S. DOT's First Responder National Standard Curriculum. Note that cognitive objectives are listed below and beside corresponding text throughout the chapter. You will also notice as you read each objective that the term Emergency Medical Responder is used. This is simply a name change and reflects the new name for the First Responder.

By the end of this chapter, you should be able to (from cognitive or knowledge information):

5–3.1 Describe the function of the musculoskeletal system. (pp. 369–371)

5–3.2 Differentiate between an open and a closed painful, swollen, deformed extremity. (pp. 374–375)

5–3.3 List the emergency medical care for a patient with a painful, swollen, deformed extremity. (pp. 380–381)

5–3.4 Relate mechanism of injury to potential injuries of the head and spine. (pp. 407–408)

5–3.5 State the signs and symptoms of a potential spine injury. (pp. 413–414)

5–3.6 Describe the method of determining if a responsive patient may have a spine injury. (pp. 414–417)

5–3.7 List the signs and symptoms of injury to the head. (p. 409)

5–3.8 Describe the emergency medical care for injuries to the head.(pp. 411–412)

By the end of this chapter, you should be able to feel comfortable enough to (by changing attitudes, values, and beliefs):

5–3.9   Explain the rationale for the feelings of patients who have need for immobilization of a painful, swollen, deformed extremity. (pp. 382, 400, 411, 429)

5–3.10   Demonstrate a caring attitude toward patients with a musculoskeletal injury who request emergency medical services. (pp. 382, 400, 411, 429)

5–3.11   Place the interests of the patient with a musculoskeletal injury as the foremost consideration when making any and all patient-care decisions. (pp. 378, 403, 407–408, 416, 417, 421, 424)

5–3.12   Communicate with empathy to patients with a musculoskeletal injury, as well as with family members and friends of the patient. (pp. 382, 400, 411, 429)

By the end of this chapter, you should be able to show how to (through psychomotor skills):

5–3.13   Demonstrate the emergency medical care of a patient with a painful, swollen, deformed extremity. (pp. 380–381)

5–3.14   Demonstrate opening the airway in a patient with suspected spinal-cord injury. (pp. 411, 412, 417)

5–3.15   Demonstrate evaluating a responsive patient with a suspected spinal-cord injury. (pp. 414–417)

5–3.16   Demonstrate stabilization of the cervical spine. (pp. 417, 418)

ADDITIONAL LEARNING TASKS

This chapter explains the functions of the muscles and bones and how they are controlled by the nervous system. You will need to understand the relationship between the system of muscles and bones (musculoskeletal system) and the nervous system, and apply the knowledge you gain to the assessment and care steps that you will provide to injured patients. As you work through this chapter and meet the objectives, you will also need to keep the following information in mind and be able to perform the skills listed.

You will learn the parts of the skeleton through the pictures in this chapter and from your instructor. As you practice your assessment skills, you must be able to:

➤ Locate and name the major bones of the skeletal system.

While performing a patient assessment, you will look and feel for signs and symptoms of injured extremities. You must be able to:

➤ Describe the signs and symptoms of a suspected fracture.
➤ Describe the signs and symptoms of an injury to the muscles, tendons, and ligaments in an extremity.

You will also practice stabilizing and immobilizing injured extremities using a variety of techniques. You must be able to:

➤ List five complications related to extremity injuries.
➤ Define the term *immobilization* and state its primary purpose.
➤ Define the term *splinting* and state its purpose.

You must handle extremity injuries carefully. There are several steps to follow when you immobilize these injuries. You must be able to:

➤ State the general principles for immobilization of a musculoskeletal injury.
➤ Define manual stabilization and describe how it is applied to an extremity prior to splinting.

Sometimes the mechanism of injury is so severe that its force causes the extremity to become deformed or bent out of its normal position. You must be able to:

➤ Describe a deformed injury and the procedures for straightening a closed deformed injury.

Emergency Medical Responders may not carry much in the way of commercial splints. Injured extremities can be immobilized with a variety of rigid, semirigid, and soft items that will support and stabilize the limb. You must be able to:

➤ List objects that can be used as splints when commercial splints are not available.
➤ Perform splinting procedures on simulated patients with extremity injuries, using improvised or commercial splints.

Depending on the mechanism of injury, bones other than the extremities can also be injured. Many vital organs are protected by bones such as the skull, spine, and rib cage. This central part of the skeleton is referred to as the axial skeleton. You must be able to:

➤ List the elements of the axial skeleton and describe their functions.

Enclosed in the skull and spinal column are the brain and spinal cord, which together form the major portion of the central nervous system. You must be able to assess and recognize injury to the central nervous system by:

➤ Identifying the parts of the central nervous system and describing their functions.
➤ Describe common mechanisms of injury that can affect the function of the axial skeleton and the central nervous system.
➤ List the signs and symptoms of head, spine, and chest injuries.

Injuries can sometimes be distracting to the rescuer. Do not let the site of an injury distract you from your priorities. You must be able to:

➤ Describe the challenges of airway management for patients with head, spine, and chest injuries.
➤ Describe and demonstrate airway management techniques for patients with head and spine injuries.

Trauma patients with head injuries may be responsive or unresponsive and, depending on the mechanism of injury, may have multiple injuries. In any case, airway management and the assessment steps must be performed carefully. You must be able to:

➤ Describe and demonstrate the steps for assessing responsive and unresponsive patients for head and spine injuries.
➤ Demonstrate the emergency care procedures for a patient with open and closed head injuries.
➤ Describe and demonstrate how to stabilize and care for injuries to the head and spine.
➤ Describe and demonstrate how to stabilize and care for injuries to the chest.
➤ Describe the problems that may result from improper care to head, spine, and chest injuries.

Emergency Medical Responders often focus on the initial assessment and the care needed for life-threatening injuries, so there may not be time to begin immobilizing less critical injuries before more advanced care providers arrive on scene. Usually, EMTs will splint extremities when they arrive, but may need Emergency Medical Responders to assist them. However, Emergency Medical Responders who learn how to assess and recognize extremity injuries and who can quickly and carefully splint them after stabilizing life-threatening problems will be able to make the patient more comfortable sooner. Your ability to assess and manage trauma patients while waiting for the EMTs will also help shorten the time patients must spend on the scene.

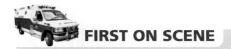

FIRST ON SCENE

Russell Sloan reached down, pushed a brightly colored golf tee into the soft ground facing the 15th fairway, and balanced his ball on it. "Okay," he said to his wife, Joan, after standing back up. "I'll bet you lunch that I get a birdie on this hole."

"You're on," she said, smiling from her seat in the golf cart. He repositioned his feet several times, drew the club back over his shoulder, and swung it in surprisingly good form, considering how the rest of his game had been going. The ball flew high and straight, moving in sharp contrast to the royal blue of the early morning sky. Joan stepped from the cart, mouth agape, and using the scorecard to shield her eyes, she followed the ball's descent to the distant green.

"Joanie! The cart!" Russell yelled, forgetting about the nearly perfect drive.

Joan turned and saw the golf cart rolling slowly backward, gaining speed as it headed for a nearby sand trap. She jogged over to it and tried to step back into the driver's seat, but just as she reached it, there was a loud snap and her right leg folded underneath her.

She fell to the ground, clutching her badly bent leg. The cart continued down the slope and overturned into the trap, sending a spray of sand up onto the dark green fairway.

Musculoskeletal System

The **musculoskeletal system** is made up of many muscles, bones, joints, connective tissues, blood vessels, and nerves. Trauma, whether minor or major, can cause a variety of injuries to the muscles, bones, and other tissues that make up the musculoskeletal system. When assessing those injuries, Emergency Medical Responders are not expected to determine whether an injury is a fractured bone, a dislocated joint, a ligament sprain, or a muscle strain. The Emergency Medical Responder's job is to carefully assess the patient, looking for signs and symptoms of injury such as pain, swelling, deformity, and discoloration. Sometimes injuries can be easily identified as fractures, dislocations, or both, simply due to the amount of deformity. However, most musculoskeletal injuries are not that obvious and often the only sign or symptom is pain.

The extremities include the many bones and joints of the arms and legs. Surrounding the bones and joints are muscles and other soft tissues such as ligaments, tendons, blood vessels, and nerves. These tissues work with the skeletal structures to nourish, support, and move those structures. Figure 11.1 shows the major blood vessels and a few of the major nerves found in the arms and legs. You do not need to remember every vessel and nerve, but you must remember that a large network of vessels and nerves are woven throughout the body. Injuries to these blood vessels and nerves can cause excessive swelling and loss of movement or function. Careful assessment and management is important for minimizing pain, further damage to vessels and nerves and blood loss. Your actions can minimize damage to the extremity and promote healing and help restore the function of the musculoskeletal system.

FIRST ➤ The musculoskeletal system has four major functions:

- *Support.* Bones support the soft tissues of the body, acting as a framework to give the body form and to provide a rigid structure for the attachment of muscles and other body parts.

musculoskeletal system ■ all the muscles, bones, joints, and related structures such as tendons and ligaments that enable the body and its parts to move and function.

REMEMBER

Medical names for bones are provided for reference. You need to remember only the common names. You will find that the medical terms become familiar as you go through the course and begin to work in the field.

5–3.1 Describe the function of the musculoskeletal system.

FIGURE 11.1 Anatomy of the extremities. (A = artery, N = nerve, V = vein)

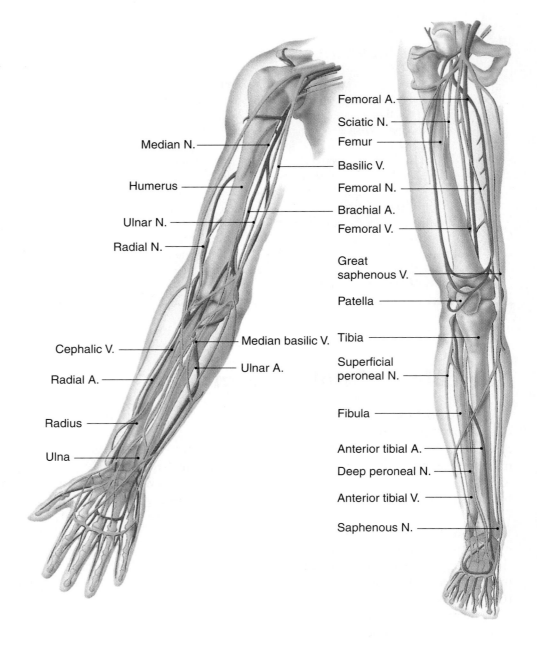

Median N.

Humerus

Ulnar N.

Radial N.

Cephalic V.

Radial A.

Radius

Ulna

Median basilic V.

Ulnar A.

Femoral A.

Sciatic N.

Femur

Basilic V.

Femoral N.

Brachial A.

Femoral V.

Great saphenous V.

Patella

Tibia

Superficial peroneal N.

Fibula

Anterior tibial A.

Deep peroneal N.

Anterior tibial V.

Saphenous N.

- *Movement.* Muscles, bones, and joints act together to allow for movement.
- *Protection.* Many of the bones in the body provide protection for vital organs: the skull protects the brain; the spine protects the spinal cord; the ribs protect the heart, lungs, liver, stomach, and spleen; and the pelvis protects the urinary bladder and internal reproductive organs.
- *Cell production.* Some bones have the special function of producing blood cells.

The bones and joints of the musculoskeletal system are what make up the **skeletal system.** Its two major divisions are the (Figure 11.2):

- **Axial skeleton.** All the bones that form the upright axis of the body, including the skull, spinal column, sternum (breastbone), and ribs, make up the axial skeleton.

skeletal system ▪ all the bones and joints of the body. The skeletal system provides body support and organ protection, enables movement, and produces blood cells.

axial (AK-si-al) skeleton ▪ bones and joints that form the center or upright axis of the body. It includes the skull, spine, breastbone, and ribs.

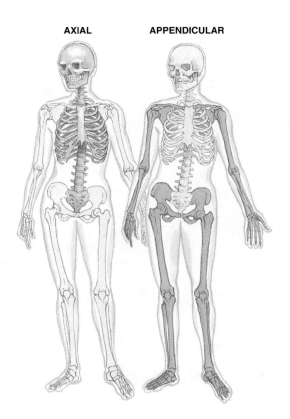

AXIAL   APPENDICULAR

FIGURE 11.2 Two major divisions of the skeletal system are the axial skeleton (see yellow on left) and the appendicular skeletal (see red on right).

- **Appendicular skeleton.** All the bones that form the upper and lower extremities, including the collarbones, shoulder blades, arms, wrists, hands, hips, legs, ankles, and feet, make up the appendicular skeleton. ■

appendicular (ap-en-DIK-u-ler) skeleton ■ bones and joints that form the upper and lower extremities.

NOTE

This chapter uses terms such as *fracture, dislocation, strain, and sprain.* This is for educational purposes only and in no way suggests that as an Emergency Medical Responder, you will be diagnosing these injuries in the field. It is not the job of an Emergency Medical Responder to diagnose an injury as a fracture, dislocation, sprain, or strain. Most of these injuries will appear to be the same. Instead, the Emergency Medical Responder should use an assessment-based approach. That is, assess the patient, identify signs and symptoms, and provide care to the patient for those signs and symptoms. For that reason, anyone with pain associated with a mechanism of injury that suggests a possible musculoskeletal injury will be cared for as though they have a fracture until proven otherwise.

Appendicular Skeleton

As stated above, the appendicular skeleton is made up of the bones that form the upper and lower extremities. The upper extremities are made up of the shoulder girdle and both arms, down to and including the fingers (Figure 11.3). Table 11–1 lists the bones of the upper extremities and the number of bones that form each structure.

The lower extremities are made up of the pelvis and both legs, down to and including the toes (Figure 11.4). Table 11–2 lists the bones of the lower extremities and the number of bones that form each structure.

FIGURE 11.3 Bones of the upper extremities.

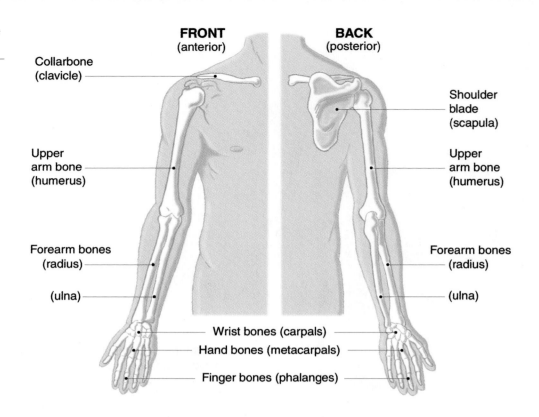

FRONT
(anterior)

BACK
(posterior)

Collarbone
(clavicle)

Shoulder
blade
(scapula)

Upper
arm bone
(humerus)

Upper
arm bone
(humerus)

Forearm bones
(radius)

Forearm bones
(radius)

(ulna)

(ulna)

Wrist bones (carpals)

Hand bones (metacarpals)

Finger bones (phalanges)

TABLE 11–1	Bones of the Upper Extremities	
COMMON NAMES	**MEDICAL NAMES**
Shoulder girdle Collarbone (1/side) Shoulder blade (1/side)	Pectoral (PEK-tor-al) Clavicle (KLAV-i-kul) Scapula (SKAP-u-lah)
Upper arm bone (1/arm, from shoulder to elbow)	Humerus (HU-mer-us)
Forearm bones (2/arm, from elbow to wrist: 1 medial and 1 lateral)	Ulna (UL-nah)-medial Radius (RAY-de-us) – lateral
Wrist bones (8/wrist)	Carpals (KAR-palz)
Hand bones (5/palm)	Metacarpals (meta-KAR-palz)
Finger bones (14/hand)	Phalanges (fah-LAN-gez)

direct force ■ a force that causes injury at the site of impact.

indirect force ■ a force that is transmitted along bones, causing injury away from the point of impact.

twisting force ■ a force that occurs when one part of an extremity remains in place while the rest moves or twists.

CAUSES OF EXTREMITY INJURIES

There are three primary forces that cause musculoskeletal injuries. They are **direct force**, **indirect force**, and **twisting force** (Figure 11.5). Extremities are often injured because of the direct force applied to a bone when a person falls and strikes an object (the edge of a step or curb) or when a person is struck by an object (the bumper of a car). Sometimes the energy of a force may be transferred up or down the extremity, which can result in an injury farther along the extremity. Such indirect force injuries can occur when one puts out the hand to break a fall and dislocates the shoulder instead of breaking the wrist.

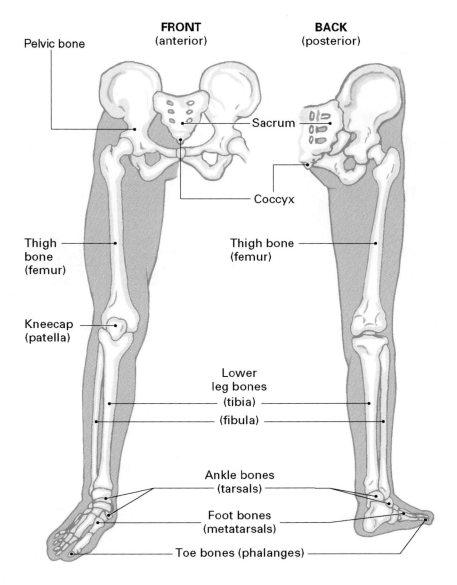

FRONT
(anterior)

BACK
(posterior)

Pelvic bone

Sacrum

Coccyx

Thigh bone (femur)

Thigh bone (femur)

Kneecap (patella)

Lower leg bones (tibia) (fibula)

Ankle bones (tarsals)

Foot bones (metatarsals)

Toe bones (phalanges)

FIGURE 11.4 Bones of the lower extremities.

TABLE 11–2	Bones of the Lower Extremities
COMMON NAMES	**MEDICAL NAMES**
Pelvic girdle (pelvis and hips)	Innominate (eh-NOM-eh-nat) or os coxae (os-KOK-se)
Thigh bone (1/leg)	Femur (FE-mer)
Kneecap (1/leg)	Patella (pah-TEL-ah)
Lower leg bones (2/leg: 1 medial and 1 lateral)	Tibia (TIB-e-ah)–medial Fibula (FIB-yo-lah)–lateral
Ankle bones (7/foot)	Tarsals (TAR-salz)
Foot bones (5/foot)	Metatarsals (meta-TAR-salz)
Toe bones (14–15/foot)	Phalanges (fah-LAN-jez)

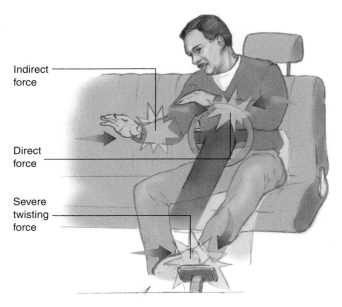

FIGURE 11.5 There are three basic types of mechanisms of injury.

Indirect force

Direct force

Severe twisting force

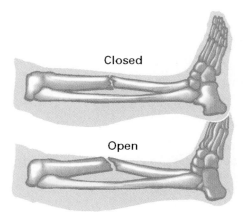

FIGURE 11.6 Closed and open musculoskeletal injuries.

Closed

Open

An example of an injury caused by a twisting force is when someone gets a hand or foot caught in a wheel or gear. The body remains stationary while the hand or foot turns in the wheel. Twisting injuries can also be caused when the body keeps moving forward while the hand or foot remains trapped.

Geriatric Focus

Aging and disease are also leading contributors to skeletal injuries. As we age, our bones can become weak and brittle, and break more easily. People with certain medical conditions such as bone cancer, kidney disease, or osteoporosis have very fragile bones and the slightest force can result in a fracture.

TYPES OF INJURIES

closed injury ■ an injury with no associated opening of the skin.

open injury ■ an injury with an associated opening of the skin. The cause of the opening may be from bone ends or fragments tearing out through the skin, a penetrating injury that has damaged a bone and surrounding soft tissue, or a shearing force that results in the tearing off of skin.

5–3.2 Differentiate between an open and a closed painful, swollen, deformed extremity.

Skeletal injuries can be categorized into one of two basic types: **closed injuries** or **open injuries** (Figure 11.6). An injury is considered closed when there is no break in the skin. In some cases, the bones and surrounding soft tissue can be damaged extensively even though the skin is unbroken.

Is It Safe ?

Scene safety is especially important at emergency scenes that involve injuries and trauma. The conditions that caused the injury for the patient may still exist even after you arrive on the scene. Pay close attention to the dispatch, and keep a close eye for both obvious and not so obvious hazards. Once you make patient contact, it will be difficult to keep an eye out for hazards. Do your best to identify and correct them before they affect you. ■

cranium (KRAY-ne-um) ▪ the bones that form the forehead and the floor, back, top, and upper sides of the skull.

An injury is considered open when the soft tissues adjacent to an injury are damaged and open. The mechanism of injury causes the bone ends or pieces of bone to tear through the skin from inside out or, in some cases, something enters and opens the skin from the outside and also breaks the bone underneath (for example, a gunshot wound).

Any strong force to the extremities can cause damage to bones and surrounding tissues (Scan 11–1). Most injuries will present with, at the very least, pain. In more severe injuries, swelling, discoloration, and deformity may also be present. Do not try to diagnose the injury as a fracture, dislocation, sprain, or strain. In most cases, the true extent of the injury cannot be determined until X-rays are taken and examined by a physician. Instead, you should assess the mechanism of injury and provide care for the injury as if it were an actual fracture.

fracture ▪ any break, crack, chip, split, or splintering of a bone.

dislocation ▪ the pulling or pushing of a bone end partially or completely free of a joint.

sprain ▪ a partial or complete tearing of a ligament.

Although you will not diagnose specific types of musculoskeletal injury, you probably should know something about each:

strain ▪ the overstretching or tearing of a muscle.

- *Fracture.* Any time a bone is broken, chipped, cracked, or splintered, it results in what is commonly referred to as a **fracture**.
- *Dislocation.* This occurs when one end of a bone that is part of a joint is pulled or pushed out of place. **Dislocations** often result in serious damage to tendons, ligaments, nerves, and blood vessels because of the way they hold a joint together or weave in and around a joint. Sometimes the force that caused a dislocation of a bone will also cause it or an adjoining bone to fracture, resulting in what is referred to as a fracture/dislocation.
- *Sprain.* The tough fibrous tissues called *ligaments* hold together the bones that make up a joint. Tendons attach muscle to bones. Excessive twisting forces can cause ligaments and tendons to stretch or tear resulting in a **sprain** injury.
- *Strain.* A **strain** is caused by overexerting, overworking, overstretching, or tearing of a muscle.

deformed injury ▪ an injury that causes a bone or joint to take on an unnatural shape or bend. Also called *angulated injury.*

sensation ▪ the ability of the skin to have feeling.

motor function ▪ the ability to move without pain or restriction.

A sign common to many serious bone injuries is angulation or deformity. **Deformed injuries** occur when an extremity is bulging, bent, or angulated where it normally should be straight. These injuries may be slight, which means that the vessels and nerves that serve the extremity will likely still be intact. In these cases, you will most likely be able to feel a distal pulse, and the patient will have normal **sensation** (able to feel your touch) and **motor function** (able to move the limb). If deformed injuries are extreme or angulated, you may not feel a distal pulse, and the patient may experience a change in sensation and/or motor function. Deformed injuries may be open or closed (Figure 11.7).

FIRST ➤ With these injuries, the signs and symptoms are typically a combination of one or more of the following: pain, swelling, discoloration, and deformity. In most cases, the emergency care that you provide as an Emergency Medical Responder will also be the same. ▪

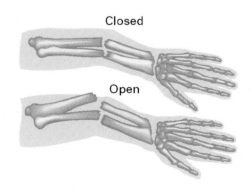

Closed

Open

FIGURE 11.7 Deformed injuries may be closed or open.

MECHANISM OF INJURY the force or forces that may have caused the patient's injury.

DIRECT FORCE energy that is transmitted directly to an extremity, causing an injury at the site of impact.

INDIRECT FORCE energy from a direct force blow that is transferred along the axis of a bone and causes an injury farther along the extremity.

TWISTING FORCE the forces caused when an extremity or part of an extremity is caught in a twisting or circular mechanism, while the rest of the extremity or the body is stationary or moving in another direction.

FORCED FLEXION OR HYPEREXTENSION
Elbow
Wrist
Fingers
Femur
Knee
Foot

DOWNWARD BLOW
Clavicle
and
Scapula

LATERAL BLOW
Clavicle
Scapula
and
Humerous

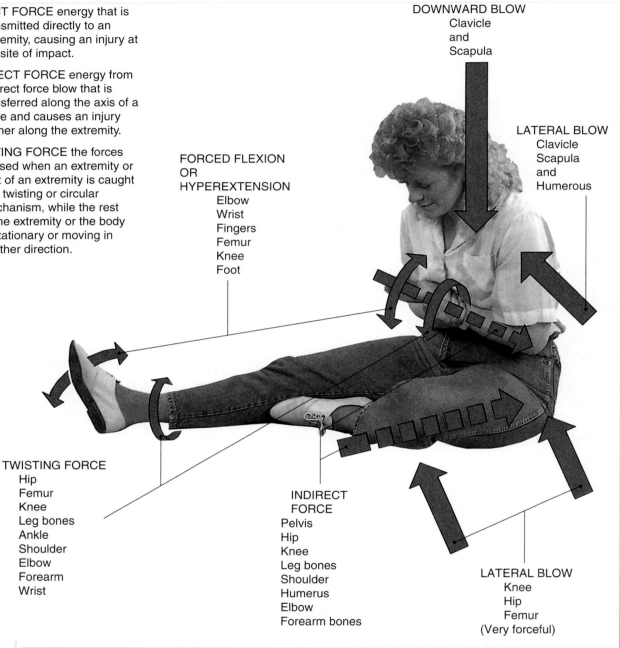

TWISTING FORCE
Hip
Femur
Knee
Leg bones
Ankle
Shoulder
Elbow
Forearm
Wrist

INDIRECT FORCE
Pelvis
Hip
Knee
Leg bones
Shoulder
Humerus
Elbow
Forearm bones

LATERAL BLOW
Knee
Hip
Femur
(Very forceful)

SIGNS AND SYMPTOMS OF EXTREMITY INJURIES

FIRST ➤ The main signs and symptoms to look for in an extremity injury include (Figure 11.8):

- *Pain.* Pain occurs when nerves surrounding the injury have been injured and are being pressed by swelling tissue or broken bone ends. Tissues near the injury site will be very tender. The patient can usually tell you where it hurts. As part of your focused assessment, gently palpate the areas above and below the injury site to help determine the extent of the pain.
- *Swelling.* The area around the injury will begin to swell because blood from ruptured blood vessels is collecting inside the tissues.
- *Discoloration.* Blood trapped under the skin may cause it to look reddish or discolored. Later, as these blood cells die, they cause the typical black-and-blue bruising, which may take 24 hours or longer to develop.
- *Deformity.* When this occurs, a part of a limb appears different in size or shape than the same part on the opposite side of the patient's body. (Always compare both arms and legs to one another.) If a bone appears to have an unusual angle, bulge, or swelling, consider this deformity to be a sign of possible fracture or dislocation. Feel gently along the patient's limbs, noting any lumps, swelling, discoloration, or ends of bones through the skin. ▪

Is It Safe ?

As an Emergency Medical Responder, you may be called on to help lift or move a patient. Doing so can put great stress on your back if you do not use good body mechanics. Use caution when lifting patients or heavy objects, and do not attempt a lift unless you have enough people to assist. Back injuries are a common cause of disability for EMS personnel. It is important to use care whenever participating in a lift. ▪

Other common signs and symptoms of an extremity injury include:

- *Inability to move a joint or limb.* Sometimes movement is possible but very painful. If the patient can move an arm but not the fingers, or if a patient can move a leg but not the toes, a fracture may have caused severe damage to

Even though most patients can tell you "where it hurts," some diabetics, spine and/or head injury patients, those with nerve damage, and patients who may be taking prescribed (or illegal) pain killers may not be able to locate or respond to pain at a suspected fracture or dislocation site.

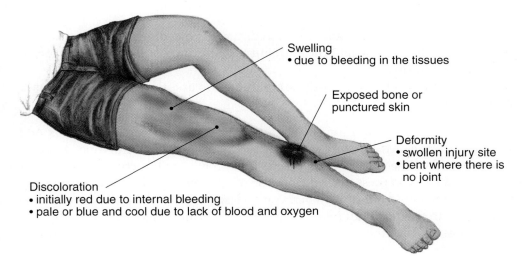

Swelling
• due to bleeding in the tissues

Exposed bone or punctured skin

Deformity
• swollen injury site
• bent where there is no joint

Discoloration
• initially red due to internal bleeding
• pale or blue and cool due to lack of blood and oxygen

FIGURE 11.8 Signs of a painful, swollen, and deformed extremity (suspected fracture).

nerves and blood vessels. The patient will often cradle, or guard, an injured arm, or hold it close to the body to stabilize it in a comfortable position. An injured person will often ask you not to touch or move the injured extremity.

- *Numbness or tingling sensation.* This can be from pressure on nerves or blood vessels caused by swelling or broken bones.
- *Loss of distal pulse.* Bone ends or bone fragments may be pressing against or cutting through an artery. Swelling from internal bleeding may be pressing against an artery. The extremity may be pale and cold because of restricted blood flow, and then turn bluish (cyanotic) because of lack of oxygen.
- *Slow capillary refill.* A decrease in perfusion may be indicated by an increase in capillary refill time.
- *Grating.* When the patient moves, the ends of fractured bones rub together, making a grating sound referred to as *crepitus* (KREP-i-tus). Do not ask a patient to move in order to confirm or reproduce this sound.
- *Sound of breaking at the time of injury.* If the patient or bystanders tell you they heard this sound, suspect a fracture has occurred.
- *Exposed bone.* In cases of open fractures, the fragments or ends of broken bones may be visible where they break through the skin.

All injured extremities should be assessed for adequate circulation, sensation, and motor function (CSM) before and after immobilization. Check circulation by assessing distal pulses and capillary refill. In the absence of a pulse, good color can be interpreted as good circulation. If necessary, compare the injured side to the uninjured side. Sensation is assessed by feeling the fingers or toes and asking if they feel tingly or numb. Determine if the patient can tell which digit you are touching without looking. Motor function can be assessed simply by the patient's ability to move the extremity. Strength testing is another way to assess motor function but may be affected by pain.

Geriatric Focus

Pain perception is often blunted in the elderly; therefore, they may not always complain of pain at the site of injury. Also, it is not uncommon for them to have referred pain. For example, they may complain of knee pain when in fact they have a broken hip. Thus, it is important to examine the entire extremity of the elderly patient to determine more precisely what is injured.

Several important signs will tell you the state of circulation to the extremity. They are:

- If the injury site is swollen and discolored, there is bleeding in the tissues.
- If there is no distal pulse and the extremity is pale and cool, there is lack of adequate blood flow.
- If the extremity is blue, there is lack of circulation and thus a lack of oxygen in the limb.

Another assessment tool for checking the circulation or perfusion status of a distal extremity is called *capillary refill time.* To assess capillary refill time, press the nail bed or pad of the finger or toe on the injured extremity between your finger and thumb. When you press, the finger or toe turns white, or blanches, because you have pressed the blood out of it. When you release pressure, the blood should flow back into the area in less than two seconds. If it takes more than two seconds, then you must suspect that there is pressure on or damage to a blood vessel and that circulation is restricted in the extremity or that there is significant blood loss in the circulatory system. This procedure is more reliable in children than it is in adults. Blood flow return time is also affected by temperature extremes of the environment. A very cold or hot environment may make the results of the capillary refill test unreliable.

While you are checking distal pulses, you can also check sensation (feeling) and motor function (ability to move). Ask the patient to tell you if he can feel your touch and where you are touching. You can also ask the patient to try to move the fingers or grasp your hand. For the foot, ask the patient to wiggle toes or press a foot against your hand. When assessing motor function of the extremity by having the patient grasp or push against your hands, be sure to assess both extremities simultaneously. This will allow for a more accurate assessment of strength between the injured and uninjured side.

Checking for sensation and motor function gives you information about the status of the nerves that supply the injured extremity. A lack of feeling or the inability to move may indicate that there is pressure on or damage to a nerve. This nerve damage may be the result of injury to the spinal cord and not just an injury to the extremity. (More later about the signs and symptoms of spine injury and the precautions to take when managing a spine-injured patient.)

TOTAL PATIENT CARE

In the scene size-up, quickly determine scene safety, take BSI precautions, and don all personal protective equipment. Note the mechanism of injury and the total number of patients. Then determine what additional assistance you may need. If the mechanism of injury suggests a possible spine injury and the scene is safe to enter, immediately stabilize your patient's head and neck.

During your initial assessment, get an impression of the environment and the patient, and determine how quickly the patient needs to be moved and transported. Do not focus on obvious injuries. Instead, assess mental status, then the ABCs. Look for and control all major bleeding. Detect and correct life-threatening problems as quickly as possible.

There is a certain order to caring for injuries. After correcting and stabilizing life-threatening injuries to the ABCs, checking for and stabilizing neck and spine injuries, and providing care for shock, then you can focus on extremity injuries. Always be sure to note the mechanism of injury because this will give you an idea of the possible extent, type, and location of the injury site.

In the order of care for skeletal injuries, first priority is given to possible injury to the spine. Next is care for possible injuries to the following:

- Skull, because it protects the brain and contains a portion of the airway.
- Rib cage, because it protects the heart and lungs and broken sections may damage the function of these organs as well as prevent adequate breathing.
- Pelvis, because it protects reproductive and urinary organs and major nerves and blood vessels.

FIRST ON SCENE

"Don't touch it, Russell. Don't touch it!" Joan shouted as he tried to gently straighten her deformed leg. It was already beginning to swell and grow purple deep below the skin, halfway between her knee and ankle.

"Listen, Joanie," Russell said, trying to maintain eye contact. "I can't feel a pulse in your foot, so I have to try to straighten your leg. It's going to hurt, but I've got to do it."

"Is everything okay?" A course groundskeeper pulled up in an electric cart stacked high with plastic bags full of freshly cut grass. At the sight of Joan's leg, he immediately grew pale and looked away.

"Can you please go call 9-1-1, and then come back and tell me what they said?" Russell asked. The man nodded, still looking away, and sped off across the fairway.

REMEMBER

Medical direction may allow you to reposition an extremity if there is no distal pulse. Follow local protocol.

- Thigh, because it takes major trauma to injure the largest, sturdiest bone (femur) in the body, which is surrounded by major nerves and blood vessels. Blood loss can be life threatening.
- Any extremity injury where no distal pulse is detected during the initial assessment.
- Injuries to the arm, lower leg, and individual ribs are considered and managed last.

Take note of the mechanism of injury, and be concerned with major bleeding and possible shock whenever there are injuries to the chest, pelvis, and thigh. A significant amount of blood can be lost internally in these areas. Monitor the patient's signs and symptoms carefully. A rapid, weak pulse, pale or blue skin color, an altered mental status, and cold extremities are signs and symptoms that should alert you to manage and transport this patient as soon as possible.

Remember the following emergency care steps when caring for a patient with musculoskeletal injuries (Figure 11.9):

5–3.3 List the emergency medical care for a patient with a painful, swollen, deformed extremity.

1. Always perform an initial assessment before focusing on a particular injury.
   - Manage life-threatening problems first.
   - Prioritize and manage other injuries second.
2. Carefully cut away clothing to expose the injury site. Control bleeding if there is an open wound. Check for distal circulation, sensation, and motor function.
3. Immobilize the extremity using manual stabilization or splints if available.
   - Immobilize the suspected fracture site.
   - Immobilize the joints above and below the suspected fracture site. Use a sling and swathe for an arm to keep it elevated across the chest. Splinted, immobilized legs may be propped up on a folded blanket or pillow if there is no indication of spine injury.
   - Recheck distal circulation, sensation, and motor function often.
4. Apply a cold pack to the injury site to help reduce the pain and swelling. Never put a cold pack directly on the skin. Wrap it in gauze or a towel first. Then place it gently over the injury site. If the patient experiences pain from this extra pressure on the injury, place the cold pack just above the site.

Care of Musculoskeletal Injuries

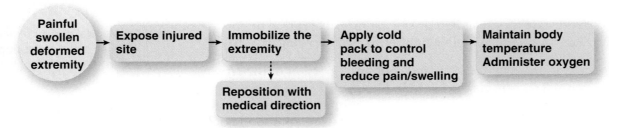

FIGURE 11.9 Algorithm for emergency care of patients with musculoskeletal injuries.

5. Administer oxygen as soon as possible as per local protocol.
6. Assess the patient's vital signs. Maintain a comfortable body temperature to help minimize the effects of developing shock.

Emotional support is important when caring for a patient with injuries. Tell the patient what you suspect may be wrong, how you will manage it, and what will be done by other emergency care providers on scene and at the hospital. You may need to remind the patient that fractures can be set at the hospital and bones will heal. Talking with the patient helps give him confidence and relieve anxiety. It may also help lower blood pressure, pulse rate, and breathing rate.

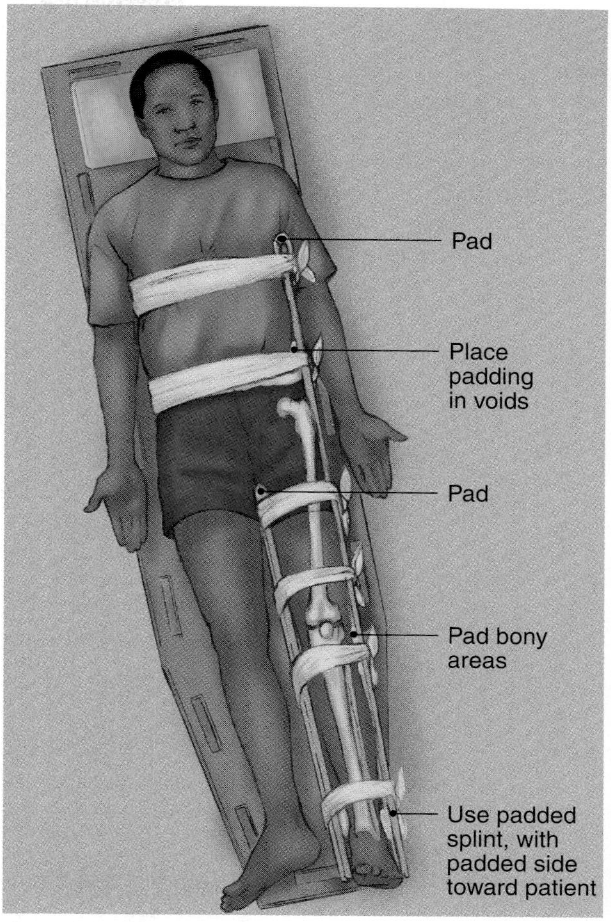

Splinting

FIRST ➤ **Splinting** is the process of immobilizing an injury using a device such as a piece of wood, cardboard, or folded blanket (Figure 11.10). Any object that can be used to restrict the movement of an injury is called a splint.

Manual stabilization is the process of restricting the movement of an injured person or body part. You can manually stabilize an injury simply by holding the part still with your hands. ■

Pad

Place padding in voids

Pad

Pad bony areas

Use padded splint, with padded side toward patient

FIGURE 11.10 Splinting immobilizes injured extremities.

WHY SPLINT?

FIRST ➤ The application of splints allows emergency care providers to reposition and transfer the patient while minimizing movement of the injury. Damage to soft tissues can cause complications and prolong recovery (Figure 11.11). Complications include:

splinting ■ applying a device that will immobilize an injured extremity.

manual stabilization ■ restricting the movement of an injured person or body part with your hands.

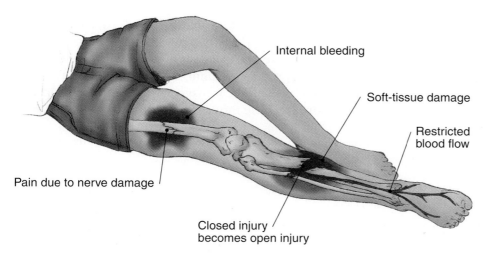

Internal bleeding

Soft-tissue damage

Restricted blood flow

Pain due to nerve damage

Closed injury becomes open injury

FIGURE 11.11 Complications associated with extremity injuries can be prevented or decreased with splinting.

REMEMBER

You cannot learn splinting without proper instruction and supervised practice. You must be trained by a qualified instructor, and you must practice splinting procedures under the guidance of that instructor.

REMEMBER

Never delay the transport of a patient with life-threatening injuries in order to splint an injured extremity.

- *Pain.* A splint can reduce much of the patient's pain because it secures the broken or dislocated bones in place and prevents them from compressing or damaging surrounding nerves and tissues.
- *Damage to soft tissues.* The movement of an injured extremity may cause blood vessels, nerves, and muscles to be crushed, ruptured, pinched, or compressed. Splinting reduces movement of the injured part; the possibility of further damage to soft tissues; and the accompanying pain, internal bleeding, and swelling.
- *Bleeding.* The initial force of injury may have caused bone ends to damage soft tissues and blood vessels. Splinting will stabilize the injury and apply a steady pressure that can reduce and control bleeding.
- *Restricted blood flow.* Dislocated joints and fractured bones and fragments also can press against blood vessels and shut off blood flow. Splinting can help relieve the pressure against blood vessels.
- *Closed injuries become open injuries.* The sharp edge of a broken bone can rip through skin to produce an open wound. Immobilizing the injured extremity by splinting it will minimize movement of the broken part and help prevent a closed wound from becoming an open wound. ▪

Geriatric Focus

Although padding is always important when splinting, it is particularly important for the elderly patient. Pressure from a hard splint could interrupt blood supply to the skin or limb and result in long-term problems well after the simple injury is healed. Be sure to add extra padding to any splint applied to an elderly patient.

EMERGENCY MEDICAL RESPONDER RESPONSIBILITIES

The primary duties of an Emergency Medical Responder are to detect and control life-threatening problems. Then, during patient assessment, attempt to find all injuries and care for the worst ones first. Most bleeding is controlled by direct pressure and elevation. Suspected fractures are cared for after neck and spine injuries, which you must stabilize. Shock is managed by administering oxygen and maintaining body temperature. In the case of major trauma, EMTs will likely arrive before you have an opportunity to apply splints.

Some patients may have indications of neck or spine injuries, and you will not be able to splint extremities until you have additional help and equipment from more advanced providers. In the meantime, this patient must not be moved but should be kept still while you stabilize his head and neck with your hands (explained later in this chapter). The process of splinting may cause you to move the patient or the injured limb, but even slight movements, without appropriate help to stabilize the body and coordinate the move, could worsen a spine injury.

FIRST ➤ For all cases involving injured extremities, alert dispatch so you may receive the appropriate assistance from EMTs. ▪

RULES FOR SPLINTING

For all cases of splinting, you will (Scan 11–2):

- Assess and reassure the patient, and explain what you plan to do.
- Splint injuries before moving the patient. Move the patient before splinting only if another injury or the environment is life threatening.

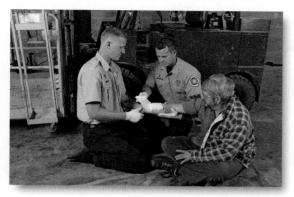

1 ■ After controlling bleeding, dress and bandage open wounds to the injured extremity.

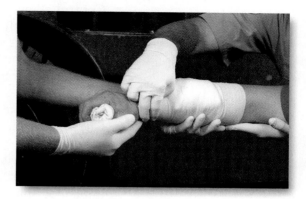

2 ■ Check distal circulation, sensation, and motor function before splinting.

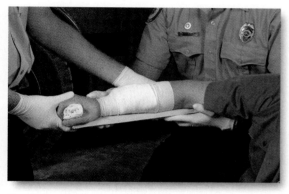

3 ■ Select an appropriate size splint for the injury and pad the splint thoroughly.

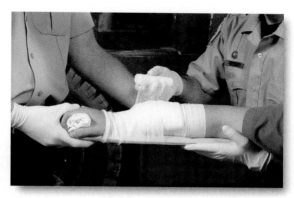

4 ■ Firmly secure the splint, leaving fingertips (or toes) exposed so you can monitor circulation.

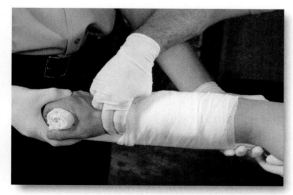

5 ■ After immobilization, reassess distal circulation, sensation, and motor function.

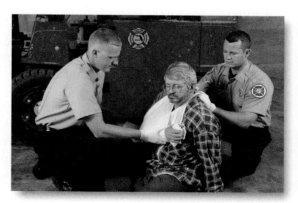

6 ■ Elevate the extremity. For an arm, use the sling to immobilize it against the chest. For a leg, prop it on a pillow or rolled blanket (if there is no indication of spine injury).

- Expose the injury site. Cut away clothing if it cannot be easily removed or folded back. Remove jewelry from the injured limb if it can be done without using force, causing pain, or repositioning the patient or the limb.
- Control all major bleeding. If necessary, use fingertip pressure. Avoid applying pressure directly over exposed bone ends. To control major bleeding, use bulky dressings secured snugly with a bandage.
- Dress open wounds. Do not push bone ends back into the wound. Do not try to pick bone fragments from the wound. If the bone ends withdraw into the wound as you care for it, report this to personnel who take over patient care so they can take steps to prevent infection in the patient.
- Check distal circulation, sensation, and motor function before and after splinting.
- Have all materials ready and at hand before splinting. Use padded splints for patient comfort and improved contact between limb and splint. Wrap unpadded splints in dressings before applying them.
- If distal circulation is absent and local protocols allow, gently attempt to realign an angulated limb in the anatomical position before splinting. Attempt to reposition the limb to regain a pulse if the limb is cold, blue, and has no pulse.
- Apply gentle manual traction (see next section), and secure the splint firmly but do not restrict circulation. Do not intentionally allow a protruding bone to re-enter the skin.
- Immobilize the suspected fracture site and the joints above and below the injury site. Secure upper extremities to the torso with a sling and swathe. Secure lower extremities to each other and assist the EMTs in transferring the patient to a spine board or similar device.
- Secure splints with cravats or roller gauze, starting at the distal end of the extremity. Leave fingertips and toes exposed so you can monitor circulation, sensation, and motor function.
- Elevate the extremity. For an arm, use a sling and swathe. For a leg, prop it on a pillow or rolled blanket if there is no indication of spine injury. Otherwise, leave the patient lying flat (supine).
- Minimize the effects of developing shock by providing oxygen as soon as possible and maintaining body temperature.

APPLYING MANUAL TRACTION

manual traction ▪ process of drawing or pulling; a stabilizing procedure that precedes the application of a splint.

FIRST ➤ The effects of splinting may be improved if you apply gentle traction to the injured extremity during the splinting process. In Emergency Medical Responder care, this traction is applied by pulling gently on the injured limb. This is called **manual traction**, which helps stabilize the injury. ▪

REMEMBER

Not all EMS systems allow Emergency Medical Responders to apply manual traction. You may only be allowed to gently reposition a limb to allow for the application of a splint. Your instructor will inform you of local guidelines.

Most EMS systems do not allow Emergency Medical Responders to straighten deformed injuries. Do only what you have been trained to do and what is allowed in your EMS system. Check your local protocols to find out what you are allowed to do if there is angulation or no distal circulation. If you find no distal pulse, and the skin in the distal extremity is pale or blue and cold, take action immediately. Notify dispatch, the responding EMTs, or the hospital and let them know the patient's status. You may be directed to gently align the limb in an attempt to restore a distal pulse. Do not force the limb if you meet resistance or if the patient complains of too much pain. Apply a soft splint and elevate the limb by propping it on a blanket roll or pillow. Provide oxygen and other appropriate emergency care interventions until the EMTs arrive.

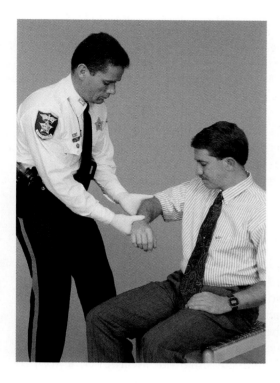

FIGURE 11.12 Manual traction of an injured limb.

When you start to apply manual traction, it may cause a temporary increase in pain for the patient. Explain this to him, but also explain that the pain caused by the injury will probably lessen once the traction and the splint are applied.

Do not release manual traction to apply a splint. Traction is of little use if it is not maintained. So, it usually takes two people to properly apply a splint: one to hold and maintain manual traction, while the other applies the splint. If you are the only trained EMS provider on scene, you may be able to direct a bystander to secure a splint while you maintain traction. (Follow local protocol.) If you are working alone, do not try to apply traction unless distal circulation is absent. Once you apply manual traction, you must maintain it until the extremity is secured to a splint.

To apply manual traction, you must (Figure 11.12):

1. Grasp the patient's limb by placing one hand above the injury site and the other hand below the injury site. Position your hands so that the splint can be applied without having to release manual traction.

2. Gently apply steady tension by pulling with your lower hand. The direction of pull should be along the long axis of the limb. If you feel resistance, stop the procedure.

3 Maintain manual traction throughout the splinting process. A **rigid splint** will maintain traction after it is secured to the patient.

STRAIGHTENING DEFORMED INJURIES

The main reason for straightening closed deformed injuries is to improve circulation. Straight limbs also make it easier for you to apply a rigid splint. If the limb cannot be straightened or if you are not allowed to straighten it, immobilize the limb in the position found. The procedure for straightening closed deformed injuries is the same as for applying manual traction:

- Attempt to straighten closed deformed injuries if there is no distal circulation.
- Make only one attempt to straighten the angulation.
- Stop if you meet resistance or if the patient complains of severe pain.

WARNING

Do not apply manual traction if the injury involves a joint. All extremity injuries that may be dislocations must be splinted in the position in which they are found. Remember, moving dislocated bones may cause further damage to surrounding tissues.

rigid splint ■ a stiff device made of a material with little flexibility (such as metal, plastic, or wood) that is long enough to immobilize an extremity and the joints above and below the injury site.

WARNING

Do only what your training and local protocols allow when caring for patients with deformed injuries.

soft splint ▪ a device, such as a sling and swathe or a pillow secured with cravats, that can be applied to immobilize a painful extremity.

triangular bandage ▪ a piece of triangular cloth material about 50 to 60 inches long at its base and 36 to 40 inches long on each side. It can be folded and used as a sling, a swathe, or a cravat.

sling ▪ a large triangular bandage or other cloth device that is applied as a soft splint to immobilize possible injuries to the shoulder girdle and upper extremity.

swathe ▪ a large cravat, usually made of cloth, used to secure a sling or rigid splint and sling to the body.

cravat ▪ a triangular bandage that is folded to a width of three or four inches and used to tie soft or rigid splints in place.

REMEMBER

As in all emergency care, providing emotional support to the patient is a significant part of total patient care.

Some jurisdictions only allow for straightening angulated injuries under certain conditions or for certain extremities. Always follow your local protocols.

TYPES OF SPLINTS

Soft Splints

There are two main types of splints: soft and rigid. When properly applied, **soft splints** such as pillows, blankets, towels, cravats, and dressings may be used to stabilize injuries. Soft splints can provide support to an injury and help decrease pain and swelling. A commonly used soft splint is the **triangular bandage**. It can be folded to any width to fit any part of the body, to secure arms to the torso and legs to each other, or to secure extremities to rigid splints. A triangular bandage is frequently used for a sling and swathe.

A **sling** is a triangular bandage used to stabilize the elbow and arm. A properly placed sling will adequately immobilize an injured elbow and provide support to the lower arm. Once the arm is placed in a sling, a **swathe** is used to hold the arm against the side of the chest and restrict movement of the shoulder. A swathe is made from a triangular bandage, which is folded to about a two-inch by four-inch width so it fits the area of the arm between the shoulder and elbow. (A triangular bandage folded to a width of three or four inches and used to tie soft or rigid splints in place is called a **cravat**.) Together, the sling and swathe work well to immobilize both the elbow and shoulder joints, which is necessary when caring for suspected fractures of the arm.

The sling and swathe are effective for injuries to the shoulder; upper arm; elbow; lower arm; wrist, hand, and fingers; and ribs. To make and apply a sling and swathe, you should (Scan 11–3):

1. Use a commercial sling, or make one from a piece of cloth or sheet. Fold or cut this material so that it is in the shape of a triangle. The ideal sling should be about 50 to 60 inches long at its base and 36 to 40 inches long on each of its sides.

2. Position the triangular material over the patient's chest. The peak of the triangle should point toward the patient's injured arm and extend beyond the elbow. The long end should be draped over the opposite shoulder. Have the patient position his arm so the hand is above the elbow. If he cannot hold his arm, have your partner or a bystander support the arm while you prepare and secure the sling.

3. Take the bottom end of the triangle and bring it up and over the patient's arm and shoulder on the injured side.

4. Draw up on the ends of the sling so that the patient's hand on the injured side is about four inches above the elbow. Tie the two ends together and be sure to position the knot so it does not rest on the back of the patient's neck. Place a flat layer of cloth (gauze pads or handkerchief) under the knot for comfort. Leave the patient's fingertips exposed so you can check for circulation, sensation, and motor function. If circulation is absent following immobilization, support the arm while the sling is removed and gently reposition it until you can feel the pulse. (Follow local protocols.) Replace the sling.

5. Take the point of the sling at the patient's elbow and fold it forward. Then tuck it in or pin it in place, or twist and tie the point. (It may be easier to tie the knot before the sling is placed on the patient.) This will form a pocket for the patient's elbow.

6. Take a second piece of triangular cloth and fold it to a two- or four-inch width. Center the widest part on the patient's injured arm. Take one end across the

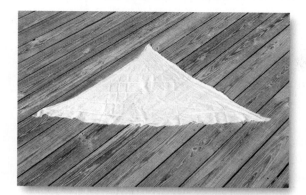

1 ■ A sling and swathe starts with a triangular bandage 50 inches at its base and about 36 inches on each side. Fold it to any width.

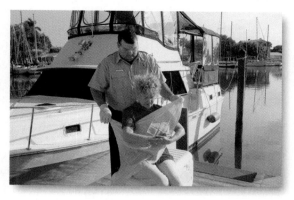

2 ■ After assessing circulation, sensation, and motor function, position the longest side of the bandage over the chest while holding on to the point and one corner.

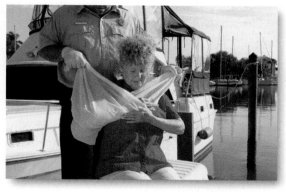

3 ■ Bring the bottom end up and over the patient's injured arm. Keep the hand elevated above the elbow.

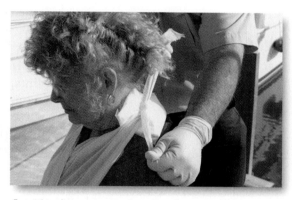

4 ■ Tie the two ends together. Pad the knot and make sure it does not rest on the patient's neck. Reassess circulation, sensation, and motor function.

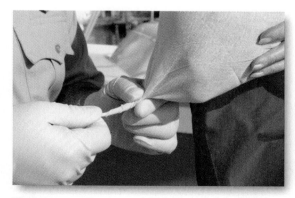

5 ■ Secure the point of the sling to form a pocket for the elbow.

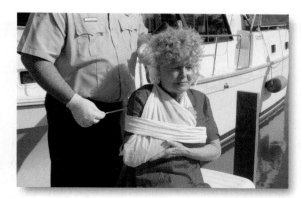

6 ■ Fold another triangular piece of material to form a swathe. Tie it around the patient to support the arm and to maintain elevation.

patient's back and one end across the chest and tie on the opposite side under the other arm. Be sure that the swathe is placed as low over the injured arm as possible. This will ensure that it stays close to the body and minimize movement of the shoulder.

Rigid Splints

Rigid splints can be made of plastic, metal, wood, or compressed cardboard and have very little give or flexibility. They are applied along an injured extremity to immobilize the suspected fracture site and sometimes the joints directly above and below the injury site.

Commercial Splints

A wide variety of commercial splints are available for emergency care. These splints are made of wood, aluminum, cardboard, foam, wire, or plastic. Some come with their own washable pads. Others require padding to be applied before being secured. Most splints are either solid rigid pieces or inflatable plastic splints. Figure 11.13 shows some of the commercially available splints. These include air splints, vacuum splints, board-and-wire ladder splints, heavy-duty cardboard splints, and flexible aluminum splints. All EMTs and many Emergency Medical Responders carry traction splints for splinting and stabilizing injuries to the femur.

Local protocols may provide guidelines for using a pneumatic antishock garment (PASG), a special device for suspected pelvic and femur fractures. You must receive training and use the PASG only as allowed by local protocols.

Inflatable Splints

Inflatable splints, or air splints, are not carried by all Emergency Medical Responder units. If you carry them and your jurisdiction allows you to use them, your instructor will teach you their application. Typically, air splints are used for patients with injuries to the arm or lower leg bones. When using an air splint, slip it uninflated over your forearm. Then grasp the patient's hand or foot and pull gentle traction while you slip the air splint onto the patient's limb. Smooth out the splint and inflate it. The splint is fully inflated and effective when you can make a slight surface indentation with your fingertip (Scan 11–4).

After inflating the splint, you must monitor the limb for changes in circulation, sensation, and motor function. Monitor the splint for changes in pressure. If the patient is moved to a warmer or colder location, the air in the splint

FIGURE 11.13 There are many types and sizes of commercial splints.

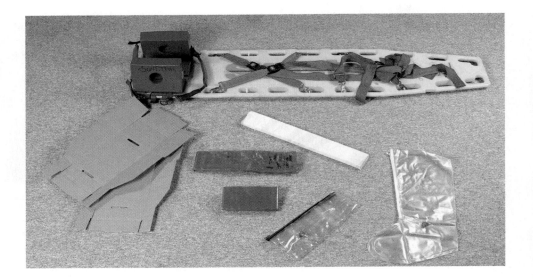

WARNING: Air splints may leak. When applied in cold weather, an air splint will expand when the patient is moved to a warmer place. Pressure also will change at different altitudes. Monitor the pressure in the splint by pressing with your fingertip. These splints may stick to the patient's skin in hot weather.

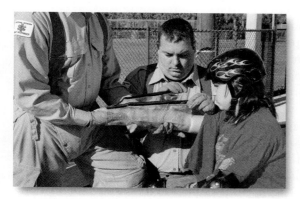

1 ■ Partially inflate the splint and slide it over the patient's extremity. Allow the fingers or toes to remain exposed at the end of the splint.

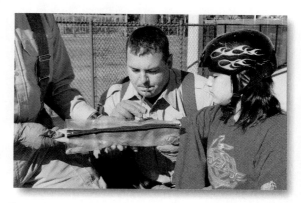

2 ■ Maintain manual stabilization of the extremity while your partner inflates the splint. Inflate so that you leave a slight dent when the splint is pressed with one finger.

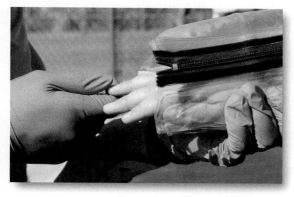

3 ■ Reassess circulation, sensation, and motor function, and monitor the pressure of the splint. Add air if necessary.

will expand or contract with the temperature change. You will have to recheck the pressure in the splint. You may have to remove increased pressure by deflating the splint slightly. The pressure in the splint also will change if the patient is moved to a different altitude. Always monitor the pressure in the splint. Periodically, check the condition of all air splints because old ones may develop leaks.

Once an air splint is applied, you may not be able to assess distal pulse. Instead, evaluate capillary refill (more reliable in pediatric patients), skin color, sensation, and motor function. The problems with air splints—the inability to check distal pulse and the potential pressure changes—have led some EMS systems to drop them from their approved equipment lists.

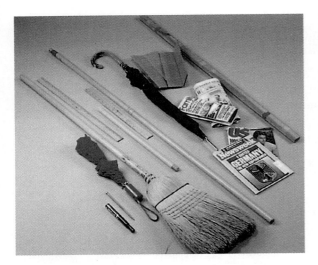

FIGURE 11.14 Improvised splints may be made from a variety of materials.

Improvised Splints

Emergency Medical Responders may arrive at the scene of an emergency without any splints, or they may use their supply of splints on one patient and have none for another patient. It is helpful to know how to make splints from materials found at the scene. Such an improvised splint may be soft or rigid and may be made from a variety of materials.

FIRST ➤ Rigid splints can be made from pieces of lumber, plywood, compressed wood products, cardboard, rolled newspapers or magazines, umbrellas, canes, broom or shovel handles, sporting equipment (shin guards are an example), and tongue depressors for fingers (Figure 11.14). Soft splints can be made from towels, blankets, pillows, and bulky clothing such as sweaters and sweat suits. Most of these items can be found at the scene of a typical incident. Many people carry some of these items in their cars. Ask people at the scene to help you find these items. Give them suggestions and ask if they have any ideas. ■

WARNING

Always wear protective gloves when providing care for extremity injuries. Face and eye shields may be necessary if injuries are spurting blood.

Management of Specific Extremity Injuries

FIRST ➤ In general, when the mechanism of injury and the patient's signs and symptoms indicate possible injuries that require splints:

- Apply rigid splints for injuries to the forearm and the lower leg. Rigid splints may be used for injuries to the thigh, but traction splints are more effective. Follow local protocol.
- Use soft splints (blanket, towel, pillow, sling and swathe) if rigid splints are not available (Figure 11.15). Provide further rigid support by securing upper extremities to the torso with a swathe and lower extremities to each other with cravats.
- Use soft or rigid splints for injuries to the arm, elbow, wrist, or hand.
- Use soft splints for injuries to the ankle or foot. ■

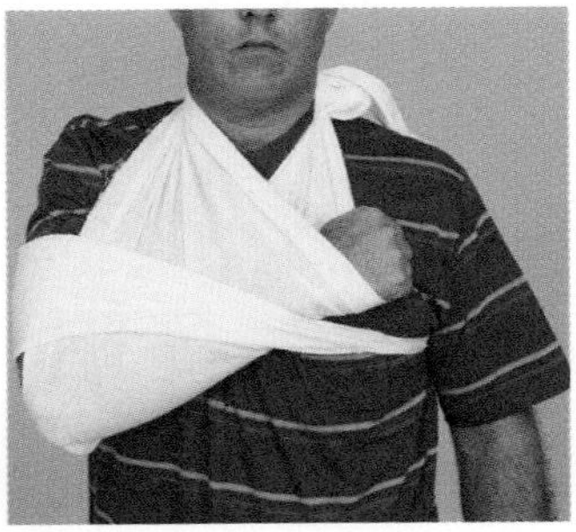

FIGURE 11.15 Sling and swathe.

Is It Safe?

If performed correctly, the application of splints will provide great comfort to the patient. However, an ill-fitting splint or a sloppy splinting job can cause great pain and discomfort for the patient. Be sure to practice your splinting skills regularly so that they will be fresh and ready when you need them. ■

For an algorithm of assessment and care of patients with specific extremity injuries, see Figure 11.16.

UPPER EXTREMITY INJURIES

Methods for splinting each type of upper extremity injury are summarized in Scan 11–5. For injuries to the upper extremities, be sure to place the hand in a **position of function**, in which the fingers are slightly flexed and the wrist is cocked slightly upward. The position of function is a normal and comfortable position for the

position of function ■ the natural position of the body part, specifically the hand or foot. In the case of the hand, the natural position is slightly flexed. In the case of the foot, the natural position is slightly extended.

Musculoskeletal Injuries to the Extremities

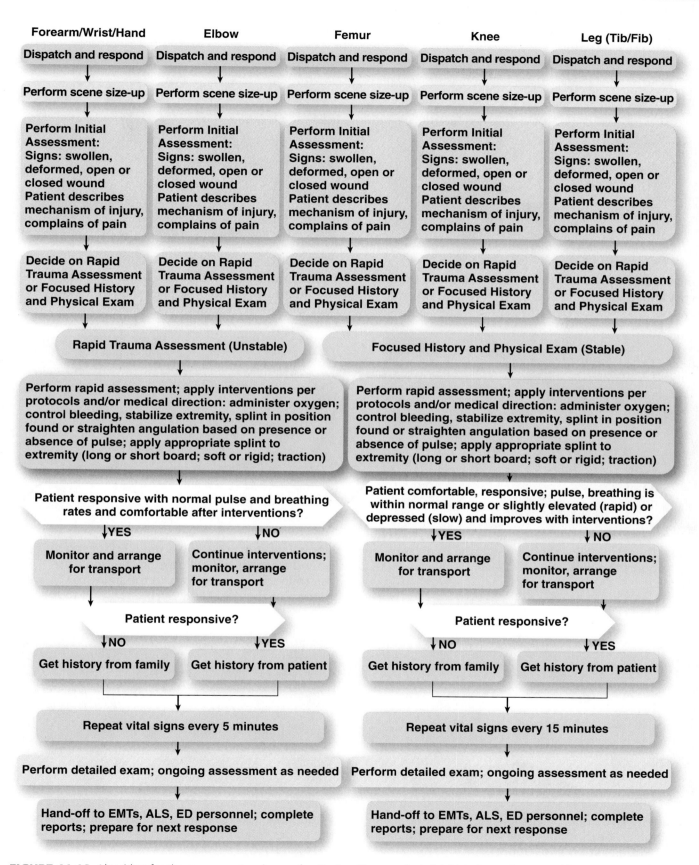

FIGURE 11.16 Algorithm for the assessment and care of patients with musculoskeletal injuries to the extremities.

NOTE: Place a roll of dressing in the hand to maintain position of function.

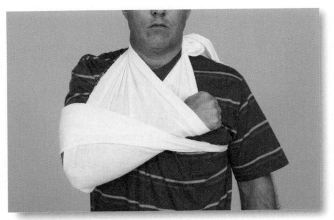

Shoulder. Apply a sling and swathe. Elevate the wrist above the elbow and support it with the swathe.

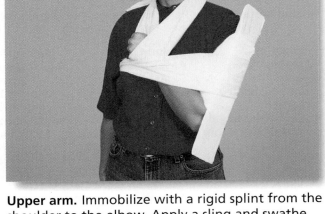

Upper arm. Immobilize with a rigid splint from the shoulder to the elbow. Apply a sling and swathe that will elevate and support the limb.

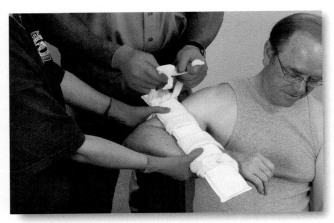

Elbow (bent). Apply a sling and swathe to elevate and support the limb.

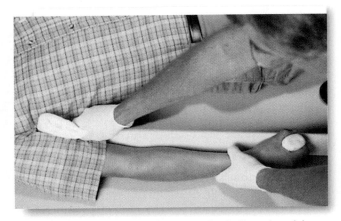

Elbow (straight). Pad the armpit. Splint should extend from the armpit beyond the fingertips. Use roller bandages to secure the splint to the arm starting at the distal end. Secure the arm to the body with cravats.

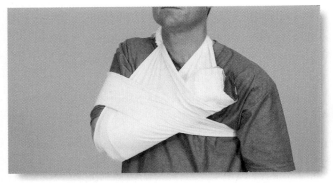

Forearm, wrist, hand. The splint should extend from the elbow to beyond the fingertips. Use a sling and swathe for elevation and support.

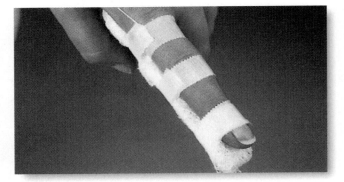

Finger. Use a tongue depressor as a splint or tape the finger to an uninjured finger.

Care of Upper Extremity Injuries

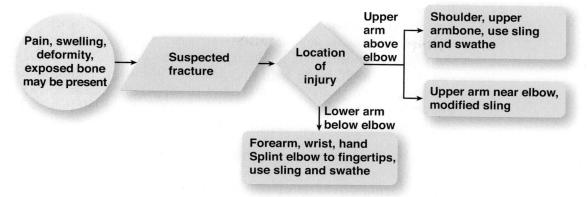

```
Pain, swelling,        →    Suspected    →    Location    Upper
deformity,                  fracture          of          arm       →   Shoulder, upper
exposed bone                                  injury      above         armbone, use sling
may be present                                            elbow         and swathe

                                                                    →   Upper arm near elbow,
                                                                        modified sling

                                              Lower arm
                                              below elbow
                                              ↓
                                    Forearm, wrist, hand
                                    Splint elbow to fingertips,
                                    use sling and swathe
```

FIGURE 11.17 Algorithm for the emergency care of patients with upper extremity injuries.

patient, especially if the extremity from forearm to hand is secured against a rigid splint. You may easily secure the hand in its position of function by placing a roll of gauze in the patient's hand before immobilizing or simply by allowing the fingers of the hand to extend over the end of the splint. (For upper extremity care, see Figure 11.17.)

Injuries to the Shoulder

A common sign of shoulder injury is a condition known as *knocked-down shoulder* or *dropped shoulder* (Figure 11.18). The patient's injured shoulder will appear to droop. The patient usually holds the arm up against the side of the chest.

Injuries to the shoulder joint often produce what is known as an *anterior* (to the front) *dislocation*. The end of the upper arm bone that forms the shoulder joint can be felt, or even seen, bulging or protruding under the skin at the front of the shoulder.

It is not practical to use a rigid splint for injuries to the collarbone, shoulder blade, or shoulder joint. Place padding between any space between the patient's injured arm and chest, use a cravat to secure the padding in place, and use a sling and swathe to secure the arm to the chest. Remember to check for distal circulation, sensation, and motor function before and after splinting. If there is no pulse, attempt to reposition to regain a pulse but do not force the arm.

FIRST ➤ When you provide care for patients with shoulder injuries, you will:

1. Take appropriate BSI precautions.
2. Care for life-threatening problems first.
3. Check distal circulation. If there is no pulse, notify the responding EMTs or notify the hospital and arrange to transport as soon as possible. Note the time that you observed the absence of the distal pulse.
4. Check for sensation and motor function of the fingers on the injured arm. If the patient has no feeling or cannot move, then there is pressure on a nerve and the patient will need transport as soon as possible.

WARNING

Do not try to realign or reposition angulations or dislocations of the shoulder. Movement in this area may cause damage to nearby blood vessels and nerves.

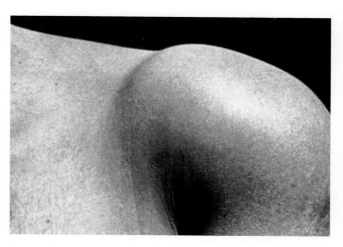

FIGURE 11.18 Deformity caused by dislocation of the shoulder joint.

5. Apply a sling and swathe. If necessary, place padding (pillow, blanket, or towel) to fill any space between the patient's arm and chest on the injured side before applying the sling and swathe.

6. Reassess the distal pulse. If the pulse is absent, you may have to gently reposition the injured arm and reapply the sling and swathe. In such cases, follow your local protocols or contact the emergency department physician for directions before repositioning the limb. Sometimes a dislocated shoulder will correct (reduce) itself. If this happens, check the distal circulation, sensation, and motor function, and apply a sling and swathe. This patient still has to see a physician. Arrange for transport, and make certain you tell the EMTs that the dislocation apparently corrected itself and the time it took place. ■

Injuries to the Upper Arm Bone

Injury to the upper arm bone (humerus) can be at its upper end (proximal end) where the shoulder joint is formed, along the midshaft of the bone, or at the lower end (distal end) where the elbow joint is formed. Care for a patient with upper arm injuries is usually the same as for all injury locations. Deformity is often a key sign of injury to this bone, but if you see no deformity, the patient will tell you the site is tender and painful when you examine it.

Emergency Medical Responders may use a soft splint (sling and swathe) or a rigid splint. If you use a sling and swathe on an injury that seems very close to the elbow, modify the full sling to minimize pressure on the elbow (Figure 11.19).

If the upper arm is angulated, check for a distal pulse. If it is present and the patient can tolerate movement, gently move the arm to the splinting position (bend the elbow with the hand elevated above the level of the elbow) and splint it. Do not force the arm to this position, and do not try to straighten the angulation. Recheck for distal pulse.

If you do not feel a pulse, attempt to straighten the angulation in the upper arm bone, if your EMS system allows you to do so. Do not force the arm. You should attempt to straighten the angulation only once and stop if there is resistance or severe pain. If straightening the limb fails to restore a distal pulse, arrange to transport the patient as soon as possible. If the pulse is restored, splint the arm and recheck the distal pulse.

If you use a rigid splint, secure it to the lateral (outside) part of the arm with roller gauze or cravats. Then apply a wrist sling and wide swathe. The swathe will secure the injured arm to the body and immobilize the joints above and below the injury site (Figure 11.20).

FIRST ➤ When you apply a splint to an upper arm injury, work with a partner. One of you will maintain manual stabilization, while the other applies the splint and the sling and swathe. To apply a splint for injuries to the upper arm bone:

1. Check for distal circulation, sensation, and motor function.
2. Select a padded splint long enough for the area between shoulder and elbow.
3. Apply manual stabilization to the injured extremity. If there is angulation or no distal pulse, gently realign and recheck for pulse.
4. Place the splint against the injured extremity.
5. Secure the splint to the patient with a roller bandage, handkerchiefs, cravats, or cloth strips. Begin securing at the distal end of the splint.
6. Maintain the hand in the position of function and apply a sling and swathe. Recheck distal circulation, sensation, and motor function.
7. Provide oxygen as soon as possible and maintain body temperature to prevent the effects of developing shock. ■

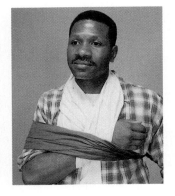

FIGURE 11.19 For an upper arm injury near the elbow joint, gently apply a modified sling so it supports only the wrist.

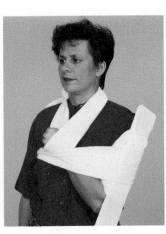

FIGURE 11.20 Wrist sling and swathe.

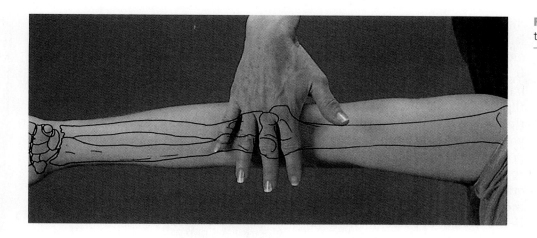

FIGURE 11.21 Consider this area to be the site of elbow injuries.

Injuries to the Elbow

The elbow is a joint (not a bone) formed by the lower, or distal, end of the upper arm bone (humerus) and the upper, or proximal, end of the forearm bones (radius and ulna). You can determine if the injury is to the elbow area by placing your hand over the back of the elbow. The elbow includes all the structures that can be covered by the palm of your hand (Figure 11.21). If the injury is above this area, the injury is to the upper arm bone. If the injury is below this area, the injury is to one of the forearm bones.

When caring for elbow injuries, immobilize the elbow in the position in which it is found. Have your partner stabilize the arm while you apply and secure the splint. Check circulation, sensation, and motor function before and after splinting.

FIRST ➤ The following methods can be used in caring for a patient with an elbow injury:

- If the elbow is found in a flexed (bent) position natural for the joint, rigid splinting is preferred. However, a simple sling and a swathe may be effective. Apply a splint as shown in Figure 11.22.
- If the elbow is found in the straight position and cannot be placed in the natural flexed position, immobilize it in the straight position. Rigid splinting is preferred,

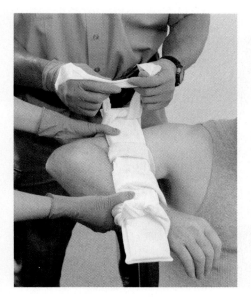

FIGURE 11.22 Splinting an injured elbow in a flexed position.

but body splinting is effective. This is done by tying the injured arm along the side of the patient's torso. If you use a rigid splint, select a padded splint that will extend from the patient's armpit past the fingertips. Place a roll of dressing in the patient's hand to maintain it in the position of function and secure the splint with roller gauze or folded cravats starting at the distal end of the arm (fingertips) (Figure 11.23).

- If the elbow appears to be dislocated and it is in an unnatural or awkward position and cannot be repositioned, place padding around the arm and between the arm and chest, if necessary. Secure the arm to the body with a sling and swathe. ■

Injuries to the Forearm, Wrist, and Hand

FIRST ➤ The most effective splint for an injured forearm, wrist, or hand is a rigid one. However, the patient can be made comfortable with a pillow splint (Figure 11.24) and a sling and swathe. A sling and swathe used alone is also effective for a forearm. Be sure to check distal circulation, sensation, and motor function before and after splinting.

To use a rigid splint for any injury to the forearm, wrist, or hand, select a padded rigid splint that extends from beyond the elbow to past the fingertips. Place a roll of dressing in the patient's hand to maintain the hand in the position of function. The steps for splinting the forearm, wrist, and hand are the same as steps 3 through 7 listed above for the upper arm. Do not apply manual traction to wrist or hand injuries.

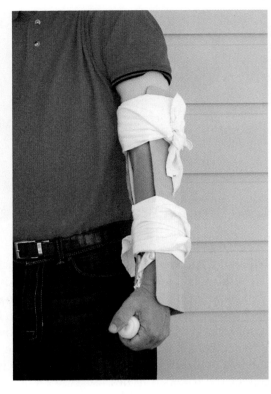

FIGURE 11.23 Splinting an injured elbow in a straight position.

FIGURE 11.24 Soft splint for wrist and hand injuries.

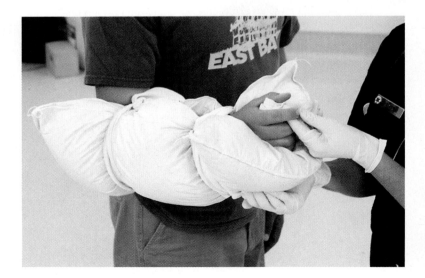

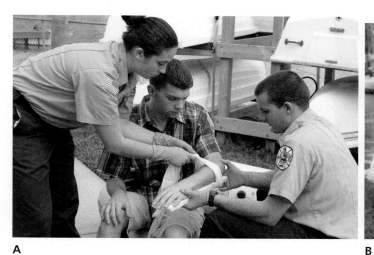
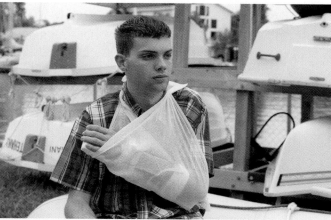

A

B

FIGURE 11.25 Rigid splinting of an injured forearm. **A.** Secure a rigid splint to the limb. **B.** Place the arm in a sling.

An alternative method for maintaining the position of function in the hand is to allow the fingers to curve over the end of the rigid splint (Figure 11.25).

Rolled newspapers, magazines, and creased cardboard make effective rigid splints for injuries to the forearm or wrist (Figure 11.26), but they still should be padded. Apply a sling after splinting to keep the forearm elevated. Add a swathe to secure the forearm to the chest and immobilize the joint above and below the injury site. ■

Injuries to the Fingers

Not all injuries to the fingers require rigid splinting. You can immobilize an injured finger by taping the finger to an adjacent, uninjured finger (Figure 11.27). You can tape the finger to a tongue depressor, an aluminum splint, or a pen or pencil. You can also make a soft splint by placing a roll of gauze in the patient's hand and wrapping more gauze around the hand and dressing. This soft-splint method immobilizes the hand and fingers and keeps them in the position of function.

Apply a sling to keep the forearm elevated. Apply a swathe to immobilize the joints above the injury site, as well as to improve circulation and patient comfort.

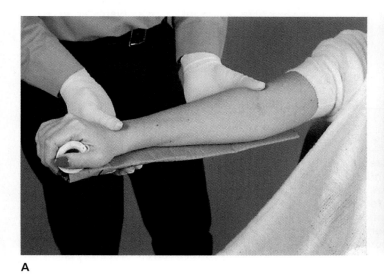
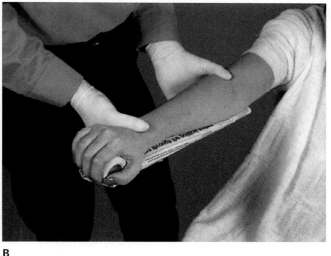

A

B

FIGURE 11.26 Rigid splints can be made from **A.** cardboard or **B.** rolled newspapers or magazines.

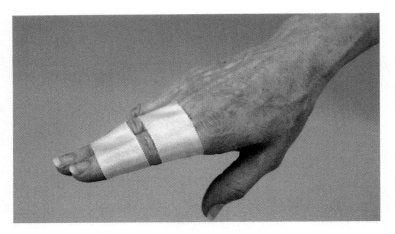

FIGURE 11.27 One way to immobilize an injured finger is to tape it to an adjacent, uninjured finger.

Do not attempt to "pop" dislocated fingers back into place. Immobilize dislocated fingers as you would an injured hand.

LOWER EXTREMITY INJURIES

When the patient has multiple injuries, it may be best to totally immobilize the patient on a long spine board or a scoop (orthopedic) stretcher rather than to try to immobilize each individual injury. However, do not attempt to use these immobilization devices unless you are trained to correctly move the patient onto them and to properly strap the patient to them.

Before moving or rolling a patient with suspected spine injury or with lower extremity injuries, be sure you have the proper equipment ready and a sufficient number of rescue personnel on hand to assist. For lower extremity care, see Figure 11.28.

Injuries to the Pelvic Girdle

FIRST ➤ The patient may have injuries to the pelvic girdle (pelvis and hip joints) if:

- Patient complains of pain in the pelvis, hips, or groin.
- Patient complains of pain when gentle pressure is applied to the sides of the hips or to the hip bones.
- Patient cannot lift the legs while lying face up (supine). The patient will usually tell you that "it hurts" or "I can't move my legs."

Care of Lower Extremity Injuries

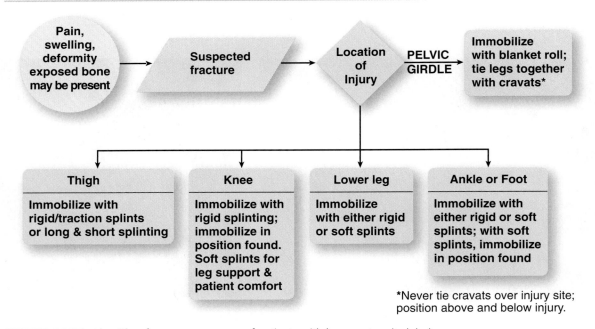

FIGURE 11.28 Algorithm for emergency care of patients with lower extremity injuries.

- The foot on the injured side turns outward (laterally) or inward (medially) more than the uninjured side.
- Injured extremity appears shorter than the uninjured side.
- Pelvis or the hip joint has noticeable deformity. ■

Pelvic injuries are serious because they can damage major blood vessels and internal organs. Injuries to these soft tissues can cause profuse internal bleeding, sterility, and infection. The force that caused the pelvic injury may also have caused spine injuries. Because of all these critical factors, it may be best to wait for more advanced care to arrive before attempting to immobilize a patient with a pelvic injury. In the meantime, provide oxygen as soon as possible and maintain body temperature to delay the onset of shock. Note the mechanism of injury so you can report it to the responding EMTs.

With certain symptoms, pelvic girdle injuries may be managed at the scene with a specialized pressure garment called a *pneumatic antishock garment (PASG)*. Your instructor will know if Emergency Medical Responders are trained and allowed to use or assist more advanced providers with PASGs in your area. Follow your local protocols or medical direction when considering the use of a PASG. Other devices and materials that are effective for immobilizing injuries to the pelvic girdle include pelvic splints (Figure 11.29), long spine boards, scoop stretchers, and blankets. If you do not carry this equipment, you may continue patient assessment while you are waiting for more advanced care to arrive.

FIRST ➤ As an Emergency Medical Responder, you can care for patients with suspected fractures to the pelvic girdle by using a soft splint. Place a blanket roll between the patient's legs and tie them together with cravats. This simple and quick immobilization method will stabilize the injury and provide patient comfort before more advanced care arrives. ■

To immobilize a pelvic injury with a blanket roll, do the following:

1. Complete a thorough assessment of the injury site.
2. Assess circulation, sensation, and motor function in both distal extremities.
3. Provide oxygen to the patient as soon as possible.
4. Place a folded blanket, large towel, or other thick padding material between the patient's legs from groin to feet.
5. Prepare four cravats (folded triangular bandages) or other strips of material.

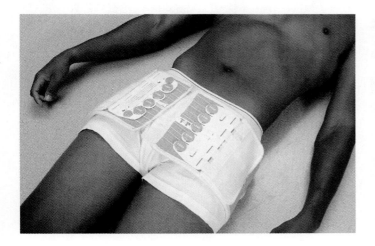

FIGURE 11.29 The application of a commercial pelvic splint helps to stabilize the pelvis and minimize bleeding.

6. Use a short splint or coat hanger and drape the ends of all four cravats over the splint or hanger. Slide them under the space behind the knees.

7. Gently slide two cravats above the knees and two below the knees.

8. Starting at the feet (distal end), tie one cravat at the ankles, one just below the knees, one just above the knees, and one just below the hips. Do not tie a cravat over or too near the injury site.

When the EMTs arrive, you can help them place the stabilized patient on a scoop stretcher or spine board. Remember to provide oxygen to the patient as soon as possible and cover the patient to maintain body temperature and to help reduce the chance of developing shock. If you suspect spine injury, do not attempt to move the patient until the EMTs arrive with additional help. In the meantime, stabilize the patient's head and neck and continue to reassure him.

Because the signs and symptoms of musculoskeletal injuries are similar, you will not be trying to determine which type of injury the patient has. Even so, there are certain signs that indicate a possible hip dislocation, and you should look for them because you do not want to attempt to move an injured leg if there is a possible hip dislocation. If you suspect a hip dislocation, there may also be injury to the thigh bone (femur). Do not try to straighten an angulated femur if the hip appears to be dislocated.

FIRST ➤ The following points describe two types of hip dislocation. Suspect the patient has a dislocated hip if you find (Figure 11.30):

- *Anterior hip dislocation.* The leg from hip to foot is rotated outward (laterally) further than the uninjured side. Leg rotation also may be an indication of hip fracture. With hip fracture, the injured leg may appear to be shorter than the other leg. You will probably see or feel the bony end of the femur under the skin at the front or side of the leg where it joins the torso.
- *Posterior hip dislocation (most common).* The leg is rotated inward (medially) and the knee is usually bent. You may see or feel the bony end of the femur under the skin at the back of the leg where it joins the buttocks.

If you suspect the hip is dislocated, wait for more advanced care to arrive. While waiting, provide oxygen as soon as possible, and cover the patient to maintain body temperature and help prevent shock. You can immobilize the injured leg

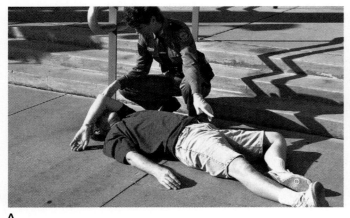

A

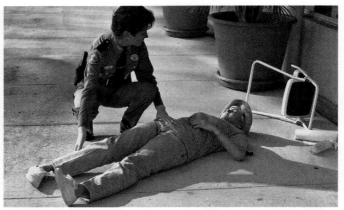

B

FIGURE 11.30 Classic signs of **A.** an anterior hip dislocation and **B.** a posterior hip dislocation.

by placing and securing pillows or folded blankets or towels around the injured leg, which will support the leg and provide comfort to the patient. Do not reposition or move the patient's leg when you place or secure pillows or blankets. ▪

Injuries to the Upper Leg

Injuries to the upper leg or thigh bone (femur) can be life threatening. Even when the injury is closed, bleeding inside the tissues can be severe. There may be a severe and obvious deformity with femur fractures. The leg below the injury site may be bent where there is no joint, or it will appear twisted.

To immobilize femur injuries, use a rigid splint or a special device called a *traction splint*. Emergency Medical Responder units may carry traction splints, and you may be trained and allowed to use them. (Your instructor will advise you if tractions splints are part of your local protocols.) Soft splints are not as effective as rigid or traction splinting, but they will stabilize the injury and provide some pain relief.

While waiting for the EMTs to arrive, provide the patient some relief from pain by securing a blanket roll between the legs in the same way you would for injuries to the pelvic girdle. This is effective once the patient is secured to a spine board or scoop stretcher, a form of rigid splinting. Provide oxygen as soon as possible, and cover the patient to maintain body warmth to help prevent shock.

An alternative approach is to immobilize the leg using a long rigid splint that extends from the patient's buttocks to past the foot. Use cravats to secure the splint. Use a splint or coat hanger to push the cravats under the patient's trunk and legs at the natural voids (lower back and knees) (Figure 11.31). Do not place a tie over the injury site, but instead place one tie above and one tie below the injury.

Injuries to the Knee

FIRST ➤ In most cases, you will not be able to tell if the knee is fractured, dislocated, or both. Because of the many nerves and blood vessels and the possibility that soft tissues were damaged, immobilize an injured knee in the position in which it is found (Figure 11.32). Do not attempt to reposition or straighten the injured knee. Some EMS systems allow Emergency Medical Responders to make one attempt at straightening the limb if there is no distal pulse. Your instructor will let you know the requirements of your local protocols. ▪

REMEMBER

Injuries to the thigh can bleed profusely. Provide oxygen as soon as possible and maintain body temperature to reduce the effects of shock. Monitor the patient's vital signs and comfort level.

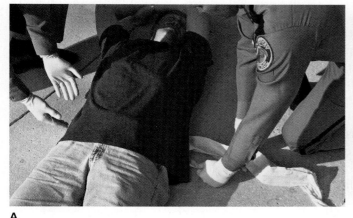
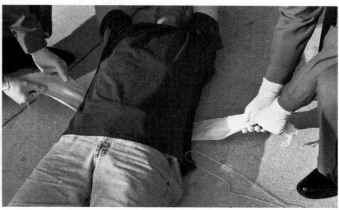

A   B

FIGURE 11.31 Safely inserting cravats under a patient. **A.** Use a coat hangar or flat splint to push the cravat under the void. **B.** Then reposition the cravat to the proper side.

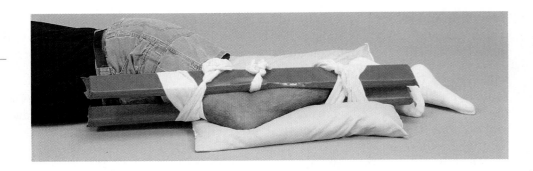

FIGURE 11.32 Splint an injured knee in the position in which it is found.

Rigid splinting is the most effective method to use when immobilizing an injured knee, but you can provide support to the leg and comfort to the patient with soft splints. Place and secure pillows or folded blankets around the knee, especially if it is found in the bent position. Do not reposition or move the patient's legs in order to place or secure pillows or blankets. If the injured knee is found in the straight position, you can effectively immobilize it with a blanket placed between both legs and secured with cravats, just as you would for a femur injury.

For rigid splinting of an injured knee in the straight position, secure a long splint behind the leg from the patient's buttocks to beyond the foot. You may also use the method described below for splinting the lower leg. In cases where the patient's leg will remain flexed at the knee, you can secure one or two shorter splints at an angle across the thigh and lower leg (A-frame) with cravats (Scan 11–6).

Injuries to the Lower Leg

You can provide care for injuries to the lower leg with either rigid or soft splints. A blanket roll between the legs is an effective soft splint. Secure it as you did for pelvic, thigh, and knee injuries described previously. Once you assist the EMTs in placing the patient on the spine board or scoop (orthopedic) stretcher, a form of rigid splinting, you have completed immobilizing all joints above and below the injury site.

If you use a rigid splint, you will need assistance. One person must maintain manual traction while you apply the splint. A single-splint method also can be used to immobilize lower leg injuries. The procedure is shown in Scan 11–7.

Before and after splinting, check for distal circulation, sensation, and motor function. If there is no pulse, remove the splint, realign or reposition the limb, and resplint.

If you live in an area where skiing is a popular sport, you may have to care for a certain kind of injury called the *boot-top injury* (Figure 11.33). This is an injury to the tibia and/or fibula (usually both) that typically occurs when a skier falls forward of the ski tips. The leg bends hard over the top of the ski boot, causing a *transverse fracture* (a break in the bone that is at a right angle to the long part of the bone) of one or both bones. The leg below the fracture is often angulated or rotated, and the fracture is quite painful. Follow these guidelines when caring for an injured skier:

- Notify the ski patrol immediately. (Send another skier to an emergency phone or lift shack.)
- Keep the patient warm with others' coats, and place something between the skier and the snow.

FIRST ON SCENE

After carefully straightening Joan's leg, Russell was able to find a strong pulse in her foot. "Now we need to splint it in this position," he said, looking at a stand of small trees that lined the course. Perhaps the branches would be strong enough for a splint.

"Why don't you use the golf clubs," Joan whispered as she tried to breathe deeply through the pain. Russell grinned and shook his head slightly, imagining his buddies at the volunteer fire station finding out that he was prepared to break down a tree to make a splint when he was surrounded by golf clubs.

"That's a great idea," he said and jogged over to the over-turned golf cart and grabbed several clubs and the shoulder straps from both bags.

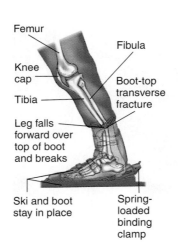

Femur
Fibula
Knee cap
Tibia
Boot-top transverse fracture
Leg falls forward over top of boot and breaks
Ski and boot stay in place
Spring-loaded binding clamp

FIGURE 11.33 Boot-top injury.

NOTE: Pillows and blankets can be used to splint injured ankles and feet.

REMEMBER: Check for distal circulation, sensation, and motor function before and after splinting.

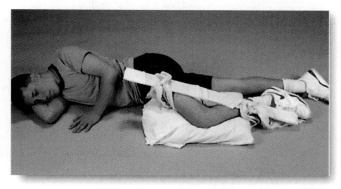

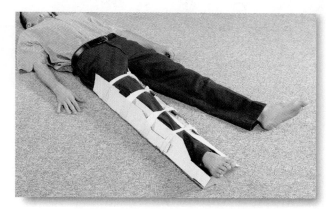

Knee

- If distal pulse present, then splint in position found.
- If no distal pulse, attempt to gently realign or reposition to regain pulse (if your EMS system allows).
- For a bent knee, secure splints behind knee, at the thigh, and at the lower leg.
- For a straight knee, splint using same steps as "Lower Leg."

Thigh. Apply a three-sided rigid cardboard splint.

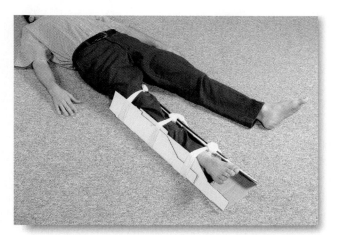

Lower Leg. Apply a three-sided rigid cardboard splint.

- Leave the leg alone or in the position found until the ski patrol arrives; or . . .
- Gently align the injury to see if that will reduce the patient's pain.
- Manually stabilize or splint the injury. A ski or ski pole will work, or use splints. Secure with scarves, handkerchiefs, or cravats.
- Do not apply snow to the injury site. Swelling is due to bleeding from the damaged soft tissues; thus, applying cold will only hasten the development of frostbite and/or hypothermia.

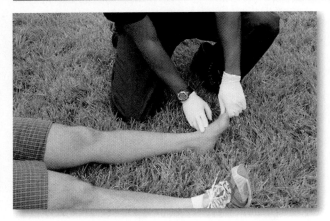

1 ■ Assess circulation, sensation, and motor function before moving or splinting the extremity.

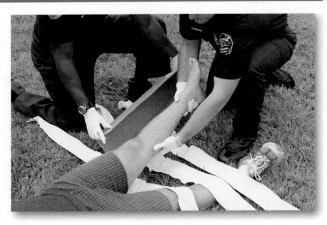

2 ■ Choose a splint that extends from the heel to well above the knee.

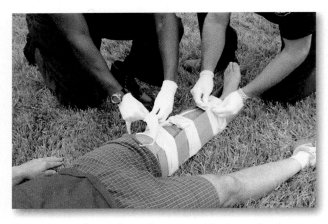

3 ■ Secure the splint above and below the knee.

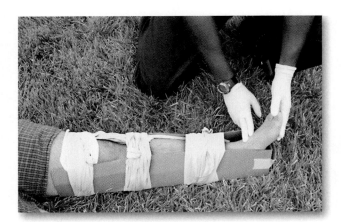

4 ■ Reassess circulation, sensation, and motor function after the splint is secure.

Injuries to the Ankle or Foot

FIRST ➤ Rigid splints may be used for injuries to the ankle or foot, but the soft splint is probably the most comfortable for the patient and the quickest for the Emergency Medical Responder to apply. If you apply a rigid splint, use one that extends from above the patient's knee to beyond the foot as described for the single-splint method for the lower leg. ■

When soft splinting an injury to the foot or ankle, immobilize it in the position found with a pillow or folded blanket. Secure the soft splint around the foot and ankle with several cravats or with roller gauze (Figure 11.34), and then elevate it by propping it on a blanket roll or pillow.

RESPLINTING

After splinting, you must always recheck distal circulation, sensation, and motor function. If absent, your protocols may direct you to remove the splint, realign the extremity until distal pulse returns, and then resplint. If you are allowed to realign an extremity, do not force the limb, and stop immediately if the movement causes severe pain. Resplint once the distal pulse returns. One reason for an absent pulse after splinting is because the gauze or cravats may have been applied too tightly. If there is still no distal pulse after removing the splint or realigning the limb, it may be that swelling and pressure have restricted circulation. Arrange for transport immediately if distal pulse does not return.

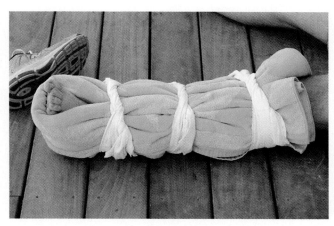

FIGURE 11.34 Soft splint of an injured ankle or foot.

Axial Skeleton

STRUCTURES OF THE AXIAL SKELETON

The axial skeleton consists of the head (skull), spinal column, and chest (sternum and ribs). It makes up the long axis of the body. Injuries to the axial skeleton can be very serious because trauma can also injure the structures protected by the bones of the axial skeleton. Your concern is not only with the bones, but also with the brain, spinal cord, airway, lungs, and heart—all vital organs protected by the axial skeleton. When the head, spine, or chest is injured, you must also assess the patient for the signs and symptoms that indicate injuries to the underlying vital organs protected by these structures.

Head

The head, or skull, is divided into two major structures: the cranium and the face (Figure 11.35). Flat, irregularly shaped bones make up the floor, back, top, and sides of the skull and the forehead. The bones are fused together into immovable joints, which form a rigid, protective case for the brain.

In infants, fusion of the skull bones is not complete. Places called *soft spots* (fontanels) can be felt at the top, sides, and back of the baby's skull. The smaller soft spots at the sides and back close in the first few months, but the largest soft spot at the top of the skull does not close completely until about 18 to 24 months. When caring for an infant with possible head injuries, avoid applying point pressure to the skull with your fingertips. Instead spread your fingers and hold or stabilize the head with your entire hand.

The face is made up of strong, irregularly shaped bones. The face bones include part of the eye sockets, the cheeks, the upper part of the nose, the upper jaw, and the lower jaw. These bones also are fused into immovable joints except for the lower jaw bone, or **mandible**, which is the only movable joint in the head.

mandible (MAN-di-bl) ■ the lower jaw bone.

cervical (SER-vi-kal) spine ■ the neck bones.

Spinal Column

The spinal column includes the neck bones and the back bones. The neck is made up of seven bones called the **cervical spine**. The rest of the spine is commonly known as the *backbone*. The spine protects the spinal cord as it runs from the brain down through the back. Many of the body's major nerves run into and out of the spinal cord and connect most areas of the body to the brain. In addition, the spine supports the entire body. The skull, shoulder bones, ribs, and pelvic bones connect to the spine.

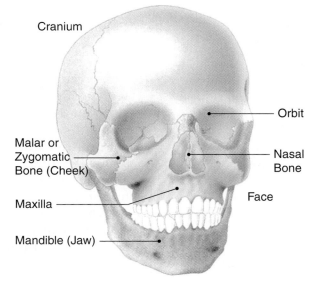

FIGURE 11.35 The head (skull) consists of the cranium and the face.

FIGURE 11.36 The chest.

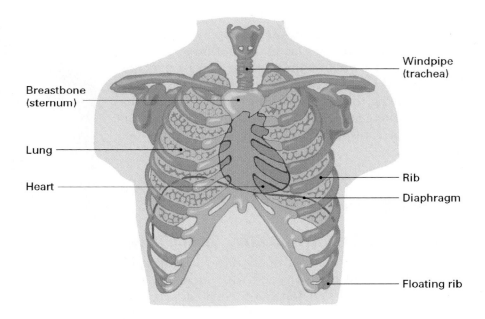

Windpipe (trachea)

Breastbone (sternum)

Lung

Heart

Rib

Diaphragm

Floating rib

Chest

There are 12 ribs on each side of the chest (Figure 11.36); the ribs connect with the spine. Most of the ribs attach directly to the sternum (breastbone) by pieces of cartilage. Some of the ribs connect to other ribs by a common cartilage strip. The bottom two ribs on each side—sometimes called *floating ribs*—do not connect to the breastbone or to other ribs. They are held in place by muscles.

The lower ribs help protect the organs in the upper part of the abdomen: the liver, gallbladder, stomach, and spleen. The upper ribs and sternum help protect the organs in the center or middle part of the chest. These organs include the heart and major blood vessels leading into and out of the heart, the trachea (windpipe) leading to the lungs, and the esophagus leading to the stomach. The upper ribs also protect the lungs, which lie on each side of the heart. The muscles of the back and chest, along with the muscles found between the ribs, give added strength to the spine and the ribs and further help protect the heart and lungs.

Central Nervous System

Injuries to the head and spine can involve much more than just the bones that make up these structures. Soft-tissue injuries to outer skin and to underlying muscles, organs, blood vessels, and nerves can occur as well.

central nervous system (CNS) ■ the brain and spinal cord.

The brain and spinal cord make up what is known as the **central nervous system (CNS)**. The brain not only takes care of thinking, but it also controls many of our basic functions, including heart activity and breathing. The brain tells muscles when to contract and relax so that we can move. It receives messages from all over the body and decides how the body will respond to these messages. Any injury to the skull could injure the brain and cause vital body functions to fail.

The spinal cord carries messages along nerves from the brain to the body and from the body back to the brain. Injury to the spine could damage the spinal cord and prevent it from carrying messages to or from a part of the body. That part of the body would no longer have contact with the brain and would be unable to function. The damage could be temporary, caused by pressure or swelling that may be corrected with proper care, or the damage could be permanent so that part of the body would never again be able to move or function. In addition, the spinal

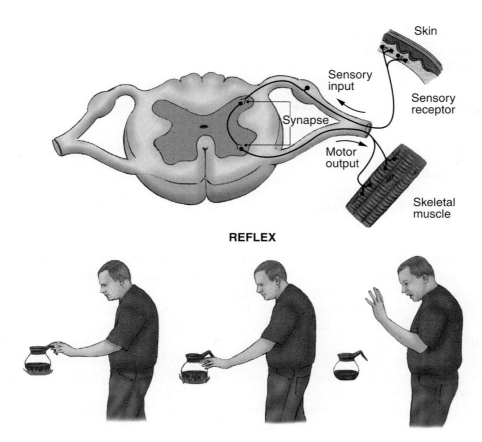

FIGURE 11.37 Reflexes allow for swift reactions to stimuli.

Skin

Sensory input

Sensory receptor

Synapse

Motor output

Skeletal muscle

REFLEX

cord is the site of many reflexes, which allow us to react quickly to such things as pain and heat (Figure 11.37). Damage to the spinal cord can take away these reflex abilities.

Geriatric Focus

As we age, our spine loses much of its flexibility due to the loss of water content in the intervertebral disks and calcification of the supporting ligaments. Sometimes the calcification can cause narrowing of the spinal canal where the spinal cord runs. What may appear to be insignificant mechanisms can cause fractures to the vertebral bodies or to the calcified ligaments, resulting in compression on the spinal cord. You should always have a high index of suspicion for spine injury in the elderly and take appropriate stabilization measures.

MECHANISMS OF INJURY

You will not always be able to find and determine all patient injuries. Most of the time, you will conclude that the patient is injured based on the mechanism of injury (MOI). Be highly suspicious of injury if the patient has been involved in or reports the following situations:

5–3.4 Relate mechanism of injury to potential injuries of the head and spine.

- Falls, diving, and motor-vehicle collisions that result in swelling or pressure on a body part.
- Direct or indirect forces that caused excessive flexion (bending) or extension (stretching) of a body part.
- Twisting forces that caused rotation or excessive twisting of a body part.
- Pulling or hanging forces that caused spinal stretching.
- Compression of the spinal column.

- Blunt trauma such as that caused by blows, a car striking a pedestrian, or a driver striking a steering wheel or windshield.
- Penetrating trauma such as that caused by gunshots or stabbings.
- Blows in assault and battery or abuse incidents and the rapid forceful shaking of infants and children.
- Any trauma situation where the patient is unresponsive.

INJURY TO THE HEAD

Types of Injuries

Injuries to the head can be caused by a variety of mechanisms that result in pain, swelling, discoloration, and deformity similar to what was described for extremity injuries. In addition, the mechanism of injury may be forceful enough to cause a patient to experience a loss of consciousness. Because the skull surrounds the brain on all sides, the force of the mechanism of injury can also be transmitted to the brain. Injury to the brain can affect the patient's ability to breathe. Because of this, airway management is always the first consideration in the care of any patient who has a head injury. Keep the airway open. In addition to skull and brain injury, there can be cuts to the scalp and other soft tissues.

There are certain signs and symptoms that will help you determine if a head injury is an open or a closed one. In an open head injury, you may be able to see or feel that the skull is cracked (fractured) or depressed (deformed), that there is blood and clear or yellow watery fluid (cerebrospinal fluid [CSF]) leaking from the ears or nose, and that the eyelids are swollen shut and beginning to discolor or bruise. The fluids that protect the brain and are normally contained within the skull are leaking out into the tissues through the crack in the skull. The brain may also be injured in open head injuries. Broken bones or foreign objects forced through the skull can cut, tear, or bruise the brain. There may be no evidence of soft-tissue damage in some cases of open head injury.

In a closed head injury, the skull is not damaged or cracked, but the brain can still be injured by the force of something striking the skull. Such a force can cause the brain to bounce off the inside of the skull. The resulting injuries to the brain include (Figure 11.38):

FIGURE 11.38 Closed head injuries.

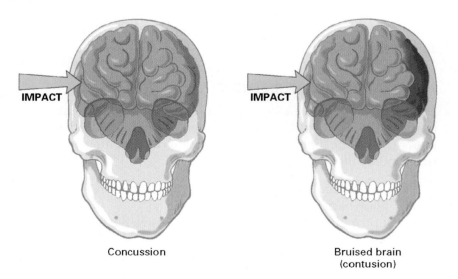

Concussion

Bruised brain (contusion)

Care for Injuries to the Cranium

FIRST ➤ When caring for patients with injuries to the cranium, always conclude that neck and spine injuries also exist. Don personal protective equipment, and then take the following steps:

1. Maintain an open airway. Use the jaw-thrust maneuver and stabilize the head.
2. Provide resuscitative measures as needed.
3. Keep the patient still. This can be a critical factor. Do not let the patient move or change position.
4. Control bleeding. Do not apply direct pressure over the injury site because you may cause further damage to the brain or soft tissues. Use a bulky dressing. Do not attempt to stop the flow of blood or cerebrospinal fluid (CSF) from the ears or nose; it needs to flow out, so as not to build up pressure inside the skull. Secure a loose dressing to absorb flow and prevent this now contaminated fluid from flowing back into the brain.
5. Talk to the responsive patient. Try to keep him calm.
6. Dress and bandage open wounds and stabilize penetrating objects. Do not remove any objects or bone fragments.
7. Provide care for shock. Maintain body warmth, but avoid overheating. Provide 100% oxygen and give nothing to eat or drink.
8. Monitor and record vital signs. Watch for and record changes.
9. Monitor the level of responsiveness.
10. Provide emotional support.
11. Be prepared for vomiting and have suction ready.
12. Arrange to transport as soon as possible. ■

Do not reposition any patient with an open head wound or any other possible serious injury to the cranium unless you must do so to provide CPR or assist ventilations. If the mechanism of injury and the patient's mental status indicate the possibility of spine injury, do not reposition the patient. Suspect that any patient who is unresponsive and has trauma above the collarbones has a spine injury. Stabilize the head and open the airway using the jaw-thrust maneuver.

For responsive patients with apparently minor closed injuries to the cranium and no sign of spine injury, you have two choices for positioning the patient. Both methods are also suitable for patients with face injuries. The methods are:

- *Option 1:* Elevate head and shoulders (Figure 11.40). Place the patient's upper body at a 45-degree angle, using several pillows or a blanket roll as needed.

5–3.8 Describe the emergency medical care for injuries to the head.

WARNING

It is a serious sign when an unresponsive patient becomes responsive and then unresponsive again. Make certain you report this to the EMTs.

REMEMBER

The two most important factors in determining the outcome in head injury are a low oxygen level in the blood (hypoxia) and low blood pressure (hypotension).

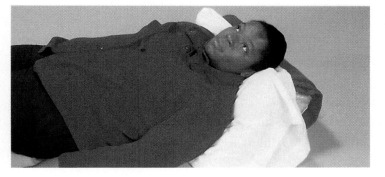

FIGURE 11.40 Head and shoulders elevated for patients with mild head injuries.

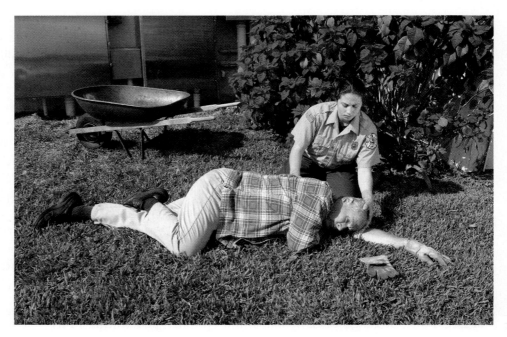

FIGURE 11.41 Recovery position for patients with mild head injuries.

- *Option 2:* Place the patient in the recovery position (on the side) as shown in Figure 11.41. Position the lower shoulder behind the patient and the hand of the upper shoulder under and supporting the cheek. Tilt the head slightly back and the face downward to allow for drainage of fluids.

Care for Injuries to the Face

FIRST ➤ As in all cases of injury to the face, make certain that the patient has an open airway. If you must assist ventilations, use the jaw-thrust maneuver and stabilize the head in case there is injury to the spine. Apply only gentle pressure to bleeding wounds. Use a bulky dressing to care for soft-tissue injuries. ■

The lower jaw can be dislocated or fractured. Because it is a joint, dislocations can occur where the lower jaw attaches to the skull just in front of the ears. Look for the mechanism of injury—a force that could have struck the jaw from the front or side. The signs and symptoms to look for include:

- Pain and tenderness.
- Swelling and discoloration.
- Deformity, distortion, or disfigurement of the face.
- Loss of use or inability to control jaw movement or to open or close mouth.
- Difficulty in speaking.
- Bleeding from the nose, mouth, or around the teeth.
- Missing or broken teeth or broken dentures.

To care for possible fracture or dislocation of the lower jaw:

1. Maintain an open airway. Be prepared to suction blood, secretions, and vomit.
2. Control bleeding and dress any open wounds. Do not tie the patient's mouth shut because there may be vomiting.
3. Keep the patient at rest and provide care for shock.
4. Closely monitor the patient and stay alert for vomiting.
5. Monitor and record vital signs.

Injuries to the face can damage teeth, crowns (caps), bridges, and dentures. Always look for and remove avulsed (dislodged) teeth and parts of broken dental appliances. Be careful not to push these down the patient's airway. When a tooth is avulsed, there is bleeding from the socket. Have the responsive patient bite down on a pad of gauze placed over the socket, but leave several inches of gauze outside the mouth for quick removal. For the unresponsive patient, hold the gauze over the socket. This will control the bleeding and prevent the airway from becoming obstructed with blood.

Wrap the avulsed tooth in a dressing. If you have a source of clean water, keep the dressing moist. (Milk can also be used.) Do not attempt to clean the tooth. Your efforts could damage microscopic structures needed to replant the tooth.

INJURY TO THE SPINE

Types of Injury to the Spine

Soft tissues of the neck can be injured by a number of mechanisms. The forces that cause soft-tissue injury can also injure underlying bones of the spinal column in the vertebrae of the neck (cervical spine). Injuries to and improper care of cervical spine injuries can impair breathing and lead to paralysis or death. Injuries along the rest of the spinal column also can cause paralysis and reduce normal body movement and function.

Spine injuries are caused by forces to the head, neck, back, chest, pelvis, or legs. Often, you will find patients with head injuries who also have cervical spine injuries. Injuries to the upper leg bones or to the pelvic bones may also cause spine injury through indirect force. Motor-vehicle crashes (including those causing whiplash), falls, diving, and skiing mishaps are common causes of spine injuries.

If a patient has numbness, loss of feeling, or paralysis in the legs with no problems in the arms, the injury to the spine is probably below the neck. If numbness, loss of feeling, or paralysis involves the arms and the legs, the injury is probably in the neck. Numbness, loss of feeling, and paralysis may be limited to only one side of the body, but usually both sides are involved.

Injuries to the spine can include fractured or displaced spinal bones (vertebrae) or swelling that presses on nerves. These injuries can produce the same signs and symptoms. In some cases, the loss of function associated with spine injuries may be temporary if the loss is caused by pressure or swelling that may eventually go away. But if the spinal cord was cut, even the best surgery and care cannot restore function.

REMEMBER

Consider every unresponsive injured patient to have a spine injury. Stabilize the patient's head and open the airway with the jaw-thrust maneuver.

Signs and Symptoms of Spine Injury

FIRST ➤ The most common signs and symptoms of spine injury include:

- Weakness, numbness, or tingling sensations, or loss of feeling in the arms or legs.
- Paralysis to arms and/or legs.
- Painful movement of arms and/or legs (or no pain or sensation).
- Pain and/or tenderness along the back of the neck or the backbone.
- Burning sensations along the spine or in an extremity.
- Deformity of the spine (the angle of the patient's head and neck may appear odd to you). You also may feel pieces of bone that have broken off the spine, although such findings are rare.
- Loss of bladder and bowel control.

5–3.5 State the signs and symptoms of a potential spine injury.

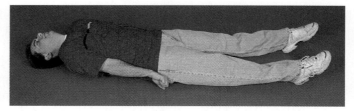

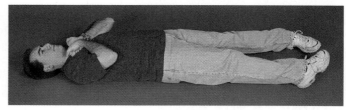

FIGURE 11.42 Suspect spine injury if you find the patient **A.** face up with arms stretched down along his sides or **B.** with arms and hands curled onto the chest (toward the midline).

A

B

- Difficult or labored breathing with little or no movement of the chest and slight movement of the abdomen.
- Positioning of the arms. You may find the patient lying face up with arms stretched out or with arms and hands curled to the chest (Figure 11.42).
- Persistent erection of the penis called *priapism* (PRY-ah-pism), which indicates spine injury affecting nerves to the external genitalia. ▪

5–3.6 Describe the method of determining if a responsive patient may have a spine injury.

FIRST ➤ As you read in Chapter 7, you should conduct a thorough patient history during your focused assessment of a responsive patient (Figure 11.43 and Scan 11–8). You may learn things about the emergency that will help determine the mechanism of injury:

- Question the patient. Do his arms or legs feel numb? Can the patient feel you touch his hands and feet? Can he squeeze your hand or push your hand with his foot? Do not ask the patient to repeat any movement that causes pain.
- Look and feel gently for injuries and deformities.

Spinal Injury Assessment

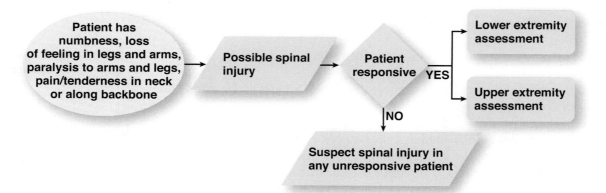

FIGURE 11.43 Algorithm for assessment of a patient with possible spine injury.

NOTE: Always consider the mechanism of injury. If it suggests a possible spine injury, then assume it is so, even if your focused assessment reveals no signs or symptoms. Also suspect spine injury in any unresponsive trauma patient.

Signs and Symptoms

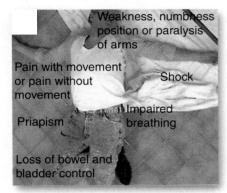

Weakness, numbness position or paralysis of arms

Pain with movement or pain without movement

Shock

Priapism

Impaired breathing

Loss of bowel and bladder control

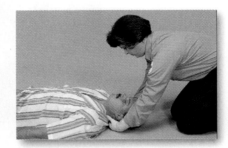

Tenderness or deformity over the cervical spine.

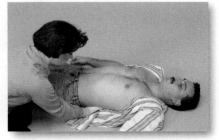

Tenderness or deformity anywhere along the spinal column.

Responsive: Lower Extremities Assessment

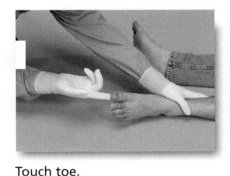

Touch toe.

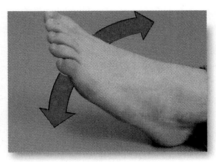

Foot movement.

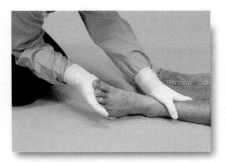

Foot push/pull.

RESULTS: If the patient can perform these tasks, there is little chance of injury to the spinal cord. However, this test does not rule out all injuries, including fractures of the spine. If the patient can perform only to a limited degree and with pain, there may be pressure somewhere on the spinal cord. When a patient is not able to perform any of the tests, suspect that there is spine injury.

Responsive: Upper Extremities Assessment

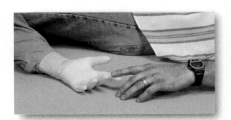

Touch finger.

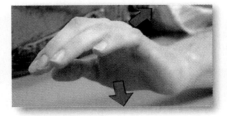

Hand movement.

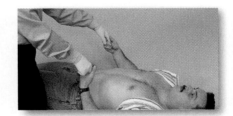

Hand squeeze.

RESULTS: If the patient can perform these tests, there is little chance of damage in the cervical area, but you cannot rule out all injuries. Limited performance and pain: pressure on spinal cord in cervical area. Failure to perform any: suspect severe spinal-cord injury in neck.

Unresponsive patients

Test the responses to painful stimuli by pinching the back of the hand, the ankle, or the top of the foot, or by squeezing a toe.

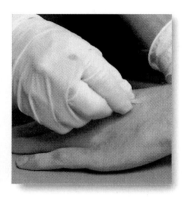 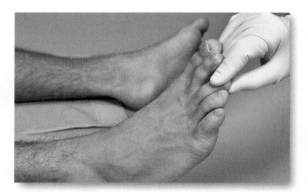

REMEMBER: It is difficult to accurately assess an unresponsive patient. If the mechanism of injury indicates possible damage to the spine, or if the patient is unresponsive, care for spine injury.

RESULTS: If slight pulling back of foot, spinal cord is usually intact. If no foot reaction, there is possible damage anywhere along the spinal cord. If hand or finger reaction, there is usually no damage to spinal cord. If no hand or finger reaction, there is possible damage to the spinal cord. Suspect damage to the spinal cord if you find no reactions, failure to perform any test, limited performance, or performance with pain.

Summary of Observations and Conclusions

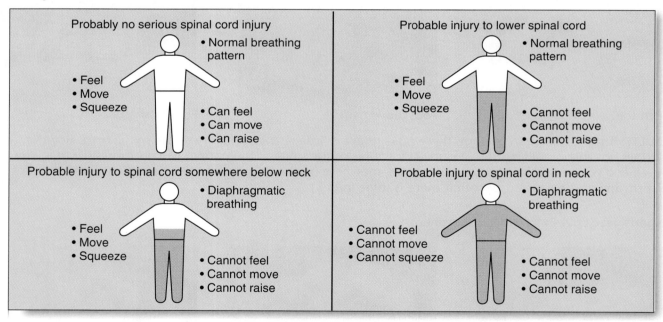

Probably no serious spinal cord injury
- Normal breathing pattern
- Feel
- Move
- Squeeze
- Can feel
- Can move
- Can raise

Probable injury to lower spinal cord
- Normal breathing pattern
- Feel
- Move
- Squeeze
- Cannot feel
- Cannot move
- Cannot raise

Probable injury to spinal cord somewhere below neck
- Diaphragmatic breathing
- Feel
- Move
- Squeeze
- Cannot feel
- Cannot move
- Cannot raise

Probable injury to spinal cord in neck
- Diaphragmatic breathing
- Cannot feel
- Cannot move
- Cannot squeeze
- Cannot feel
- Cannot move
- Cannot raise

WARNING: If the patient is unresponsive or the mechanism of injury indicates spine injury, provide care for spine injury.

- See if the patient can move his arms and legs. Do not do this if you have noted any mechanism of injury or other signs that indicate possible injury to the spine.

For the unresponsive patient, remember to:

- Ask bystanders for information on the emergency and what they saw happen to the patient. This may help you determine the mechanism of injury.
- Look and feel for injuries and deformities.
- See if the patient responds to pressure on or pinching of the feet and hands. Never probe palms and soles with sharp objects. ■

Rules for Care of Spine Injury

FIRST ➤ Always follow these rules for Emergency Medical Responder care of patients with possible spine injuries:

- Make certain the airway is open. Assist ventilations or perform CPR as needed, even though the patient may have spine injuries. Use the jaw-thrust maneuver when ventilating the patient.
- Attempt to control serious bleeding. Avoid moving the injured part of the patient and any of the limbs when applying dressings.
- Always conclude that an unresponsive trauma patient has spine injuries.
- Do not attempt to splint long-bone injuries if there are indications of spine injuries until you have appropriate help.
- Never move a patient with suspected spine injuries unless you must do so to provide CPR or assist ventilations, need to reach and control life-threatening bleeding, or must protect yourself and the patient from immediate danger at the scene.
- Keep the patient still. Tell him not to move. Position yourself to stabilize the patient's head, neck, and as much of the body as possible.
- Continuously monitor patients with possible spine injury. These patients will often go into shock. Sometimes, their chest muscles will be paralyzed and they will go into respiratory arrest. ■

Stabilizing the Patient's Head and Neck

Suspect that any patient with head injury also has a spine injury. Suspect that a patient with chest trauma has injuries to the neck. Work carefully and gently as you immobilize the patient. Do not apply traction to the patient's head and neck. Just grip the head with your hands as you would to perform the jaw-thrust maneuver. Do not try to place an extrication collar on the patient or position the patient on a spine board unless you have had training in these procedures and there is enough help to move the patient properly.

Is It Safe ?

It is important to understand the priorities of care when dealing with a patient with suspected spine injury. At no time does a suspected spine injury become a higher priority than airway, breathing, and circulation. You *must* ensure an open airway and adequate breathing, even if you suspect a spine injury. Manage the airway first, while always being mindful of a possible spine injury. When moving the patient's head to open the airway, be gentle and only move the head as far as necessary to ensure an open airway. ■

WARNING

Stabilize the patient's head and neck and wait for more advanced care to arrive before attempting to immobilize further.

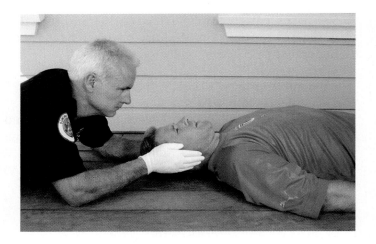

FIGURE 11.44 Manual in-line stabilization of the patient's head and neck.

A patient with spine injuries may be able to move his head, neck, arms, trunk, or legs but movement can cause more injury. For this reason, keep the patient from moving by verbally reassuring him and by physically stabilizing the head and neck.

FIRST ➤ Follow these guidelines when you manually stabilize a patient's head and neck (Figure 11.44):

1. Kneel at the top of the patient's head.
2. Place your hands on each side of the head and position your fingers under the lower jaw.
3. Keep the patient's head and neck steady (stable) in this position. Do not allow the patient to move his head and neck. Explain your actions to the patient and offer reassurance while you are keeping his head stable. Do not apply traction or turn or lift the patient's head.
4. Maintain your position until a rigid cervical or extrication collar is applied. (See Chapter 5, Scans 5–12 through 5–15, for application steps, but do not attempt to apply a collar to a patient until you have received proper training from your instructor.)

It is best to stabilize a patient's head and neck and wait for the EMTs to arrive before trying to proceed any further in immobilizing the patient. Immobilizing a patient on a backboard is not a required Emergency Medical Responder skill. However, your jurisdiction may require that you learn this skill. If so, your instructor will teach you the proper techniques. Do not attempt to place a patient on a backboard without proper training. ■

Helmet Removal

Helmets are designed to absorb energy forces and prevent injury to the head. However, well-fitting helmets—even the most modern ones—cannot prevent the brain from striking the interior of the skull in extreme or high-speed crash forces. When the brain rapidly and repeatedly strikes the inside of the skull, brain tissue is bruised and blood vessels tear and bleed. The patient can suffer a concussion, a contusion, or develop a hematoma (blood clot) in the brain tissue or under one of the layers of tissue that protects the brain.

For an unresponsive athlete (or any injured patient wearing a helmet), suspect a spine injury, properly immobilize the spine, and initiate safe transport to the hospital. When it is necessary to assess the patient's face to manage the airway, to assist breathing, or to provide CPR, it is recommended that only the face guard of the football helmet should be removed. Removing the face guard gives emergency care providers access to the face and airway and allows them to assess vital signs, provide care for face injuries, or begin resuscitation. The helmet should be removed only if the rescuers are unable to gain access to the airway by any other means.

For football players who are wearing shoulder pads, the helmet left in place keeps the cervical spine in a midline position. Removing the helmet but keeping the shoulder pads in place causes the head to hyperextend or fall back in an overextended position, which pulls the spinal column out of alignment. Helmets do not prevent neck injuries. The majority of sports-related neck injuries are caused by flexing of the neck either too far forward (hyperflexion) or too far backward (hyperextension), or by a sudden compressing force to the top of the head, which compacts the spinal column.

There are many types of helmets (Scan 11–9). They are made in half-size, three-quarter size, and full-size. Full-size helmets cover the mouth and sometimes part of the nose and usually have a face shield. Bicycle helmets are usually half-size and open in the front and have no face shield or face guard. Football helmets are full-size and have face guards. Motorcycle helmets are available in all three sizes, with the full-size helmets having a clear face shield or visor that moves up and down and is easy to remove. Motorcyclists who wear the half-size or three-fourths size helmets will usually wear glasses or goggles to protect their eyes. If the helmet has a face guard or face shield, remove it to gain access to the patient's airway. If any patient who is not breathing is wearing a helmet with a face guard or face shield that cannot be removed, remove the helmet to gain access to the airway. If a helmet is removed, it must be done cautiously and by two people.

Before removing a helmet, perform the following steps:

1. Remove the face piece or face shield while your partner stabilizes the head. Do not cut the chin strap. Remove glasses or goggles.

2. Check to see if the patient is breathing by placing your ear and/or hand in front of the nose and mouth. Even with full-size, snugly fitting helmets, there is room to slip your hand under the protective face portion to check breathing.

3. If the patient is breathing, check the helmet for fit. An Emergency Medical Responder can stabilize the head by grasping the patient's lower jaw under the helmet while a partner gently pulls on the helmet.

   An alternative method is to have a partner stabilize the head by placing her hands on either side of the helmet while you slide both hands under the helmet on either side of the jaw to check the helmet for fit and snugness. A well-fitting helmet can stay in place as long as the patient is breathing.

4. Determine if you can gain access to the patient's airway without removing the helmet if airway care and breathing assistance are necessary.

5. If you cannot gain access to the airway and you must clear the airway or assist the patient with breathing, remove the helmet. If the patient is wearing shoulder pads, leave them in place. While your partner is maintaining the head in line with the body, place a similar amount of padding under the patient's head to help your partner keep the patient's head in line with the body while you perform airway, ventilation, or resuscitation measures.

Check local protocols for helmet removal procedures. Work with local coaches to learn and practice them. Check with helmet vendors to become familiar with the types of helmets and their fit. Note that the half-size and three-quarter size helmets give easy access to airway and breathing, but if they are left in place, you may have to place extra padding behind the patient's shoulders.

To be effective, all helmets must fit the wearer properly, be worn correctly, and meet helmet criteria based on testing by the Snell Memorial Foundation, the only helmet-testing lab accredited to ISO 25 in the United States by the American Association for Laboratory Accreditation. Snell also tests helmets for removability. Emergency care providers must be able to quickly remove headgear from injured patients in order to check for vital signs and to perform emergency procedures.

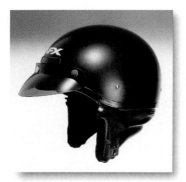

Half-size motorcycle helmet. Provides head protection from impact but may not provide face and eye protection, even with a face shield. Easier to remove than a full helmet. *(AFX North America, Inc.)*

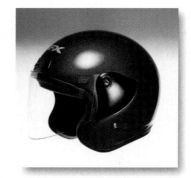

Three-quarter size motorcycle helmet. Provides head protection from impact and may provide face and eye protection. Somewhat easier to remove than the full-size helmet. *(AFX North America, Inc.)*

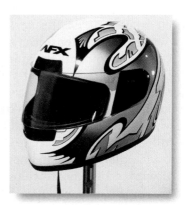

Full-size motorcycle helmet. In addition to head impact protection, provides a measure of protection to the face with a face shield. Properly fitting helmets have room beneath the chin bar for a hand to slide under and check for airway and breathing. *(AFX North America, Inc.)*

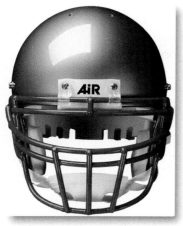

Football helmet. Provides a measure of protection to the face with a face shield in place as well as head impact protection. *(Schutt Sports)*

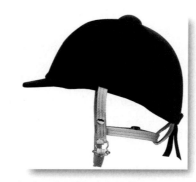

Horseback riding helmet. Provides head protection from impact but may not provide face and eye protection. *(International Riding Helmets)*

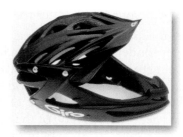

Mountain bike helmet. Provides head protection and, with a chin bar, some face protection. *(Giro Sport Design)*

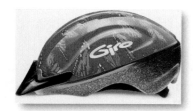

Youth's bicycle helmet. Provides head protection if it fits properly and is worn correctly. *(Giro Sport Design)*

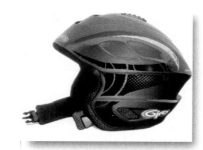

Snowboarding helmet. Provides head protection and, with a chin bar, some face protection. *(Giro Sport Design)*

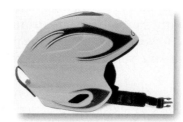

Downhill skiing helmet. Provides head protection and, with a chin bar, some face protection. *(Giro Sport Design)*

Provide care to any unresponsive patient as if there is a spine injury. When you find any helmeted patient face down or on one side, log roll him onto his back (supine). Your instructor will show you how to log roll a patient if Emergency Medical Responders are allowed to do this in your jurisdiction.

Leave the helmet in place if you find or suspect the following:

- Helmet fits well, and the patient's head does not move (or moves very little) inside of it. A well-fitting helmet keeps the head from moving and should be left on if there are no airway or breathing problems and the helmet does not interfere with assessment and management of the airway and breathing.
- Patient is breathing adequately and has no airway problems (fluids, obstructions).
- Patient can be placed in a neutral, in-line position for immobilization on a spine board.
- Helmet does not interfere with your ability to reassess and maintain the patient's airway or assist breathing.
- Patient is wearing shoulder pads. If the helmet is removed, place a similar amount of padding under the head or remove the shoulder pads. However, removing the shoulder pads may cause further harm to the patient.

Remove the helmet if you find the following:

- Helmet interferes with your ability to assess or manage the patient's airway and breathing.
- Helmet does not fit snugly, and the patient's head moves inside the helmet.
- Helmet interferes with placing the patient on a spine board in a neutral, in-line position. When the helmet rests on the spine board, its size may force the patient's head forward (hyperflexion) and close the airway. Padding can be placed under the patient's shoulders to prevent hyperflexion and maintain an in-line position.
- Patient is in cardiac or respiratory arrest. Quickly remove the helmet while a partner stabilizes the head. Proceed with CPR steps, using the jaw-thrust maneuver.

If you must remove the helmet, consult with medical direction and remove it according to local protocol. The steps listed below provide general directions for removal of full-size helmets (Scans 11–10 and 11–11). Your instructor will demonstrate them. Practice with all three sizes of helmets.

1. Rescuer 1 will kneel at the head of the patient and stabilize the patient's head by placing his hands on each side of the helmet, with fingers on the patient's jaw to prevent movement.

2. Rescuer 2 will kneel on one side of the patient at the patient's shoulders, unfasten the chin strap, remove the face guard or face shield (if not yet done), and remove the patient's glasses or goggles if present.

3. Rescuer 2 will place one hand on the mandible at the angle of the jaw and the other hand behind the neck at the base of the skull and stabilize the head while rescuer 1 removes the helmet.

4. Rescuer 1 will pull sides of the helmet apart and slowly and carefully slip the helmet halfway off the patient's head until rescuer 2 can reposition the hand behind the head and neck.

5. Rescuer 2 will maintain the hand position that is stabilizing the jaw. Reposition the hand at the back of the neck a little higher on the back of the head to maintain stabilization of the head and its in-line position of the body, particularly if the patient is wearing shoulder pads.

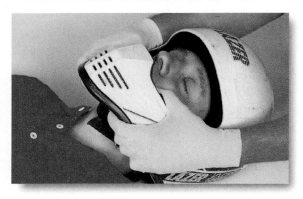

1 ■ Rescuer 1: kneel at the head of the patient. Stabilize the patient's head.

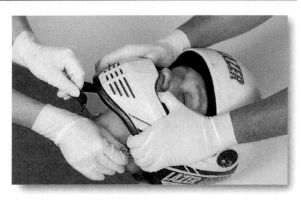

2 ■ Rescuer 2: kneel at the side of the patient's shoulders. Unfasten the chin strap. Remove the face guard, face shield, goggles, or glasses, if present.

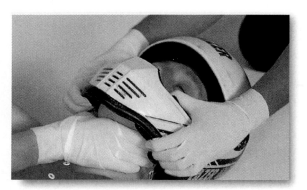

3 ■ Rescuer 2: place one hand on the mandible at the angle of the jaw and the other hand behind the neck at the base of the skull to stabilize the patient's head.

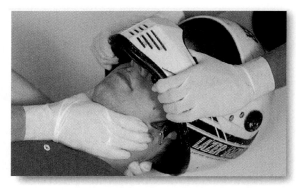

4 ■ Rescuer 1: pull sides of helmet apart and carefully slip helmet halfway off.

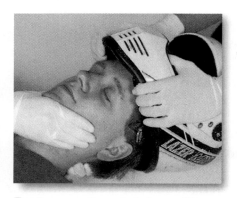

5 ■ Rescuer 2: maintain position of hand stabilizing the jaw. Reposition at the back of the neck slightly higher on the back of the head to maintain in-line stabilization.

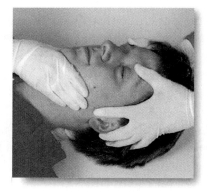

6 ■ Rescuer 1: finish removing the helmet and then place hands on either side of the patient's head to take over in-line stabilization.

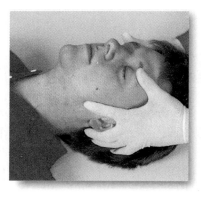

7 ■ Rescuer 2: check and clear airway, provide ventilations, and apply a collar.

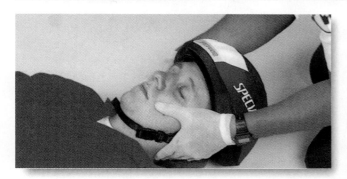

1 ■ Apply steady stabilization to the neck in neutral position.

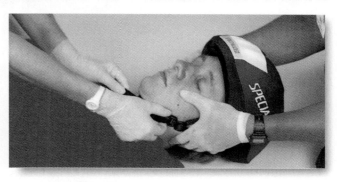

2 ■ Remove the chin strap.

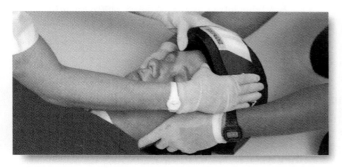

3 ■ Remove helmet by pulling the sides apart (laterally).

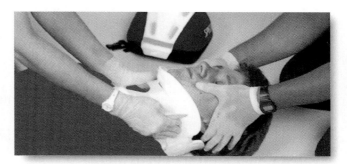

4 ■ Apply a suitable cervical spine immobilization collar and secure the patient to a long board.

6. Rescuer 1 will finish removing the helmet, place padding under the patient's head as needed (if the patient is wearing shoulder pads), and then place his hands on either side of the patient's head to take over in-line stabilization.

7. Rescuer 2 will check and clear the airway, provide ventilations with supplemental oxygen, and apply a collar.

Remember that you do not have to remove a helmet from a patient if the patient has an airway and is breathing, if the helmet is snug, and if the patient can be secured to a spine board with the helmet on and the head in a neutral, in-line position with the spine.

INJURIES TO THE CHEST

Chest injuries can damage the lungs, heart, major vessels, and upper abdominal organs protected by the ribs. Ribs can be fractured or crushed, or the sternum may become fractured or completely separated from the ribs. Broken and crushed ribs and sternum can cause punctures and tears to organs and vessels underneath. The force of the trauma may also directly or indirectly damage the section of the spine where the ribs are attached. Because of these problems, it is important to stabilize the head and neck of a chest trauma patient. Wounds to the chest need immediate attention and care.

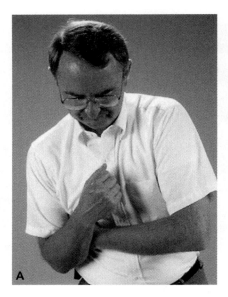
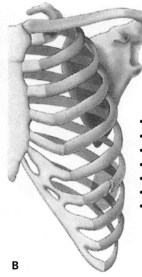

- Tenderness
- Local pain
- Deformity
- Shallow breathing
- Coughing
- Painful movement
- "Crackling" sensation in skin if lung is punctured

A   B

FIGURE 11.45 Possible fractured ribs. **A.** Characteristic stance. **B.** Other signs and symptoms.

Rib Injuries

FIRST ➤ Signs and symptoms of suspected fractured ribs include (Figure 11.45):

- Pain and tenderness at the site of the injury.
- Deformity at the site of the injury, which may be slight swelling or obvious rib displacement.
- Increased pain at the site on moving or breathing.
- Shallow breathing, sometimes with the patient reporting a crackling sensation at or near the site of injury.
- Characteristic stance. Often, the patient will lean toward the side of the injury, with a hand or forearm pressed over the injury.
- Guarding the injury site. Often the patient will hold his hand across the injured side to help support and stabilize the injury. This is called *self-splinting*. ▪

If it appears that no underlying organs have been damaged, you do not need to take any immediate action other than keeping the patient at rest in a comfortable position. But if there are signs that the lungs have been damaged by the fractured rib (for example, frothy blood in the mouth) or several ribs are apparently fractured, you must provide additional care for the patient.

FIRST ➤ The care for injured ribs requires you to wear personal protective equipment and:

1. Ensure an open airway. Suction or clear the mouth, if necessary. Keep the patient at rest and monitor breathing.
2. Provide oxygen as soon as possible as per local protocols. Maintain body temperature to help minimize the possibility of shock.
3. Place the forearm of the injured side in a sling so that it rests across the patient's chest. Apply a swathe to provide additional support (Figure 11.46).
4. Initiate transport to the hospital to be examined by more highly trained personnel. ▪

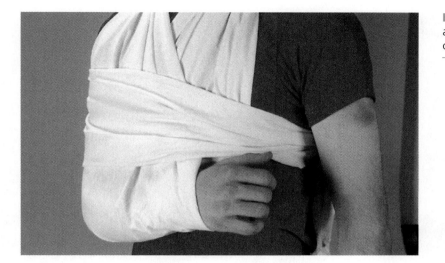

Flail Chest

When two or more consecutive ribs on the same side of the chest are fractured in two or more places, it can create a section of chest that moves in the opposite direction of the rest of the chest wall during breathing. The same type of chest wall movement is seen when the breastbone is broken away from the ribs. This type of injury is referred to as a **flail chest** (Figure 11.47). Emergency Medical Responders see flail chests most often at motor-vehicle collisions, where the patient, who is not wearing a seat belt, is thrown against the steering wheel during sudden deceleration (sudden stop).

FIRST ➤ The signs and symptoms of flail chest include (Figure 11.48):

- Same signs and symptoms as fractured ribs.
- Section of the chest wall that moves in the opposite direction of the rest of the chest when the patient is breathing. This motion may be slight and can be seen as you watch the patient inhale (the chest expands), when the flail section will slightly depress or sink inward. As the patient exhales (chest relaxes), the flail section will slightly push out from the rest of the chest wall.

flail chest ■ the condition that results when there are two or more ribs fractured in two or more places, or the breastbone separates from the chest and produces a loose segment of the chest wall. This segment will move in the opposite direction of the chest during breathing.

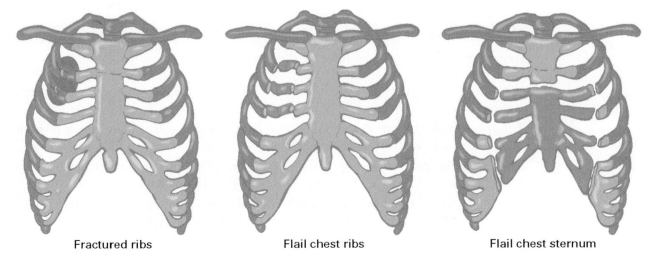

Fractured ribs   Flail chest ribs   Flail chest sternum

FIGURE 11.47 Rib fractures and a flail chest.

FIGURE 11.48 Signs and symptoms of a flail chest.

MECHANISMS OF INJURY

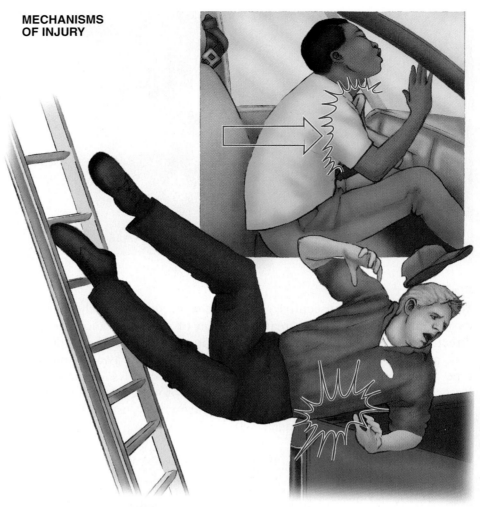

SIGNS OF FLAIL CHEST

- Pain
- Shallow breathing
- Deformity
- Painful movement

- Tenderness
- Crackling sensation
- Irregular chest movement

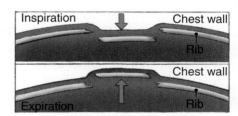

To care for a flail chest and stabilize the loose segment (Figure 11.49):

1. Locate the flail section by gently feeling the injury site. In the majority of cases, the injury will be at the side of the chest.

2. Apply a bulky pad of dressings, several inches thick, over the site or use a small pillow that is soft and lightweight.

3. Use large strips of tape to hold the pad in place. Do not tape entirely around the chest; it would restrict breathing efforts. If you do not have tape:
   - Position the patient on the injured side. Body weight against the surface will help splint the injury. (Do not do this if spine injuries are suspected.)

   OR . . .
   - Hold the pad in place by hand. When doing so, position your body so that you will not have to shift your weight and move the pad.

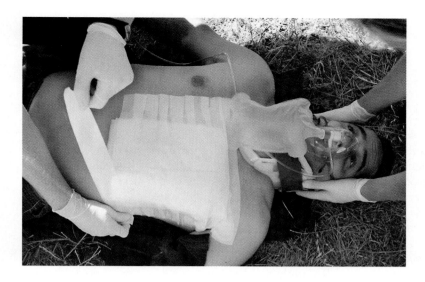

FIGURE 11.49 Emergency care of a patient with flail chest.

4. Provide 100% oxygen via nonrebreather mask as soon as possible if allowed by your local protocols and maintain body temperature to minimize the effects of shock.

5. Monitor vital signs, ensure adequate breathing, and look for signs of heart and lung injury. ■

When the ribs and breastbone are injured, the lungs and the heart can also be injured. Always look for frothy blood in the patient's mouth and signs of difficult or labored breathing, which indicate injury to the lungs. In cases of flail chest, make certain to examine the patient for the following:

- Distended (bulging) neck veins.
- Blue coloration of the head, neck, and shoulders.
- Bulging, bloodshot eyes.
- Blue coloration and swelling of the lips and tongue.
- Obvious chest deformity.

These signs indicate that the heart has been injured and that blood has been forced back out of its right side and up through the major veins that lead to the heart from the neck. These patients need oxygen as soon as possible and must be transported immediately.

FIRST ON SCENE WRAP-UP

Russell had just finished splinting Joan's leg with a putter and a sand wedge when the ambulance approached them, moving slowly across the grass. The EMTs complimented Russell on straightening and splinting Joan's injured leg and decided to transport her with the makeshift splint. Just before the ambulance crew shut the doors, Russell patted Joan's uninjured leg and said, "Let me just get this golf cart figured out, and I'll meet you over at the E.D."

"Russell," she looked at him sternly, her voice muffled by the oxygen mask. "Don't you dare finish the game without me!"

Summary

When caring for patients with suspected musculoskeletal injuries, remember that scene safety and the mechanism of injury are important factors to consider before patient care may begin. Assess and care for all life-threatening problems first. Before focusing on extremity injuries, provide care for injuries to the head and spine, open injuries to the chest and abdomen, and all serious burns. Provide oxygen, and maintain body temperature to help prevent shock.

The musculoskeletal system provides body support and movement, protects organs, and produces blood cells. Soft tissues such as muscles, nerves, and blood vessels are damaged when bones are injured. Manage them as part of total patient care.

An open injury occurs when a bone tears through the skin or the mechanism of injury causes a puncture to the outer skin and damages the bone inside. If the bones do not tear through the patient's skin, the injury is called a *closed injury*. Apply sterile dressings to all open injuries. A bone that is broken and bends at a place other than a joint is called a *deformed or angulated injury*.

Typical signs and symptoms for musculoskeletal injuries include pain, swelling, discoloration, and deformity. Other signs and symptoms include loss of use, tenderness, guarding, loss of distal pulse, slow capillary refill (in pediatric patients), numbness, tingling, grating, the sound of breaking bone, and exposed bone.

Some special signs to look for with injured extremities include guarding of the injured extremity, bulging where there is a joint or where the extremity joins the torso, pelvic pain on compression of the patient's hips, and leg rotating outward or inward.

Emergency care procedures for injured extremities include applying a rigid or soft splint. When in doubt about the extent of a musculoskeletal injury, use a splint. All splinting must immobilize the injured extremity and the joints directly above and below the injury site.

Soft splinting can effectively immobilize an injured extremity without rigid splints. Use a sling and swathe for:

- Injuries to the collarbone or shoulder blade.
- Dislocation of the shoulder. Add padding in the space between arm and chest and the sling and swathe.
- Injuries to the upper arm bone and forearm. Modify the full sling to a wrist sling if the injury is in the elbow area. Add a swathe.
- Injuries to the elbow. Use a wrist sling and a swathe.
- Injuries to the wrist, hand, or fingers. NOTE: Always place the hand in the position of function.

Use padding such as folded blankets or towels for injuries to the pelvis or hip, thigh, knee, or leg. Secure the blanket or towels with four cravats, two above and two below the knees. Then, with EMT assistance, place the patient on a spine board or scoop (orthopedic) stretcher.

Use a pillow for injuries to the ankle or foot. Secure the pillow with cravats and elevate.

Applying a splint can prevent or reduce complications, such as pain, soft-tissue damage, bleeding, and restricted blood flow, and can prevent closed injuries from becoming open injuries.

To apply a splint, first cut away or remove clothing from the injury site. Control bleeding and dress open wounds. Check for distal circulation, sensation, and motor function before and after splinting. If there is no distal pulse, realign deformed (angulated) injuries or reposition extremities until pulse is regained, if allowed to do so by your EMS system.

Pad all rigid splints before they are secured to the patient. Manual traction is applied by pulling gently on an injured limb along its long axis. If manual traction is applied, maintain it until the rigid splint is secured.

Emergency Medical Responders may use noncommercial splints, such as lumber, plywood, rolled newspapers and magazines, compressed wood products, sporting equipment, canes, umbrellas, cardboard, and tool handles.

Open head injuries involve fractures of the skull. There can be direct injury to the brain in open head injuries such as cuts, tears, and bruising. In closed head injuries, the skull is not damaged, but injuries to the brain can occur and include concussions (brain shaking or bouncing), contusions (brain bruises), and hemorrhage (bleeding inside skull).

Head injuries may be obvious, or they may be difficult to detect. Always look for wounds to the head, deformity of the skull, bruises behind the ear, black eyes, sunken eyes, unequal pupils, and blood or clear fluids flowing from the ears and/or nose. Brain injury can occur with head injuries. Look for signs of possible skull fracture, loss of awareness, confusion, unequal or unresponsive pupils, and paralysis.

When caring for a patient with injuries to the head, maintain an open airway using the jaw-thrust maneuver and manually stabilize the head. Assist ventilations or provide CPR if needed. Keep the head injury patient at rest and talk to him. Control bleeding but avoid pressure over the site of the injury. Do not remove impaled objects, bone fragments, or other objects from head wounds.

Face injuries often cause airway obstruction. Maintain an open airway with the jaw-thrust maneuver. The mechanism of injury that causes injuries to the face can also cause spine injury. Be sure to stabilize the head when managing the airway.

Spine injuries can be very serious and can result in permanent paralysis or disability. Keep the patient from moving. Suspect that all unresponsive trauma patients have spine injuries. If the mechanism of injury indicates possible spine injuries, proceed as if they are present.

The focused assessment is very important in determining if the patient has spine injuries. Always look for weakness, numbness, loss of feeling, pain, or paralysis to the limbs of a patient. Remember to press or pinch the feet and hands of the unresponsive patient and look for reactions.

Follow certain rules when caring for a patient who may have spine injuries. Even though a patient has spine injuries, provide ventilations or CPR, if needed, and control bleeding. Do not attempt to splint suspected fractures without help. Never move a patient with spine injuries without help unless absolutely necessary. Stabilize the patient's head and neck and as much of the body as possible. Continuously monitor the patient.

Injuries to the chest can include soft-tissue injuries, crushing injuries, and penetrating injuries that can cause fractured ribs, flail chest, spine injuries, lung injuries, and heart injuries. Pain at the site may indicate rib fractures; apply a sling and swathe, placing the forearm of the injured side across the chest. Opposite motion in the ribs or breastbone may indicate flail chest; apply a thick pad over the site and tape it in place.

Remember and Consider

When you are at the scene of any injury, listen to what other care providers are saying and how they care for the emotions of their patients. When people are injured, they are concerned with the pain and how soon you can relieve it. Children want to stop hurting and want you to make the pain go away.

➤ Think about what you will tell your injured patients as you provide care for their injuries.

Sometimes when you have to move a patient during the assessment or while you dress a wound or splint an extremity, the movement will cause additional pain. You must let your patients know what you are doing and why, if it will hurt and for how long, and what the result will be when you are finished.

➤ Keep in mind that most patients will cooperate with your care if they know what to expect. You must respect their concerns, answer their questions, and provide them with as much information about their injury as possible.

Investigate

If you have not had a chance to look through your Emergency Medical Responder vehicle and see what equipment and supplies are carried, take some time to do so. Ask someone you know in fire services or the rescue squad to work with you to show you where splinting items are kept, or to suggest to you what items can be used as improvised splints.

➤ What materials for securing splints are carried on the unit?

➤ Are the splinting materials in places where they are easily reached, or will you have to take a few minutes to access them?

Practice using items in your unit for splinting. Work with other department members or with friends.

➤ As you hold traction, can you direct your friends to properly apply a commercial or an improvised splint?

➤ As you work with more experienced department members, can you follow their directions to hold traction or to splint while they hold traction?

Quick Quiz

1. All of the following are functions of the musculoskeletal system EXCEPT:

   a. strength.
   b. support.
   c. protection.
   d. cell production.

2. An injury that is characterized by broken bone ends protruding through the skin is commonly described as a(n) _____ wound.

   a. open
   b. closed
   c. complex
   d. superficial

3. Which one of the following would NOT be considered appropriate when caring for a suspected fracture?
   a. Cut away clothing to expose the injury site.
   b. "Pop" possible dislocations back into place.
   c. Assess circulation, sensation, and motor function.
   d. Immobilize the joint above and below the injury site.

4. When caring for patients who have sustained a significant mechanism of injury, the Emergency Medical Responder must:
   a. place in the recovery position.
   b. identify the medical problem.
   c. provide low-flow oxygen.
   d. suspect spine injury.

5. Numbness, tingling, loss of feeling, and weakness in the extremities are symptoms of a(n):
   a. severe allergic reaction.
   b. head injury.
   c. open fracture.
   d. spine injury.

6. All of the following are signs and symptoms of a head injury EXCEPT:
   a. altered mental status.
   b. deformity of the skull.
   c. discoloration of the nose.
   d. clear fluid exiting the ears.

7. A _____ occurs when one end of a bone that is part of a joint is pulled or pushed out of place.
   a. fracture
   b. dislocation
   c. concussion
   d. rotation

8. A thorough assessment of an extremity injury includes an evaluation of distal CSM. What does CSM stand for?
   a. circulation, sensation, motor function
   b. color, sensation, motor function
   c. color, strength, manual movement
   d. circulation, strength, motor function

9. All of the following are common signs and symptoms of an extremity injury EXCEPT:
   a. pain.
   b. swelling.
   c. deformity.
   d. lengthening.

10. Which one of the following injury locations has the highest priority for care?
    a. chest
    b. skull
    c. lower leg
    d. upper arm

11. The process of immobilizing an injury using a device such as a piece of wood, cardboard, or folded blanket is called:
    a. immobilization.
    b. traction.
    c. splinting.
    d. manual stabilization.

12. You are caring for a patient who has an injury characterized by an open wound, severe deformity, and bleeding. Your highest priority is:
    a. straightening the deformity.
    b. covering the open wound.
    c. splinting the extremity.
    d. controlling bleeding.

13. The straightening of an angulated injury is indicated when:
    a. the distal pulse is absent.
    b. there is an open wound.
    c. a splint is unavailable.
    d. directed by your partner.

14. A triangular bandage used to stabilize the elbow and arm is called a:
    a. cravat.
    b. dressing.
    c. bandage.
    d. sling.

15. When properly applied, a sling and swathe will adequately immobilize a:
    a. wrist.
    b. forearm.
    c. shoulder.
    d. knee.

16. It is important to maintain the hand and foot of an injured extremity in a normal and comfortable position during splinting. This is called the:
    a. recumbent position.
    b. position of function.
    c. position of comfort.
    d. resting position.

17. In most cases, injuries to a joint will be managed by:

   a. splinting in position found.
   b. manual stabilization.
   c. traction splinting.
   d. long spine board.

18. When caring for a patient with multiple injuries, it may be best to:

   a. splint all injuries before moving.
   b. splint only deformed injuries.
   c. immobilize on a long spine board.
   d. immobilize using a soft stretcher.

19. You are caring for a patient who has one leg that is shortened with the foot rotated to one side. These are likely signs of a possible:

   a. fractured pelvis.
   b. dislocated hip.
   c. dislocated knee.
   d. sprained ankle.

20. Which one of the following is the most efficient method of immobilizing an injured ankle?

   a. short spine board
   b. traction splint
   c. cardboard splint
   d. folded blanket

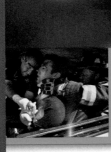

CHAPTER 12

Caring for the Geriatric Patient

This chapter introduces the special considerations necessary in assessing and providing care for geriatric patients. Because there are currently more than 35 million elderly persons in the United States, with that number expected to more than double in the next two decades, Emergency Medical Responders will commonly find themselves providing care for these older patients. It is important to understand that although people are living longer and healthier lives than ever before, age-related changes in anatomy and physiology do make these patients more susceptible to certain illnesses and injuries. Geriatric patients also tend to respond differently to medical emergencies than younger patients do, so Emergency Medical Responders should expect their assessment findings to differ—sometimes significantly—the older the patient is.

OBJECTIVES

There are currently no National Standard Objectives for First Responders that address the care of geriatric patients.

ADDITIONAL LEARNING TASKS

This chapter introduces many of the reasons why geriatric individuals are unique when compared to other age groups. The text and your instructor will help you understand how to treat elderly patients in a variety of emergency situations. Caring for geriatric patients requires that you understand not only the physical differences, but also the emotional and social ones. As you read this chapter, think about and be able to:

➤ State the unique challenges that may arise when caring for the geriatric patient.
➤ Describe changes in the approach to care when dealing with elderly people.

Although elderly people are all unique individuals, they share some commonalities. Think about these similarities and be able to:

➤ List the general characteristics of elderly patients.
➤ Identify some of the most common age-related physical changes found in geriatric patients.

After reading the text and working with your instructor, you will be able to provide competent care for geriatric patients. As you are practicing patient assessments and care, focus on being able to:

➤ Describe the general assessment considerations for elderly patients.
➤ List the considerations of performing a physical exam on a geriatric patient.
➤ Identify the common medical problems of geriatric patients.

 FIRST ON SCENE

Security Officer Hal Bergstrom tapped the steering wheel of his small car and waited for the light to turn green. He had less than seven minutes to get over to the Meadow Glen Apartments and lock up the pool area or else he was going to be running behind on his nightly route. Just then he heard the roar of a motorcycle engine from somewhere, loud enough to drown out the music on his car radio, followed by the squeal of tires. He had just started to look around at the other cars waiting on different sides of the intersection when his small car shuddered with the sound of crushing metal. "What in the heck?"

He looked over his right shoulder and saw a small woman on a large, black motorcycle wobble past his passenger window and slide sideways into the middle of the intersection, showering bright sparks into the air. The motorcycle came to rest on its side with the woman crumpled next to it. Hal grabbed his orange Emergency Medical Responder jump bag, hurried into the intersection, and shut off the still blaring motorcycle.

"Are you okay?" he said to the rider who had her face buried in the crook of her leather-clad elbow. Her shoulders shook as if she was sobbing, making her black helmet—painted with Egyptian hieroglyphics—tap on the ground. He noticed that the woman's left leg was resting at an odd angle on the pavement as he gently touched her shoulder. At his touch, she lifted her face from the sleeve of her leather jacket and turned toward him. She was very old, and she was not crying. She was laughing.

Introduction

There is a common misconception among EMS professionals that most **elderly** people are usually ill, hard of hearing, and altered in their mental state to the point of not being able to provide reliable information to caregivers. You should understand that this is not true. The vast majority of the elderly lead healthy, active lives and are able to communicate clearly and effectively with those around them (Figure 12.1). Why the misconception, then? It is probably because people who are healthy and active rarely require EMS assistance. So when EMS providers are summoned to help an elderly person, the calls frequently come from extended-care facilities where chronically ill and/or mentally altered geriatric patients are cared for. You should not let frequent calls to these types of facilities distort your view of the geriatric population as a whole.

elderly ■ a person age 65 or older.

NOTE

There are two terms commonly used when referring to geriatric patients. The term "elderly" commonly refers to those individuals between 65 and 85, and the term "aged" is used to refer to those individuals over the age of 85.

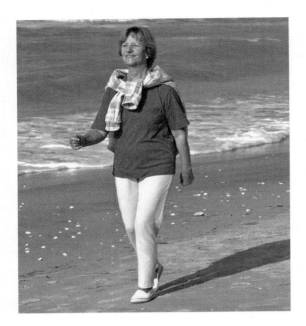

FIGURE 12.1 Many older adults live active lives.

lucid (LOO-sid) ▪ clear perception or understanding.

Although you should now understand that the majority of elderly patients are as healthy and **lucid** as you are, there are some important differences that you should keep in mind when dealing with older people. These range from unique life experiences and the accompanying concerns that younger people may not really understand (such as the fear or distrust of ambulances and hospitals) to actual anatomical and physiological differences caused by age.

FIRST ➤ Successful treatment of elderly patients involves understanding the physical, emotional, and financial difficulties commonly experienced by persons in the 65 and older age group. ▪

Characteristics of Geriatric Patients

Even though geriatric patients, their bodies, and their specific illnesses grow more unique as they age, there are certain generalizations that are fairly consistent across this segment of the population. As an Emergency Medical Responder, you will not need to know the specifics of their development or disease processes, but being familiar with the following general areas will greatly assist you in understanding your geriatric patients.

MULTIPLE ILLNESSES

Elderly patients are just as likely to suffer from the same illnesses and disorders as everyone else, but their bodies are less able to defend against them and recover afterward. This results in multiple simultaneous illnesses. Elderly persons commonly have at least four to six illnesses or diseases at one time. This number tends to increase as the elderly patient ages. Multiple illnesses create a unique challenge for the medical responder who is assessing the geriatric patient. The patient may be displaying signs and symptoms from a variety of illnesses, with none of them appearing to be anything specific. Do not worry. It will not be your job to diagnose the patient. It usually takes a physician examining the geriatric patient and ordering a battery of lab tests before a diagnosis can be made.

MEDICATIONS

toxic (TOK-sik) ▪ poisonous.

Related directly to the presence of multiple illnesses, you will also find that elderly patients take numerous prescription and over-the-counter (OTC) medications each day. Actually, patients age 65 and older take an average of 4.5 medications per day. Incorrect medication usage (sometimes caused by forgetfulness or confusion about instructions) can create numerous problems, from overdosing to underdosing. Overdosing will result in **toxic** medication levels in the patient's system, and underdosing can cause the patient's illness or disease process to get worse (Figures 12.2 and 12.3). Another common cause of medication misuse is due to the cost of prescription medications. The elderly patient on a fixed income may cut their medications in half or take them only every other day in an attempt to get them to last longer than prescribed.

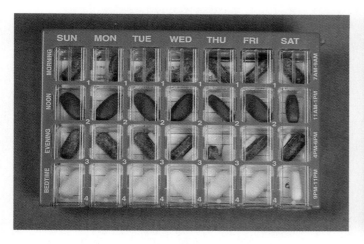

FIGURE 12.2 Many elderly people use a pill organizer to help them remember when to take their medications.

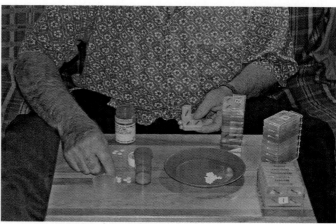

FIGURE 12.3 There are many kinds of devices that help elderly people keep track of medications.

FIRST ➤ When taking an elderly patient's medical history, make sure to ask if the patient is taking a prescribed medication as directed. Just because the patient states that he has medications does not mean that he has been taking them as prescribed. ▪

MOBILITY

Regular exercise is very important to keeping aging patients healthy and mobile, but it is common for some elderly persons to live sedentary lifestyles. This can be due to illnesses such as arthritis, fears (falling, being assaulted, and so on) or even medications that cause excessive tiredness. Having limited **mobility** can cause many problems for the elderly person, such as (Figure 12.4):

mobility (mo-BIL-i-tee) ▪ ability to move.

- ▪ Isolation.
- ▪ Poor nutrition.
- ▪ Depression.

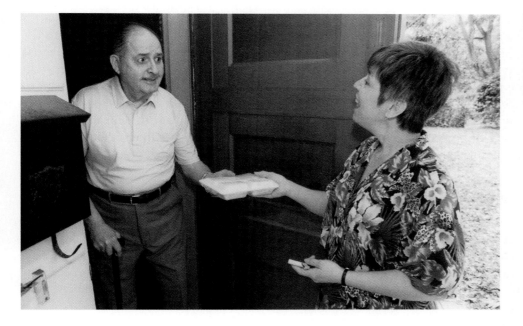

FIGURE 12.4 Meals-on-Wheels helps ensure that elderly people receive adequate nutrition by providing from one to three meals a day. *(© Craig Jackson/In the Dark Photography)*

Table 12–1	Age-Related Difficulties with Communication
DIFFICULTY	**STRATEGY**
Poor vision	Position yourself directly in front of the patient so you can be seen. Put your hand on the arm of a blind patient so he knows where you are. Locate the patient's glasses, if necessary.
Decreased hearing	Speak clearly. Check hearing aids. Write notes. You might even try letting the patient wear a stethoscope and speak into the head like a microphone.
Inability to speak clearly	Ask patient to put dentures in (or adjust them), if possible.

- Difficulty using the bathroom.
- Loss of independence.
- Higher likelihood for falls or other injuries.

DIFFICULTIES WITH COMMUNICATION

You will find that many geriatric patients have some age-related sensory changes. It is normal for elderly people to experience a lower sensitivity to pain or touch, an altered sense of smell or taste, a certain amount of hearing loss, and impaired vision or blindness. Any of these can affect your ability to assess and communicate with the patient. See Table 12–1 for some ideas about how to effectively communicate with an elderly patient.

INCONTINENCE

incontinence (in-CON-ti-nents)
- inability to retain urine or feces due to loss of muscle control.

Not necessarily caused by aging, several factors predispose elderly persons to the inability to retain urine or feces. Diseases such as diabetes, illnesses that cause diarrhea, and certain medications can all contribute to **incontinence**. Studies indicate that between 15% and 60% of all elderly persons suffer from some form of incontinence. You should also understand that it is important that you *not* make a big deal out of a geriatric patient's incontinence. The need to help maintain the dignity of any patient is important, but for elderly patients, in particular, respect and dignity is extremely vital.

CONFUSION OR ALTERED MENTAL STATUS

The most important thing to remember when you encounter an elderly patient who seems confused or appears to present with an altered mental status is to try to determine if the patient is always like that. You want to avoid placing too much importance on a patient's confused state if they are usually like that and not placing enough importance on it if the patient is normally clear thinking.

Is It Safe ?

Confused or altered geriatric patients can become belligerent, argumentative, or sometimes even physically abusive. When treating these patients, keep your own safety and the safety of others at the scene in mind. Do not let the patient's attitude or words upset you. Understand that the patient is not acting as he normally would. Do not allow yourself to be in a position where the patient can easily assault you. ▪

Age-Related Physical Changes

Although aging seems determined by genetics and begins at the cellular level, it is greatly affected by lifestyle and environment. As anyone can see by looking around in his or her own community, the aging process can differ greatly from person to person. There are, however, some general age-related changes that will be fairly consistent throughout the older population. It is important for Emergency Medical Responders to understand the basics of these changes and how they can impact the assessment and care process (Figure 12.5).

RESPIRATORY SYSTEM

Without regular exercise, the lungs will begin the aging process with decreased ability to ventilate properly as early as the age of 30. Aging creates many changes in the respiratory system. For example, the mechanism that helps the body detect low levels of oxygen in the blood becomes increasingly less efficient over time. This means that a geriatric patient may become severely **hypoxic** before the body even realizes it and attempts to compensate. Aging also leads to a decrease in the number of **cilia** in the airway, exposing the elderly person to more respiratory illnesses, such as pneumonia. Other respiratory changes due to aging include:

hypoxic (hi-POX-ik) ▪ state of having inadequate oxygen.

cilia (SILLY-uh) ▪ tiny hair-like structures that help sweep mucus and foreign particles upward in the respiratory system.

- Reduced strength and endurance of respiratory muscles.
- Decreased chest wall flexibility.
- Loss of lung elasticity.
- Collapse of smaller airway structures.

As with any patient, it is important that you continually assess and maintain the geriatric patient's airway.

CARDIOVASCULAR SYSTEM

Much of what affects the cardiovascular system seems related to lifestyle, but aging does seem to affect it to a certain degree. Some of the age-related changes in the cardiovascular system include:

- Enlargement of the left ventricle, which can decrease the amount of blood moved by the heart.
- Stiffening and elongation of the aorta, making it more susceptible to tearing.
- Degeneration of the heart's electrical system, causing **dysrhythmias.**
- Loss of elasticity in the blood vessels, which can result in high blood pressure and poor circulation.

dysrhythmias (dis-RITH-mee-uhs) ▪ a disturbance in heart rate or rhythm.

In addition, medications prescribed to elderly patients for heart conditions may prevent effective compensation for blood loss. Geriatric trauma patients who

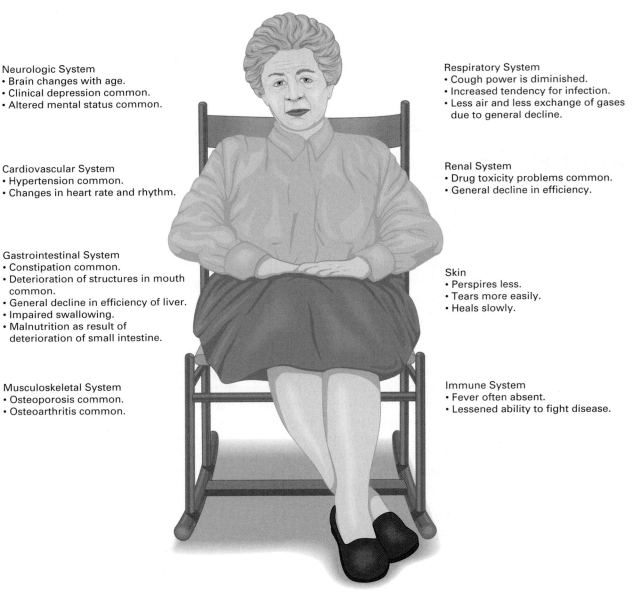

Neurologic System
- Brain changes with age.
- Clinical depression common.
- Altered mental status common.

Cardiovascular System
- Hypertension common.
- Changes in heart rate and rhythm.

Gastrointestinal System
- Constipation common.
- Deterioration of structures in mouth common.
- General decline in efficiency of liver.
- Impaired swallowing.
- Malnutrition as result of deterioration of small intestine.

Musculoskeletal System
- Osteoporosis common.
- Osteoarthritis common.

Respiratory System
- Cough power is diminished.
- Increased tendency for infection.
- Less air and less exchange of gases due to general decline.

Renal System
- Drug toxicity problems common.
- General decline in efficiency.

Skin
- Perspires less.
- Tears more easily.
- Heals slowly.

Immune System
- Fever often absent.
- Lessened ability to fight disease.

FIGURE 12.5 Common changes in the body systems of the elderly.

have lost a good amount of blood should be treated for shock even if their signs and symptoms do not indicate it.

NERVOUS SYSTEM

Aging has been shown to affect a person's nervous system in a few key areas. First, the brain loses about 10% of its overall weight between the ages of 20 and 90 years. Although this does *not* mean that elderly patients are less intelligent than younger ones, because no relationship between brain size and intelligence has ever been found, it does mean that there is more room for destructive bleeding inside the skull following a blow to the head. Also, aging causes a substantial decrease in the overall number of nerve fibers and the speed at which the impulses travel across them. These deteriorations mean that elderly patients may experience some of the following changes over time:

- Decreased reaction times.
- Difficulty with recent memory.
- Psychomotor slowing.
- Forgetfulness.

As you examine the geriatric patient, assess for sluggishness, confusion, or any mental status that appears below the level of full coherence. An altered mental status can indicate a wide range of illnesses and injuries, from infection and medication overdose to brain attack (stroke) and head trauma, all of which are very serious conditions. It is important that you summon advanced medical care for any elderly patient who presents with an abnormally altered mental status.

Although it may not be uncommon for an elderly person to seem agitated, confused, or have a decreased level of consciousness, always assume that he or she is normally coherent and mentally sharp until you can determine otherwise by questioning caregivers, spouse, or family members.

Although not directly related to the physical effects of aging on the nervous system, it is worth mentioning here that depression is a common condition found among elderly patients. In fact, suicides, or suicide attempts, are not unusual in the 65 and older segment of the population, especially among males. Be alert for signs of depression, such as poor hygiene, poor eating habits, and disorderly living environments.

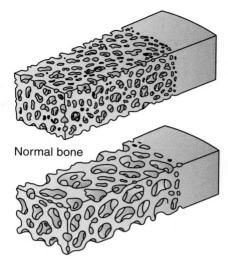

FIGURE 12.6 During the aging process, osteoporosis causes a reduction in the quality of bone, making the skeletal tissue more brittle and less elastic.

Normal bone

Osteoporotic bone

Is It Safe ?

Not only is suicide somewhat common for elderly patients, the use of firearms seems to be the preferred method. Be alert to your surroundings and always have a high index of suspicion when the patient exhibits any signs of depression. Some suicidal patients will wait until rescuers are present before attempting anything, usually to avoid being discovered by a family member. ■

osteoporosis (AH-stee-oh-pore-osis) ■ softening of bone tissue due to the loss of essential minerals, principally calcium.

MUSCULOSKELETAL SYSTEM

Age-related changes in the musculoskeletal system can lead to changes in posture, range of motion, and balance. Some elderly people can even lose up to three inches of overall height due to deterioration of the discs between the vertebrae and **osteoporosis** (Figure 12.6). Osteoporosis is the loss of minerals from bones, which causes the bones to soften and become weak. Because of these changes in the musculoskeletal system, the elderly are more susceptible to falls; once they fall, the injuries can be very severe. Also keep in mind that age-related changes in the spine may result in curvatures that can affect your ability to manage the patient's airway or effectively immobilize them following an injury.

FIRST ON SCENE

"Did you see that?" The woman's smile stretched from one helmet strap to the other. "I got that thing up to 80!"

"Ma'am," Hal placed his hands on either side of the black helmet and tried to hold the woman's bobbing head in place. "You may have injured yourself. Please don't move." He could hear sirens growing louder from down Porter Street.

"The leg's a bit sore, but other than that I feel just as right as rain! I didn't hit anybody did I?"

"Well, I think you actually hit my car."

Her eyes narrowed and she lowered her voice, "Don't you worry, my Frank always kept plenty of insurance on the vehicles."

"Ma'am, right now I'm just worried about you. Please just lie there and hold still. I can hear help coming."

The woman exhaled roughly and let her head rest on Hal's gloved hand. "You know," she touched her left leg with a shaky hand. "This leg is really starting to smart quite a bit. Can you straighten it out for me?" Hal looked over and saw that the woman's pants were growing dark over the spot where her leg appeared to be angulated.

INTEGUMENTARY SYSTEM (SKIN)

Because of its prominence on the body, age-related changes to the skin are going to be the most obvious to you as an Emergency Medical Responder. As people grow older, their skin loses its elasticity and thickness, causing it to be easily torn or injured. You may also notice dark areas of pigment on the skin, usually called "age spots" or "liver spots." The skin of a geriatric patient may be dry and flaky due to a decrease in the production of oils, and the ability to perspire tends to decrease as well, making heat-related emergencies more common and the onset of shock harder to recognize. As skin grows thinner and weaker, cell reproduction slows down so that not only are skin injuries worse among the elderly, but healing times also can be greatly extended.

Assessment of the Geriatric Patient

SCENE SIZE-UP

Your assessment of a geriatric patient will follow the same basic path as any other patient assessment with a few additional considerations. As always, make sure you begin by taking appropriate BSI precautions.

FIRST > Due to an increased risk of tuberculosis in nursing home patients, consider using a HEPA mask as part of your personal protective equipment (PPE). ▪

You will then want to complete your scene size-up, not only ensuring that it is safe to enter, but also looking for the following:

- Inadequate food, shelter, or hygiene.
- Lack of a working heating or cooling system.
- Potential fall hazards.
- Conditions that suggest abuse or neglect (Figure 12.7).

FIRST > Most states have laws that require Emergency Medical Responders to report suspect cases of geriatric abuse and neglect. Make sure that you are familiar with your local requirements. ▪

When you approach the patient, focus on her instead of caregivers or family members who may be present. This will show the patient that you respect her as a person and will give her a sense of control over the situation. If the patient is seated or lying on a bed, position yourself at the patient's level and make eye contact before introducing yourself (Figure 12.8). Another way to show respect to the patient is to use her title and last name, such as "Mrs. Becker," for example. Avoid using generic nicknames such as "dear," "sweetie," or "honey." Also avoid using an elderly person's first name (unless you are asked to use it); doing so could be considered rude or disrespectful. If appropriate, offer to shake the patient's hand during the

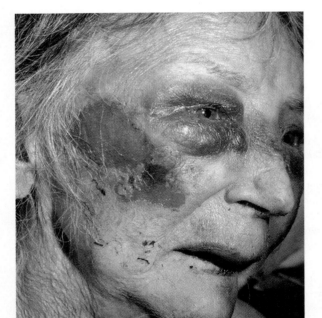

FIGURE 12.7 When you encounter evidence of trauma, consider the possibility of abuse until proven otherwise.

introduction. This builds rapport while also giving you the ability to check the patient's skin signs and mobility in an unobtrusive way.

FIRST ➤ Geriatric patients often do not reveal problems behind the chief complaint because they either fear the loss of independence or they consider the illness "normal" for their age. The best way to determine the patient's chief complaint without getting too much information about unrelated conditions is to ask, "Why did you call today?" or "What is different about how you feel today?" ▪

OBTAINING A HISTORY

Unlike the majority of younger patients, gathering a medical history on an elderly person may take quite a bit of time. You will find it helpful to first obtain the patient's medications (prescription and over-the-counter) and then ask why each is taken. Also be aware of the patient's surroundings. Are there medical identification tags or stickers? Oxygen supplies? Is there anything else that would indicate a medical condition? If you are unsure about a patient's answers to your questions, try to verify the information he or she gives you with a reliable source such as a caregiver, but do this when the patient will not be able to hear you.

THE PHYSICAL EXAM

The following considerations are important when examining a geriatric patient:

- Handle elderly patients gently.
- Histories and exams can easily tire elderly patients.
- Always explain what you are going to do before you do it.
- Anticipate numerous layers of clothing (due to problems with temperature regulation).
- Respect the modesty and privacy of elderly patients.

You should also remember that some geriatric patients may deny or minimize symptoms during the physical exam because they fear being institutionalized and losing their self-sufficiency if the extent of their condition is "discovered."

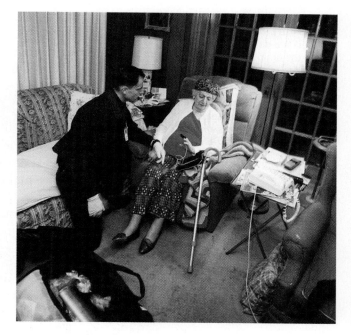

FIGURE 12.8 Position yourself at the patient's level, make good eye contact, and speak slowly and clearly.
(© *Craig Jackson/In the Dark Photography*)

REMEMBER

Speak slowly and clearly if your patient is hard of hearing. Refer to elderly patients as "Mr." or "Mrs." to show your respect.

Common Medical Problems of Geriatric Patients

ILLNESSES

Common illnesses among the elderly include pneumonia, chronic obstructive pulmonary diseases (**bronchitis**, **emphysema**, and so on), lung cancer, heart attacks, heart failure, dysrhythmias, **aneurysm**, high blood pressure, brain attack (stroke),

bronchitis (bronk-I-tus) ▪ inflammation of the bronchi; a form of chronic obstructive pulmonary disease (COPD).

emphysema (emf-a-ZEE-muh) ▪ disease that causes a loss of elasticity in the lungs; a form of chronic obstructive pulmonary disease (COPD).

aneurysm (ann-YER-ism) ▪ a ballooning of a weakened section of an artery.

dementia, **Alzheimer's disease, Parkinson's disease**, diabetes, bleeding in the stomach or esophagus, bleeding in the intestines, urinary tract infections, and reactions to medications. Due to the thinning of skin, a decreased ability to perspire, and muted physical sensations, heat- and cold-related emergencies are also common among geriatric patients.

INJURIES

Trauma caused by falls is the leading cause of injury death among the elderly. The weakening of bones, deterioration of skin integrity, and loss of blood vessel flexibility all combine to make injuries much more severe for geriatric patients. Add to that the medications taken by many elderly persons that can prevent clotting and make controlling bleeding extremely difficult, and you can have a relatively minor injury for a young patient actually causing serious injury or even death for an elderly one.

FIRST ➤ When assessing an elderly fall patient, remember that a fall often has more than one cause. ■

Is It Safe ?

An elderly patient who has suffered an injury has a greater likelihood of developing hypothermia, even in an environment that you would consider mild or warm. Ensure that the patient is kept warm at all times. ■

As an Emergency Medical Responder, you should be an advocate for injury prevention among the elderly. As you are responding to the homes of geriatric patients, you should always be looking for potential dangers, such as unsecured rugs, loose handrails, unsafely stacked items, and so on, and make a caregiver or family member aware of the safety concerns.

 FIRST ON SCENE WRAP-UP

Within minutes, the intersection was bustling with firefighters in turnout pants and dark T-shirts, along with several serious-looking police officers. The ambulance arrived moments later, its siren trailing off to silence about two blocks before it reached the scene. A bald firefighter with a large mustache took over holding the patient's head while several others began gently straightening her body on the pavement. Hal stood and stretched his back before quickly pointing at the patient's leg. "I think it looks broken. Make sure to be careful with it."

"We've got it, thanks," came the reply from one of the firefighters. By now the patient was no longer smiling, but biting her lower lip and clawing at the pavement each time the group of firefighters straightened body parts.

Once the woman was secured to the board and being lifted onto the ambulance gurney, the bald fireman walked over to where Hal stood giving information to a police officer. "You did a real good job by taking care of the C-spine right away," he patted Hal on the shoulder. "A lot of people would've jumped right to dealing with the busted leg."

"Thanks," Hal smiled, feeling his face redden. He wanted to say more but before he could think of anything, the firefighter had already disappeared into the fire truck across the intersection. About 20 minutes later, Hal got back into his car, intent on finally locking up the pool area at the Meadow Glen Apartments. Only now, as he rested his hand on the jump bag in the passenger seat, he wasn't quite so concerned about running behind.

Summary

The assessment and emergency care of geriatric patients can sometimes be challenging due to normal age-related changes in the human body. For example, you may find it more difficult to communicate with some elderly patients due to poor eyesight and hearing or confusion and an altered mental status. It is important, though, not to assume that just because a patient is elderly he will have these problems with communication. It can be insulting to an elderly person if you speak loudly, assuming a hearing problem, or if you speak in direct, simple terms, assuming that he is confused. Start with each patient as if he has no problems with communication and is perfectly lucid, and only adjust your approach if you find that you need to in order to communicate more effectively.

Also remember that there are specific age-related characteristics shared by many geriatric patients, such as the tendency to have multiple illnesses, to be taking numerous prescription and OTC medications, to have problems with mobility, and to have issues of incontinence.

In addition to general characteristics of the elderly, there are also specific ways that an increase in years will affect the patient's body systems.

- The respiratory system can experience a reduction in strength and endurance of the muscles that assist in breathing, a loss of lung elasticity, and collapsing of the smaller airway structures, all of which contribute to respiratory challenges.
- The circulatory system can be affected by a thickening of the walls of the heart, a reduction in the effectiveness of the heart's conduction system, and a loss of elasticity of the blood vessels, which can cause everything from reduced cardiac output and dysrhythmias to aneurysms that can burst.
- Age-related deterioration of the nervous system can cause slowing of psychomotor functioning, decreased reaction times, forgetfulness, and loss of sensation and coordination, which is often the cause of falls among the elderly.
- Osteoporosis and degeneration of the musculoskeletal system can cause bone weakness and general instability, which can lead to falls and serious injuries. You will also

notice degeneration-related curvature of the spine in some elderly patients, which makes immobilization and airway maintenance a challenge.
- Age changes the skin in several important ways also. It becomes thinner and weaker, more susceptible to tears and injuries, and yet due to sluggish cellular regeneration, it can be very slow to heal.

When assessing a geriatric patient, remember to look for things in the patient's environment such as unsafe conditions, nonworking heating and cooling systems, and signs that may indicate abuse or neglect. Also expect to spend extra time gathering the patient's medical history because many older patients have extensive histories of illness and injury. If you are unsure about the information provided by the patient, confirm the information with a caregiver or family member where the patient cannot hear you and be insulted. Also look for clues to the patient's history in the medications that he takes and the environment that he lives in.

Be respectful when physically examining a geriatric patient, ensuring modesty and privacy. Keep in mind that some patients can become fatigued easily during the exam. You should also handle elderly patients gently, explain what you are going to do before doing it, and anticipate that the patient may be wearing numerous layers of clothing.

Keep in mind that elderly persons commonly suffer from many of the same illnesses, such as pneumonia, COPD, heart attacks, high blood pressure, brain attack (stroke), dementia, diabetes, and reactions due to medication overdosing, underdosing, or mixing.

Finally, remember that trauma is the leading cause of death among the elderly. Injuries that rarely prove fatal to younger patients commonly cause the deaths of older patients. This is due in part to the age-related changes in the musculoskeletal and circulatory systems. Falls or blunt force injuries can easily cause breaks and blood vessel tears. Those injuries, along with commonly prescribed cardiac medications, can prevent both clotting and changes in the patient's vital signs. An elderly person can go into shock quickly, with few signs or symptoms to warn the Emergency Medical Responder.

Remember and Consider

➤ If you began assessing an elderly patient who seemed confused about your questions and gave several inappropriate answers, how would you establish a "baseline" mental status for this patient?

Question caregivers or family members to determine if the patient is responding as he normally does.

➤ If you are called to assist an unresponsive elderly patient who was found alone in an apartment by a maintenance worker, how might you determine the patient's medical history?

Observing the patient's environment can provide valuable clues about his medical history. What medications can you locate? Does the patient have a MedicAlert pendant? Is there a Vial-of-Life sticker on the refrigerator? Do you see oxygen administration equipment? These things will help you gather information that can be very helpful in treating the patient.

➤ What are some of the types of injuries you expect to encounter among the elderly?

➤ What would you want your life to be like when you are elderly? What can you do right now to help ensure that you will have that lifestyle when you are older? How would you like to be treated by responders if you called for medical assistance as an elderly patient?

➤ If you work for an emergency response agency, try to find out how many and what type of geriatric calls your organization responded to last year.

These topics will help prepare you in several ways. You will develop a general idea about injuries among the elderly and what types of illnesses/injuries are common in your community. You will also begin building empathy toward geriatric patients by imagining yourself as one of them. Many responders are uncomfortable with very old patients until they understand that they are unique individuals, just like themselves. Just because someone is old, does not mean he has lost dignity, dreams and aspirations, and personality. You may be surprised at how much you come to enjoy interacting with the elderly.

Investigate

➤ The majority of calls to assist elderly patients come from long-term care facilities and residential care homes.

Familiarize yourself with the long-term care facilities and residential care homes in your community. Get to know the staff members, the general layouts of the facilities, and spend time visiting with the elderly residents. You will find yourself seeing older people as unique individuals and becoming more adept at relating to them, regardless of their particular communication challenges.

➤ Many elderly patients live alone and depend on others for assistance.

Check with organizations such as Meals-on-Wheels or visiting nurse associations to get an idea about the elderly population in your community. How many are there? Are they active and social? Are there many shutins? Ask the workers about their personal experiences with the elderly. Consider volunteering.

Quick Quiz

1. Geriatric patients are often less able to defend against illness and may take much longer to recover when they do become ill. This often results in:

   a. multiple simultaneous illnesses.
   b. forgetting doctor appointments.
   c. taking the wrong medications.
   d. hearing loss.

2. The average geriatric patient takes _____ medications per day.

   a. 2.5
   b. 3.0
   c. 4.5
   d. 10.0

3. Which one of the following can cause a patient's illness or disease process to become worse?

   a. overdosing
   b. underdosing
   c. dementia
   d. incontinence

4. The loss of mobility is a common complaint among the elderly and can lead to other problems such as:

   a. better nutrition.
   b. independence.
   c. depression.
   d. nearsightedness.

5. The inability to retain urine or feces is called:

   a. dementia.
   b. aphasia.
   c. priapism.
   d. incontinence.

6. When assessing a geriatric patient who has an altered mental status, you must:

   a. do your best to keep him awake and alert.
   b. determine if his mental state is normal.
   c. determine if he has had any recent surgeries.
   d. find out from family if he can walk or not.

7. All of the following are ways the respiratory system is affected by the aging process EXCEPT:

    a. increased strength of respiratory muscles.
    b. decreased flexibility of the chest.
    c. collapse of the smaller airways.
    d. loss of elasticity.

8. The aging process can cause a degeneration of the heart's electrical system, which can lead to:

    a. hearing loss.
    b. vision loss.
    c. dysrhythmias.
    d. stroke (brain attack).

9. Age-related changes in the musculoskeletal system can lead to changes in posture, range of motion, and:

    a. awareness.
    b. medication usage.
    c. mental status.
    d. balance.

10. Most states have laws that require Emergency Medical Responders to report suspected cases of:

    a. dementia.
    b. abuse and neglect.
    c. Alzheimer's disease.
    d. overdose.

MODULE 6

Childbirth and Children

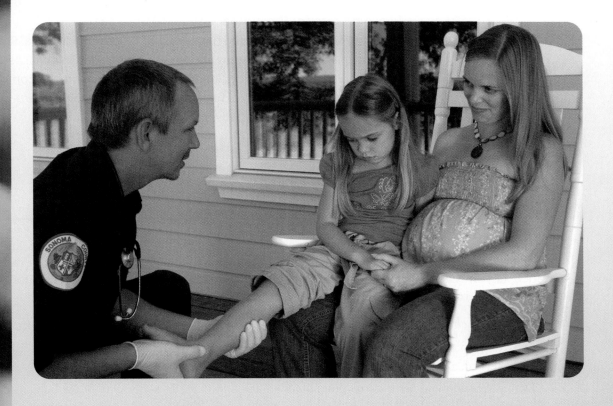

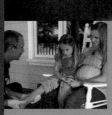

CHAPTER 13

Childbirth

Most expectant mothers know that they need to care for themselves and for their unborn infants during pregnancy. Usually, expectant mothers are under the care of a physician, so they do not often have to call for emergency services to assist with the delivery of their babies. Sometimes, though, physiological or environmental situations cause birth to occur unexpectedly or with complications and before the mother can get to the hospital. In addition, trauma to the mother also affects the fetus; therefore, providing care for the mother also helps the infant.

When the unexpected happens, the Emergency Medical Responder must recognize signs and symptoms and know what to do. This chapter introduces you to the normal terms, events, and stages, as well as to the complications of pregnancy and childbirth, the steps for delivery, and how to care for the mother and fetus during and after delivery.

OBJECTIVES

This chapter is based on the objectives of the U.S. DOT's First Responder National Standard Curriculum. Note that cognitive objectives are listed below and beside corresponding text throughout the chapter. You will also notice as you read each objective that the term Emergency Medical Responder is used. This is simply a name change and reflects the new name for the First Responder.

By the end of this chapter, you should be able to (from cognitive or knowledge information):

6–1.1 Identify the following structures: birth canal, placenta, umbilical cord, and amniotic sac. (pp. 451–452)

6–1.2 Define the following terms: crowning, bloody show, labor, and abortion. (pp. 451–452, 469)

6–1.3 State indications of an imminent delivery. (pp. 456, 457)

6–1.4 State the steps in the predelivery preparation of the mother. (pp. 454–457)

6–1.5 Establish the relationship between body substance isolation and childbirth. (pp. 453, 454, 457, 469, 479)

6–1.6 State the steps to assist in the delivery. (pp. 457–461)

6–1.7 Describe care of the baby as the head appears. (p. 460)

6–1.8. Discuss the steps in delivery of the afterbirth. (p. 461)

6–1.9. List the steps in the emergency medical care of the mother post-delivery. (pp. 461, 467–468)

6–1.10 Discuss the steps in caring for a newborn. (pp. 461–467)

By the end of this chapter, you should be able to feel comfortable enough to (by changing attitudes, values, and beliefs):

6–1.11 Explain the rationale for attending to the feelings of a patient in need of emergency medical care during childbirth. (pp. 454–455, 456, 457, 460, 467, 468, 470, 474, 476)

6–1.12 Demonstrate a caring attitude toward patients during childbirth who request emergency medical services. (pp. 454–455, 456, 457, 460, 467, 468, 470, 474, 476)

6–1.13 Place the interests of the patient during childbirth as the foremost consideration when making any and all patient care decisions. (pp. 456, 461, 464, 466, 474)

6–1.14 Communicate with empathy to patients during childbirth, as well as with family members and friends of the patient. (pp. 454–455, 456, 457, 460, 467, 468, 470, 474, 476)

By the end of this chapter, you should be able to show how to (through psychomotor skills):

6–1.15 Demonstrate the steps to assist in the normal cephalic delivery. (pp. 457–461)

6–1.16 Demonstrate necessary care procedures of the fetus as the head appears. (p. 460)

6–1.17 Attend to the steps in the delivery of the afterbirth. (p. 461)

6–1.18 Demonstrate the post-delivery care of the mother. (pp. 461, 467–468)

6–1.19 Demonstrate the care of the newborn. (pp. 461–467)

ADDITIONAL LEARNING TASKS

EMS providers assist with the delivery of thousands of babies each year in the United States. You must be able to remember the steps involved in childbirth and assist in the delivery. The mother will go through several stages of labor, which may happen very quickly. You must recognize these stages and, if needed, prepare the mother for delivery. You must be able to:

➤ Define and describe the three stages of labor.
➤ List and explain the use of the supplies needed for preparation and delivery.

The mother is not the only patient. If the baby arrives before the mother can get to the hospital, you must also know what to do for the newborn. Be able to:

➤ Describe assessment steps for an infant and how to determine the need for resuscitation.

Sometimes the mother will go through a prolonged birth process, which is not only distressing to the mother, but also stressful for the baby. You must be able to:

➤ Recognize meconium staining in the birth fluids, understand its seriousness, and know what to do for the baby.
➤ Discuss the significance of a stressful birth in which meconium is present.

In an emergency involving a pregnant woman, you will care for most medical and trauma situations as you would for any other patient, but you must be aware of special problems that some expectant mothers may have. Be able to:

➤ List basic care procedures for predelivery emergencies, including seizures, vaginal bleeding, and trauma.

Most mothers will progress through the birth process without any problems. Others will have medical or physical problems that will cause an unusual or complicated birth. Be able to:

➤ Describe common delivery complications, including prolapsed cord, breech birth, limb presentation, premature births, miscarriages, and stillbirths, and state the care for each.

Even more unusual than delivering an infant in the field is delivering two. Once you have delivered one baby, you need to recognize the signs of another delivery, which are slightly different. Be able to:

➤ Describe Emergency Medical Responder steps for delivery in multiple-birth situations.

Trauma is critical for anyone, especially for an expectant mother. Pregnancy conditions may mask signs and symptoms of shock. Not only is the mother an injured patient, but so also is the fetus. In the event of a trauma or any type of assault, be able to:

➤ Describe the care for shock and explain reasons for starting early care.
➤ Describe special care considerations for patients who have been victims of trauma or sexual assault.

As you practice skills with classmates, frequently review and practice the steps for neonatal resuscitation. You must practice these skills frequently so that you can perform them automatically and effortlessly when needed. Be able to:

➤ Demonstrate resuscitation steps for an infant with an inadequate respiratory and/or heart rate.

 FIRST ON SCENE

The first thing that Doug could see other than the blinding white of the snow swirling across the hood of his truck was the red and blue flashing lights of a state trooper's car. The heavily bundled officer had blocked both lanes with his patrol car and was waving traffic toward the snow-packed off ramp. Doug rolled his window down and a wave of cold air instantly filled the cab, numbing his face and arms. "What's going on?" he shouted above the howling afternoon wind.

"Interstate's closed!" the trooper shouted back, his voice blurred by the mask that he wore. "Pull off here and find a place to park."

Doug sat for a moment, trying to quickly calculate another route to Denver, and then sighed, rolled the window up, and followed the officer's order.

The end of the off ramp opened up into the parking lot of a small, crowded travel stop. As he crept up and down each aisle of the lot, looking for a space where his pickup would fit in the field of car-shaped snow mounds, he began to regret not flying to the MERT conference.

He was just backing into a slim opening between an overflowing garbage dumpster and an idling semi when he heard a man yelling for help. The man was poorly dressed for the extreme weather and running up and down between vehicles, shouting for help and knocking on snow-blinded windows.

"My wife!" the man shouted in a heavy foreign accent, his breath exploding out in thick white clouds. "I think she's having her baby! Somebody please help!"

Understanding Childbirth

You may have noticed that this chapter is called "Childbirth" and not "Emergency Childbirth." As a culture, we have arrived at the point where any birth away from a hospital delivery room is considered an emergency, which is just not true. In many parts of the world, babies are born away from medical facilities. Birth is a natural process. The anatomy of the human female, the unborn child, and the structures formed during pregnancy enable the birth process to occur with few problems. Assistance from the medical community reduces the chances of problems for the mother and the child, but in most deliveries, high-tech medical skills and equipment are not needed.

FIRST ➤ Mothers do all the work of delivering their babies. Emergency Medical Responders assist. Your role, then, will be one of helping the mother as she delivers her child. ▪

The presence of an Emergency Medical Responder at the scene of a birth that takes place away from a medical facility can be the key factor in a baby's survival if something should go wrong. The mother may need the skills of an Emergency Medical Responder during the birth process to ensure safe delivery if there are complications. The care provided after delivery is just as important. The first hour of life after birth can be a difficult time for some babies and mothers. Your assistance can make a difference.

ANATOMY OF PREGNANCY

An unborn baby is called a **fetus** as it develops and grows inside of the mother. The average period of development for the fetus is from 36 to 40 weeks, or approximately nine months. This development period is divided into three-month segments called *trimesters*. The fetus develops inside a muscular organ called the womb, or **uterus** (Figure 13.1). The mother and the developing fetus are normally physiologically ready to deliver sometime after 37 weeks of pregnancy. Then labor will begin.

During labor, the muscles of the uterus contract and push the baby down through the neck of the uterus, which is called the **cervix**. As the cervix expands to allow the head of the fetus through, the mother may notice a slight staining of blood or blood-tinged mucus. This is called "bloody show" and is normal. The fetus passes through the cervix and enters the birth canal, or **vagina**, through which it moves to the outside world to be born. During your assessment of the mother, you must examine her for crowning. **Crowning** is the showing of the baby's presenting part, normally the head. However, any part of the baby may present first, including the buttocks or feet. Once the baby passes into the birth canal, more of the head (or other presenting part) will show, or appear to grow larger, with each contraction. This means that birth is *imminent* (about to occur).

6–1.1 Identify the following structures: birth canal, placenta, umbilical cord, and amniotic sac.

6–1.2 Define the following terms: crowning, bloody show, labor, and abortion.

fetus (FE-tus) ▪ the developing unborn baby. The fertilized egg is an embryo until the eighth week after fertilization, when it becomes a fetus.

uterus (U-ter-us) ▪ the womb. The muscular structure in which the fetus develops.

cervix (SUR-viks) ▪ the neck of the uterus; the lower portion of the uterus, where it enters the vagina.

vagina (vah-JI-nah) ▪ the birth canal.

crowning ▪ the bulging out of the vagina caused by exposure of the baby's head or other presenting part during contractions.

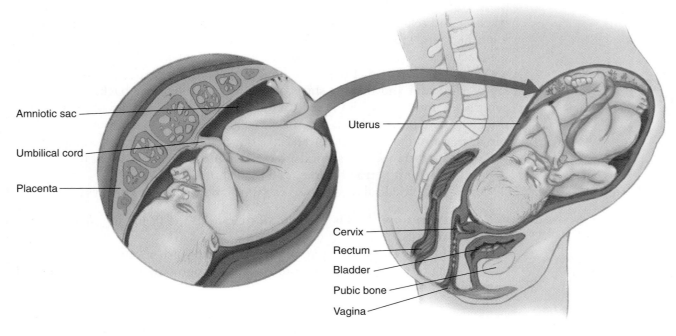

Amniotic sac

Umbilical cord

Placenta

Uterus

Cervix

Rectum

Bladder

Pubic bone

Vagina

FIGURE 13.1 Structures of pregnancy.

amniotic (am-ne-OT-ik) sac ▪ the fluid-filled sac that surrounds the developing embryo and fetus.

placenta (plah-SEN-tah) ▪ an organ of pregnancy that is composed of maternal and fetal tissues by which exchange between the circulatory systems of the mother and fetus can take place without the mixing of their blood.

umbilical (um-BIL-i-kal) cord ▪ the structure that connects the fetus to the placenta. It contains fetal blood vessels.

afterbirth ▪ the tissues that deliver after the birth of the baby; consists of placenta, umbilical cord, tissues from the amniotic sac, and some tissues from the lining of the uterus.

contraction time ▪ the period of time that a contraction of the womb lasts during labor. It is measured from the start of the uterus contracting until it relaxes.

interval time ▪ the period of time from the start of one contraction until the beginning of the next.

The fetus grows inside a special sac, the **amniotic sac,** which is filled with fluid (amniotic fluid) that surrounds and protects the baby. Although the sac may have ruptured earlier, it usually breaks during labor, and the fluid, or water, flows out of the vagina. This is called the *rupture of membranes* and is an important milestone in the birthing process. When you are assessing the mother, you will ask her if her "water has broken." She will usually know and be able to tell you if it has or not. Sometimes the sac will break very early in the labor process. Sometimes it will break much later. The fluids help lubricate the birth canal for the passage of the baby.

During pregnancy, a special organ called the **placenta** develops in the womb. Oxygen and nourishment from the mother's blood pass through the placenta and enter fetal circulation through the **umbilical cord.** Fetal wastes pass back through the umbilical cord and the placenta to the mother's circulation to be eliminated.

STAGES OF LABOR

On average, the process of labor lasts about 16 hours for the first-time mother. In some cases, labor may take longer, or it may take a much shorter time. The time will vary with each mother. You may also expect that, typically, the labor process will be shorter with each successive birth. There are three stages of labor:

- First stage begins with contractions and ends when the cervix is fully dilated so the baby can enter the birth canal.
- Second stage begins when the baby enters the birth canal and ends when he is born.
- Third stage begins when the baby is born and ends when the placenta, commonly referred to as the **afterbirth,** is delivered.

It is normal to have vaginal discharges throughout labor. During the first stage of labor, the first type of discharge to appear should be a watery, bloody mucus. Later, the discharge will appear as a watery, bloody fluid. This is normal and not the same as bleeding. If there is bleeding from the vagina prior to delivery, rather than the normal bloody fluids, then something is wrong. This could be a serious problem, which requires assistance from a higher level of EMS provider and transport as soon as possible.

Contractions of the uterus cause labor pains, and they occur in cycles of contraction and relaxation. At first, contractions are far apart. However, as the fetus is pushed into the birth canal and the time of birth gets closer, the time between contractions becomes shorter. The first contractions are about 30 minutes apart and become closer and closer until they are three minutes apart or less. Pain during labor is normal and usually starts as an ache in the lower back. Then, as labor progresses, the pain is felt in the lower abdomen. As the muscles of the uterus contract, the pain begins. When the muscles relax, the pain is usually relieved. During the relaxation time, the mother rests. Labor pains normally come at regular intervals and last for about 30 seconds to one minute. It is not unusual for these pains to start, stop for a period of time, and then start again.

Emergency Medical Responders can time labor pains in two ways (Figure 13.2):

- **Contraction time.** This is the span of time from the beginning of a contraction until it relaxes.
- **Interval time.** This is the span of time from the start of one contraction to the beginning of the next contraction. As labor progresses, the interval time will become shorter.

Sometimes the mother will experience light, painless, irregular contractions throughout her pregnancy, which may increase gradually in intensity and frequency during the third trimester. About four weeks prior to delivery, as the uterus

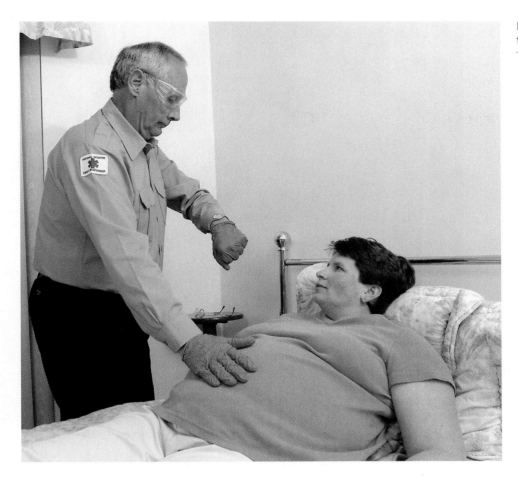

FIGURE 13.2 Determining contraction and interval times.

begins to change its size and shape, some women begin to experience these types of contractions and have the sensation that labor has begun. This is known as *false labor*, also referred to as *Braxton Hicks contractions*. False labor pains are not as regular and rhythmic as true labor contractions.

It may be difficult for you and the mother to distinguish false labor pains from true labor. Even when you are certain that the patient is having false labor, it is still recommended that you arrange for EMTs to transport the patient. Any pregnant woman who is having contractions should be evaluated by her doctor.

Remember that your primary role is to help the mother deliver the baby if birth is imminent. You will need to make sure that you have the necessary supplies and materials to do this.

SUPPLIES AND MATERIALS

Is It Safe ?

The delivery of an infant in the field setting presents a significant risk of exposure to blood and other potentially infectious materials to the Emergency Medical Responder. This is one of the rare occasions when you would actually don full BSI precautions, including gloves, face mask, and gown. ■

6–1.5 Establish the relationship between body substance isolation and childbirth.

The items you will need for preparing the mother for delivery and initial care are provided in a commercial *obstetric (OB) kit* (Figure 13.3). If your response unit does not carry a commercial OB kit, assemble and store the required items in a

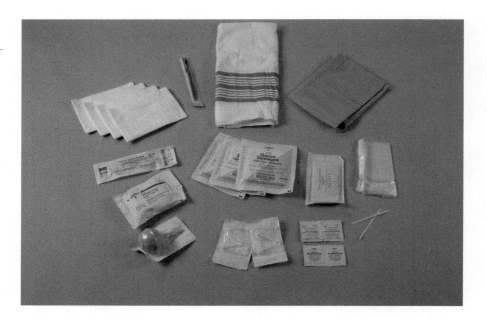

FIGURE 13.3 Contents of a commercial obstetric (OB) kit. All items are disposable.

special kit and keep it on your unit. Some of these items are available at the patient's home, but during the emergency is not the time to find supplies. The items that you will need include the following:

- Personal protective equipment such as protective gloves. Face masks, eye shields, and gowns are also included.
- Towels, sheets, and blankets for draping the mother, for placing under her, and for drying and wrapping the baby.
- Gauze pads for wiping mucus from the baby's mouth and nose.
- A rubber bulb syringe for suctioning the baby's mouth and nose.
- Clamps and ties for use on the umbilical cord before cutting.
- Sterile scissors or a single-edged razor for cutting the cord.
- Sanitary pads or bulky dressings for vaginal bleeding.
- A basin and plastic bags for collecting and transporting the placenta.
- Red, plastic biohazard bags for storing and disposing soiled linens and dressings.

Your initial and focused assessments will help you determine if the mother is ready to deliver. If birth appears likely before EMTs can transport her to the hospital, place supplies so they are within your reach during the delivery process, don your personal protective equipment, and prepare the mother for delivery.

Delivery

PREPARING FOR DELIVERY

6–1.4 State the steps in the predelivery preparation of the mother.

Due to the nature of childbirth, it is important for you to wear appropriate face and eye protection, in addition to protective gloves, to minimize exposure to the mother's body fluids during delivery. Make sure that EMS (9-1-1) has been activated. Let the mother know that you have called for additional assistance and that you will stay with her to help if she starts to deliver the baby. Provide emotional support throughout the entire process of birth. Talk with the mother to help her remain calm and, if needed, remind her that birth is a natural process.

If the expectant mother complains that she feels as if she needs to go to the bathroom, tell her that this is normal and that it is caused by pressure on her bladder and lower intestine. Encourage her to remain lying down. Explain that her body is reacting

454   Module 6 Childbirth and Children

normally to all the changes taking place. It is important that you keep her calm and begin assessing her status as soon as possible. Place layers of newspaper covered with layers of linens under her. If she does have a bowel movement or urinates, tell her that this is normal. Remove soiled linens and replace them with fresh ones.

Fear of delivering away from a hospital can lead some people to try to delay birth. The mother, family, or onlookers may suggest the mother hold her knees together, which you should not allow. It will not slow delivery, but it may complicate the birth or harm the fetus. Have unneeded family members find supplies if you are at the home. Have unneeded onlookers form a privacy shield with blankets, coats, or their bodies facing away if you are in a public place. Your task is to reassure the mother, begin your assessment, and provide care.

FIRST ➤ Begin to evaluate the mother by asking for the following information (Figure 13.4):

- Her name, age, and expected due date.
- If she has been seeing a doctor during her pregnancy. If so, ask for the contact phone number.
- If this is her first delivery, labor will typically last about 16 hours. Labor time is usually shorter for subsequent deliveries.
- If she has any known complications, particularly a multiple birth.
- If she has discharged any watery or bloody mucus.
- How long she has been having labor pains.
- How frequent are her contractions.
- If her water has broken, when, and what color (clear, which is normal, or cloudy or green, which indicates a stressed fetus and requires immediate transport).
- If she feels strain in her pelvis or lower abdomen, if she feels as if she needs to move her bowels, and if she can feel the baby beginning to move into her vaginal opening.
- If she has any significant medical information such as a history of seizures, diabetes, or vaginal bleeding during the pregnancy. ■

Assisting in a Normal Delivery

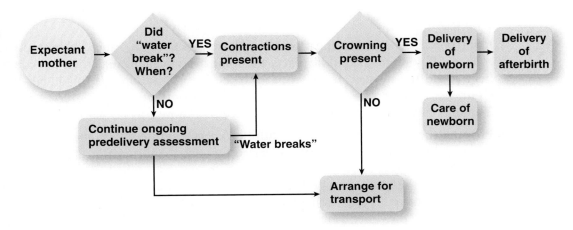

FIGURE 13.4 Algorithm for assisting a mother in a normal delivery.

If the mother says she feels the baby trying to be born or that she has the urge to bear down, birth will probably occur before the EMTs arrive. If the mother is having contractions about two minutes apart, birth is near. Should she also be straining, crying out, and complaining about having to go to the bathroom, prepare to deliver very shortly. Even a first-time mother will have some understanding of what is going on. When she says she feels the baby coming, believe her.

Find out if she has taken a childbirth preparation class or natural childbirth classes. In these classes, the expectant mother works with someone she chooses to be her coach. Use her coach if this person is present or tell her that you will work with her to help her follow the procedures she learned in her class with her coach or partner. Although you must follow standard EMS system practices for assisting with the delivery and for providing care afterward, you or her coach can help the mother with breathing and timing contractions as she was taught in her classes. In addition, you or her coach can also offer the encouragement and support she will need throughout labor. You or her coach can make suggestions on how she can breathe and when to push or relax. Following are a few simple coaching steps:

- As each contraction begins, have the mother take a deep breath and encourage her to gently bear down, or push. She can push with several breaths during each contraction.
- The mother should rest until the next contraction.
- As the baby's head emerges, ask the mother to stop pushing and to start panting so that the baby's head can slide slowly out of the birth canal.

Is It Safe ?

It is important to understand that when the baby enters the birth canal, he is causing downward pressure on the rectum. This pressure will feel to the mother as if she needs to have a bowel movement. She may insist on using the bathroom during the delivery process. Be prepared for this, and never allow a mother in active labor to use the restroom.

FIRST ➤ After evaluating and examining the mother and finding that birth may occur shortly, immediately prepare her for delivery. You will:

1. Take BSI precautions. Put on your personal protective equipment (gloves, mask with eye shield, gown), if you have not already done so.
2. Control the scene so that the mother will have privacy. Ask unneeded bystanders to leave. If you are in a public place, ask some bystanders to turn their backs and help shield the mother. If she appears to be in early labor and this is her first child, her labor pains typically will have long contraction and interval times. You may have to move her a short distance to a more private place.
3. Position the mother on her back with her knees bent, feet flat, and legs spread wide apart. If this position causes her to feel dizzy and faint, it is because the weight of the baby is pressing on the inferior vena cava, the vessel that returns blood from the lower part of the body to the heart, and restricting blood flow back to the heart. If the mother feels dizzy and faint, position her slightly on her left side with one knee bent and foot flat, the other leg extended, and her legs spread wide apart. Place pillows or blankets under her right side to support the pelvis in the raised position.

4. Feel the abdomen for contractions when the patient says she is having labor pains. Explain what you are going to do and place the palm of your hand on her abdomen above the navel. It is not necessary to remove any of the patient's clothing to feel for contractions. If the mother says that she can feel the baby coming, skip this step. Do not delay other procedures to wait for a contraction. Feel for and time several contractions to help determine if birth is near. As birth nears, the interval time will decrease, and you will feel the uterus and the abdomen become more rigid. If the interval time between contractions is five minutes or less, consider that birth may be imminent.

5. Prepare the mother for examination. Tell her that you need to see if her baby has entered the birth canal. Help her remove clothing or underclothing that obstructs your exam of her vaginal opening. Use clean sheets, towels, or tablecloths to cover the mother. If you have a commercial obstetrical (OB) kit, use the materials provided. Make sure you have enough light to see what you are doing. It may be necessary to supply portable lighting or to move lamps in the home to enable you to evaluate the mother and to assist in delivering the baby.

6. Check for crowning. See if any part of the baby is visible at the vaginal opening. In a normal cephalic (head-first) birth, you will see the top of the baby's head. As you learned previously, this is called *crowning*, although any part of the baby may present first. The area of the head (or other presenting part) that you see on your first inspection may be less than the size of a dollar coin. If more of the baby's head (or presenting part) becomes visible with each contraction, birth is occurring. The mother is now in the second stage of labor because the baby is in the birth canal. Do not try to transport the mother yourself in your first response unit. Wait for EMT or ALS personnel to respond.

   The mother, father, or anyone assisting may be embarrassed when you check for crowning. You can minimize this embarrassment by maintaining your professional manner and by explaining what you are going to do and why before you begin. Your professional appearance and approach will generate confidence and trust.

7. Do not attempt any type of internal or vaginal exam. Touch the vaginal area only as necessary during the delivery process. ■

NORMAL DELIVERY

During the delivery, talk to the mother. Ask her to relax between contractions. If her water breaks, remind her that this is normal. Consider the delivery to be normal if the baby's head appears first.

FIRST ➤ Perform the following steps when assisting the mother in a normal delivery (Figure 13.5 and Scan 13–1):

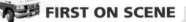

FIRST ON SCENE

"Hey! Buddy!" Doug pushed his door open, scraping it on the dumpster next to him. "Where is she?"

The man, drawn by a response to his cries for help, began running toward Doug, shaking his clasped hands in front of him as if begging. "She is in my car," the man breathed heavily. Sparkling strands of ice hung from his mustache and beard. "Please help her. I do not know what to do."

"Well, for starters we've got to get her inside," Doug said as he pulled on his heavy jacket and wool gloves. "Take me to your car." The man quickly shook Doug's hand with both of his, turned and jogged back through the cars, continually looking back over his shoulder to make sure that Doug was following.

Like many of the other vehicles in the lot, the man's car looked like a snow sculpture. The rising exhaust smoke and the dull red glow of the buried taillights were the only clues that there was actually a vehicle there. The man knocked a clump of white powder from the handle and pulled the door open wide, exposing the warm interior of the car and his very pregnant, very terrified wife.

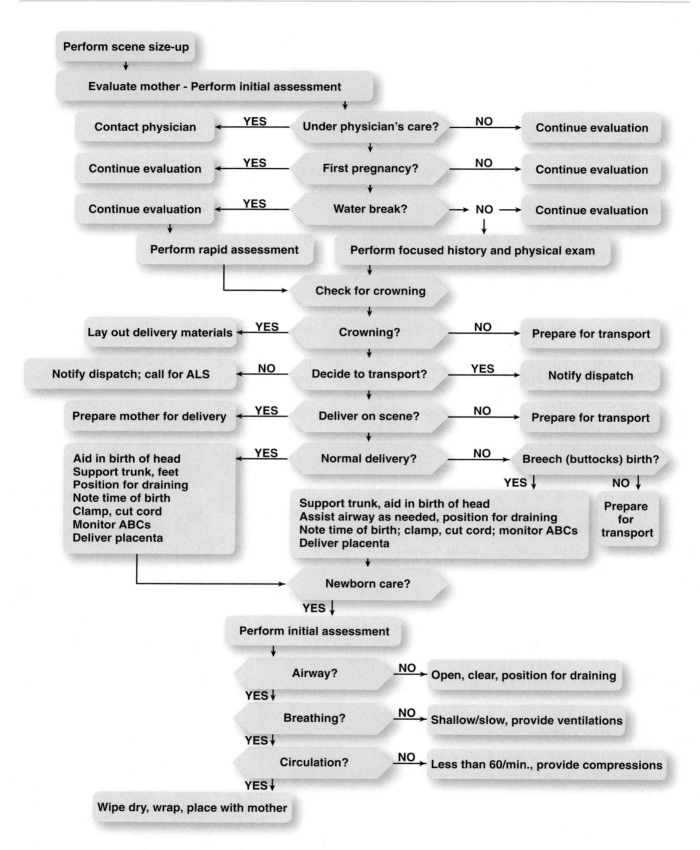

FIGURE 13.5 Algorithm for step-by-step assistance in childbirth.

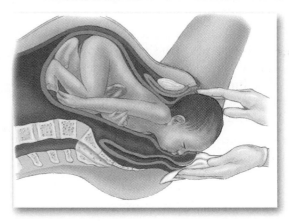

1 ■ Support the head.

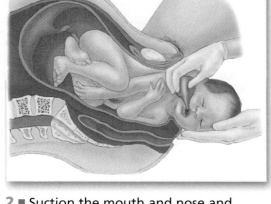

2 ■ Suction the mouth and nose and check for the position of the cord.

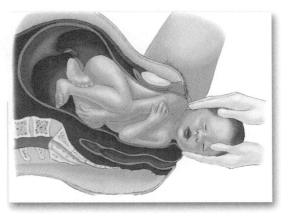

3 ■ Assist in the birth of the head and shoulders.

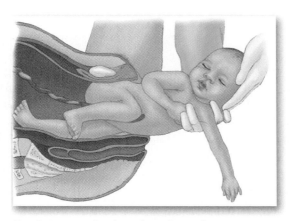

4 ■ Support the head and trunk.

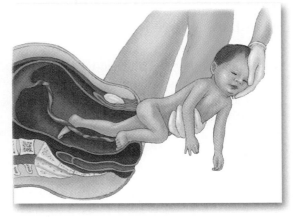

5 ■ Support the head, trunk, and legs.

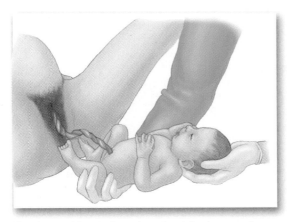

6 ■ Keep the infant level with the vagina until the umbilical cord stops pulsating.

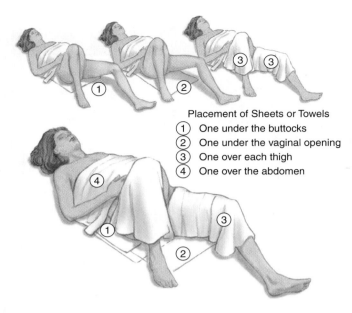

Placement of Sheets or Towels
1. One under the buttocks
2. One under the vaginal opening
3. One over each thigh
4. One over the abdomen

FIGURE 13.6 Preparing the mother for delivery.

6–1.6 State the steps to assist in the delivery.

6–1.7 Describe care of the baby as the head appears.

REMEMBER

Tearing of the perineum is normal.

REMEMBER

Maintain support of the baby throughout the birth process.

1. Wash your hands with soap and water, or use a commercial hand wash. Don personal protective equipment (gloves, mask with eye shield, gown), if you have not already done so.

2. Drape the mother and place her on top of layers of newspapers and clean sheets or towels (Figure 13.6). Place a folded blanket, towels, or sheets under her buttocks to lift her pelvis about two inches. You may place a pillow under her head and shoulders for comfort.

3. Place someone near the mother's head or use the mother's coach to reassure and offer her encouragement and to turn her head in case she vomits. If no one is on hand to help, talk with the patient during the delivery process and be alert for vomiting.

4. Place one hand below the baby's head as it delivers. Spread your fingers evenly around the head to support it but avoid pressing the soft areas at the top, back, and sides of the baby's skull. Apply a slight pressure on the baby's head as it emerges to control the delivery speed. Sometimes the head can "pop out" too quickly from the birth canal, which can badly tear the skin at the vaginal opening. (Some stretching and tearing is normal.) Use your other hand to help cradle the baby's head. Do not pull on the baby.

   As the baby's head emerges, you may notice that it has caused the skin area between the vaginal and rectal openings (called the perineum, per-i-NE-um) to tear. This is normal and will be treated at the hospital. After the delivery, place a sanitary pad at the vaginal opening, which will also help control bleeding from torn tissues. Replace sanitary pads as needed.

5. If the amniotic sac has not yet ruptured, use a cord clamp or your gloved fingers to tear the membrane and pull it away from the baby's mouth and nose. An unbroken sac will prevent the baby from breathing.

6. If the umbilical cord is wrapped around the baby's neck, place your finger under the cord and gently pull it over the baby's head.

   You will have some time before the shoulders emerge. If it is possible for you to do so, clear the airway of fluids by suctioning the baby's mouth first, and then the nose (see step 8). It is especially important that you suction the airway if meconium staining (green or brownish-yellow discoloration) was present in the amniotic fluid.

7. Most babies are born face down as the head emerges, and then they rotate to the right or left. The upper shoulder (usually with some delay) delivers next, followed quickly by the lower shoulder. Continue to support the baby throughout the entire birth process. Gently guide the baby's head downward, which will assist the mother in delivering the baby's upper shoulder. Scan 13–1 illustrates hand placement during delivery.

8. Once the baby's feet deliver (the end of the second stage of labor), lay the baby on his side with his head slightly lower than his body. This position will enable blood, other fluids, and mucus to drain from the mouth and nose. Wipe the baby's mouth and nose with gauze pads. If you have not yet cleared the airway, suction the mouth first, then the nose.

Standard procedures call for clearing the baby's airway once the head delivers, but Emergency Medical Responders may not carry the rubber bulb syringe (unless it is in an OB kit) for this procedure. Even if you have one, do not try to stop the birth process or release your support of the baby to clear the airway. Because you will not be delivering babies every day, it is normal to lack the confidence to try to assist with the birth and clear the airway at the same time. Most babies can wait the few more seconds of delivery to have their airways cleared.

9. Note the exact time of birth. In many systems, the normal procedure is to notify dispatch or medical direction, where time of birth is recorded.

10. Keep the baby at the level of the vagina until the cord is cut.

11. Clamp or tie the umbilical cord. It should be clamped or tied first at about 10 inches from the baby's belly and again about three inches closer to the baby. (More about this later.) Then cut the cord between the ties. If you do not have sterile equipment, do not cut the cord. Simply clamp it. (Some jurisdictions may not allow Emergency Medical Responders to cut the cord. Follow local protocol.)

12. Monitor and record the baby's and mother's vital signs (ABCs).

13. Watch for more contractions, which signal the delivery of the placenta. The placenta is a part of the afterbirth, and it is important to save it for examination. If any part of it remains attached inside the uterus, it can cause bleeding and an infection. Wrap it and other birth tissues in a towel, place them in a plastic bag, and give it to EMT or ALS personnel to transport to the hospital.

6-1.8 Discuss the steps in delivery of the afterbirth.

14. Place a sanitary pad over the mother's vaginal opening. Lower her legs, and place them together. Label the bag with the mother's name. ■

6-1.9 List the steps in the emergency medical care of the mother post-delivery.

NOTE

Babies in the process of being born are slippery. Make certain you have a good but gentle grip and provide proper support throughout the delivery process. Some deliveries can be uncontrolled and rapid, sometimes referred to as an "explosive" delivery. Do not squeeze or counterpush the baby too much. Remember, you can use one hand to place slight pressure on the baby's head to help prevent an explosive delivery.

CARING FOR THE BABY

6-1.10 Discuss the steps in caring for a newborn.

FIRST ➤ As you assist the mother with the delivery of her baby (Figure 13.7):

1. Clear the baby's airway. Position the baby on his side with head slightly lower than his body to allow for drainage. Keep the baby's body at the level of the vagina until the cord is clamped. Use a sterile gauze pad or a clean handkerchief to clear mucus and blood from around the baby's nose and mouth (Figure 13.8). Use a rubber bulb syringe, if one is available, to clear the airway. The correct steps for using the bulb syringe are as follows:
   – Squeeze the bulb first.
   – Insert the tip about one inch into the baby's mouth.
   – Gently release the pressure to allow the syringe to take up fluids from inside the baby's mouth (Figure 13.9).

Assessment of the Newborn

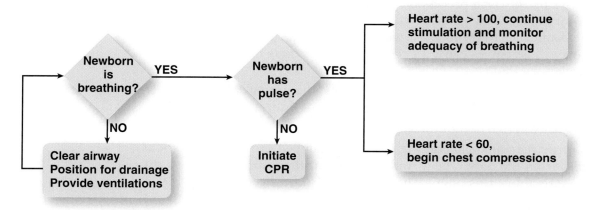

FIGURE 13.7 Algorithm for the assessment of the newborn.

- Remove the tip of the filled syringe from the baby's mouth and squeeze out any fluids onto a towel or gauze pad.
- Repeat this process two or three times for the mouth and for each nostril.

Throughout the rest of your care steps, be sure that the baby's nose is clear. Babies are nose breathers. Plugged nostrils may prevent adequate breathing.

2. Make certain that the baby is breathing. Usually the baby will be breathing on his own by the time you clear the airway, which will take about 30 seconds.

   If the baby is not breathing, then you must encourage him to do so. Begin by vigorously but gently rubbing the baby's back. If this fails to stimulate breathing, snap one of your index fingers against the soles of the baby's feet (Figure 13.10). (Care for the nonbreathing newborn is covered later in this chapter.)

3. Once you are sure the baby is breathing, perform a quick assessment. Note skin color (blue, pale), any deformities, the strength of his cry (strong or weak), and whether he moves on his own or just lies still. After a few minutes, note if there

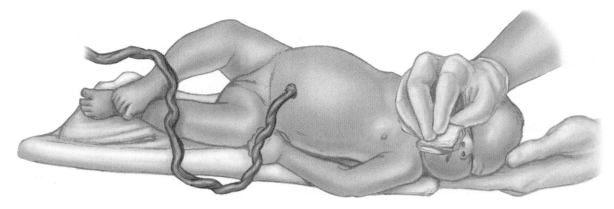

FIGURE 13.8 Use a sterile pad or clean handkerchief to wipe blood and mucus from around the baby's mouth and nose.

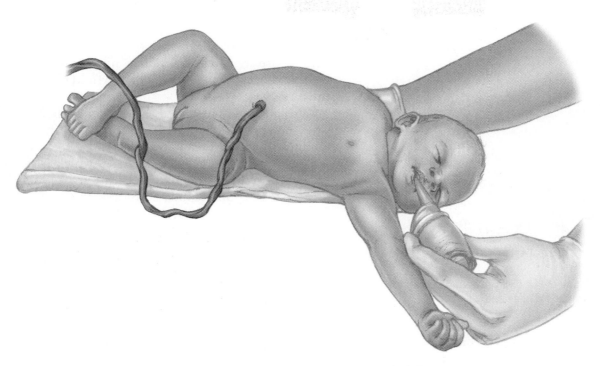

FIGURE 13.9 If you have an OB kit, use the rubber bulb syringe to clear the baby's airway.

are any changes in these conditions. It is important to give this information to the transport personnel for relay to the hospital physician, who will base the baby's subsequent exam on the original assessment.

4. Clamp or tie off the cord, if protocols allow. (Details are provided later in this chapter.)

5. Keep the baby warm. Dry the baby and discard the wet material in a biohazard bag. Wrap the baby in a clean, dry towel, sheet, or baby blanket and place him on the mother's abdomen. Keep the baby's head covered to help reduce heat loss.

   The mother may want to nurse the baby. You may suggest and encourage the mother to do so because it helps contract the uterus and control bleeding.

6. If tape is available, write on a long piece of it the mother's last name and the delivery time. Place a slightly shorter piece of tape on the back of the first one so the adhesive does not come in contact with the baby's skin. Leave an end exposed to tape to itself in a loop. Place it loosely around the baby's wrist. ■

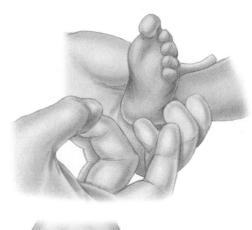

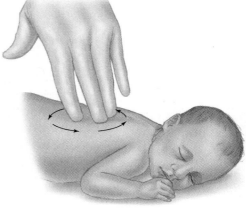

FIGURE 13.10 It may be necessary to stimulate the newly born baby to breathe.

Caring for the Nonbreathing Newborn

In step 2 above, you helped the baby breathe. If you are unsuccessful, provide two gentle but adequate breaths using a mouth-to-mask or bag-valve mask technique (Figure 13.11). Then assess breathing and heartbeat. To check the heartbeat of a newborn, listen at the chest with your ear or a stethoscope (Figure 13.12) or feel for a pulse by lightly grasping the base of the umbilical cord. Do not use a bag-valve mask or airway adjuncts designed for older children or adults to resuscitate a newborn. Do not use any

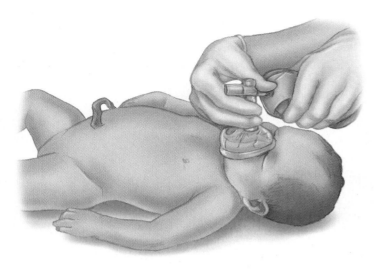

FIGURE 13.11 Resuscitate the newly born baby with bag-valve mask resuscitator that is an appropriate size.

device unless you have been trained and your jurisdiction allows Emergency Medical Responders to use it. Be careful not to hyperextend the head and neck of the baby, which would close off the airway.

Provide ventilations if breaths are shallow, slow, or absent. Ventilate at 40 to 60 breaths per minute (about one breath every second) with 100% oxygen. Watch for the chest to rise, which is the best indication of adequate ventilation. Reassess breathing after 30 seconds of assisted ventilations. The next step depends on the heart rate:

- If the heart rate is 100 beats per minute or greater and the infant is breathing adequately, stop ventilations but continue to provide gentle stimulation (rub the back) to help maintain and improve the baby's breathing. Continue to provide oxygen.
- If the baby's heart rate is below 100 beats per minute and respirations are inadequate, continue to assist ventilations with a bag-valve mask.
- If the heart rate is less than 60 beats per minute, continue to assist ventilations and begin chest compressions. Perform infant CPR with either your fingertips or your thumbs with your hands encircling the chest, not the heels of your hands.

IF THERE IS A PULSE, BUT YOU SEE THIS:	THEN DO THIS:
Breathing rate is inadequate.	Ventilate at 40 to 60 breaths per minute for 30 seconds and reassess breathing.
Heart rate is at least 100 beats per minute and spontaneous breathing is present.	Stop ventilations but continue to gently stimulate the baby by rubbing the skin.
Heart rate is less than 60 beats per minute.	Continue to assist ventilations. Start chest compressions.

Is It Safe ?

Do not be fooled into thinking that an infant with a pulse is doing okay. Infants have a much higher baseline heart rate than children or adults. Take time to assess the rate accurately, and if the rate is below 60 beats per minute, begin chest compressions. ▪

Continue resuscitation until the baby has spontaneous heart and lung actions or when a higher level of EMS provider relieves you. Alert dispatch to the baby's status. Dispatch will contact and send appropriate assistance. Your instructor will advise you if protocols allow you to provide oxygen to the baby.

If you are allowed to provide oxygen to the baby, do not blow a stream of oxygen directly into the baby's face. This may cause him to react by holding his breath. In addition, the rich oxygen supply can cause other medical problems. Instead, direct a stream of oxygen toward the baby's face, either through a face mask or by passing an oxygen tube through the bottom of a paper cup. Hold the mask or cup several inches from the baby's face (Figure 13.13).

Research has found that withholding oxygen may be more damaging than delivering too much. Follow local protocols for delivering oxygen, but never withhold oxygen from a sick baby or one who is struggling to breathe in the prehospital setting. If your response unit does not carry oxygen, notify EMT or ALS personnel through dispatch that the infant will need it.

The above ventilation and chest compression steps will usually revive the baby, but it is still important to have him and the mother transported as quickly as possible to the hospital.

Most first response units are not designed for transport. Protocols in some states do not allow Emergency Medical Responders to transport. Check your protocols about transporting childbirth patients.

The primary role of the Emergency Medical Responder during such an emergency is to provide basic life support until EMT or ALS units arrive. If you are asked to assist during transport and the afterbirth has not delivered yet, carefully move mother and baby as a unit. Keep the mother on her back and the baby between her legs. If you are resuscitating the baby, coordinate your moves so you do not have to stop resuscitation while moving them. Continue to monitor the baby's breathing and pulse during transport and continue resuscitation as needed. Do not stop resuscitation to tie and cut the umbilical cord; someone else can do this. If you have cut the cord, monitor both ends for bleeding.

If you are assisting EMTs during transport, keep in mind that the mother may still be in labor if she has not delivered the afterbirth. She still carries the placenta,

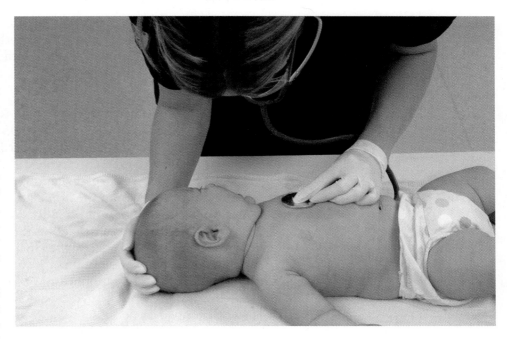

FIGURE 13.12 Check the apical (over the chest) pulse for a neonate.

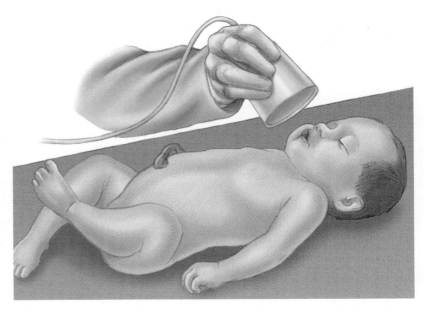

FIGURE 13.13 Place a face mask or a paper cup attached to oxygen tubing several inches from the baby's face to "blow by" oxygen.

which has the other end of the umbilical cord attached to it. Move the mother carefully. If you have not tied and cut the cord, both mother and baby are still connected as a unit, and they have to be moved with great care to avoid tearing the afterbirth from the uterine wall.

Umbilical Cord

Your instructor will tell you if local protocol allows Emergency Medical Responders to clamp and cut the umbilical cord. If you are allowed to do so, remember that the baby can get an infection through the cord, so cut it only if you have sterile conditions. If you must cut the cord, you will need a sterile pair of scissors, a single-edged razor blade, or a sharp-edged knife. If you do not have sterile items from an OB kit, gather them from the home and soak them in isopropyl alcohol for 20 minutes or sterilize them in boiling water. There will be plenty of time to sterilize these items while you are delivering the baby. Do not touch the cutting edges or lay them on unsterile surfaces after they have been sterilized.

Cutting the umbilical cord is usually a low priority and Emergency Medical Responders may provide other care until EMT or ALS personnel arrive. In most cases, if dispatch has alerted EMT or ALS personnel, they should arrive before the cord needs to be clamped or tied.

Usually, it is not necessary to tie and cut the cord until the afterbirth is delivered and the cord is empty of blood and stops pulsating. If you see or feel the cord pulsating, it is still delivering oxygen to the baby from the mother. The baby will benefit from this oxygen.

However, if during the delivery, you see that the umbilical cord is around the baby's neck, you must either slip one or two fingers under the cord and try to slip it back over the infant's head or you must cut it. If the cord cannot be slipped over the head, then quickly place clamps or ties on it and cut it. If this is not done and the infant delivers, the cord may strangle him.

If you are allowed, take the following steps in a normal delivery when the cord has stopped pulsating (Figure 13.14):

1. Use sterile clamps or umbilical tape found in the OB kit. If you do not have a kit, then use clean shoelaces. Never use wire or string because it is too narrow and will slice the cord rather than clamp it. Tie the umbilical tape or shoelace in a square knot.

2. Apply one tie or clamp to the cord about 10 inches from the baby's belly.

3. Place a second tie or clamp about three inches closer to the baby.

4. Cut between the two ties or clamps. Never untie or unclamp a cord once it is cut. Examine the cut ends of the cord. After trapped blood drains, bleeding should stop if the clamps or ties are secure. If bleeding continues, apply another tie or clamp as close to the original as possible.

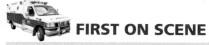

FIRST ON SCENE

The loud talking at the travel stop's small restaurant grew silent and the crowd instinctively parted as Doug and the other man crashed through the doors, carrying the pregnant woman.

"What's wrong with her?" an elderly woman holding a steaming cup of coffee with both hands asked, peering over the tops of her glasses.

"She's having a baby," Doug grunted as he grabbed a tablecloth from an empty table and handed it to a trucker wearing a puffy down vest. "Lay that out flat on the floor, please. Quick." The trucker complied and within moments the crying woman was resting on the floor with her head propped up by a hastily gathered pile of jackets.

"Could you get me some towels and a couple more table cloths?" Doug asked a waitress who absent-mindedly scribbled his request onto a notepad and disappeared into the wall of people surrounding them. "And could you all turn around and give the lady some privacy?"

"Please, do something for my wife," the husband said, grabbing at Doug's jacket sleeves.

"I am. I am. Just stay calm," he said before turning his attention to the panting woman. "Everything's going to be okay. Just relax. What's your name?"

"Silvia," the woman growled. As her face contorted in pain, she grabbed her large stomach with both hands.

"Okay, Silvia," Doug said, getting a handful of towels and tablecloths from the waitress. "I'm going to cover you up and then I need to look down there to see how close the baby is, okay?"

The woman, her face now shining with sweat, glanced at the circle of people—all with their backs to her—and nodded rapidly at Doug before clenching her teeth with another strong contraction.

If the afterbirth delivers while you are still providing care to the baby and you are not allowed to cut the cord, then place the afterbirth at the same level as the baby, or slightly higher. The placenta is still the baby's blood source, and blood can continue to flow to him if the placenta is positioned as described. If the placenta is placed lower than the baby, blood can also flow away from him back into the placenta.

If the afterbirth delivers and you are allowed to clamp and cut the cord, do so. Advise dispatch and medical direction of the baby's delivery status.

CARING FOR THE MOTHER

Care for the mother includes helping her deliver the afterbirth (the placenta and other birth tissues), controlling vaginal bleeding, making her as comfortable as possible, and providing reassurance.

Delivering the Placenta

The delivery of the placenta (afterbirth) is the third stage of labor. It delivers anywhere from a few minutes to 20 minutes or longer after the baby is born. Some women want to get up or assume a seated position after they deliver their babies. You may have to remind them that they will have to remain at rest until they deliver the afterbirth. Make the mother as comfortable as possible and wait for the delivery. You will both know it will be soon when she begins to have more contractions. These contractions will be milder with little discomfort.

FIRST ➤ Save the placenta, all attached membranes, and all soiled sheets and towels. A physician must examine these items to ensure the entire organ and its membranes were expelled from the uterus. Try to position a basin or container at the vaginal opening so the afterbirth will deliver into it (Figure 13.15). Once you collect it, place the container in a biohazard bag. If no container is available, allow the afterbirth to deliver directly into a biohazard bag and place the bag into another biohazard bag. Always label the bag with the mother's name. ∎

Controlling Vaginal Bleeding After Delivery

Bleeding from the uterus is normal after the mother has delivered the afterbirth. Blood is discharged through the vagina, is seldom a problem, and is usually easy to care for.

FIRST ➤ Perform the following steps to care for vaginal bleeding after delivery:

1. Place a sanitary pad or clean towel over the vaginal opening. Do not place anything in the vagina.
2. Have the mother lower her legs and keep them together. (She does not have to squeeze them.) Elevate her legs.
3. Feel the mother's abdomen until you find a grapefruit-size object. This is the uterus. Gently, but

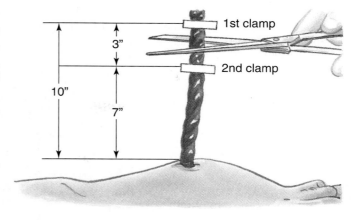
FIGURE 13.14 Cutting the umbilical cord.

6–1.9 List the steps in the emergency medical care of the mother post-delivery.

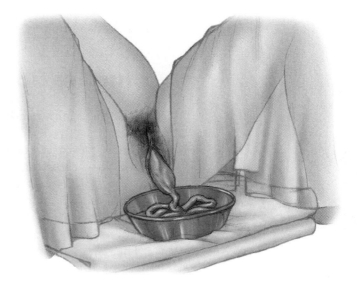
FIGURE 13.15 Collect the afterbirth and have it transported with the mother and infant. A physician must examine the placenta.

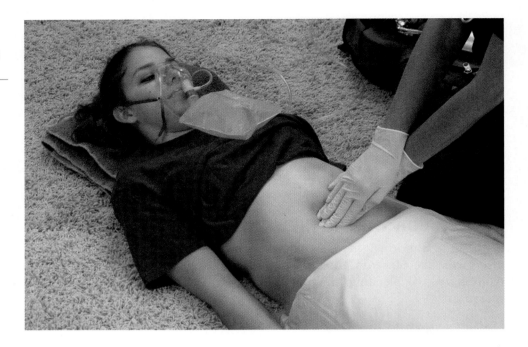

firmly massage from the pubis bone at the front of the pelvis upward only and toward the naval (Figure 13.16).

4. If bleeding continues, provide oxygen and maintain normal body temperature to reduce the effects of shock. Arrange transport as soon as possible and continue to massage the uterus. If the mother wants to nurse, allow her to do so. Nursing stimulates contraction of the uterus and helps control bleeding. ▪

Providing Comfort to the Mother

Talk with the mother throughout the entire birth process, explaining what you are doing and what is happening. She will especially want to know about the baby. Once you have completed your duties with the afterbirth, replace any soiled towels or sheets with clean, dry ones. If possible, wipe and dry the mother's face and hands. Make sure that both she and the baby remain warm and comfortable.

Complications and Emergencies

Some of the common complications and emergencies of childbirth include bleeding and other predelivery emergencies, miscarriages, prolonged labor, abnormal deliveries, premature deliveries, multiple births, and stillbirths. Keep in mind that most births are normal. Those births that produce complications often do not present with immediate problems at the scene. Emergency Medical Responders can often care for some of the difficulties that arise with unusual deliveries. However, some severe complications must be handled by ALS personnel and require immediate transport to a medical facility.

The risk of complications before, during, and after delivery increases when the patient has one or more of the following factors:

- Younger than 18 or older than 35 years of age.
- First pregnancy or more than five pregnancies.
- Swollen face, feet, or abdomen from water retention.

- High or low blood pressure.
- Diabetes.
- Illicit drug use during pregnancy.
- History of seizures.
- Predelivery bleeding.
- Infections.
- Alcohol dependency.
- Injuries from trauma.
- Premature rupture of membranes (water broke more than a few hours before delivery).
- Use of medications such as lithium carbonate, magnesium, or reserpine.

You will find out this information when you gather the patient's history during the focused history and physical exam. As you assess the patient, ask her the questions necessary to see if she is in a high-risk group.

FIRST ➤ Some pregnant patients develop medical problems long before they are ready to deliver. Some patients will require care for these problems before they show any outward signs of pregnancy. You may improperly assess the patient if you do not know she is pregnant. Be certain to ask the patient if she is pregnant when the patient tells you, or you notice, any of the following:

- Any new medical complaint in women of childbearing age.
- Unusual vaginal bleeding or missed menstrual period(s).
- Swelling of the face, hands, and feet.
- Headache, visual problems, apprehension, and shakiness along with upper abdominal pain.
- Nausea, vomiting, or severe abdominal pain that had a sudden onset.

Other pregnancy-related medical emergencies may present as:

- Chest pain.
- Difficulty breathing.
- Seizure. ▪

Infections of the reproductive organs, especially infection by sexually transmitted diseases (STDs), may be transmitted to the baby and to you during birth. Remember to take BSI precautions and wear all personal protective equipment, which will protect you as well as the mother and the infant. Report to the hospital any information you receive from the mother about a history of infection.

PREDELIVERY EMERGENCIES
Prebirth Bleeding

FIRST ➤ When a pregnant woman has vaginal bleeding early in pregnancy, it may be that she is having a **miscarriage** (spontaneous **abortion**). Light, irregular discharges of blood, called *spotting,* are normal in early pregnancy but may concern the patient. If bleeding occurs late in pregnancy or while the patient is in labor, the problem may be with the placenta. Regardless of the cause of bleeding or stage of pregnancy, you will:

1. Make certain that dispatch has been advised of the situation and that additional resources are on the way.
2. Take BSI precautions if you have not already done so.

miscarriage ▪ the natural loss of the embryo or fetus before the twenty-eighth week of pregnancy. Also called a *spontaneous abortion.*

abortion ▪ a spontaneous miscarriage or induced loss of the embryo or fetus.

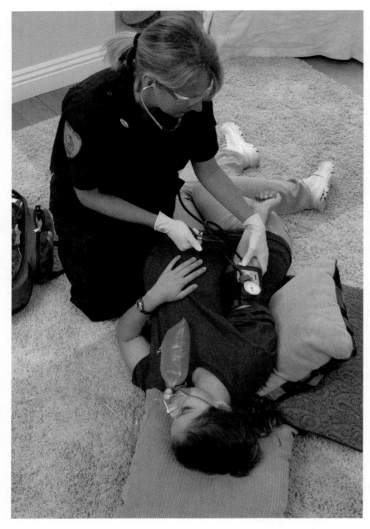

FIGURE 13.17 Position the patient to control excessive prebirth bleeding.

3. Place the patient on her left side, but do not hold her legs together (Figure 13.17).

4. Provide care for shock, monitor the patient's airway, and administer oxygen as per local protocol.

5. Place a sanitary pad or bulky dressings over the vaginal opening.

6. Replace pads or dressings as they become soaked. Do not place anything in the vagina.

7. Save all blood-soaked pads and dressings, as well as any tissues that the mother passes. Place them in a biohazard bag for transport to the hospital and examination by a physician.

8. Monitor and reassure the patient while you wait for EMT or ALS personnel. ▪

Miscarriage and Abortion

If the fetus delivers before it can survive on its own (before the twenty-eighth week), it is considered a miscarriage. The correct term for a miscarriage is a *spontaneous abortion*. However, because the word *abortion* has other meanings in our society, never use the word with a woman who is having a miscarriage or premature signs of labor.

FIRST ➤ Miscarriage and abortion patients typically have abdominal cramps and pains. Vaginal bleeding is to be expected and can be mild to severe. In many cases, there will be vaginal discharges of bloody mucus and tissue particles.

When caring for a woman having a suspected miscarriage or from vaginal bleeding following an elective abortion, first get a general impression of the environment and the patient, perform an initial assessment, and then focus on the physical exam and patient history. Take the following steps to care for the patient:

1. Place the patient on her side, provide care for shock, and administer oxygen per local protocols.

2. Take an initial set of vital signs and repeat them every few minutes.

3. Place a sanitary pad or bulky dressing over the vaginal opening. Do not place anything in the vagina.

4. Save all blood-soaked pads and any tissues that are passed. Place them in a biohazard bag.

5. Provide emotional support.

6. Arrange for EMT or ALS personnel to transport immediately. ▪

Regardless of the cause of the emergency, the patient will need emotional support. Provide professional care, show concern, and reassure the patient.

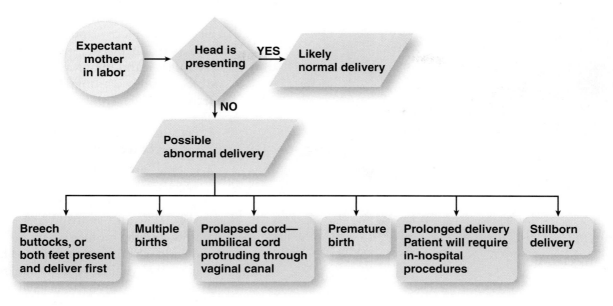

FIGURE 13.18 Algorithm for complications of childbirth.

ABNORMAL DELIVERY

See Figure 13.18 for the steps to take in the assessment of a mother in labor with signs of a complication of childbirth.

Meconium Staining

A stressful or difficult delivery affects both the mother and the baby. When the baby is stressed during delivery, he may defecate (empty the bowel). The fecal material is called *meconium*. When this material mixes with amniotic fluid, the normally clear fluid is stained green or brownish-yellow and is called **meconium staining.** If the baby inhales this fluid on his first attempt to breathe, he will develop aspiration pneumonia, a lung infection caused by aspirating (breathing in) the meconium.

Sometimes the amniotic sac will rupture many hours before delivery. You will have to rely on information from the mother to determine if the fluids were clear or stained. Ask the mother if she noticed the color of the fluid when her water broke. If you witness the rupture, look for meconium staining. Be prepared to wipe the baby's mouth and nose and to suction.

Breech Birth

In a **breech birth,** the buttocks or both feet (not just one) present and deliver first. Even in this position, the baby can be born without complications. As the buttocks and trunk deliver together, place one hand and forearm under the baby for support. Be sure to also support the head as it delivers. A breech birth can be a complication if the baby's head will not deliver.

REMEMBER

In your focused history and physical exam, ask about and look for meconium staining after the amniotic sac has ruptured.

meconium staining ▪ amniotic fluid that has a green or brownish-yellow color from fetal fecal contamination, which occurs when the fetus is stressed.

breech birth ▪ a birth in which the buttocks or both feet deliver first.

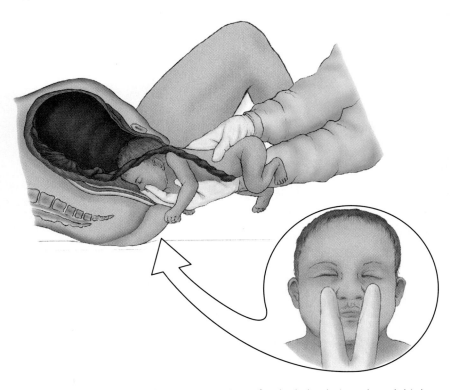

FIRST ➤ In a breech birth, when the baby's head does not deliver within three minutes after the buttocks and trunk, you must immediately notify dispatch to alert responding EMT or ALS personnel. They must transport the mother and infant as soon as possible. While waiting for them to arrive, do the following:

1. Place the mother on a high concentration of oxygen.

2. Create an airway for the baby because the umbilical cord will be compressed between the infant and vaginal wall, shutting off blood flow. Tell the mother what you must do and why. Insert your gloved hand into the vagina, with your palm toward the baby's face. Form a "V" by placing one finger on each side of the baby's nose (Figure 13.19). Push the wall of the birth canal away from the baby's face. If you cannot complete this process, then try to place one fingertip into the infant's mouth and push away the birth canal wall with your other fingers.

FIGURE 13.19 Create and maintain an airway for the baby during a breech birth.

3. Maintain the airway. Once you have created an airway for the baby, keep the airway open. Do not pull on the baby. Allow delivery to take place while you continue to support the baby's body and head.

4. If the head does not deliver in three minutes after you have created an airway, it is necessary to have the mother and infant transported to a medical facility immediately. Maintain the airway throughout all stages of care until higher-level EMS personnel relieve you.

REMEMBER

Call for immediate ALS assistance and transport for all limb presentations.

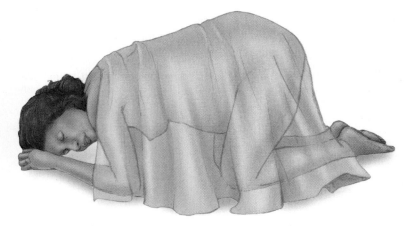

FIGURE 13.20 Place the mother in the knee-chest position, which will help keep pressure off the umbilical cord in a limb presentation birth.

Limb Presentation

The presentation of an arm or a single leg is not a breech birth. It is called a *limb presentation* and is an emergency requiring EMT or ALS personnel to transport the mother to a medical facility immediately. Ask dispatch to notify EMT or ALS responders of the emergency. Do not pull on the limb or try to place your gloved hand into the birth canal. Do not try to place the limb back into the vagina. Place the mother in the knee-chest position (Figure 13.20) to help reduce pressure on the fetus and the umbilical cord. Medical direction and protocols may instruct you to keep the mother in the typical delivery position. Follow your protocols.

Prolapsed Cord

FIRST ➤ When you examine the mother for crowning, you may find the umbilical cord protruding from the vaginal opening. When the umbilical cord delivers first, this is called a **prolapsed cord** and is common in a breech birth. Call for EMT or ALS personnel to transport the mother with a prolapsed cord to a medical facility immediately.

A prolapsed cord endangers the life of the baby. As the baby emerges through the vaginal opening, his head presses the umbilical cord against the vaginal wall, reducing or completely cutting off blood flow and oxygen. When oxygen flow through the cord is obstructed, the baby will try to breathe. But because the baby's face is pressed against the wall of the birth canal, the mouth and nose cannot take in air. To help the baby breathe, provide an airway, using the same methods described for breech birth. That is, place your fingers into the vaginal opening in front of the infant's face and make a "V." Do not try to push the cord back into the birth canal.

In addition, take the following steps. (Check with medical direction or your protocols to find out what Emergency Medical Responders are allowed to do.)

- Place the mother in a knee-chest position to reduce pressure on the cord.
- Try to maintain a pulse in the cord.
- Place wet dressings (use sterile water or saline if it is available) over the cord to keep it moist.
- Wrap the cord in a towel or dressings to keep it warm.
- Provide the mother with a high concentration of oxygen as soon as possible.
- Monitor vital signs and arrange for transport immediately. ▪

prolapsed cord ▪ a potential birth complication in which the umbilical cord presents through the vaginal opening before the baby's head. It is a birth complication if pressure from the baby's head compresses the cord during birth and cuts off oxygen and blood to the baby.

NOTE

The baby's chances for survival improve if you can keep the head from pressing on the umbilical cord and keep the cord pulsating. Check with your instructor to see if protocols allow you to insert several fingers into the mother's vagina and gently push up on the baby's head to keep pressure off the cord.

Multiple Births

Multiple births are not necessarily abnormal. However, they do frequently involve premature delivery. Premature infants may not be fully developed and often have respiratory complications. If the mother is giving birth to more than one infant, she will have contractions begin again shortly after the birth of the first baby. These contractions may deliver the afterbirth of the first or another baby. If more than one baby is in the uterus, the mother's abdomen will remain rather large. Ask the mother if she has been told to expect twins (or more).

The procedures for assisting the mother remain the same. Normally, you will tie or clamp the cord of the first baby before the second baby is born, if the umbilical cord has stopped pulsating. Check with your instructor about the protocols in your area for caring for the cords in multiple baby births. Once the babies are delivered and they are breathing, assess each one, noting skin color (blue, pale), any deformities, strength of their cries, and whether they move on their own or just lie still. After a few minutes, note if there are any changes in these conditions. Perform resuscitation, if necessary. Document the time of birth for each baby. Call for assistance as soon as possible.

Premature Births

Any baby weighing less than 5.5 pounds at birth or any baby born before the thirty-seventh week (prior to the ninth month) of pregnancy is considered a

premature baby ■ any baby
that is born with a birth weight
of less than 5.5 pounds or before
the thirty-seventh week (prior to
the ninth month) of pregnancy.

premature baby. If the mother tells you the baby is early by more than two weeks, play it safe and consider the baby to be premature.

In addition to the procedures for normal births, you must take special steps to keep a premature baby warm. It is important to dry the baby. Wrap him in a blanket, sheet, towel, or aluminum foil. (Fold the edges of the foil to avoid cutting the baby.) A blanket covered with foil is ideal. There are also commercial wraps available, which your unit may carry or your department may purchase. Cover the baby's head, but keep his or her face uncovered. Transfer the baby to a warm environment (90°F to 100°F, 32°C to 37°C), but do not place a heat source too close to the baby. Ventilate a premature baby who needs resuscitation using a mouth-to-mask technique or an appropriately sized bag-valve mask (see Appendix 2). Wipe or suction blood and mucus from the mouth and nose first before ventilating.

Stillborn Deliveries

Some infants are born dead and are called *stillborn*. Some die shortly after birth. Either event is very sad for the mother and father, family members, and care providers. Do not feel embarrassed to show your emotions, but be prepared to continue to act professionally and provide comfort to the mother, father, and other family members who are present.

If the infant shows no signs of life at birth (no attempts to breath and move) or goes into respiratory or cardiac arrest, provide the resuscitation measures described earlier in this chapter and in Chapter 8. Do not stop resuscitation until the baby regains respirations and a heartbeat, other emergency care providers relieve you, or you are too exhausted to continue.

There are cases in which a baby has died hours or longer before birth. Do not attempt to resuscitate a stillborn infant that has large blisters and a strong unpleasant odor. There may be other indications that the infant died earlier in the uterus such as a very soft head, swollen body parts, or obvious deformities.

OTHER EMERGENCIES

Trauma

Vital signs of a pregnant woman are usually different from a woman who is not pregnant. A pregnant woman's blood volume increases up to about 30% to 45%, a natural protection and preparation for the mother who will lose blood during delivery. Her heart rate increases by about 15 beats per minute, and her blood pressure falls 10 to 15 mmHg. Do not mistake the high pulse rate and low blood pressure for signs of shock in the normal nontrauma pregnant woman. But in a trauma situation, the larger blood volume allows the mother's body to compensate for blood loss and may not show early signs of shock.

A pregnant woman can lose almost 40% of her blood volume before she shows any signs of shock. In shock, the mother's body shunts blood away from the uterus first. Less blood to the uterus affects the fetus, causing harm well before the mother shows any signs. Blood loss may be internal and not obvious to the Emergency Medical Responder. Always suspect internal bleeding in any pregnant trauma patient, even if she seems to be initially unharmed and shows normal vital signs for a pregnant woman. Even if the mother is not injured, the fetus may be injured in an advanced pregnancy.

During the scene size up, look carefully at the environment, the patient, and the mechanism of injury. Try to determine what injuries might have been caused (Figure 13.21). Two common types of trauma that can cause significant harm to the mother and the fetus are blunt force and penetrating injuries:

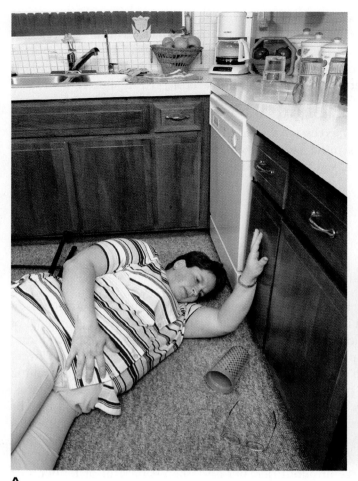

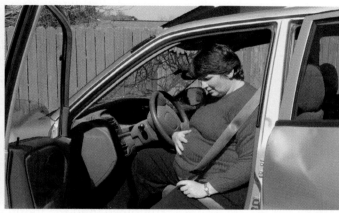

A   B

FIGURE 13.21 Look at the mechanism of injury to try to determine the possible injuries the mother may have received and the forces to which she was exposed.

- *Blunt force injuries*, which are common in falls, vehicle crashes, abuse, and assaults.
- *Penetrating injuries*, which are usually a result of gunshot wounds and stabbings or punctures from the debris of the auto wreckage.

During the early months of pregnancy when the fetus is small, the fluids in the amniotic sac provide some protection from blunt force trauma. As the fetus grows, and especially in the last two months of pregnancy, blunt force trauma can cause more damage to the fetus. As a result, Emergency Medical Responders should provide direct care for the mother and indirect care for the fetus.

The greatest danger to both the mother and the baby is bleeding and shock. First ensure an open airway and adequate breathing and look for and control external bleeding. Provide a high concentration of oxygen as soon as possible and keep the patient warm but do not overheat her. The steps that prevent or care for shock will assist the fetus also. Arrange for immediate transport, and while waiting for EMT or ALS personnel to arrive, provide appropriate care based on the mechanism of injury, such as immobilization for possible spine injuries, splinting for possible fractures, and dressing wounds.

In advanced pregnancies, the large fetus can press on the mother's inferior vena cava when she is lying on her back (supine) and restrict blood return to the heart, causing a condition called *supine hypotensive syndrome* (low blood pressure). This condition greatly affects the fetus. If you immobilize an injured pregnant woman on a spine board, raise the right side of the board slightly and support it with rolled blankets or pillows. The weight of the fetus will shift to the left and off the vena cava, allowing better blood flow (venous return) to the heart.

Vaginal Bleeding

There are many reasons for excessive vaginal bleeding during pregnancy. Emergency Medical Responders must be aware of them and look carefully for the mechanism of injury that caused them, including the following:

- Blunt force and penetrating trauma.
- Intercourse.
- Sexual assault.
- Reproductive organ problems.
- Abnormal pregnancy.
- Placental tears and uterine rupture.

There are two types of placenta tears: placenta previa and placenta abruptio. In *placenta previa*, the placenta lies low in the uterus and attaches itself over the opening of the cervix, meaning it would have to emerge before, or previous to, the fetus during birth. In this position, the placenta tears and bleeds when the cervix dilates during labor. *Placenta abruptio* can occur in a trauma situation when the force of the trauma abruptly tears the placenta partially or completely away from the wall of the uterus. The pregnant woman may have major internal blood loss because blood can be trapped between the placenta and the uterine wall. She may also lose blood vaginally.

The only indications you may have of internal blood loss and developing shock are changes in vital signs, feeling a hard uterus when examining the abdomen, and the mother's complaint that her abdomen is painful or tender. Get a set of baseline vital signs as soon as possible in your assessment, and monitor the vital signs by retaking them every few minutes. Provide her with a high concentration of oxygen as soon as possible and maintain body temperature to help reduce the effects of shock. Arrange for immediate transport.

It is possible that the uterus will rupture in a rapid deceleration injury (vehicle crash) or with a direct compression injury (vehicle crash or blunt force injury). A ruptured uterus is almost always fatal to the fetus. The mother will bleed severely, and she will have a tender abdomen that is no longer large and evenly round but asymmetrical. When you palpate the abdomen, the mother complains of tenderness, and you may feel the head, arms, or legs of the fetus through the abdominal wall. The mother will quickly lose blood and go into shock. Provide a high concentration of oxygen and arrange for immediate transport.

The care for controlling vaginal bleeding includes the following:

- Place sanitary pads or bulky dressings over the vaginal opening.
- Replace pads or dressings as they become soaked.
- Do not place anything in the vagina.
- Save all blood-soaked pads and dressings. Place them in a biohazard bag for transport to the hospital and examination by physician.

Sexual Assault

Sexual assault or rape is always a psychologically and physically traumatic experience. The Emergency Medical Responder's professional manner, attitude, and emotional support are important steps in the care of the expectant mother who has been assaulted.

As the woman struggles or resists the attacker, and as the attacker uses force to make her submit, she can receive many types of injuries to the external soft tissues, the vaginal canal and the internal organs, and the musculoskeletal system. The fetus is also a victim in the assault. The injuries that the fetus receives may be direct from blows to the abdomen, or indirect as a result of injuries to the mother. The emotional trauma to the woman may be greater initially than the physical trauma.

You may have multiple roles to perform as an Emergency Medical Responder who is caring for a pregnant woman. You may have to provide care for injuries, including spinal immobilization, extremity splinting, and wound dressing. In sexual assault cases, you will need to provide emotional support and protect the patient from embarrassment from onlookers. Do not clean the vaginal area. Do not let the patient wash. Do not let her go to the bathroom. If she insists on cleaning herself and changing clothes, you cannot stop her. You should advise her that hospital personnel would be able to collect evidence from her that will help identify and convict the rapist. Emergency Medical Responders should collect clothing and any items that were used during the assault for examination and legal needs. Transport evidence in a paper container or wrap them in a towel. Do not place them in plastic.

For any emotional, violent, or traumatic injury and for complicated deliveries, provide care that will prevent or manage shock and arrange transport as soon as possible. Promote patient confidence by providing emotional support and physical comfort. Listen to your patient and talk to her throughout all procedures. You will find that some roles come easily. Other roles will take knowledge, practice, and skill.

 FIRST ON SCENE WRAP-UP

As snowflakes continued to fall in gentle arcs and swirls outside the steamed windows of the restaurant and the bundled trooper kept directing the occasional car or big rig down the exit ramp, the cries of the pregnant woman were replaced by the small wails of a newborn.

"It's a boy," Doug said, wiping his forehead with the back of one trembling hand as the child's father stood proudly smiling down at the small, bloody infant.

"You did a great job," the waitress said, her breath smelling faintly of spearmint gum as she leaned in close to see the baby. "The ambulance said they couldn't get here for an hour or more, though."

"That's fine," Doug said as he finished wiping the baby down and wrapping him in several clean, warm towels. "There's absolutely nothing wrong with this little guy." He gently passed the bundled child to his parents and stood to stretch his back.

While watching the husband and wife in their unguarded amazement of the tiny person in their arms, Doug was suddenly very glad that he hadn't taken that plane to Denver after all.

Summary

Begin caring for the pregnant mother by letting her know that you are an Emergency Medical Responder. Alert dispatch and gather all supplies and materials needed for delivery and for post-delivery care of the mother and baby.

Perform initial and focused assessments and determine if the mother is about to deliver. Ask if this is her first labor and how far apart the contractions are. Ask if she feels pressure or if she has the urge to move her bowels. Ask if her water has broken and if there was green or brownish-yellow discoloration (meconium staining). Ask if she feels the urge to push.

If you believe that birth may occur before the mother can be safely transported to the nearest hospital, provide the mother with as much privacy as possible. Position her on her back with her knees bent, feet flat, and legs spread apart. If this position makes her feel dizzy, position her slightly on her left side. Ensure your own protection by wearing gloves, mask, eye shield, and a gown. Remove any clothing obstructing your view of the vaginal opening. See if any part of the baby is visible or becomes visible (crowning) during contractions.

Assist the mother as she delivers her baby. It is normal if the skin between the vaginal and rectal openings (perineum) tears during delivery. Carefully support the baby's head as it is born. Spread your fingers flat around the baby's head. A slight, evenly distributed pressure will prevent an explosive birth. Provide support for the baby's entire body and head as birth proceeds.

If the umbilical cord is around the baby's neck, gently loosen the cord with your fingers and slip it over the baby's head. If the amniotic sac has not ruptured, puncture the sac and pull it away from the baby's mouth and nose.

For care of the newly born baby, clear the airway and be sure that he is breathing. If he is not breathing, encourage him to do so by rubbing his back or by snapping your index finger on the soles of his feet. For non-breathing babies, provide ventilations at 40 to 60 breaths per minute. If using a bag-valve mask, only use one that is an appropriate size. After ventilating for 30 seconds, check the heart rate. If the heart rate is 100 beats per minute or greater, gradually reduce assisted ventilations. Gently rub the baby's back to maintain and improve his breathing and continue to provide oxygen. If the baby's respirations are inadequate or the heart rate is below 100 beats per minute, assist ventilations with a bag-valve mask. If the heart rate is less than 60 beats per minute, continue to assist ventilations and begin chest compressions. Perform CPR with either your fingertips or your thumbs with your hands encircling the chest.

Continue resuscitation until the baby has spontaneous heart and lung actions.

Your local protocols may require you to tie or clamp the cord. Do not tie, clamp, or cut the cord until the baby is breathing on his own (unless you must start CPR).

Assist the mother as she delivers the afterbirth (placenta). Save all tissues for transport. Control vaginal bleeding by placing clean pads over the vaginal opening and massaging her abdomen from the pubic bone upward. Allow the mother to nurse her baby. Replace wet towels and sheets with clean, dry ones. Wipe clean the mother's face and hands.

Throughout the birth process, provide emotional support to the mother.

Be ready for complications during a delivery. Look for meconium staining. Provide an airway with your fingers in cases of breech birth and prolapsed cord. Maintain this airway until the baby is born or until you turn the mother over to more highly trained professionals. The EMS system should transport all mothers when there are emergencies that pose immediate life threats to the baby (prolapsed umbilical cord or limb presentation). If there is severe bleeding before delivery, place pads at the vaginal opening, provide care for shock, and arrange for transport as soon as possible.

Expect a multiple birth if the abdomen is still large and contractions of the same intensity continue after a first baby is born. When possible, tie or clamp the umbilical cord of the first baby before the next baby is born.

Keep all babies warm. It is especially critical to keep premature babies warm. Be prepared to resuscitate premature babies.

In cases of a possible miscarriage, provide emotional support to the mother. Place pads at her vaginal opening if there is bleeding. Save all blood-soaked pads and any passed tissues and place them in a biohazard bag for transport and examination. Provide care for shock.

For stillborn infants, remain professional and provide emotional support to the mother, father, and other family members.

When the mother is involved in trauma, sexual assault, or is bleeding heavily from the vagina, care for injuries and provide emotional support. The greatest danger to both mother and baby is bleeding and shock. The pregnant mother's increased blood volume compensates for blood loss and masks the signs of shock. Provide a high concentration of oxygen and maintain body temperature. Transport as soon as possible.

Remember and Consider

➤ Does your response unit carry any supplies for assisting in childbirth?

Check your station or department and your unit or Emergency Medical Responder kits. Find out where the supplies are kept. Do you have a commercial package or have company members created a special "jump bag" or OB kit for childbirth incidents? What would you put into a childbirth jump bag or kit? Find out how many births your unit or personnel have responded to in the past year. Why do you think there are so few, or so many, in your area? Will obstetric patients go to the local hospital or to a specialized one? Are there separate birthing centers in your area? Do they handle only normal deliveries or complicated ones as well? Visit a birthing center and obtain additional information on childbirth and delivery.

Investigate

➤ After you have checked for childbirth supplies, ask your supervisor or supply officer about the procedure for replacing used items. Many childbirth items, such as gauze pads and trauma dressings, are used for wound care and trauma management as well. Ask if it would be practical to keep childbirth items in a separate cabinet, jump bag, or kit. Offer to set up, stock, and monitor supplies and replace them as needed. When extra dressings are needed for trauma emergencies, the childbirth dressings will be used, and supplies that were set aside for childbirth may be overlooked when personnel replace items after an incident.

➤ Assisting childbirth in the field is rare, but Emergency Medical Responders must be ready for the event. If you have a training officer, ask if he or she is planning a drill or refresher class on childbirth. Find out what you can do to help prepare for or present the program. County and state training agencies will have films you can borrow. Health departments will have materials and information for handouts. Obstetricians from local hospitals will be interested in speaking to emergency personnel who will be responsible for assisting childbirth in the out-of-hospital situation.

Quick Quiz

1. The structure that is only present during the development of a fetus is the:
   a. placenta.
   b. uterus.
   c. vagina.
   d. cervix.

2. The rupturing of membranes is an important milestone in the birthing process. It is the:
   a. first contraction the mother is aware of.
   b. widening of the cervical opening.
   c. rupturing of the amniotic sac.
   d. detachment of the placenta.

3. The organ that delivers oxygenated blood and nourishment to the fetus and removes fetal wastes is the:
   a. pubis.
   b. placenta.
   c. vagina.
   d. cervix.

4. A vaginal discharge occurs:
   a. only during the first stage of childbirth.
   b. during the first and second stages of childbirth.
   c. throughout the different stages of childbirth.
   d. only during abnormal childbirth.

5. Which one of the following statements about labor pains is most accurate?
   a. They come at the same time intervals during all stages of labor.
   b. They come at longer time intervals as the birth of the child nears.
   c. They come at shorter time intervals as the birth of the child nears.
   d. They come at regular time intervals during all stages of labor.

6. For your personal safety during a field birth, it is best to have gloves and:
   a. face mask, eye shield, and gown.
   b. face mask, gown, and red biohazard bags.
   c. gown, red biohazard bags, and basin.
   d. face mask, red biohazard bags, and basin.

7. When evaluating the mother before delivery, all of the following information is important to have EXCEPT:
   a. her name, age, and expected due date.
   b. if she has been under a physician's care during pregnancy.
   c. if her water has broken and, if so, when and what color.
   d. when she expected to begin labor contractions.

8. All of the following are signs that the birth of the baby is imminent EXCEPT the mother:
   a. has the feeling that the baby is trying to be born.
   b. is experiencing labor contractions that are two minutes apart.
   c. is experiencing labor contractions at five-minute intervals.
   d. is straining, crying out, and complaining of the urge to go to the bathroom.

9. It is essential that you take BSI precautions for your safety as well as the mother's:
   a. during both assessment and delivery.
   b. while you are assessing the patient.
   c. only if you determine as necessary.
   d. as the baby delivers only.

10. You should consider the delivery normal if the:
    a. baby's feet appear first.
    b. baby's head appears first.
    c. mother is experiencing irregular contractions.
    d. mother tells you the baby is about to be born.

11. During a normal delivery, you should do all of the following EXCEPT:
    a. support the head, trunk, and legs.
    b. suction the baby's mouth, nose, and the cord.
    c. support the head and assist in the birth of head and shoulders.
    d. keep the baby level with the vagina until the cord stops pulsating.

12. When preparing to cut the umbilical cord, clamp the cord:
    a. 10 inches from the baby's belly.
    b. 5 to 10 inches away from the baby's belly.
    c. only if your jurisdiction allows you to do so.
    d. at 10 inches from the belly and then 3 inches closer to the belly.

13. The placenta, or afterbirth:
    a. does not concern you because it will deliver at the hospital.
    b. needs to be delivered by you and saved for further examination at the hospital.
    c. needs to be delivered by you and discarded into a red biohazard bag.
    d. needs to be delivered and examined by you before being discarded.

14. When caring for the baby you MUST do all of the following immediately after the birth EXCEPT:
    a. clear the baby's airway.
    b. make sure the baby is breathing.
    c. perform a quick assessment of the baby.
    d. clamp off the cord and cut it.

15. During the assessment of the infant, remember that the heart rate is:
    a. slower than that of a child or an adult.
    b. the same as that of a child or an adult.
    c. faster than that of a child or an adult.
    d. dependent on the weight of the newborn.

Caring for Infants and Children

This chapter introduces methods used in providing care for medical and trauma emergencies that involve the pediatric patient. Pediatric patients must be managed and cared for differently than adults, because of their age, physical and mental development, personalities, and experiences. Children respond well to familiar, normal routines. They have difficulty handling strange situations and unfamiliar adults, including Emergency Medical Responders, who suddenly arrive in their environment to look at them and handle them.

Seriously ill and injured children also provoke strong emotions in those who must provide care. Through proper training and ample practice, Emergency Medical Responders can increase their professional confidence and manage the pediatric emergency calmly and effectively. As a result, pediatric patients will find an empathetic care provider in the Emergency Medical Responder.

OBJECTIVES

This chapter is based on the objectives of the U.S. DOT's First Responder National Standard Curriculum. Note that cognitive objectives are listed below and beside corresponding text throughout the chapter. You will also notice as you read each objective that the term Emergency Medical Responder is used. This is simply a name change and reflects the new name for the First Responder.

By the end of this chapter, you should be able to (from cognitive or knowledge information):

6–2.1 Describe differences in anatomy and physiology of the infant, child, and adult patient. (pp. 489–495)

6–2.2 Describe assessment of the infant or child. (pp. 495–499)

6–2.3 Indicate various causes of respiratory emergencies in infants and children. (pp. 499–503)

6–2.4 Summarize emergency medical care strategies for respiratory distress and respiratory failure/arrest in infants and children. (pp. 502–503)

6–2.5 List common causes of seizures in the infant and child patient. (pp. 503–504)

6–2.6 Describe management of seizures in the infant and child patient. (p. 504)

6–2.7 Discuss emergency medical care of the infant and child trauma patient. (pp. 509–523)

6–2.8 Summarize the signs and symptoms of possible child abuse and neglect. (pp. 518–523)

6–2.9 Describe the medical-legal responsibilities in suspected child abuse. (pp. 518–523)

6–2.10 Recognize the need for Emergency Medical Responder debriefing following a difficult infant or child transport. (p. 518)

By the end of this chapter, you should be able to feel comfortable enough to (by changing attitudes, values, and beliefs):

6–2.11   Attend to the feelings of the family when dealing with an ill or injured infant or child. (pp. 484–485, 488, 490–491, 495, 499, 502, 506)

6–2.12   Understand the provider's own emotional response to caring for infants or children. (pp. 489, 518, 520, 522, 524, 525)

6–2.13   Demonstrate a caring attitude toward infants and children with illness or injury who require emergency medical services. (pp. 484–485, 488, 490–491, 495, 499, 502)

6–2.14   Place the interests of the infant or child with an illness or injury as the foremost consideration when making any and all patient-care decisions. (pp. 492, 494, 501, 505, 518–523)

6–2.15   Communicate with empathy to infants and children with an illness or injury, as well as with family members and friends of the patient. (pp. 484–485, 488, 490–491, 495, 499, 502)

By the end of this chapter, you should be able to show how to (through psychomotor skills):

6–2.16   Demonstrate assessment of the infant and child. (pp. 495–499)

ADDITIONAL LEARNING TASKS

This chapter describes some of the many characteristics that make children different from adults. The text and your instructor will help you understand how to handle children in a variety of emergency situations. No emergency is routine, but with some experience you will become confident with what to do. With pediatric patients, though, you will find you may have to adjust your approach and care. As you read this chapter, think about and be able to:

➤ State the unique challenges that may arise when caring for the pediatric patient.
➤ Describe the changes in the approach to care when dealing with infants and children.

As children develop, their physical and emotional characteristics change. As they grow and get older, they also want to be treated differently. However, their behavior may regress when faced with a frightening emergency. Think about children you know and how they act in different situations. Then talk with classmates and members of your agency about the response of children in different age groups and how to handle them. Be able to:

➤ List the developmental age categories of infants and children.
➤ List some methods to use that will help in interacting with pediatric patients.

Emergency Medical Responder units may or may not carry oxygen. If your unit does, you will want to learn how to administer it. Your instructor will show you the equipment, demonstrate how to use it, and let you practice. Once you have learned how to operate the equipment, also be able to:

➤ Describe the methods and devices used for delivering oxygen to pediatric patients.

Children are afraid of strangers, and they can be most uncooperative when frightened by an emergency. Think about how children might respond, recall your patient assessment steps, and discuss how you could approach children to gain their confidence. Be able to:

➤ List the steps for performing a scene size-up, initial assessment, focused history and physical exam, detailed physical exam, and ongoing assessment for both infant and child patients.

You will provide emergency care to infants and children that is similar to the care you would provide to an adult. Recall some emergency situations and be able to:

➤ List assessment and care concerns for the pediatric patient who has signs and symptoms of fever, hypothermia, vomiting, and diarrhea.
➤ Describe the care you will provide to the patient in suspected child abuse situations.

- List the signs and symptoms of shock and describe emergency care.
- List the causes and signs of altered mental status.
- Describe the steps to take with an infant and his parents when managing a suspected sudden infant death syndrome (SIDS) incident.
- Define shaken baby syndrome and describe its signs.

By the time you finish reading the chapter and working with your instructor and other classmates, you will feel comfortable with what you know. In class, you will begin to practice the skills you need to perform when responding to infant and child emergencies. Take every opportunity to practice in and out of class so you can:

- Demonstrate the emergency care for trauma emergencies, including care for shock, burns, and spine injuries.
- Demonstrate the emergency care for medical emergencies, including airway obstruction, respiratory infection, fever, asthma, seizures, altered mental status, poisoning, near-drowning, and sudden infant death syndrome (SIDS).
- Discuss how to work with the parents of children who are attached to technical medical equipment at home and need emergency care.

 FIRST ON SCENE

City police officer Jenny Baker backed the cruiser into an empty parking space and opened her laptop, hoping to catch up on paperwork for what is turning out to be a very busy swing shift. It seems to her that as the sun sinks behind the city's well-known skyline, the streets are filling with people up to no good. "Bizarre," she thinks. "Maybe it's the full moon."

Just as she gets connected to the department's server, the radio blares to life. "Adam eight, priority call on tach three." The dispatcher's voice is monotone, bordering on mechanical.

Jenny hit the radio's channel button several times and announced that she was ready for the call. "Adam eight."

A different, yet just as emotionless, voice answers. "Respond priority one for shots fired at the 43rd Street subway station entrance. We're trying to clear a backup unit for you, but for now, you're it."

"Adam eight copy." Jenny slid the laptop back into its black nylon case and shifted the car into drive. Her stomach was immediately tense and nauseous, and she had to force herself to breathe evenly while maneuvering the patrol car in and out of the Friday night traffic.

As she navigated the final turn to the scene, she saw that the street was in chaos. People were crouching against buildings, laying flat on the pavement, and running hunched over in all directions. The front windows to several businesses were shattered and large shards of broken glass hung in the frames like jagged teeth. A woman who had been huddled next to a low concrete wall bordering the subway station stairs saw Jenny's patrol car, scrambled to her feet, and ran directly toward her. As Jenny climbed from the car, gun drawn and ready, the woman reached her and screamed about an ambulance.

"Who was shooting?" Jenny demanded, looking directly into the woman's terrified eyes.

"I don't know. It was from a, a car!" The woman was bordering on hysteria.

"So the shooter drove away?" Jenny noticed that blood was dripping at the feet of the crying woman.

"Yes!" She screamed. "It was a green van-type thing, and they just kept shooting, and then they, they drove that way. Please! I need help for my baby!" The woman moved a dark blanket that she had been carrying and Jenny's stomach dropped as she saw the small, pale face spattered with bright red drops of blood.

Caring for the Pediatric Patient

Responding to a call for a child's illness or injury can be stressful for the Emergency Medical Responder. Some situations will make you feel sad or angry. You will not be able to express your emotions in front of the child or parent. When faced with the assessment and care of an infant or a child, you may at first feel that you do not know what to do or where to start. An anxious, fretful, or frightened child who cannot be comforted may further add to your stress level and reduce your confidence. Remember that many of the assessment and care techniques used for adults are the same for children, with some modifications. These modifications take into account the child's age, physical development, and emotional response.

After caring for the child and dealing with the parents, be aware of how you feel. Do not hesitate to talk with other care providers, support groups, or your family about your feelings. You will not have to go through the tough, stressful calls by yourself. Knowing that others have gone through the same emotions can help you become more comfortable with your own.

Emergency Medical Responders who are unsure of what to do in pediatric emergencies are likely to have a stronger emotional response during and after an incident than those who are prepared and confident in their actions. By training, practicing, and drilling to prepare for pediatric incidents, you will not only improve your confidence and decrease your stress but improve patient outcome as well.

Following are some methods that will help you understand and care for pediatric patients.

Characteristics of Infants and Children

Everyone has some fear of the unknown. Because so many things are unknown to a child, it is easy to see why emergencies can be so frightening for them. A severe illness or injury is a new and unknown experience for children, and it is an experience that increases their anxiety, especially if parents are not there. For most children, security comes from their parents. Wanting parents may be a child's first priority, even above having you offer help, comfort, or relief of pain.

FIRST ➤ When you are dealing with children, you need to gain their trust. You can attempt to calm and reassure them by using the following techniques:

- Approach them slowly, establish contact from a safe distance, and ask permission to get closer. Offering them something (a toy of their own or one you brought) may help prevent them from feeling threatened by your approach. (Many first response units carry new teddy bears for their pediatric patients.)
- Let them know that someone will call their parents.
- Sit down with them so you are at their level. Standing makes you appear large and frightening.
- Let them see your face and expressions. You want to appear friendly, yet concerned and willing to listen. Speak directly to them. Speak clearly and slowly so that they can hear and understand you. Keep your voice gentle and calm even when you need to be firm. Try not to raise your voice or talk loudly to a crying or screaming child. Some children are bashful or uncomfortable with strangers and may not look at you. Try to maintain eye contact (Figure 14.1).

- Pause frequently to find out if they understand what you have said or asked. Even if you communicate easily with your own children, never assume that other children understand you. Find out by asking questions.

- Quickly determine if there are any life-threatening problems and care for them immediately (Scan 14–1). If there are no immediate life threats, continue with patient assessment at a relaxed pace. Avoid moving children, if possible. Movement may cause unexpected pain or, with certain medical problems, extreme responses. Children may be frightened by a rapid-pace exam and a stranger's questions. Responsive, alert young children may become frightened if you start your exam with their head and face. If children show fear as you reach out to touch them, begin the physical examination at the feet and slowly work your way up to the head if they are not critically injured. While you are performing this toe-to-head assessment, look for the same signs of illness and injury as you do when assessing the adult patient. Take time, though, to consider special assessment needs based on the anatomy of the child (Figure 14.2).

- Always tell children what you are going to do before each step of the patient assessment. Do not try to explain the entire procedure at once. Explain one step, do it, and then explain the next step.

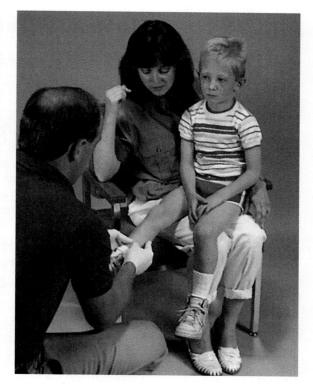

FIGURE 14.1 Let the child see your face and speak directly to him. Try to maintain eye contact.

- Never lie to children. Tell them if it will hurt when you are examining them. If children ask if they are sick or hurt, tell the truth, but reassure them by saying that you are there to help and other people also will be helping. While you talk and work with them, smile. It carries a lot of weight with most children.

- Offer comfort to children by stroking their foreheads or holding their hands. Children will let you know if they do not want to be touched. Most children have learned from parents and teachers that they should not let strangers touch

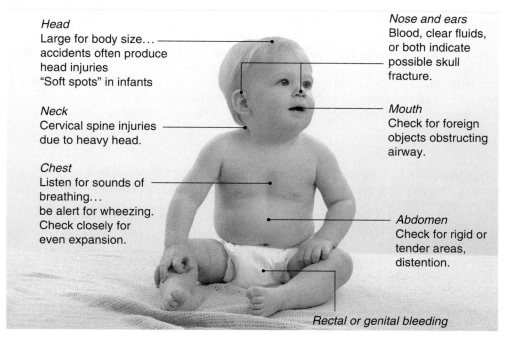

FIGURE 14.2 Special assessment considerations.

Head
Large for body size...
accidents often produce
head injuries
"Soft spots" in infants

Neck
Cervical spine injuries
due to heavy head.

Chest
Listen for sounds of
breathing...
be alert for wheezing.
Check closely for
even expansion.

Nose and ears
Blood, clear fluids,
or both indicate
possible skull
fracture.

Mouth
Check for foreign
objects obstructing
airway.

Abdomen
Check for rigid or
tender areas,
distention.

Rectal or genital bleeding

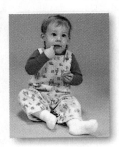

INFANTS

Birth to One Year

- Perform a scene size-up. In your initial assessment, establish your general impression from a distance.
- Ensure an adequate airway. If needed, provide ventilations.
- Protect the head and spine.
- Control your emotions and facial expressions to help reduce the child's fear.
- Provide care to prevent shock. (A small amount of blood loss can cause shock.)

Establishing Responsiveness: The infant should move or cry when gently tapped or shaken. Is he alert, responsive to voice or to pain stimulus, or unresponsive?

Opening the Airway: Use slight head-tilt, chin-lift. (Use the jaw-thrust for possible spine injury.)

Evaluating Breathing: If the infant is responsive but cyanotic, struggling to breathe, or has inadequate breathing, arrange for immediate transport. If the infant is unresponsive, look, listen, and feel for breathing. If there is no breathing, provide rescue breaths.

Providing Breaths: Provide two ventilations while watching for chest rise and fall. Ventilate with the mouth-to-mask technique, using an appropriate pediatric-size mask or a pediatric bag-valve mask. If there is evidence of airway obstruction, clear the airway.

Clearing the Airway

- Make certain that you have not overextended or underextended the neck. Place a folded towel under the shoulders to keep the head in a neutral position. If this does not open the airway, then ...
- Place the infant over the length of your arm face down with the head lower than the trunk. Support the head with your hand placed around the jaw. Support your forearm by placing it on your thigh.
- Deliver five back blows between the shoulder blades with the heel of your free hand.
- Place your free arm on the infant's back and support the back of his head with that hand. Sandwich him between your arms and hands and turn him over. Support your arm on your thigh. Keep the head lower than the trunk and deliver five chest thrusts. If the airway remains obstructed, but the patient is responsive, continue back blows and chest thrusts.
- If the airway remains obstructed and the patient is unresponsive, open the mouth to look for an obstruction.
- Do not attempt blind finger sweeps. You must see the object before you sweep the mouth with your little finger.
- Even if you did not see or dislodge an obstruction, attempt to ventilate. If unable to ventilate, begin chest compressions. After 30 compressions, look for and remove visible obstructions, and attempt to ventilate again. Repeat sequence of compressions and ventilations until the object is removed or EMS arrives.

Continuing Rescue Breathing

- If patient is still not breathing but you gave two successful breaths, check for a brachial pulse.
- If there is a pulse, but no breathing, continue to provide rescue breaths at a rate of one breath every three to five seconds. If there is no pulse, start CPR.

Performing CPR

- If the patient is unresponsive and not breathing, open the airway and look, listen, and feel for breathing for no more than 10 seconds. If there are no breaths, provide two initial breaths. (Ensure the chest rises.) If there is no indication of obstruction, but the patient is unresponsive and is not breathing, check pulse.
- Check for the presence of a brachial pulse for no more than 10 seconds. If there is no pulse and no breathing, start CPR. If you are alone, do CPR for one minute before calling dispatch.

- Start compressions. For the infant, the compression site is one finger-width below an imaginary line drawn across the nipples. Compress with the tips of two or three fingers approximately one-third to one-half the depth of the chest at a rate of at least 100 per minute. For two rescuers, use overlapping or side-by-side thumbs and compress on the middle third of the sternum just below the nipple line. The remaining fingers encircle the chest and support the back.
- For a single rescuer, deliver two ventilations following each set of 30 compressions. For two rescuers, deliver two breaths every 15 compressions.

Controlling Bleeding

- Use direct pressure as a primary method to control bleeding.
- If bleeding is not controlled, use elevation combined with direct pressure. If bleeding is still not controlled, use pressure points combined with elevation and direct pressure.
- A small amount of blood loss (25 milliliters) is serious. Care for shock.

CHILDREN

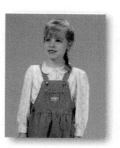

One Year to the Onset of Puberty

- Perform a scene size-up. In your initial assessment, establish your general impression from a distance.
- Ensure an adequate airway. If needed, provide ventilations as you watch for the chest to rise.
- Protect the head and spine. A child's head is proportionately larger than her body.
- Control your emotions and facial expressions to help reduce the child's fear.
- Evaluate blood loss. Provide care to prevent shock. (A small amount of blood loss can cause shock.)

CAUTION: A child's size and weight may be more important than age when providing care.

Establishing Responsiveness: The child should move or cry when gently tapped or shaken.

Opening the Airway: Use slight head-tilt, chin-lift or jaw-thrust maneuver, as appropriate.

Evaluating Breathing: If the child is responsive but cyanotic or struggling and failing to breathe, arrange for immediate transport. If the child is in respiratory arrest, open the airway and look, listen, and feel for breathing. If there is no breathing, provide breaths.

Providing Breaths: Provide two ventilations while watching for chest rise and fall. Ventilate with the mouth-to-mask technique, using an appropriate pediatric-size mask or a pediatric bag-valve mask. If there is evidence of airway obstruction, clear the airway.

Clearing the Airway

- Make certain that you have the proper head-tilt for an unresponsive child. Place a folded towel under shoulders to keep the head in a neutral position. If this does not open the airway, then …
- If the airway remains obstructed and the patient is responsive, perform abdominal thrusts.
- If the airway remains obstructed and the child is unresponsive, begin CPR.
- Do not attempt blind finger sweeps. You must see the object before you sweep the mouth. Use your little finger.
- Even if you did not see or dislodge an obstruction, attempt to ventilate. If unable to ventilate, begin chest compressions. After 30 compressions, look for and remove visible obstructions, and attempt to ventilate again. Repeat sequence of compressions and ventilations until the object is removed or EMS arrives.

Continuing Rescue Breathing

- If patient is still not breathing but you gave two successful breaths, check for a carotid pulse.
- If there is a pulse, but no breathing, continue to provide breaths at a rate of one breath every five to six seconds. If there is no pulse, start CPR.

(continued next page)

Performing CPR

- If the patient is unresponsive and not breathing, open the airway and look, listen, and feel for breathing. If there are no breaths, provide two initial breaths. (Ensure the chest rises.) If there is no indication of obstruction, but the patient is unresponsive and is not breathing, check pulse.
- Check carotid pulse. If there is no pulse and no breathing, start CPR. Have someone call dispatch. If you are alone, do CPR for one minute before calling.
- Start compressions with the heel of one hand.
- Depress the sternum approximately one-third to one-half the depth of the chest.
- Deliver compressions at a rate of 100 per minute.
- Deliver two ventilations every 30 compressions.

Controlling Bleeding

- Use direct pressure as a primary method to control bleeding.
- If bleeding is not controlled, use elevation combined with direct pressure. If bleeding is still not controlled, use pressure points combined with elevation and direct pressure.
- A blood loss of one-half liter (about one pint) is serious. Care for shock.

them. Special child safety programs make children aware of what kind of touching is allowable and what is a "good touch" or a "bad touch." Children will show their acceptance of you by their reactions to your touch. Do not expect rapid acceptance. Use your smile and gentle words to provide comfort.

- Do not direct all your conversation to the parents. Talk to the child. If you are at the scene of an emergency in which the parents are also injured, let the child know that people are caring for their parents, too. ■

While assessing and caring for children, you will have to consider and work with the reactions of the parents or other adults who care for them. Usually, the responses of a parent or guardian are positive and helpful even while they are concerned. Sometimes parents will react with strong emotional responses that can hinder your care of the child. Both types of reactions are natural.

Ask the anxious parent or guardian to help you with tasks, such as holding and reassuring the child, holding the dressing in place, holding the oxygen mask, or assisting with any other device you need to use in your care of the child. If this does not work to calm the parent, have a friend, neighbor, or other Emergency Medical Responder distract the parent with questions about the child's history or with getting the child's toy, favorite blanket, or clean clothes. Last, have someone gently and tactfully guide the parent away from the scene while you evaluate the child.

Some children who are seriously ill or injured are recuperating or being cared for at home while attached to medical equipment. These children may be on special monitors, have special tubes in their throats or abdomens, have intravenous drips containing medications, or be in special traction units. The parents have been trained by the child's doctors and nurses to operate the child's special equipment, but these children still have emergencies, and the parents will call EMS for help.

You do not have to learn how to operate all the different types of special equipment, nor are you expected to. The parent will know how to manage the equipment. Your concern will be how to help the child, and the parent can assist you in providing care. However, some parents may hesitate, especially when EMS personnel arrive. Some may be nervous or unsure about working the equipment. Encourage them to go ahead and do what they have been trained to do, and explain that they are more familiar with the equipment than you are. Ask the parents what they need you to do and how. Then help the parents do it.

Sometimes this special equipment malfunctions and, again, the parent may be anxious and unsure. Calm the parents, and remind them that they have had training and that you will do what you can to help as they give you instructions. If the parents still hesitate, ask them to contact the child's doctor or the medical supply company that provided the equipment. Most of these companies will have emergency contact numbers and staff on call 24 hours a day, seven days a week to assist with equipment emergencies. After you and the parents have managed the child's emergency and the special equipment, call for EMT or ALS personnel to transport, if necessary.

Take advantage of public education or public relations opportunities to encourage families to notify local emergency responders of children with special needs in the community. Arrangements can then be made to make sure the proper personnel and equipment are dispatched to them when emergencies occur.

AGE, SIZE, AND RESPONSE

FIRST ➤ You will find that you instinctively treat infants and children differently from adults. You will know that an infant needs to be handled and cared for differently than a toddler, and that a toddler is spoken to and cared for differently than a school-age child or a teenager. Through proper training and with experience, you will become familiar with the age ranges, mental and physical development, and varying personalities of pediatric patients so you can assess and care for them appropriately.

6-2.1 Describe differences in anatomy and physiology of the infant, child, and adult patient.

You already learned that for the purpose of performing CPR, pediatric patients are classified as infants (up to one year) and as children (one year up to the onset of puberty). After that, CPR is performed on them the same as it is performed on an adult.

However, in general, when assessing and caring for pediatric patients, you must keep the following developmental categories in mind (Table 14–1):

- Infants are those from birth to one year old.
- Toddlers are from one to three years old.
- Preschool children are three to six years old.
- School-age children (usually in elementary school) are six to 12 years old.
- Adolescents (usually in middle and high school) are 12 to 18 years old. ■

Each of these developmental stages requires a slightly different approach to assessment. However, there will be times when you are unable to determine the age of an infant or a child. Some are large or small for their age, and parents may not be there to help you. You will have to estimate age based on the physical size, emotional responses, interaction with you, and language skills.

SPECIAL CONSIDERATIONS

You already realize that infants and children are not the same as adults in size, emotional maturity, and responses. You need to be aware that there are important anatomical differences as well. Because of these differences, your care will sometimes be somewhat different than it is for adults. Consider the following important differences and comparisons.

| TABLE 14-1 | Developmental Characteristics of Infants and Children |

AGE GROUP	CHARACTERISTICS	ASSESSMENT AND CARE STRATEGIES
Newborns (birth to one month)	Infants do not like to be separated from their parents.	Have the parent hold the infant while you examine him or her.
Infants (birth to one year)	They have minimal stranger anxiety. They are used to being undressed but like to feel warm, physically and emotionally. The younger infant follows movement with his or her eyes. The older infant is more active, developing a personality. They do not want to be "suffocated" by an oxygen mask.	Be sure to keep the infant warm. Also, warm your hands and stethoscope before touching the infant. It may be best to observe the infant's breathing from a distance, noting the rise and fall of the abdomen for normal breathing and the chest for respiratory distress, the level of activity, and the infant's color. Examine the heart and lungs first and the head last. This is perceived as less threatening and therefore less likely to cause crying. A pediatric nonrebreather mask may be held near the face to provide blow-by oxygen.
Toddlers (one to three years)	Toddlers do not like to be touched or separated from their parents. They may believe that their illness is a punishment for being bad. Unlike infants, they do not like having their clothing removed. They frighten easily, overreact, and have a fear of needles and pain. They may understand more than they communicate. They begin to assert their independence. They do not want to be "suffocated" by an oxygen mask.	Have a parent hold the child while you examine him or her. Assure the child that he was not bad. Remove an article of clothing, examine the toddler, and then replace the clothing. Examine in a toe-to-head approach to build confidence. (Touching the head first may be frightening.) Explain what you are going to do in terms he can understand. (Taking the blood pressure may be a "squeeze" or a "hug on the arm.") Offer the comfort of a favorite toy. Consider giving him a choice: "Do you want me to look at your belly first or your feet first?" A pediatric nonrebreather mask may be held near the face to provide blow-by oxygen.

TABLE 14–1 | *(Continued)*

AGE GROUP	CHARACTERISTICS	ASSESSMENT AND CARE STRATEGIES
Preschool (three to six years)	Preschoolers do not like to be touched or separated from their parents. They are modest and do not like their clothing removed. They may believe that their illness is a punishment for being bad. They have a fear of blood, pain, and permanent injury. They are curious, communicative, and can be cooperative. They do not want to be "suffocated" by an oxygen mask.	Have a parent hold the child while you examine him. Respect the child's modesty. Remove an article of clothing, examine him, and then replace the clothing. Have a calm, confident, reassuring, and respectful manner. Be sure to offer explanations about what you are doing. Allow the child the responsibility of giving the history. Explain as you examine. A pediatric nonrebreather mask may be held near the face to provide blow-by oxygen. Do not lie. Explain that what you do to help may hurt.
School age (six to 12 years)	This age group cooperates but likes their opinions heard. They fear blood, pain, disfigurement, and permanent injury. They are modest and do not like their bodies exposed.	Allow the child the responsibility of giving the history. Explain as you examine. Present a confident, calm, and respectful manner. Respect the child's modesty. Do not lie. Explain that what you do to help may hurt.
Adolescent (12 to 18 years)	Adolescents want to be treated as adults. They generally feel that they are indestructible but may have fears of permanent injury and disfigurement. They vary in their emotional and physical development and may not be comfortable with their changing bodies.	Although they want to be treated as adults, they may need as much support as children. Present a confident, calm, respectful manner. Be sure to explain what you are doing. Respect their modesty. You may consider assessing them away from their parents. Have the physical exam done by an Emergency Medical Responder of the same sex as the patient if possible. Do not lie. Explain that what you do to help may hurt.

REMEMBER

Children are more vulnerable to spine injuries than adults because of the larger, heavier head and the underdeveloped neck muscles and bone structure.

Head and Neck

A child's head is proportionately larger and heavier than her body. The body will catch up with the size of the head at about age six. Because of the size and weight of the head, the child can be considered top heavy and is likely to land head first in a sudden fall or stop. Common examples include falls from shopping carts and unrestrained children who are propelled head first through windshields in motor-vehicle collisions. Both incidents result in severe head injuries to pediatric patients. Be especially suspicious of a mechanism of injury (MOI) that suggests a possible fall from a height taller than the child.

Is It Safe?

The fontanels of a young infant are soft spots where the bones of the skull have not grown together. These areas are not quite as fragile as some may believe. Although you certainly should not poke and prod or apply firm pressure to these areas, they can be gently palpated without causing harm to the infant.

Always handle the head of the newborn with caution because of the fontanels (soft spots). The largest soft spot, the one on top of the head, does not close completely until about 18 months of age. This soft spot is flat when the infant is quiet, and you may see it pulsate with each heartbeat. If the soft spot is sunken, the child may have lost a lot of fluids (dehydration) because illness has caused inadequate fluid intake and/or diarrhea and vomiting. If the soft spot is bulging, it may indicate that there is increased pressure inside the skull. This can be due to brain swelling from trauma or from an illness such as meningitis. Because the fontanels can also bulge when the infant is agitated and crying, they should be assessed when the infant is quiet. Again, consider the mechanism of injury or nature of the illness during your assessment and care.

In any head injury, look for blood and clear fluids leaking from the nose and ears, just as you would in adults.

When infants and small children suffer head injuries and also show signs of shock, suspect and assess for internal injuries as well. A head injury alone is seldom a cause of shock.

The Airway and Respiratory System

The airway and respiratory systems of the infant and child have not developed fully. The tongue is large relative to the size of the mouth, and the airway is narrower than the adult airway and thus more easily obstructed. In addition, because the muscles in the neck are not fully developed, it may be difficult for a child to hold his head in an open-airway position when sick or injured.

When a child is lying on his back, the large head may cause the airway to flex forward and close. So place a towel that is folded flat under the child's shoulders to help keep the head in line with the body (a neutral position) and the airway open (Figure 14.3). For infants and small children, use a slight head-tilt.

There are some unique points to remember about children's breathing. Infants are generally nasal breathers. That is, if the nose is obstructed, the infant will not immediately open his mouth to breathe as an adult would. Make sure the nostrils are clear of secretions so the patient can breathe

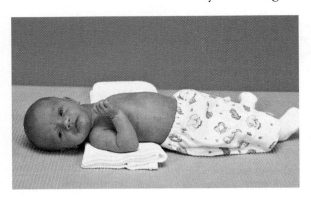

FIGURE 14.3 Use a folded towel to keep the infant's head in a neutral position, neither hyperflexed nor hyperextended.

freely. Remember that the child's windpipe (trachea) is also softer, more flexible, and narrower than an adult's windpipe, and it will obstruct easily. For this reason, you must be careful when opening the airway.

REMEMBER

Infants are primarily nose breathers. They will not automatically open the mouth when the nose is obstructed.

Chest and Abdomen

Because the diaphragm is the major breathing muscle for normal respirations in the infant and child, you will see more respiratory movement in the abdomen than in the chest. But the chest is more elastic, so when the child's breathing is labored or distressed, chest movement is obvious in the muscles between the ribs and in the muscles above the sternum around the neck and shoulders. The use of these accessory muscles for breathing is important to note and indicates the child is in urgent need of medical care.

The child's less developed and more elastic chest may have an advantage over an adult's chest. In a crushing mechanism of injury, the bones of the child's chest may not break, but they will flex. The disadvantage of this is that the more flexible chest offers less protection to the vital organs underneath (the heart and lungs). In your physical exam, the mechanism of injury is important and will help you determine possible internal injury, especially if there is no obvious external injury. Some signs to look for are loss of symmetry (unequal appearance on both sides of the chest), unequal chest movement with breathing, and bruising over the neck and/or ribs.

Injury to the abdomen can result in tenderness, distention, and rigidity just as it can in adults. The abdominal muscles are not as well developed as they are in the adult and offer less protection. The abdominal organs (especially the liver and spleen) are large for the size of the cavity and are more susceptible to injury. A child who has a blunt abdominal injury can bleed out within minutes. Injury that causes distention or swelling can restrict movement of the diaphragm muscle and make it difficult for the child to breathe.

Pelvis

The child can lose a large amount of blood into the pelvic cavity as a result of trauma to the pelvic girdle. If you suspect hip or pelvis injury, monitor vital signs for shock just as you would in the adult and arrange for transport to a medical facility as soon as possible. Check for bleeding or bloody discharge from the genital area. Do not rock the hips to check for instability.

Extremities

Assess for circulation, sensation, and motor function at the distal ends of all extremities. Assess circulation by checking the pulse and capillary refill. Capillary refill is checked by pressing briefly and gently on the hand, foot, forearm, or lower leg. You do not have to press the tiny nail bed. Pressing on the skin will push blood out of the area, cause it to briefly whiten (blanch), and then suddenly refill when pressure is released. Capillary refill time should be less than two seconds.

Injuries that cause soft-tissue swelling or displaced or broken bones can restrict circulation. Always check both pulses and capillary refill in injured extremities. If Emergency Medical Responders perform splinting or other immobilization procedures in your area, recheck circulation, sensation, and motor function after the splint is in place. The EMTs will recheck it regularly en route to the hospital.

Adult bones may fracture in a trauma situation. Children's bones are less developed and more flexible, and will bend and splinter before they break. Provide care for injury sites where there are signs and symptoms of painful, swollen, and deformed extremities, especially at any joint (fingers, wrists, elbows, ankles, knees, hips).

Children have growth plates at the ends of each long bone. A growth plate is developing tissue and the weakest area of a growing skeleton. A child who seriously injures a joint is likely to damage the growth plate, which determines the future length and shape of the mature bone. Growth-plate injuries may be the result of falls, competitive sports, recreational activities (biking, skateboarding), and even from overuse. Pay special attention to a child who complains of pain or who has swelling or deformity in any joint.

Body Surface Area

Infants and children have a large amount of total surface area (skin) in proportion to total body mass. The large surface can easily lose heat and cause the pediatric patient to become chilled, or hypothermic, even in an environment in which an adult feels comfortable. It is important to keep infants and children covered and warm, especially if there is trauma and blood loss or illness and fluid loss.

Blood Volume

The smaller the patient, the less blood volume the patient has. The newborn may have slightly less than 12 ounces, or about a cup and a half of blood, and cannot afford to lose many drops. As children grow, their blood volume increases. By age eight, they will have about two liters (roughly one-half gallon) of blood. Moderate blood loss in an adult may not concern you if it is easily controlled, but the same amount of blood loss in an infant or small child can be life threatening.

Vital Signs

Pulse and respiratory rates vary with the size of the child. The smaller the child, the higher these rates are. Table 14–2 lists pulse and respiratory rates for infants and children.

Is It Safe ?

Never make an assumption that a child is stable or otherwise healthy based on just one set of vital signs. The signs and symptoms of children and infants must be continually assessed for changes. These changes will reveal important trends in the child's condition.

TABLE 14–2	Pulse and Respiratory Rates	
AGE	AVERAGE PULSE RATE (PER MINUTE)	AVERAGE RESPIRATORY RATE (PER MINUTE)
Newborn (birth to one month)	120–160	30–50
Infant (one month to one year)	80–140	25–30
Toddler (one to three years)	80–130	20–30
Preschool (three to six years)	80–120	20–30
School age (six to 12 years)	70–110	15–30
Adolescent (12 to 18 years)	60–105	12–20

Blood pressure also varies in children and depends on their gender, age, and height. Boys have slightly higher blood pressure than girls do. Taller children have higher blood pressure than shorter children. The following factors will also influence blood pressure readings:

- *Time of day.* Blood pressure fluctuates during waking hours and is lower during sleeping hours.
- *Child's physical activity.* Blood pressure is higher during and immediately after exercise or activity, such as running, playing ball, or jumping rope, and it is slower during inactive periods, such as reading, coloring, or watching television.
- *Child's emotional moods or feelings.* Blood pressure fluctuates when the child is afraid, angry, stressed, or happy.
- *Child's physical condition.* The blood pressure will rise or fall based on the type of illness or an injury.

If you are trained to take blood pressure, use the appropriate size cuff when you take a child's blood pressure. It should cover about one-half of the child's upper arm. Cuffs that are too small or too large may give inaccurate readings. Although there are so many factors that can affect a child's blood pressure, you can still determine an appropriate systolic range by using some simple calculations:

- To determine the upper limit of a child's systolic blood pressure, multiply the child's age in years by two and add 90 (age $\times$ 2 + 90 = upper limit of systolic blood pressure).
- To determine the lower limit of a child's systolic blood pressure, multiply the child's age in years by two and add 70 (age $\times$ 2 + 70 = lower limit of systolic blood pressure).

It is not necessary to measure a blood pressure on a child younger than the age of three in the prehospital setting.

Assessment of Infants and Children

You may want to review Chapter 7 at this time.

SCENE SIZE-UP

FIRST ➤ Size up the scene involving a pediatric patient just as you would a scene involving an adult, but approach slowly so you do not frighten the child. Determine scene safety and the number of patients involved in the emergency. Determine the mechanism of injury or the nature of illness. Prepare for patient care by putting on appropriate personal protective equipment. If you think you may need additional resources, call for them immediately. ▪

INITIAL ASSESSMENT
General Impression

6–2.2 Describe assessment of the infant or child.

FIRST ➤ Forming a general impression involves looking at the child and the environment as you approach. Quickly gather critical information that will help you decide whether to hurry or take your time. From a short distance or from across a room, you can see if the child is alert, struggling to breathe, crying, quiet and listless, or unresponsive to your approach. Is the skin pale, bluish, or flushed? How is the child interacting with the environment, with those around him, and to you as you approach? What is the child's body position? From these clues, you can get a general impression of the child's status. In children, the general impression is an important indicator of the severity of illness.

Once you reach the child, you can quickly determine mental status using the AVPU scale. Is the child alert? Is he responsive to your voice or only to a painful stimulus, such as squeezing his shoulder? Or is he unresponsive? Is he oriented to person, place, and time? An infant or a very young child is not able to answer questions about his name, where he is, or what day it is; however, parents or caregivers can explain if the child's actions are as they would normally expect them to be.

Next, quickly assess the child's ABCs. You may assume that the crying child has an airway, breathing, and circulation. For the quiet or unresponsive child, check the airway. Is it open? Check breathing. Is the child breathing normally or with effort? What is the rate? Is chest expansion adequate and equal? Are there noises such as grunting or a high-pitched sound (stridor) associated with the child's respiratory efforts? Is the skin blue (cyanotic), indicating low oxygen levels? Check circulation. Is the pulse strong and regular? Is there any bleeding?

For all children, you will want to find out: Is the skin warm and dry, indicating normal circulation? Or is it cool and clammy, suggesting blood loss and shock? What skin areas are most accessible for you to determine cool and clammy skin? Is capillary refill time less than two seconds? Care for the life-threatening conditions that affect the ABCs first. Remember that the unresponsive child needs immediate care.

When you determine priority of transport, you will recognize the high-priority infant or child patient as one who:

- Displays a poor general impression.
- Has an altered mental status.
- Has an airway problem.
- Is in respiratory arrest, or has inadequate breathing or respiratory distress.
- Has a possibility of developing shock.
- Has evidence of uncontrolled bleeding that may soon result in shock.

FIRST ON SCENE

After radioing for an ambulance and notifying dispatch of the description and direction of the suspect vehicle, she quickly flipped the car radio to the loudspeaker mode. "Attention! This is the police! Is anyone injured?" She spoke clearly into the mic. Her voice bounced off the surrounding buildings and echoed into the distant man-made canyons of the city's west side. People were cautiously standing up all around the intersection, looking around with wide eyes.

There was no indication of other injuries, so Jenny turned her attention to the baby. She gently removed the child from the arms of the sobbing woman and set the bundle onto the hood of her patrol car. The baby cried weakly as she unwrapped the blanket and examined the little pale body. There was a ragged wound to the child's lower abdomen and a small round hole in the lower back. Blood flowed steadily from both wounds and Jenny cradled the baby in one arm as she ran to the trunk of the patrol car to get the Emergency Medical Responder bag.

Managing the Airway

The airway is your first concern in the care of any patient. Always ensure that the airway is open and clear and that the patient is breathing adequately or is receiving appropriate ventilations and supplemental oxygen when necessary. (You may want to review airway care techniques for infants and children in Chapter 6 at this time.)

Opening the Airway

FIRST ▶ When a child lies on his back, the tongue will fall to the back of the throat as it does in adults. Remember, though, that in an infant or child the tongue is larger and can more easily obstruct the airway. Also, when lying on the back, the larger head of the infant may cause the head to flex or bend too far forward and close off the airway. In small children, if you are not careful when opening the airway, you may cause hyperextension or bend the head too far back, which also can close off the airway. You must be sure to align the head and neck or place it in a neutral position so that the airway is open. As noted previously in this chapter, you can easily position the infant or small child correctly by placing a towel under the shoulders. Check for breathing before repositioning the head. Then, if necessary, perform a slight head-tilt or a jaw-thrust maneuver (for trauma) to assess breathing and provide ventilations. ■

Clearing and Maintaining the Airway If air does not enter easily or the chest does not rise when providing artificial ventilation, reposition the head and try again. If you still have no success in ventilating the patient, give back blows and chest thrusts on an infant (younger than one year of age) and abdominal thrusts for children older than one year. Then check the mouth to see if there is an obstruction. If you see one, sweep the mouth with the little finger of your gloved hand. Do not perform blind finger sweeps.

If there are fluids in the airway, clear them by sweeping the mouth with a gauze pad or by suctioning. Check with your instructor to see if Emergency Medical Responders are allowed to use suctioning equipment in your area. If so, your instructor will provide you with training. You also may be able to use nasopharyngeal and oropharyngeal airways in the infant and child patient. Again, your instructor will let you know and give you appropriate training.

Providing Oxygen In some jurisdictions, and for some EMS agencies, training Emergency Medical Responders in oxygen delivery is optional. If you are allowed to provide oxygen to patients, your instructor will have the appropriate equipment and train you how and when to use it with pediatric patients.

The oxygen requirement for children is twice that of adults. Children must receive a high concentration of oxygen when they are in respiratory distress, have inadequate respirations, or have blood loss that can result in shock. A low oxygen level (hypoxia) causes serious physical reactions in children. It can affect the heart rate, slowing the pulse and reducing oxygen circulating to tissues. This in turn affects the brain, decreasing oxygen to cells and causing altered mental status and tissue death. Always follow the rule: "If they are blue, give O$_2$."

Providing oxygen may be a vital part of the emergency care procedures used in caring for children. However, it may be difficult to deliver in the prehospital setting. Many adults are not comfortable wearing an oxygen mask because it feels confining and suffocating. Children also will fear having a mask placed over the face, and the flow of oxygen may even cause children to hold their breath. The Emergency Medical Responder can still provide enriched oxygen to children who need it by using a blow-by technique.

To perform the blow-by technique, hold, or have the parent hold, the oxygen tubing or the pediatric nonrebreather mask about two inches from the child's face. The oxygen will enrich the area in front of the face as it blows by and the child inhales (Figure 14.4). Oxygen tubing can be plugged into the bottom of a colorful paper cup and provide oxygen effectively. The advantage to this method is that the child will likely be curious about the cup and hold it to his face to examine it or try to drink from it. At the same time, the child is receiving oxygen, he will also calm down because he has something of interest to keep his attention. You have provided a toy and gained confidence so your exam can proceed more smoothly. You may also use a paper cup for blow-by oxygen. Do not use a Styrofoam cup because it will crumble and particles can blow into the child's face, eyes, and airway.

REMEMBER

An infant's tongue, as well as a hyperflexed or hyperextended head, can easily obstruct the airway.

REMEMBER

Do not perform blind finger sweeps when trying to clear an airway obstruction.

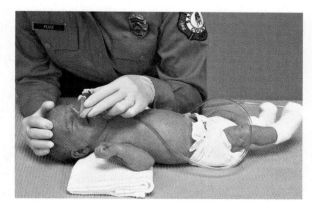

FIGURE 14.4 You can deliver oxygen by using the blow-by method.

If the patient is not breathing, provide artificial ventilation. For infants, provide rescue breaths at a rate of one breath every three to five seconds using a pediatric-size pocket face mask or a bag-valve mask ventilator of the correct size. Remember the following steps when ventilating:

- Breathe less forcefully through the pocket face mask. Watch for the chest to rise. Ventilate slowly so as not to cause stomach distention.
- Excessive force is not needed with the bag-valve mask ventilator. Watch for the chest to rise.
- Use a properly sized face mask to get a good mask-to-face seal.
- Do not use flow-restricted, oxygen-powered ventilation devices (demand valve).
- If ventilations are not successful, perform the procedures for clearing an obstructed airway. Then try to ventilate again.

FOCUSED HISTORY AND PHYSICAL EXAM

FIRST ➤ After completing your initial assessment, focus on getting a history and conducting a physical exam. These steps may be done at the scene with the responsive patient and while you are waiting for the ambulance to arrive. Normally, infants or very young children will not respond to your questions, but children older than two or three years will be able to answer questions that require a yes-or-no answer, and they can tell you or point to where it hurts. Otherwise, parents or other responsible adults, such as babysitters or teachers, will have to give you information about the child's history and how he became sick or hurt.

While you are getting a general impression of the child, decide if he is seriously injured or sick. For any child who is critically injured or sick, perform a rapid assessment, as you would do for an adult:

- *Patient with significant MOI.* Check ABCs first, with manual in-line stabilization of the head and spine. Inspect and palpate each body area. Get baseline vital signs and, if possible, get a history.
- *Unresponsive patient.* Perform any medical interventions, such as opening and clearing the airway, ventilating the patient, and starting CPR. Inspect and palpate each body area. Get a history, or as much information as possible, about the events leading to the illness. Get baseline vital signs.

If you decide from your general impression that the child is responding or acting normally, then perform the appropriate focused assessment:

- *Trauma patient with no significant MOI.* Find out the chief complaint, or what hurts. Inspect and palpate the area. Get baseline vital signs. Gather a history that focuses on events that caused the injury and the injury itself.
- *Responsive medical patient.* Find out the chief complaint, or the nature of illness. Gather a history of the events leading up to the illness and the illness itself. Focus your physical exam on the area of complaint, or inspect and palpate the part of the body involved. Get baseline vital signs. ■

DETAILED PHYSICAL EXAM

FIRST ➤ Now that you have completed a focused assessment, you may have time to perform a more detailed physical exam. This exam will be similar to what you do for the adult, except it is performed in reverse order (toe to head) when you examine the alert but frightened or crying infant or young child. This will give the child an opportunity to get used to you and your touch, if he has not done so during the short focused assessment.

In a medical situation, you can examine the child in more detail from toe to head, while he is in the parent's lap or being held by someone else he knows well. In a trauma situation with no significant MOI, you can again let the parent or other known adult help comfort the child while you begin your detailed toe-to-head physical exam and assess for DCAP-BTLS and crepitus (grating noise or sensation).

Always explain to the child and parent what you are doing and make sure that both understand. Most young children are used to being dressed and undressed and examined by their doctors and will not be embarrassed. As they get older, children are more modest and have learned that strangers should not touch them. Adolescents are concerned about body changes and wonder if they are normal. Remove or rearrange only the necessary clothing during your exam. Then replace it when you have examined that part of the body.

Trauma patients with a significant MOI or unresponsive medical patients who require a rapid assessment are usually unresponsive or too critically injured or ill to know or care where you start your assessment. Stabilize the head and neck before you reposition the head to assess the ABCs in a trauma case, and then follow the steps described above. ■

ONGOING ASSESSMENT

FIRST ➤ You are never finished with your patient until he has been turned over to an equal or higher level of medical care. This means that when you finish your detailed physical exam, you will start again. This is called the *ongoing assessment*, and it will continue until EMT or ALS personnel arrive. The status of a child can change rapidly and frequently, so you will need to reassess mental status, maintain airway, monitor breathing, check pulse, and re-evaluate skin color, temperature, and condition. Take and record vital signs every five minutes for unstable patients and every 15 minutes for stable patients. Continue to monitor the effects of interventions, provide appropriate care, and give emotional support. ■

Managing Specific Medical Emergencies

Many of the specific medical emergencies listed here have been described in detail in other chapters. Much of the care you will provide to infants and children is similar to what you would provide to adults.

RESPIRATORY EMERGENCIES

Emergency Medical Responders do not usually receive the in-depth training for determining different respiratory illnesses and causes of airway and breathing problems in pediatric patients. This section lists some common causes, cover general signs and symptoms, and describe management of respiratory emergencies in pediatric patients.

Guidelines for the assessment and emergency care of a pediatric patient with any respiratory emergency are summarized in Figure 14.5. It is important to note that the most common cause of cardiac arrest in infants and children is respiratory arrest. Identifying and caring for a respiratory problem early can minimize the chances of cardiac arrest.

6–2.3 Indicate various causes of respiratory emergencies in infants and children.

Pediatric Respiratory Emergencies

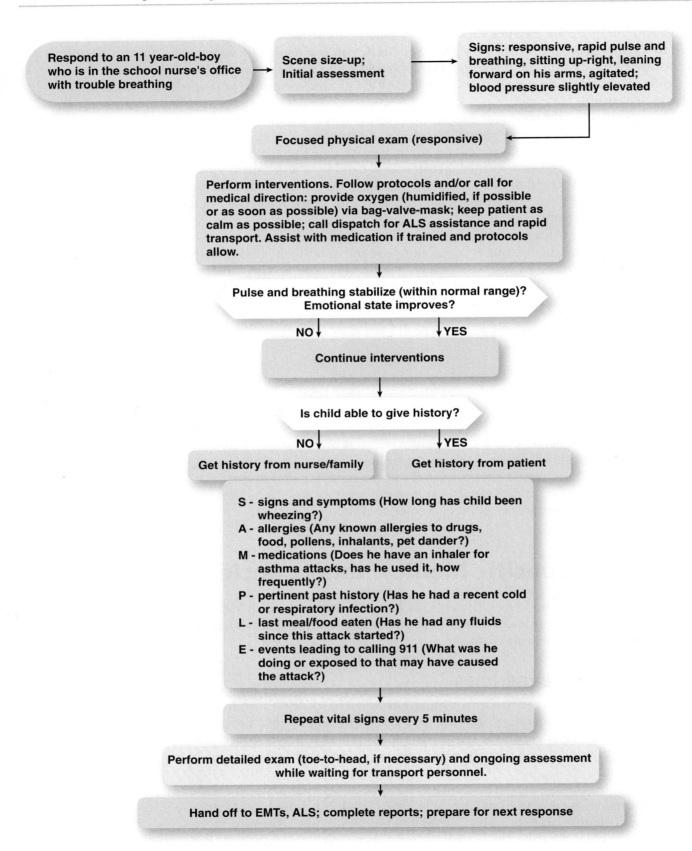

FIGURE 14.5 Algorithm for the emergency care of pediatric patients with respiratory emergencies.

Airway Obstruction

You may want to review the signs and symptoms and the management of partial and complete airway obstruction for pediatric patients in Chapter 6. Continue to review and practice them during and after your training. This will enable you to act quickly to ensure an open airway and adequate breathing for all patients. Because the steps of relieving an obstructed airway in infants are different than for adults, practice the steps of back blows and chest thrusts frequently so that you can perform them quickly and effectively. Remember that the unresponsive child needs immediate care.

Difficulty Breathing

There are many types of airway and respiratory infections and conditions that cause airway and breathing problems. A simple cold can plug the nose and make breathing difficult, but the nose can be easily cleared by blowing or suctioning. A respiratory infection can cause swelling of the respiratory tract or blocking by mucous secretions, making it difficult to breathe.

Another respiratory problem that occurs in some infants involves periods of time when they will stop breathing and then start up again on their own. This period of interrupted breathing is known as **apnea**. In almost all cases, apnea occurs while sleeping. For this reason, it is called *sleep apnea*. Some cases of sleep apnea are related to airway obstruction, while others are associated with failure in the central nervous system to stimulate respiration during sleep. The relationship between apnea and sudden infant death syndrome (SIDS) is still under study.

apnea (ap-ne-ah) ▪ absence of breathing.

Respiratory Infections

Upper respiratory tract infections are very common in infants and children. One such infection is known as croup. Any infant or child with noisy respiration and a hoarse cough may have **croup**. Croup is an infection caused by a virus and affects the larynx (voice box), trachea, and bronchi. It usually causes the tissues in the upper airway to become swollen, which restricts airflow.

A less common problem that can affect the respiratory status of a pediatric patient is known as **epiglottitis**. This occurs when the epiglottis (the flap that closes over the trachea while swallowing) becomes inflamed. Epiglottitis can have a sudden onset in what seemed to be an otherwise healthy child. Suspect this respiratory emergency if the child develops a rapid fever, has cold-like symptoms, has difficulty swallowing, and is drooling. Children with epiglottitis will also sit upright in a **tripod position** (leaning forward with arms braced on the edge of the bed or chair) with the chin thrust out and the mouth wide open. You will notice that they will use the muscles in their upper chest and those around their shoulders and neck to breathe. This effort to breathe is very tiring for the child. The Emergency Medical Responder must act quickly. Although rare, epiglottitis is considered life threatening.

croup (KROOP) ▪ acute respiratory condition found in infants and children, which is characterized by a barking type of cough or stridor.

epiglottitis (ep-i-glot-I-tis) ▪ swelling of the epiglottis that may be caused by a bacterial infection. It can obstruct the airway and is potentially life threatening.

tripod position ▪ leaning forward with arms braced on the edge of the bed or chair.

Is It Safe ?

When caring for a patient with suspected croup or epiglottitis, *do not* attempt to examine the mouth by placing a tongue blade or bite stick in the mouth. Doing so could cause rapid swelling of the tissues of the throat and upper airway. This could lead to complete airway obstruction. If you see a child presenting with signs and symptoms of croup or epiglottitis, call for transport immediately and keep the child comfortable and calm. ▪

Because it may be difficult to determine what type of respiratory emergency an infant or a child is having, consider any airway problem or breathing difficulty a life-threatening emergency and call for transport immediately. Provide oxygen as soon as possible using a blow-by technique if you cannot get the child to accept a face mask or a nasal cannula. Do not place anything in the mouth, such as a tongue depressor, in an attempt to examine the airway. Probing the mouth can cause spasms that will further close the airway. Avoid any actions that might agitate or stimulate the child.

FIRST ➤ Signs and symptoms of respiratory distress include the following:

- Wheezing or a high-pitched harsh noise, or grunting.
- Exhaling with abnormal effort.
- Breathing that is faster or slower than normal is inadequate and requires assisted ventilations and oxygen.
- Use of accessory muscles to breathe.
- Child is in a tripod position.
- Drooling.
- Nasal flaring.
- Cyanosis (late sign).
- Capillary refill of more than two seconds (late sign).
- Slow heart rate (late sign).
- Altered mental status (late sign). ▪

Asthma is also a respiratory condition common to children. It can become life threatening if left untreated. Most children who have asthma use a medication or inhaler prescribed by their doctors. Parents or caregivers call for assistance for a child with asthma if the signs and symptoms are new and unfamiliar, do not respond to at-home care, or the child is not responding to the usual prescribed treatment. Signs and symptoms of asthma occur when the small airways in the lungs go into spasm and constrict, or become too narrow for air to pass through. Something the child eats or breathes or unusual excitement may trigger the attack.

FIRST ➤ Signs and symptoms of asthma include:

- Shortness of breath.
- Wheezing that can be heard with a stethoscope and possibly without.
- Obvious respiratory distress with easy inhalation and forced expiration.
- Cough.
- Faster than normal breathing rate.
- Increased heart rate.
- Sleepiness or slowed response.
- Bluish (cyanotic) tint to the skin, especially around the lips and eyes. ▪

FIRST ➤ Provide emergency care to the pediatric patient who has difficulty breathing and the above signs and symptoms by following these steps:

1. Act calmly and with assurance, which will help calm and reassure the child and the parents or caregiver. For mild distress, the child will be agitated. For severe distress, the child will be exhausted and unable or unwilling to move. Signs of sleepiness and slow response mean low oxygen levels.
2. Place the child in a sitting position. The child will likely have taken a position of comfort that makes it easy for him to breathe, usually a tripod position, leaning forward and bracing himself on his forearms.

WARNING

Whenever possible, listen for evidence of wheezing. A child with a history of asthma who is in respiratory distress and who is not wheezing is at serious risk of respiratory failure.

6–2.4 Summarize emergency medical care strategies for respiratory distress and respiratory failure/arrest in infants and children.

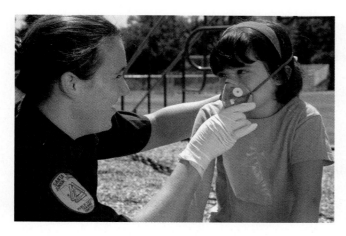

FIGURE 14.6 For respiratory distress, provide oxygen with a correctly sized pediatric nonrebreather mask placed on the child or use the blow-by method.

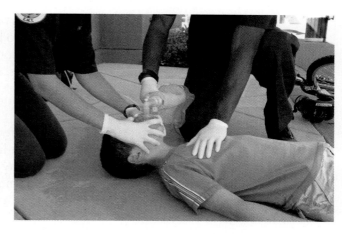

FIGURE 14.7 For severe distress and respiratory arrest, provide assisted ventilations with a pediatric-size bag-valve mask ventilator and supplemental oxygen.

3. Administer oxygen (follow local protocols). Ask the child to breathe in normally but to blow out air forcefully, as if blowing out the candles on a birthday cake or blowing up a balloon. Show the child how and breathe with him.

4. If you are allowed to assist in giving medications, help the parents or caregiver administer the child's medication. Check local protocols and always call for medical direction before assisting a patient with medications (see Appendix 3).

5. Have the parents or caregiver contact the child's physician.

6. Arrange for transport by ambulance. If the signs and symptoms are not relieved with your care and the child continues to worsen, call for transport. A severe and ongoing asthma attack that is not relieved by medication and oxygen may be status asthmaticus, a very serious and life-threatening condition. ▪

In cases of respiratory distress, provide oxygen by a pediatric-size nonrebreather mask (Figure 14.6) or by using the blow-by technique. For severe distress and respiratory arrest, provide assisted ventilations with a pediatric-size bag-valve mask ventilator and supplemental oxygen and call for support (Figure 14.7).

Always allow the child to assume a comfortable position. The alert child will naturally find the position in which it is easiest to breathe. Remember, if you are not trained to use oxygen or do not carry it, call for transport at the first sign of respiratory distress in children.

SEIZURES

FIRST ➤ A seizure will cause a sudden change in mental status as well as sensation, behavior, or movement. The more severe forms of seizure cause violent muscle contractions called *convulsions*. Seizures may be the result of high fever, epilepsy, infections, poisoning, low blood sugar (hypoglycemia), or head injury. They may also occur when the brain does not receive enough oxygen because of inadequate blood circulation (shock) or inadequate oxygen in the blood (hypoxia). In some cases, there is no known cause. Many children suffer seizures, but they are rarely life threatening. Seizures caused by fever (febrile seizures) should be taken seriously. If a child is having prolonged or multiple seizures and has an altered mental status, consider these conditions as a life-threatening emergency and call for transport immediately.

WARNING

Emergency Medical Responders should consider all respiratory disorders in children as serious and take action immediately. Respiratory distress and low oxygen levels in children are the primary causes of cardiac arrest not related to trauma.

6–2.5 List common causes of seizures in the infant and child patient.

In many cases, a patient's seizures stop before EMS arrives. After a seizure, it is normal for children to be either lethargic (drowsy) and difficult to arouse or agitated and combative. Look for signs of illness or injury and question the child or family about symptoms. Also get the following information. Ask:

- Has the child had prior seizures? How long did they last? What part of the body was affected?
- Has the child had a fever?
- Has the child had an injury or fall in which the head may have been struck?
- Is the child taking any medications, specifically medication for seizures?
- Did the child's skin (nail beds and mucous membranes) change from its normal color to bluish or grayish, indicating low oxygen (hypoxia)?

6–2.6 Describe management of seizures in the infant and child patient.

Any child who has had a seizure must have a medical evaluation. Arrange for transport as soon as possible. In the meantime, provide the following emergency care steps:

1. Maintain an open airway and insert nothing in the mouth.
2. Look for evidence of injury suffered during the seizure.
3. If you do not suspect spine injury, position the child on his side.
4. Be alert for vomiting.
5. Provide oxygen or assisted ventilations with supplemental oxygen, if allowed to do so.
6. Monitor breathing and altered mental status. ▪

ALTERED MENTAL STATUS

Any medical or trauma emergency that affects the brain can cause an altered mental status. Examples include low blood sugar (hypoglycemia), poisoning, infection, head injury, decreased oxygen levels, shock, and seizures. As you assess the child, note the mechanism of injury or nature of illness, which will give clues to causes of the child's mental status. Look for signs of poisoning (ingested, inhaled, or absorbed) and ask family members or teachers if there is a history of diabetes or seizure disorder. Take and monitor vital signs, which can indicate shock as a cause. While observing and examining the child, you may notice signs of sleepiness, confusion, agitation, or listlessness.

As you gather information, perform the following emergency care steps:

1. Maintain an open airway, but protect the spine in cases of trauma. If necessary, ventilate the patient.
2. Provide oxygen as soon as possible by nonrebreather mask, or assist ventilations with a bag-valve mask ventilator and supplemental oxygen.
3. Place the patient in the recovery position if there is no indication of spine injury. Care for shock.
4. Arrange to transport as soon as possible.

SHOCK

Common causes of shock in infants and children include losing large amounts of fluid from diarrhea and vomiting, blood loss, and abdominal injuries and other trauma. Shock from fluid loss occurs quickly in infants and is a serious emergency; call for transport immediately. Although not as common, shock can also be caused by allergic reactions, poisoning, and, rarely, cardiac-related problems.

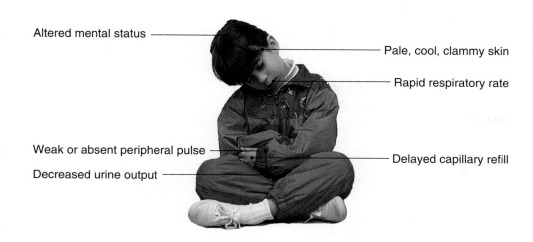

FIGURE 14.8 Signs of shock in an infant or a child.

Altered mental status

Pale, cool, clammy skin

Rapid respiratory rate

Weak or absent peripheral pulse

Decreased urine output

Delayed capillary refill

The child's body can compensate for shock for a long time, but the body's compensating mechanisms can suddenly fail. This failure is called *decompensated shock*. It occurs when the body can no longer function or compensate for low blood volume or lack of perfusion of oxygenated blood to the brain. As a result, the child has an altered mental status and the blood pressure drops (hypotension). When a child goes into the decompensated shock stage, signs and symptoms of shock can develop rapidly.

NOTE

In the adult, shock typically develops more gradually, and the signs tend to be easier to recognize. In the child, you must suspect and anticipate shock and begin caring for it immediately, even before you see definite signs of it.

FIRST ➤ Signs and symptoms of shock include (Figure 14.8):

- Rapid heart and respiratory rate. (Both heart rate and respiratory rate will reflect the course of shock.)
- Weak or absent pulse.
- Delayed capillary refill.
- Decreased urine output (information from parents), which indicates dehydration.
- Altered mental status.
- Pale, cool, clammy skin.
- Sunken fontanels.

Provide the following care in your management of the sick or injured infant or child who has evidence of shock (Figure 14.9):

1. Ensure an open airway, but protect the spine in cases of trauma. Provide ventilations, if necessary.
2. Provide oxygen by nonrebreather mask or assist ventilations by bag-valve mask ventilator with supplemental oxygen as per local protocols.
3. Control any bleeding and dress wounds.
4. Elevate the legs if there is no trauma or suspected spine injury.
5. Maintain body warmth but do not overheat.
6. Arrange to transport as soon as possible.
7. While waiting for EMT personnel to arrive or while en route, continue to monitor airway, breathing, and vital signs and continue any care. ◼

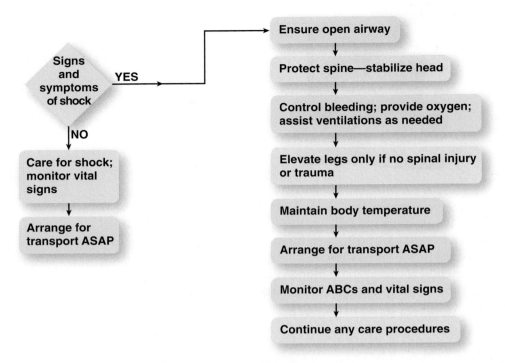

FIGURE 14.9 Algorithm for the emergency care of pediatric patients with signs of shock.

SUDDEN INFANT DEATH SYNDROME

In the United States, sudden infant death syndrome (SIDS) claims thousands of infants each year. It is the sudden unexplained death during sleep of an apparently healthy baby in the first year of life—even a baby who is receiving proper care and has just passed a physical exam. Possible causes and theories are still being investigated. It is known that SIDS is not caused by external methods of suffocation, by vomiting, or by choking.

When Emergency Medical Responders arrive, they may see distraught parents with their infant in respiratory and cardiac arrest during the scene size-up. Because Emergency Medical Responders cannot diagnose SIDS, you must immediately start emergency care as you would for any patient in cardiac arrest. Provide resuscitation and arrange transport to the hospital. Assure the parents that everything is being done for the baby. Normally, Emergency Medical Responders will not begin resuscitation if there is obvious stiffening of the body (rigor mortis) or if blood has pooled (lividity) along whatever side the child was lying on. Check with your instructor to find out what your protocols require for this situation. In either case, be sure to provide emotional support to the parents.

FEVER

The body's normal response to many childhood diseases and infections is a high temperature or fever. But the rise in body temperature may also be caused by heat exposure, by a noninfectious disease problem, and even by childhood immunization shots. The parents probably monitored their child's temperature and can report the temperature readings taken before you arrived. Try to find out how

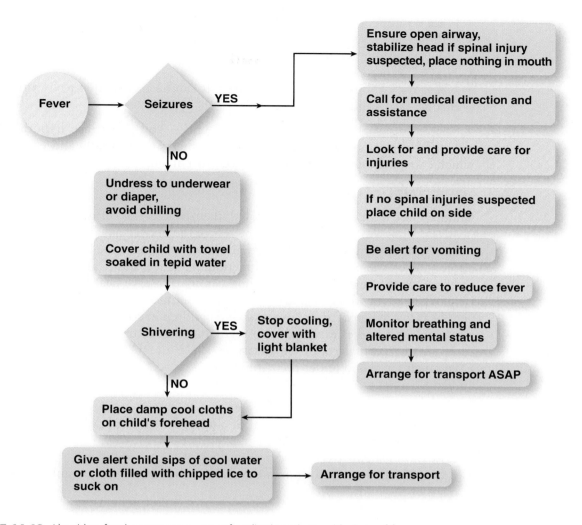

Fever → Seizures — YES →

Ensure open airway, stabilize head if spinal injury suspected, place nothing in mouth

↓

Call for medical direction and assistance

↓

Look for and provide care for injuries

↓

If no spinal injuries suspected place child on side

↓

Be alert for vomiting

↓

Provide care to reduce fever

↓

Monitor breathing and altered mental status

↓

Arrange for transport ASAP

Seizures — NO ↓

Undress to underwear or diaper, avoid chilling

↓

Cover child with towel soaked in tepid water

↓

Shivering — YES → **Stop cooling, cover with light blanket**

Shivering — NO ↓

Place damp cool cloths on child's forehead

↓

Give alert child sips of cool water or cloth filled with chipped ice to suck on → **Arrange for transport**

FIGURE 14.10 Algorithm for the emergency care of pediatric patients with signs of fever.

high the fever is and how rapidly it rose. Increased temperature is not necessarily what causes a seizure, but a rapid rise in body temperature can cause one.

A fever with a rash, long bouts of diarrhea and vomiting, little intake of fluids, or a fever that rose rapidly with or without seizure are all indications that a potentially serious medical condition may be present. Call for transport as soon as possible.

It is not necessary to try to take a temperature. If the skin feels very warm to touch, report this finding along with skin color and condition. A child with a high fever will likely be flushed (red) and dry. A mild fever may quickly elevate to a high fever and become a life-threatening problem.

If the child is hot to the touch and there is a history of fever reported by the parent or caregiver, take the following steps if your local protocols allow (Figure 14.10):

- Undress the child down to underwear or diaper, but do not allow him to become chilled. Many parents still believe that feverish children must be bundled up so they will not become chilled or so they will sweat out a fever. All this clothing retains the heat of the fever.

- Cover the child with a towel soaked in tepid (not cold) water if the fever is the result of heat exposure. If the child starts to shiver, stop the cooling process and cover with a light blanket.
- Place damp, cool cloths on the child's forehead.
- Call for the transport of any child who has had a seizure. If the child is seizing, monitor airway and breathing.
- *Never* submerge a child in cold water.
- *Never* use rubbing alcohol for cooling. It can be absorbed in toxic amounts through the child's skin.

Be cautious about cooling a fevered child. You can cause hypothermia or reduced body temperature. Wet towels and sheets cool rapidly and become cold, which causes the child to shiver and become chilled.

HYPOTHERMIA

Children lose a lot of body heat through their heads. The surface area of the child's head is proportionately larger than the rest of the body. The large head radiates and loses heat when it is uncovered. When the head is exposed, the body will make every effort to keep the brain warm and functioning, so it sends heat from other parts of the body to the head. Because the child cannot conserve heat well, it will not take long to use up any reserves and develop hypothermia. Keep the head covered to prevent heat loss when caring for infants and children in cool environments.

Children's bodies are unable to regulate temperatures as well as adult bodies can, even in normal room temperatures (68°F or 20°C). Most children do not have much fat stored under their skin and cannot conserve heat. They can become chilled through the environment, injury, or illness, including:

- Exposure to cool weather and water.
- Damp or wet clothes, or removal of clothes for medical evaluation.
- Alcohol or drugs, which dilate peripheral vessels.
- Low blood sugar (hypoglycemia).
- Brain disorder or head trauma that affects the temperature regulation mechanism of the body.
- Severe infection.
- Shock.

When you look for a mechanism of injury or try to determine the nature of illness, also think about conditions that can cause overcooling of the child. In a cold environment, warm the child by stripping off any wet clothing and by wrapping him in a blanket. Be sure the head is covered.

DIARRHEA AND VOMITING

The child can lose large amounts of needed body fluids through vomiting and diarrhea, which are normal reactions to illness (and sometimes to certain ingested poisons). This fluid loss is called **dehydration**. Infants are more susceptible to dehydration than adults are because the infant has such a small circulating blood volume to start with. For example, think about losing one cup of fluid during an illness. This would be insignificant to an adult, whereas the total circulating blood volume in a newborn is only a cup and a half.

Suspect that a child is dehydrated if he has been feverish for some time, if he has been vomiting without taking in any fluids, or if he has had diarrhea for several days. As the child loses fluids through vomiting and diarrhea and cannot replace them, the fluid balance in the body is disturbed. A balance of fluids-in to fluids-out is needed to maintain muscle and organ function. Shock can result when large amounts of fluids are lost, even if the fluid is not blood.

dehydration ■ excessive loss of body water (fluids).

If you suspect a child is dehydrated, do the following:

1. Monitor the airway.
2. Position the child so the airway will not be obstructed if the child vomits. Elevating the legs may help if the patient is showing signs of shock.
3. Monitor respirations and administer blow-by oxygen as per local protocols.
4. Check vital signs. If they indicate shock, arrange to transport immediately.
5. If possible, save some vomit for hospital personnel to examine.

POISONING

Part of a child's learning experience includes exploring and tasting things. This can sometimes lead to exposure to or ingestion of poisonous substances. Poisons can affect any or all of the body's systems and can rapidly threaten the life of a child. Much of your assessment and care will be the same as for an adult. Know your local protocols for contacting medical direction or a poison control center if there is any indication or suspicion that a child has been exposed to a poison. Be aware that some poisons may be considered hazardous materials, which will require response by specialized personnel trained to handle them.

NEAR-DROWNING

The child who has been submerged in water may still be alive or clinically dead (no breathing and no heartbeat), but not biologically dead (brain cells are still alive). Many patients have been revived after more than 30 minutes of submersion in cold water. Children have been successfully revived more often than adults in these situations. When caring for a possible near-drowning patient:

1. Make sure the airway is clear and free of fluids.
2. Provide artificial ventilations or CPR as necessary.
3. Protect the spine in cases where the near-drowning was the result of a diving or boating incident.
4. Get the patient to a warm and dry environment away from wind to prevent or care for hypothermia. Remove wet clothing.
5. Place the child in the recovery position to prevent aspiration. Administer high-concentration oxygen (as per local protocols).
6. Obtain a baseline set of vital signs.
7. Arrange to transport all near-drowning patients, even if they have recovered and are breathing on their own. It is possible that they will deteriorate hours after they have recovered.

Managing Trauma Emergencies

GENERAL CARE OF THE CHILD TRAUMA PATIENT

Because of their size, curiosity, and lack of fear due to their inexperience, infants and children are frequent victims of trauma. It is the number one cause of death in people one to 18 years of age—as a result of motor-vehicle crashes, drowning, burns, firearms, falls, blunt and penetrating trauma, abuse, entrapment, crushing, and various other mechanisms of injury (Figure 14.11).

6–2.7 Discuss emergency medical care of the infant and child trauma patient.

When performing a physical exam on a stable, responsive child, you may reverse your assessment order and do a toe-to-head physical exam. For unresponsive or unstable patients, perform the head-to-toe assessment, focus on the ABCs, and determine priority of transport.

FIGURE 14.11 Look for the mechanism of injury.

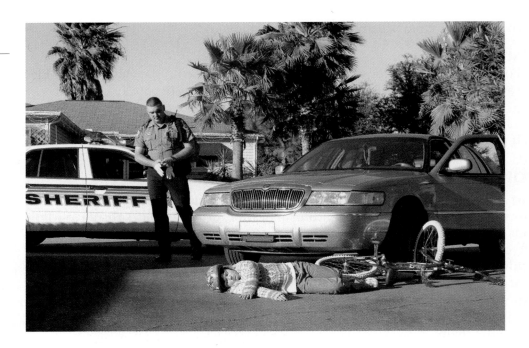

When managing injuries in children, keep in mind that their larger head size and weight will make them more prone to head and neck trauma in motor-vehicle collisions, especially if unrestrained. This is also true of bicycle mishaps if children are not wearing helmets, in mishaps in which they are struck, in swimming and diving mishaps, and in sports mishaps. Suspect abdominal and pelvic injuries in vehicle crashes in which the child is restrained, and extremity injuries in falls of three times their height or greater.

FIRST ➤ General emergency care steps for the infant or child trauma patient include the following (Figure 14.12):

1. Ensure an open airway. Manually stabilize the head and neck. Use a jaw-thrust maneuver to open the airway and protect the spine. Place a folded towel under the shoulders to maintain a neutral position for the airway and alignment of the head.

2. Make sure the airway is clear. Suction, if local protocols allow. If necessary, provide ventilations.

3. Provide oxygen by nonrebreather mask or assist ventilations with a bag-valve mask ventilator with supplemental oxygen as per local protocols.

4. Control bleeding by applying appropriate dressings.

5. Stabilize suspected fractures.

6. Maintain manual stabilization of the patient's head and neck until the ambulance arrives.

7. Arrange for transport as soon as possible.

8. While waiting for the EMTs to arrive or while en route, perform your detailed and ongoing assessments. ▪

For a summary of the assessment and emergency care of pediatric patients with specific musculoskeletal injuries, see Figure 14.13. For assessment and care of bleeding, shock, and specific soft-tissue injuries, see Figure 14.14.

FIRST ON SCENE

"Ma'am, you need to help me!" Jenny shouted at the woman who had now sunk to the pavement and was crying loudly. The woman climbed unsteadily to her feet and approached the back of the patrol car where her hands flew up to cover her mouth at the sight of the baby's injuries. "Ma'am," Jenny said firmly. "I need you to hold these dressings in place while I get a bandage on!" The crying woman took a step toward Jenny and had to force her shaking hands out to hold the white gauze onto the baby's torso while the police officer unrolled the bandage.

"Now I need you to hold your baby close and talk to him." Jenny helped the woman hold the crying baby up to her chest. "Keep talking to him, do you understand?"

The woman nodded, trying to curb her own sobs as she gently rocked the small child. Jenny sighed with relief as she heard the quickly approaching sirens of both medical aid and police backup.

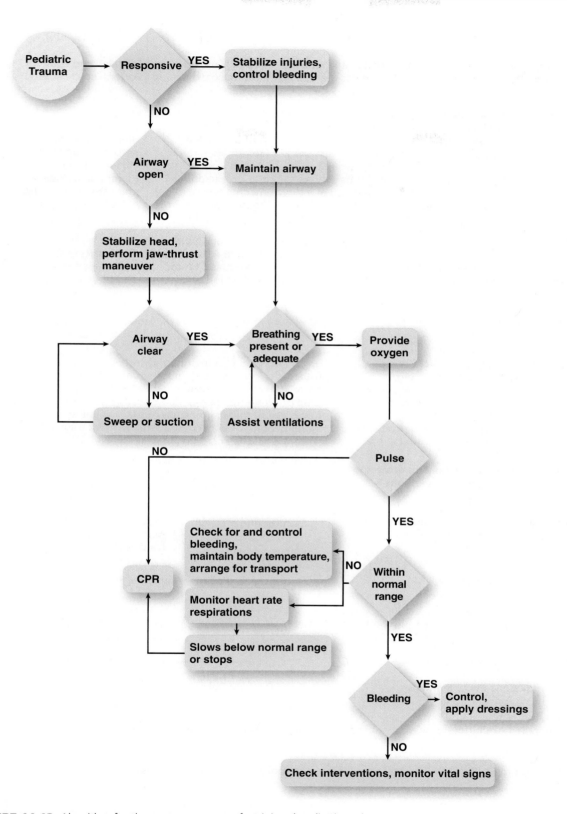

FIGURE 14.12 Algorithm for the emergency care of an injured pediatric patient.

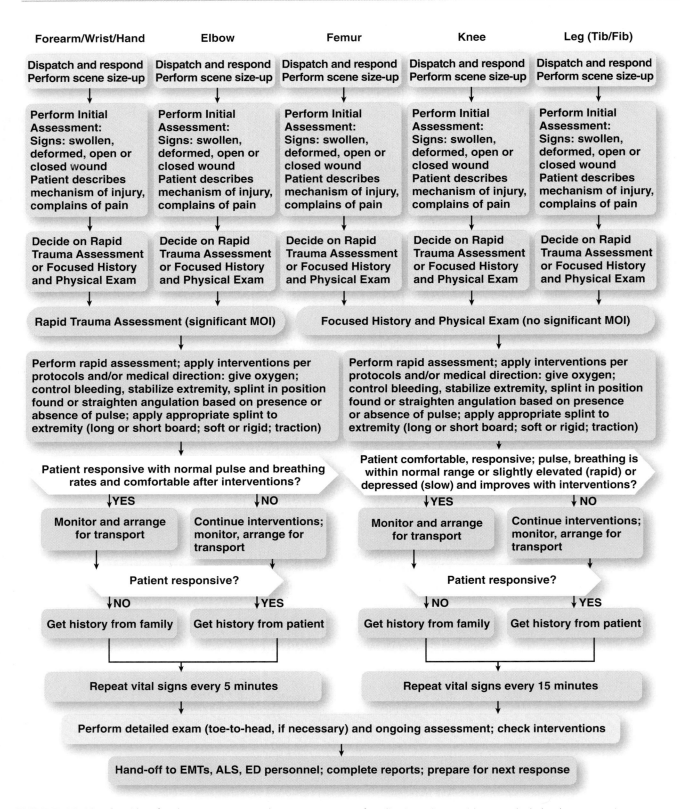

FIGURE 14.13 Algorithm for the assessment and emergency care of pediatric patients with musculoskeletal emergencies.

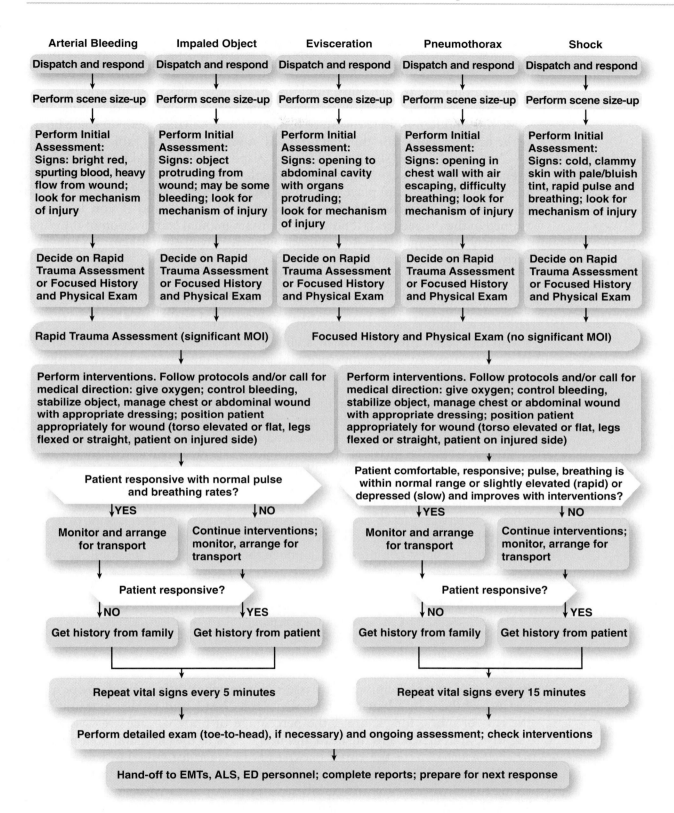

Arterial Bleeding	Impaled Object	Evisceration	Pneumothorax	Shock
Dispatch and respond	Dispatch and respond	Dispatch and respond	Dispatch and respond	Dispatch and respond
Perform scene size-up	Perform scene size-up	Perform scene size-up	Perform scene size-up	Perform scene size-up
Perform Initial Assessment: Signs: bright red, spurting blood, heavy flow from wound; look for mechanism of injury	Perform Initial Assessment: Signs: object protruding from wound; may be some bleeding; look for mechanism of injury	Perform Initial Assessment: Signs: opening to abdominal cavity with organs protruding; look for mechanism of injury	Perform Initial Assessment: Signs: opening in chest wall with air escaping, difficulty breathing; look for mechanism of injury	Perform Initial Assessment: Signs: cold, clammy skin with pale/bluish tint, rapid pulse and breathing; look for mechanism of injury
Decide on Rapid Trauma Assessment or Focused History and Physical Exam	Decide on Rapid Trauma Assessment or Focused History and Physical Exam	Decide on Rapid Trauma Assessment or Focused History and Physical Exam	Decide on Rapid Trauma Assessment or Focused History and Physical Exam	Decide on Rapid Trauma Assessment or Focused History and Physical Exam

Rapid Trauma Assessment (significant MOI)

Focused History and Physical Exam (no significant MOI)

Perform interventions. Follow protocols and/or call for medical direction: give oxygen; control bleeding, stabilize object, manage chest or abdominal wound with appropriate dressing; position patient appropriately for wound (torso elevated or flat, legs flexed or straight, patient on injured side)

Perform interventions. Follow protocols and/or call for medical direction: give oxygen; control bleeding, stabilize object, manage chest or abdominal wound with appropriate dressing; position patient appropriately for wound (torso elevated or flat, legs flexed or straight, patient on injured side)

Patient responsive with normal pulse and breathing rates?

Patient comfortable, responsive; pulse, breathing is within normal range or slightly elevated (rapid) or depressed (slow) and improves with interventions?

↓YES — Monitor and arrange for transport
↓NO — Continue interventions; monitor, arrange for transport

↓YES — Monitor and arrange for transport
↓NO — Continue interventions; monitor, arrange for transport

Patient responsive?
↓NO — Get history from family
↓YES — Get history from patient

Patient responsive?
↓NO — Get history from family
↓YES — Get history from patient

Repeat vital signs every 5 minutes

Repeat vital signs every 15 minutes

Perform detailed exam (toe-to-head), if necessary) and ongoing assessment; check interventions

Hand-off to EMTs, ALS, ED personnel; complete reports; prepare for next response

FIGURE 14.14 Algorithm for the assessment and emergency care of pediatric patients with bleeding, shock, and soft-tissues injuries.

SAFETY SEATS

Too many safety seats are not installed correctly, and children often are not secured properly by the safety straps and harnesses. Any movement of the seat or the child can throw both forward in a crash. As a result, the child receives internal injuries, which emergency care providers may not be able to initially detect. Usually, the child's body will compensate for these internal injuries and bleeding, which can lull the rescuers into thinking the child is unharmed and stable.

Based on crash-result studies over recent years, it has been determined that removing children from their safety seats and immobilizing them on spine boards is the best procedure for children involved in vehicle crashes (Table 14–3).

Any vehicle crash should lead you to suspect that the child has been injured, even if you do not see any damage to the safety seat. Carefully extricate the child from the safety seat and place him on a spinal immobilization device, if local protocols allow Emergency Medical Responders to do so (and if you have been trained in the procedures). If not, then maintain manual stabilization of the child's head in neutral alignment and maintain an open airway until other EMS providers arrive to take over patient care.

There are many types of child safety seats, but each provides the same safety functions if properly used. Emergency Medical Responders should not hesitate to act to immobilize and provide initial airway care for a child, even if they are not familiar with the safety seat they find at a crash site. Use the following guidelines if you must extricate an infant or a child from a safety seat, but do not perform these steps unless you have learned and practiced them under the supervision of your instructor:

- Do a quick visual inspection of the vehicle interior. Did the crash force the safety seat from its position, even slightly? Was the safety seat in the rear or front vehicle seat? Was the safety seat a rear-facing or forward-facing seat? Is there structural damage to the seat?
- Throughout the assessment and immobilization process, be sure that someone maintains manual stabilization of the infant's or the child's head.
- Assess the patient for the ABCs. Assess for injuries.
- If the safety seat has a protection plate over the patient's chest, remove it (cut the straps securing it, if necessary) in order to assess the chest. (Before performing chest compressions, remove the infant onto an immobilization device.)
- As you assess the patient, check for loose straps, which would have provided little protection. Extricate the child onto an immobilization device, which can then be secured to the ambulance stretcher (Scan 14–2).

BURNS

Burns in infants and children are assessed somewhat differently than for adults because of the child's larger surface area, larger head, and smaller extremities. In the rule of nines, for example, the percentage of body surface area assigned is slightly different: 18% to the head and neck, 18% to the chest and abdomen, 9% to each arm, 18% to the entire back, 14% for each leg, and 1% to the genital area. If you find it is difficult to do the estimations with accuracy while you are trying to quickly care for and stabilize the patient, do not worry about precision. The safest procedure is to estimate quickly and overestimate rather than underestimate the body surface area burned. The younger the child, the more important it is that he is seen in a burn center because of concerns about abuse and long-term morbidity.

TABLE 14–3	Child Safety Seats
ISSUES	**FACTS**
Installation and child security	Too many safety seats are not installed correctly, and children are often not secured properly by the safety straps and harnesses.
Restrictions on care	Emergency Medical Responders and other emergency care providers cannot adequately provide airway management care, maintain an open airway, or provide bag-valve mask resuscitation on a child who is immobilized in a safety seat.
Position of the child	A child's torso in a safety seat is in a flexed position because the seat is designed that way. Spinal immobilization straightens and extends the spine from the cervical spine (the neck) to the sacrum (the part of the spine between the hip bones). Leaving the child in a safety seat continues to stretch the spine in a curved position rather than in a straight, extended position.
Injuries to the child	If an infant or small child of any age is riding in the forward-facing position, the crash forces likely caused the child's body to flex forward extremely (hyperflexion), especially if the seat was installed improperly or the harness securing the child was too loose. This sudden forward flexion causes injury to the cervical spine.
Protection for the child	Children up to age four and up to 40 pounds may be too large for the child safety seat to support the head and protect them properly. If the child's head extends above the top edge of the seat back, the head may hyperextend (be forced extremely backward) in a crash. At the same time, the body is thrust forward. All this sudden and extreme motion stretches the ligaments and muscles of the spinal column, causing severe injuries.
Car seat damage and stability	The safety seat (especially an improperly installed one) involved in a vehicle crash is likely to be damaged, although the damage may not be noticed even on close inspection. A damaged seat will not adequately immobilize and support the child. Furthermore, manufacturers state that child safety seats are not designed to be used as immobilizing devices. Using the safety seat for purposes other than the manufacturer intended places the liability for further patient injury on emergency care providers.
Transport considerations	Safety seats cannot be properly secured in the ambulance. Furthermore, if the ambulance is involved in a collision en route to the hospital, the safety seat cannot endure the forces of another crash. There are enough reports of ambulance crashes while en route to the hospital with patients to cause concern. A second crash may further weaken the effectiveness of the safety seat and leave the child, who is immobilized in it, unprotected. However, many ambulances are now carrying child safety seats in the event they must transport uninjured children to the hospital with their injured parents. The child safety seats are secured in the captain's chair.

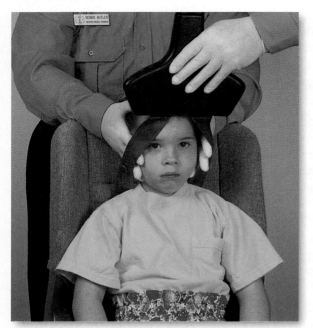

1 ■ Rescuer 1 stabilizes car seat in upright position and applies manual head/neck stabilization. Rescuer 2 prepares equipment, then loosens or cuts the seat straps and raises the front guard.

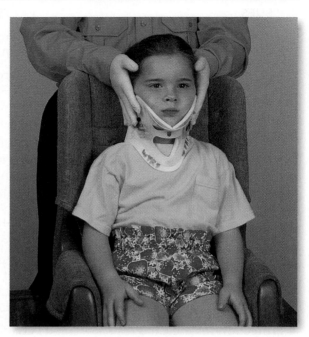

2 ■ Cervical collar is applied to patient as Rescuer 1 maintains manual stabilization of the head and neck.

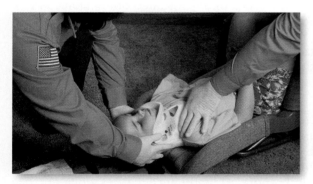

3 ■ As Rescuer 1 maintains manual head/neck stabilization, Rescuer 2 places child safety seat on center of backboard and slowly tilts it into supine position. Both rescuers are careful not to let the child slide out of the chair. For the child with a large head, place a towel under area where the shoulders will eventually be placed on the board to prevent head from tilting forward.

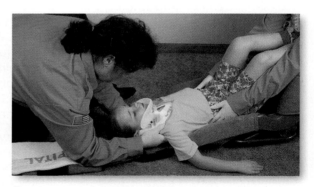

4a ■ Rescuer 1 maintains manual head/neck stabilization and calls for a coordinated long axis move onto the backboard.

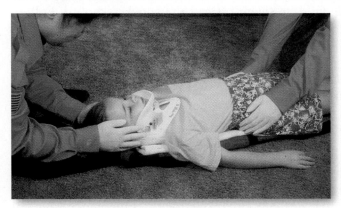

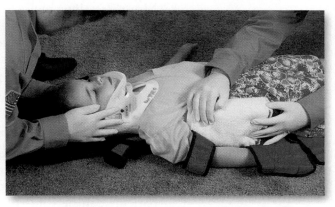

4b ■ Rescuer 1 maintains manual head/neck stabilization as the move onto board is completed, with the child's shoulders over the folded towel.

5 ■ Rescuer 1 maintains manual head/neck stabilization. Rescuer 2 places rolled towels or blankets on both sides of the patient.

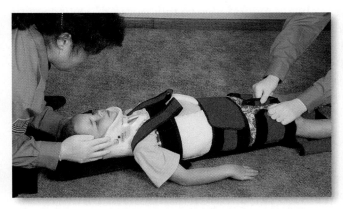

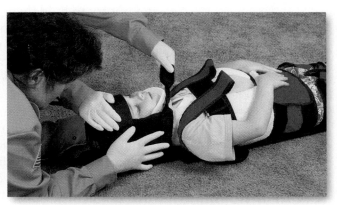

6 ■ Rescuer 1 maintains manual head/neck stabilization. Rescuer 2 straps or tapes patient to board at level of upper chest, pelvis, and lower legs. Do not strap across abdomen.

7 ■ Rescuer 1 maintains manual head/neck stabilization as Rescuer 2 places rolled towels on both sides of head, then tapes head securely in place across forehead and maxilla (jaw bone) or cervical collar. Do not tape across chin to avoid putting pressure on neck.

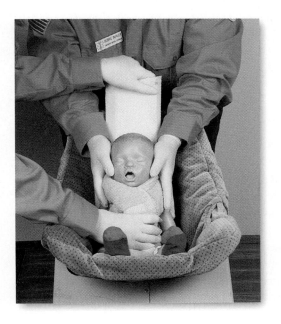

■ The infant procedure is exactly the same as for a child, except that an arm board is inserted behind the infant in step 2. If the infant is very small, the arm board may actually be used as the spine board.

Carefully and quickly care for the burned area with dry, sterile, and nonadherent dressings or sheets. Dry dressings will keep air and foreign materials or dirt off the burn and will help keep the child warm, which will help in preventing shock. Moist dressings may chill the child and could speed the shock response. Follow local protocols for burn management. Arrange to transport the burned child as quickly as possible. Check local protocols for determining the type of cases (degree of severity, respiratory burns) that should be transported to a burn center. Burns are excruciatingly painful, and children are likely to be frantic. Rapid transport is important for obtaining pain relief for the child and care of the burns.

SUSPECTED NEGLECT AND ABUSE

6–2.10 Recognize the need for Emergency Medical Responder debriefing following a difficult infant or child transport.

The news media have been reporting more stories of child neglect and abuse in recent years. These events are not something new. Rather, they have always existed but are now more recognized and reported. Calls involving pediatric patients can be some of the most difficult situations for the Emergency Medical Responder to handle both during and after the call. It is normal to experience strong emotions following a difficult call, but calls involving pediatric patients can be especially difficult emotionally. It is very important to recognize these feelings and not try to hold them in. It is always a good idea to talk out your feelings with those who can offer support and understanding. If given the opportunity, it is highly recommended that you participate in a formal debriefing for any difficult call. Remember to maintain patient confidentiality. You cannot name the child or family to anyone but medical or juvenile authorities or the police.

6–2.9 Describe the medical-legal responsibilities in suspected child abuse.

You must collect information, perform your assessments, and provide care without making a judgment or expressing your suspicion, distaste, or disbelief. Keep in mind that the abuser also needs help. Remember that your suspicions may be unfounded and that not every injury or sign of possible abuse to a child is the result of actual abuse. It is not your place to accuse the parents or caregiver because they may not even be the abuser. You will need to check for patterns in responses and reports to confirm your suspicions. Report your concerns and impressions to ambulance personnel, medical direction, or social services, the health department, or law enforcement, as required by local protocols. In most jurisdictions, there is a legal obligation to report suspected child abuse. Be aware of your local laws and protocols regarding reporting abuse.

6–2.8 Summarize the signs and symptoms of possible child abuse and neglect.

FIRST ➤ There are several different forms of child abuse, and they frequently occur in combination (Figure 14.15):

- Psychological abuse.
- Neglect.
- Sexual abuse.
- Physical abuse. ▪

Psychological Abuse

It may be rare that Emergency Medical Responders are called to care for a patient who has been psychologically abused because there is no physical injury. However, there may be emotional signs and symptoms that may be difficult to assess unless you know the patient.

psychological abuse ▪ persistent emotional or verbal abuse that affects a child's positive emotional development, self-esteem, and emotional well-being.

Psychological abuse includes emotional or verbal abuse that seriously affects the child's positive emotional development, well-being, and self-esteem. Children exposed to psychological abuse may feel rejected, degraded, or terrified. They may be forced into isolation with limited freedom or contact with others. They may be

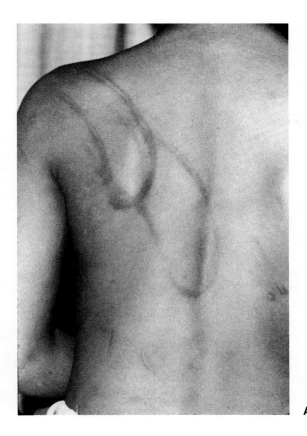

A

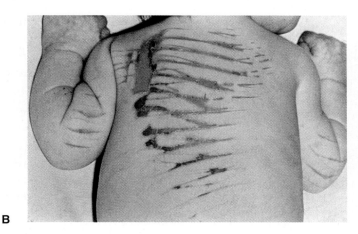

B

FIGURE 14.15 Examples of injuries caused by abuse and neglect: **A** cord bruise to the back. *(© Robert A. Felter, MD)*, and **B** cigarette lighter burns to the back *(© Robert A. Felter, MD)*.

exploited or corrupted and forced to accept the beliefs of another, such as a cult or gang leader. Verbal abuse that affects emotional well-being and self-esteem and causes feelings of rejection or degradation in children includes phrases such as, "You're stupid," "You are no good," "You are not like your sister," "I wish you were never born," or "I hate you." Some parents isolate their children, locking them in closets or not letting them attend school. Cult and gang leaders often exploit the emotions of vulnerable teenagers, making them believe that the cult loves them or the gang gives them power and freedom and their parents do not.

Although psychological abuse can occur alone, victims often suffer other forms of abuse with it, such as sexual and **physical abuse**. The victims of psychological abuse, as well as other forms of abuse, are those with the least power and resources—children and women. Possible signs of psychological abuse include the following:

- Depression.
- Withdrawal.
- Extreme anxiety.
- Low self-esteem.
- Feelings of shame and guilt.
- Fear.
- Lack of normal social skills because of isolation.
- Avoidance of eye contact.
- Extreme passiveness or compliance.
- History or indications of self-harm.
- Substance abuse.
- Increased tension or anxiety when the abuser is present.

Provide care and emotional support by listening to and believing what the child tells you and by expressing your understanding. Let the child know that

physical abuse ■ inflicting any type of physical injury or performing any physical act that harms or disfigures the child.

there are people who will help and that you can get help. Arrange to have the child transported to get him away from the abuser, if necessary. Be sure to report your findings to the transport personnel and to social services, the health department, or the police, as required by your protocols.

Neglect

Emergency responses are usually for the obvious traumas that occur in physical and sexual abuse, not for neglect. However, long-term neglect may result in physical deterioration and injury or medical problems. Child **neglect** occurs when parents or caregivers do not provide for any or all of the following basic needs of the child: food and water, appropriate shelter and clothing, medical care, and education.

On arrival, your scene size-up may reveal obvious signs of neglect, such as a child who is dressed inappropriately for the weather; a child who is lean, lethargic, and has signs of dehydration; or an environment with unclean living conditions, particularly where the child sleeps or is confined.

Consider also the circumstances of the family. They may not be able to financially afford to provide for the basic needs of the child or even themselves, and the entire family may need help from social services. Provide appropriate care for the child's illness or injuries and arrange to transport. Follow your protocols for reporting your concerns.

Sexual Abuse

There are many forms of **sexual abuse**, including physical sexual contact or exposure and sexual exploitation by displaying or photographing children for sexual purposes or with sexual intent. Emergency Medical Responders usually receive a call for sexual abuse if the child is injured or showing signs of a sexually related medical condition. A child can be the victim of sexual abuse from a parent or other relative and sometimes from a neighbor, teacher, or other trusted individual.

Do not expect the abuser to admit that sexual abuse is the reason for the call. Many excuses and reasons are given for the child who has genital injuries or who has signs and symptoms of sexually transmitted diseases. Continue to act professionally and control your emotions.

When providing care, avoid embarrassing the child or making him feel guilty. Let the child know that you and the people at the hospital will help. Some signs of sexual abuse include:

- Obvious injuries to the genital area, including burns, cuts, bruises, and abrasions.
- Rashes or sores around the genitals, discharges (such as seminal fluid), and bleeding from the genital openings or on underclothing.
- Information from the child that he was exposed, touched, or assaulted.

FIRST ➤ Be sure to report your suspicions and findings to ambulance personnel or to the appropriate agency, as per local protocols. Use these emergency care steps:

1. Dress wounds and provide other appropriate care for injuries.
2. Save any evidence of sexual abuse, such as soiled or stained clothing. Do not let the child use the bathroom to urinate or defecate. If the child must go to the bathroom, try to collect it in a container for hospital examination. Do not let the child drink any fluids or eat anything. Do not wash the child or let the parent wash the child or change his clothes. (The parent may insist on washing the child and changing his clothing; the child may insist that he must use the bathroom. Be aware that you cannot prevent them from doing so.)
3. Minimize embarrassment by covering the child with a blanket, if necessary.

neglect ■ failure of the parents or caregivers to provide for the child's basic physical, social, emotional, medical, and/or medical needs.

sexual abuse ■ physical sexual contact with or exposure to children and sexual exploitation of children by exposing, displaying, or photographing them for sexual purposes or with sexual intent.

4. Arrange for transport as soon as possible.

5. Provide emotional support and reassurance. Remember, you are still caring for a child. Try to engage him with toys or age-appropriate conversation or games. ▪

Physical Abuse

Any form of violent, harmful contact with a child or any disfiguring act performed on the child is physical abuse, no matter what the intent of the adult. Some of the indications of physical abuse include the following:

- Outline of marks or bruises that are the size or shape of the object used to strike the child, such as the hand, a belt, strap, rope, or cord.
- Areas of swelling, black eyes, loose or missing teeth, split lips.
- Lacerations, incisions, abrasions.
- Any unexplained bruises, broken bones, or burn marks.
- Broken bones, signs of injuries healing incorrectly (misshaped limbs), or a history of numerous broken bones.
- Head injuries or indications of closed head injuries that could be the result of violent shaking (bulging fontanels, unresponsiveness), especially in infants and small children.
- Bruises—old and new—in various stages of healing.
- Abdominal injuries with signs of bruising, distention, rigidity, or tenderness that could be the result of punching or kicking.
- Genitalia injuries with lacerations, avulsions, or bleeding.
- Bite marks showing the pattern and size of an adult mouth.
- Burn marks or patterns caused by cigarettes, hot irons, stove burners; water burns or scalding marks on the legs, such as stocking burns from dipping in hot water, or a hand mark on the buttocks where the child's skin was protected from immersion. The creases at the knees and thighs are also protected when the child flexes his legs while being dipped in hot water.

The child's relationship with the parents or a parent's attitude toward the child or the situation may be a clue to abuse. However, these will not always be reliable indicators of the family relationship. Look for the following:

- Story of how the injury occurred that does not match the injury found.
- Child who seems afraid to say how the injury occurred.
- Child who is obviously afraid of a parent or other person at the scene.
- Child who seems to expect no comfort from the parent.
- Child who has no apparent reaction to pain.
- Parent who does not want to leave you alone with the child.
- Parents who tell conflicting stories or change explanations.
- Parent who blames the child for being clumsy or accident prone.
- Parent who seems inappropriately concerned or unconcerned.
- Parent who is angry and is having trouble controlling it.
- One parent who appears depressed or withdrawn while the other parent is expressing anger or giving explanations.
- Any signs of alcohol or drug abuse.
- Any expression of suicide or seeking mercy for their children.
- Parent who is reluctant to give the child's history or to permit transport or who refuses to go to the nearest hospital.

You must be the child's advocate and convince the parents that the child needs to be seen by a physician because of "the difficulty of determining the seriousness of injuries in the field." Do not accuse anyone of any wrongdoing.

You may respond to a call for an injured child and have no idea that the injury is related to abuse. You may observe that the child and parents relate well and that there is a strong bond between them. There are still abuse indications that will make you suspicious over time. Be alert for:

- Repeated responses for the same child or children in the same house.
- Signs of past injuries during your assessment.
- Signs of poorly healing wounds.
- Signs of burns that are fresh or in various stages of healing.
- Many types of injuries on numerous parts of the body.

Obvious abuse situations can trigger strong emotions in you. Most people feel it is their duty to protect young children. Your first reactions to an abuse situation may be anger and disgust. However, you should not display these feelings while caring for the child or dealing with the parents or other caregivers. Providing necessary care for the child's injuries, clearly documenting objective findings, and alerting the proper authorities of your suspicions are appropriate actions.

If you suspect abuse and the parent or caregiver will not allow the child to be transported, call for law enforcement assistance.

Shaken Baby Syndrome

Another type of abuse is shaken baby syndrome. It is a group of signs and symptoms that usually occur in children younger than two years but may be seen in children as old as five years. The syndrome results from the trauma caused by an angry or an extremely frustrated parent or caregiver who shakes the baby as a punishment or as an attempt to quiet him. The intent, usually, is not to harm the baby. Rarely, the syndrome may be caused accidentally by tossing the baby in the air or jogging with the baby in a backpack. It is not a result of gentle bouncing.

Infants and children have large heavy heads, weak and not fully developed neck muscles, and space between the brain and the skull to allow for growth. The skull is also soft and pliable and not yet strong enough to absorb much force. During violent shaking, the brain will rebound against the inside of the skull and bruise, swell, and bleed, which causes increased pressure. Shaking also can cause injury to the neck and spine and to the eyes, causing loss of vision.

If you are called to the scene of a sick or injured child, ask the parent or caregiver questions to obtain a history. Look for signs and symptoms of illness or injury in your assessment. A shaken baby may have no obvious signs of trauma, such as bruising, bleeding, or swelling. The history and some of the signs and symptoms of shaken baby syndrome may include the following, which may also be indications of other illnesses:

- Change in behavior.
- Irritability.
- Lethargy or sleepiness.
- Decreased alertness.
- Unresponsiveness.
- Pale or bluish (cyanotic) skin.
- Vomiting.
- Convulsions (seizures).
- Not eating normally.
- Not breathing.

Shaken baby syndrome is a serious emergency. Call for transport immediately for any child with the above signs and symptoms. While waiting for them to arrive, ensure that the baby has an airway, is breathing, and has a pulse. Perform rescue breathing or CPR as needed and provide oxygen, if you are trained and allowed to do so. If the child is vomiting, protect and clear the airway. Be sure to turn the infant as a unit, keeping the head in line with the body. If the infant is having seizures, protect him from further injury.

 FIRST ON SCENE WRAP-UP

The scene was suddenly awash with flashing emergency lights, and both police officers and firefighters scattered around the intersection checking on people and securing the area. Jenny described the child's wounds to the medical crew, who quickly gave the mother an oxygen mask to hold near the baby's face and ushered her to the back of the ambulance.

"It's good that he's crying," the paramedic said to the mother as he helped her into the ambulance. "But we need to get him over to the university right away."

He then turned to Jenny, just before closing the back doors, and said, "You did a great job, officer. You did perfect." Jenny nodded and waved weakly.

As the ambulance moved quickly across 43rd Street and down Buchanan, Jenny sat down on the bumper of her patrol car. "We caught the shooters, you know," a voice said, startling her. She looked up and saw the shift sergeant standing on the sidewalk, looking at her and the bloody exam gloves that she wore.

"How's the little one going to be?" he asked, stepping closer and putting a hand on her shoulder.

"I hope he'll be okay," she answered, standing up. "I mean, I think I did everything that I was supposed to."

"You did just fine," he smiled. "Go ahead and head back to the station and relax. We'll all debrief when we're done here."

Summary

Assessment and emergency care of infants and children is basically the same as for adults. However, you must consider the special characteristics of the pediatric patient's anatomy, physiology, and emotional responses when assessing and caring for them. For example, to help keep an infant or a child calm, reverse the order of the physical exam. Begin at the toes and work toward the head. Infants and children may also be examined while sitting on a parent's lap.

One example of a child's different anatomy compared to that of an adult's is the head. In infants and children, the head is larger and heavier in proportion to the rest of the body. Be suspicious of mechanisms of injury that have the potential to cause head and spine injury. Also, carefully handle the head of an infant up to 18 months; do not apply any pressure to the fontanels (soft spots).

Infants breathe through the nose. If it is obstructed, they may not immediately open their mouths to breathe. Be sure to clear the nostrils of secretions. Remember also that because the tongue is larger in infants and children, it can cause airway obstruction. When managing the airway of an infant, make sure the large head is in a neutral position, neither hyperflexed nor hyperextended. Place a folded towel under the infant's or the child's shoulders to maintain the spine and the airway in neutral alignment.

Care for respiratory distress in infants and children immediately. For respiratory distress, provide oxygen with a pediatric-size nonrebreather mask or by using the blow-by technique. For severe distress and respiratory arrest, provide assisted ventilations with the appropriate device, such as a pocket face mask or pediatric bag-valve mask ventilator and supplemental oxygen. Do not place anything in the mouth of the infant or child unless you see an obstruction. Arrange for transport immediately.

Children tolerate high fevers better than adults do, but a fever that rises rapidly can cause seizures. Arrange to transport the feverish child as soon as possible. Also arrange to transport the child who is vomiting and has diarrhea.

The surface area of a child's body is large in proportion to weight. This makes infants and children more vulnerable to hypothermia. Covering the patient, especially the head, will help maintain warmth.

Care for shock early. In an infant or child, signs and symptoms of shock mean it has progressed and is in the late stages. If you suspect that shock may result from the mechanism of injury or nature of illness, provide emergency care immediately.

Because of their size, curiosity, and a lack of fear due to their inexperience, infants and children are frequent victims of trauma. When assessing and providing emergency care, keep in mind that their larger head size and their weight make pediatric patients more prone to head and neck trauma. In addition, be calm, professional, and discreet about suspicions of abuse or neglect in the presence of caregivers. Be an advocate for the child, and remember your obligation to report any suspicions to the proper authorities.

Remember and Consider

Children are curious and daring, and they like to have fun. Sometimes they get into fights or into situations in which they get hurt. Many result in bumps and scrapes that are easy for a parent to care for, but sometimes an illness or injury is serious enough, or frightening enough to the child or parent, that EMS is needed.

➤ What are some of the types of injuries you expect to see in certain age groups?

➤ What can you do to help calm a crying and frightened child?

➤ Think about the many activities that children are involved in today. How do they compare with what you did as a child? Do children have more opportunities, freedom, and choices of activities today? Do these activities bring a higher potential for illness or injury?

➤ Find out how many pediatric calls your department or agency had this past year and what types they were. Were there more responses to illnesses or to injuries?

With this information, you can get an idea of where you will want to concentrate your learning and practice. Many emergency responders are nervous about caring for children. It may be because they have little experience with children who are healthy and much less experience with those who are seriously ill or injured. It may also be because children appear small and helpless, and care providers are often afraid of causing more pain while trying to help. Many children are afraid of strangers, and the care provider will find it hard to communicate with them, which may make you uncomfortable. As a result, you may not know what to do. This is normal, but you cannot allow it to interfere with your ability to care for these patients. If you never have the opportunity to work with or be around children, it is, of course, more difficult to work with them in an emergency. If you have the time to work with children as a babysitter, coach, camp counselor, or tutor, you will learn more about their personalities and feel more comfortable working with any child.

Investigate

➤ Locate the schools and day-care centers in your area.

Find out if the schools have health rooms and school nurses. Are the nurses on duty every day? What does the school or day-care center do when a child is taken seriously ill or is injured? Are parents or EMS called first? Will you be able to provide care for or transport a child without a parent present? (You may want to review legal and consent issues in Chapter 2.) Ask other EMS providers to tell you about their experiences.

➤ Locate the ball fields, parks, and playgrounds in your area.

During what seasons are these areas the most populated by children? What sports do they play, who supervises them, and what policies are followed if a child is hurt at an organized game? What injuries would you expect to find at a baseball or softball game; at a field hockey or ice hockey game; at a soccer, basketball, or football game? Are the coaches trained in providing care for sports injuries? If the parents are not at the game, how can they be contacted? Will you care for the child without consent?

Quick Quiz

1. The techniques used for the assessment and care of children are the same as for adults with certain modifications. Those modifications reflect the patient's differences in age and:
   a. physical and intellectual development.
   b. physical development and emotional response.
   c. emotional response and sex of the child.
   d. emotional response and language skills.

2. The most appropriate approach when assessing the pediatric patient is to:
   a. remain at eye level, explain each step of the exam, be truthful.
   b. remain at eye level, move to a quiet location, perform the exam.
   c. move to a quiet location, perform the exam, call parents.
   d. remain at eye level, perform the exam while telling jokes.

3. When assessing infants younger than one year, ensure an adequate airway and:
   a. protect the head, provide care to prevent shock.
   b. protect the head and spine, provide care to prevent shock.

   c. protect the head and neck, do not become too emotional.
   d. protect the head and trunk, do not become too emotional.

4. If you need to clear the airway of an unresponsive infant:
   a. open the mouth and perform a finger sweep.
   b. provide chest thrusts as quickly as possible.
   c. open the mouth, give two slow breaths, and perform a finger sweep.
   d. open the mouth, look for obstructions, perform a finger sweep if you see one.

5. If you need to perform CPR on an infant, the proper location for chest compressions is:
   a. two finger widths below the imaginary nipple line.
   b. one finger width below the imaginary nipple line.
   c. three finger widths below the imaginary nipple line.
   d. in the center of the chest between the nipples.

6. You are caring for a responsive child who is cyanotic and struggling to breathe. You should FIRST:
   a. perform a finger sweep.
   b. arrange for immediate transport.
   c. begin rescue breathing.
   d. give two breaths and begin CPR.

7. If parents or guardians are present and their emotional response to the child's injury hinders your ability to properly care for the child, do all of the following EXCEPT:

    a. ignore them.

    b. ask them to assist you with your tasks.

    c. have someone tactfully remove them from the scene.

    d. have a friend, neighbor, or other EMS responder distract them with questions.

8. When examining a child, the strategy that may be perceived by the child as LEAST threatening is first examine the:

    a. head and neck and then the rest of the body.

    b. head, neck, chest, and then the rest of the body.

    c. heart and lungs, and then the rest of the body.

    d. legs and chest, and then the neck and head.

9. All of the following statements are true for a child from three to six years of age (preschool) EXCEPT they:

    a. do not like to have their clothing removed.

    b. have a fear of blood, pain, and permanent injury.

    c. believe illness or injury is punishment for being bad.

    d. do not care if they are separated from their parents.

10. All of the following are characteristics of a child from six to 12 years of age EXCEPT they:

    a. are cooperative but like to have their opinions heard.

    b. are modest and do not like to have their bodies touched.

    c. have a fear of blood, pain, disfigurement, and permanent injury.

    d. believe that their illness or injury is a punishment for being bad.

11. The fontanels on an infant's head do not completely close until about ___ months of age.

    a. 15

    b. 16

    c. 18

    d. 12

12. All of the following are unique to a pediatric patient's breathing EXCEPT:

    a. infants are generally nasal breathers.

    b. there is more respiratory movement in the chest than abdomen.

    c. they have a less developed and more elastic chest than adults have.

    d. the trachea is softer, more flexible, and narrower than an adult's.

13. All of the following are true about children EXCEPT:

    a. they have a larger skin surface area in proportion to total body mass.

    b. they have a constant blood volume regardless of age.

    c. normal vital signs vary with the size of the child.

    d. blood pressure will vary depending on age, sex, and height.

14. All of the following are common medical emergencies for the pediatric patient EXCEPT:

    a. respiratory emergencies.

    b. altered mental status.

    c. heart attacks.

    d. seizures.

15. Several different forms of child abuse that usually occur together are sexual, physical, and:

    a. psychological.

    b. neglect.

    c. social.

    d. mental.

MODULE 7
EMS Operations

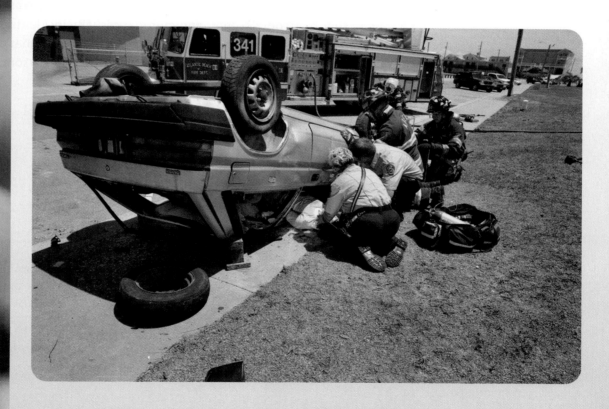

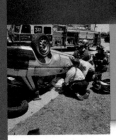

CHAPTER 15

EMS Operations

Emergency Medical Responders are just one component of an EMS system that functions and responds 24 hours a day every day of the year. These operations include many services involving a wide range of skills. Emergency Medical Responders provide basic services, such as responding to minor illnesses and injuries. They are also prepared for more serious medical and trauma incidents, such as helping EMT and ALS personnel in monitoring and providing care for critically injured patients at vehicle crashes, building fires and other hazardous scenes, and multiple-casualty incidents.

Learning what steps to take, what care to provide, what assistance to give, and performing these tasks in cooperation with other personnel and services in the system are all part of EMS operations.

OBJECTIVES

This chapter is based on the objectives of the U.S. DOT's First Responder National Standard Curriculum. Note that cognitive objectives are listed below and beside corresponding text throughout the chapter. You will also notice as you read each objective that the term Emergency Medical Responder is used. This is simply a name change and reflects the new name for the First Responder.

By the end of this chapter, you should be able to (from cognitive or knowledge information):

7-1.1 Discuss the medical and nonmedical equipment needed to respond to a call. (pp. 531–532)

7-1.2 List the phases of an out-of-hospital call. (pp. 531–533)

7-1.3 Discuss the role of the Emergency Medical Responder in extrication. (pp. 533–542)

7-1.4 List various methods of gaining access to the patient. (p. 537)

7-1.5 Distinguish between simple and complex access. (p. 537)

7-1.6 Describe what the Emergency Medical Responder should do if there is reason to believe that there is a hazard at the scene. (p. 530)

7-1.7 State the role the Emergency Medical Responder should perform until appropriately trained personnel arrive at the scene of a hazardous materials situation. (pp. 547–549)

By the end of this chapter, you should be able to feel comfortable enough to (by changing attitudes, values, and beliefs):

7–1.11 Explain the rationale for having the unit prepared to respond. (pp. 531–532)

ADDITIONAL LEARNING TASKS

This chapter explains the operations of the EMS system and how all system services and personnel coordinate their activities to rescue and provide care in multiple-casualty or disaster situations. As you work through the chapter to meet the above objectives, there is some additional information that will be essential to consider and act on at the scene of certain critical incidents.

One of the most common critical incidents for an Emergency Medical Responder may be a motor-vehicle collision, especially if you are a police officer. You should be able to:

➤ State what elements you must evaluate at the scene of a motor-vehicle collision or incidents involving multiple vehicles.

➤ Describe safety steps to take at a motor-vehicle collision scene before you gain access to patients.

➤ Describe how to stabilize a vehicle that is on its side.

➤ State how you would gain access to patients who are in a stabilized vehicle that is on its side.

➤ State how you would free patients trapped in a vehicle.

If your training agency provides old vehicles for practicing extrication skills, your instructor will teach you how to use simple tools to gain access to the patient. If so, you should be able to:

➤ Demonstrate the steps of evaluating and making the scene safe.

➤ Demonstrate how to stabilize an upright vehicle.

➤ Demonstrate how to stabilize an overturned vehicle.

➤ Demonstrate how to gain access to patients in vehicles, using simple tools.

Many Emergency Medical Responders are firefighters who often discover, report, or arrive first at structure fires. Firefighters wearing appropriate protective gear may be assigned to find victims in the building and to care for patients brought from a building. You should be able to:

➤ Describe the basic ways to gain access to patients found in a variety of structures.

➤ Identify those hazards that are unique to a fire scene.

➤ State what you should do if electrical or gas hazards exist at the scene.

Hazardous materials training is a separate and special program. Many jurisdictions require all emergency services personnel to complete the awareness level of hazardous materials training before they respond on any emergency call. For any emergency incident involving possible hazardous materials, you should be able to:

➤ State how to recognize a possible hazardous materials incident.

➤ Describe Emergency Medical Responder duties at hazardous materials incidents.

➤ List the types of information that must be gathered from and reported on a hazardous materials scene.

"Okay, people, we're rolling!" Robert Ellis, safety supervisor for Legend Studios, shouted into the bullhorn. "Fire in the hole!"

The small army of technicians and pyrotechnicians all donned safety goggles and squinted against the anticipated propane explosion. It was a cool, dark night and once the flood lights were doused, shrouding the five-story tall, fabric blue screen in total darkness, the only light still visible on the film set was the bobbing tip of somebody's cigarette.

After a full minute of dark silence, somebody swore loudly and yelled for the lights. The generators coughed and sputtered to life, and as the flood lights warmed, they grew steadily brighter until the entire set was illuminated in harsh, white light.

"What's the problem, Reed?" Robert walked over to the pyrotechnician who was hovering above the control box.

"I don't know," the man wearing a baseball cap pulled low over his receding hairline said. "It should have gone." He was interrupted by a deafening rushing sound, like a tornado passing directly overhead, and jets of flame erupted like large, boiling clouds from the pressure valve at the far end of the pipe system.

The explosion immediately superheated the night air and sent crew members scattering in all directions as the monstrous blue screen caught fire. The flames raced up the fabric, sending burning bits fluttering down behind them.

"Shut it off!" Robert shouted as he tried to avoid the flames that were floating down from the sky like glowing snowflakes. "Everybody run!"

The lead pyrotechnician succeeded in shutting the main propane valve, but it was too late and the blue screen was fully engulfed and raining fire down onto a bank of large propane tanks on a nearby concrete pad. Robert dialed 9-1-1 on his cell phone as he and the crowd of technicians ran east along the main studio access road.

7–1.6 Describe what the Emergency Medical Responder should do if there is reason to believe that there is a hazard at the scene.

standard operating procedures (SOPs) ■ written directions that define how one should act given specific situations.

Safety

Your first consideration at any emergency scene is your own safety. To ensure it, you must learn to follow **standard operating procedures (SOPs)**, limit your actions to your training level, and use the proper equipment and the required number of trained persons for any task (Figure 15.1).

There are always risks, but EMS personnel must minimize them and learn which ones can be controlled before acting. For example, you have no control over the chance that a drunk driver could crash into you as you provide care at the scene of a traffic collision. But by using proper warning devices to divert traffic (for example, flares) and by positioning your own vehicle or response unit a proper distance from the scene, you can minimize your risks of being injured by passing cars (Figure 15.2). At any emergency scene, you must always:

REMEMBER

When you are restricted to following SOPs, you must follow a procedure that may not fit every variable encountered on an incident. However, a guideline provides some leeway for decision making for trained and experienced EMS providers.

- Before you approach the patient, make certain that you will be in no danger while you work on the patient. If there is a hazard, make sure you can control it before you approach. If you cannot control a hazard, wait for assistance.
- Use the protective gear appropriate for the situation and for which you are certified or qualified to wear. Examples include firefighting turn-out gear, hazmat suit, reflective vest, eye protection, and gloves.
- Legally and ethically, you are limited by your level of training. If you attempt to act beyond your level of training, you may risk injury to yourself, cause harm to the patient, or add to the extent of the incident.
- When you call dispatch, describe the incident so that the needed personnel and equipment may respond as soon as possible.

Preparing for the Call

Emergency Medical Responder responsibilities at motor-vehicle collisions will vary, depending on the type of agency, jurisdiction requirements, regulations, and standard operating procedures (SOPs). You must be prepared to perform your duties on any emergency call (Figure 15.3).

All EMS responses progress through several phases. These phases may differ slightly, depending on the level of care you provide. For Emergency Medical Responders, the phases of an emergency call include the following.

PHASE 1: PREPARATION

Being prepared means having the proper training, tools, equipment, and personnel.

- *Medical supplies.* Make sure your unit is stocked with medical supplies such as BSI equipment, airways, suctioning equipment, artificial ventilation devices (pocket face masks, bag-valve masks), and basic wound-care supplies (dressings, bandages).
- *Nonmedical supplies.* Check for other necessary items such as personal safety equipment (helmets), flares, flashlights, fire extinguisher, blanket, simple tools (screwdrivers, hammer, spring-loaded punch), and area maps.
- *Equipment.* Be sure to check that all special equipment is on your unit and operating properly, that any malfunctioning equipment is

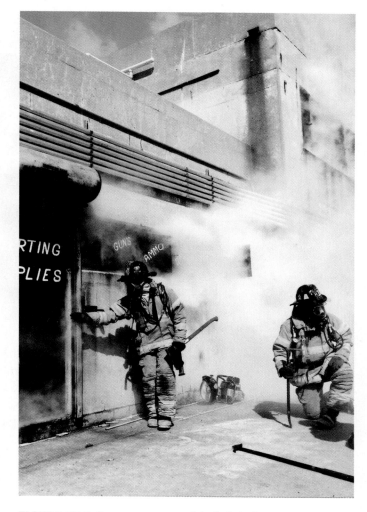

FIGURE 15.1 Ensure your own safety first at all emergency scenes. (*© Craig Jackson/In the Dark Photography*)

7–1.1 Discuss the medical and nonmedical equipment needed to respond to a call.

7–1.2 List the phases of an out-of-hospital call.

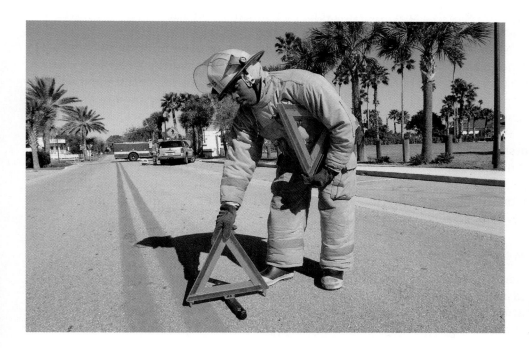

FIGURE 15.2 Make the scene safe before approaching.

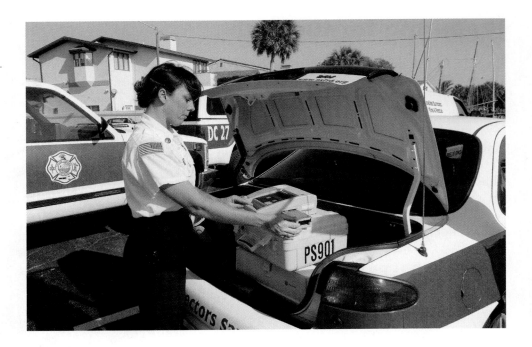

FIGURE 15.3 Always be prepared to perform your duties on any incident.

replaced or repaired, and that all supplies are restocked. Check the engine compartment and fluid levels of your vehicle (fuel, oil, transmission, windshield washer). It is also important to check the emergency equipment, including flashing lights, sirens, and radios, at the beginning of every shift or on a daily basis.

- *Personnel.* Ensure that the appropriate number of personnel are on duty and will be able to respond with you or can be dispatched to assist you, if necessary.

PHASE 2: DISPATCH

Be familiar with your dispatch or communications system and what procedures you follow when dispatched. Note any information the dispatcher gives you about the call.

Most dispatch systems have a central dispatch or communications center with 24-hour access. Dispatch centers are staffed with personnel especially trained to dispatch the most appropriate units. Many dispatch centers are training their personnel in Emergency Medical Dispatch programs so they may provide pre-arrival instructions to the caller over the telephone while EMS personnel are responding.

All dispatchers are trained to gather as much information from the caller as possible and relay that information to responding units. The nature of the call, the location of the incident and/or the patient, the number of patients, and the severity of illness or injury, as well as any other special problems that responders might encounter at the scene, are all important pieces of information and must be relayed to responding personnel.

PHASE 3: EN ROUTE TO THE SCENE

Emergency Medical Responder duties continue while en route to an emergency and include more than finding the location on the map. You must fasten your seat belt and be sure you have personal protective equipment ready. Then contact dispatch and let them know you are en route. Be sure you have the essential information on the call, such as location, potential hazards, and number of patients. Do not hesitate to check back with the dispatcher if you need more information.

PHASE 4: ARRIVAL AT THE SCENE

When arriving at the scene, be extra alert and approach cautiously. Look for hazards. Position your response unit where you have access to it but where it will not interfere with traffic flow. Activate emergency lights or flashers. Remember to always keep your eye on traffic. Do not become a victim yourself.

Notify the dispatcher of your arrival. Because dispatchers can only communicate what they are given from the reporting party, you may have to provide additional information once you arrive on scene, such as:

- Actual location of the incident if it is different from what was given on dispatch.
- Type of incident and the need for additional resources (engine company, Air Medical helicopter, rescue squad).
- Number of victims or an estimate if there are many.

Size up the scene to ensure that it is safe and contains no hazards. Put on your personal protective equipment, including reflective vests. If you wear dark clothing, other drivers may not see you. As you approach, look for the mechanism of injury in trauma scenes or determine if it is a medical emergency.

Always stabilize vehicles before entering them or attempting to extricate any patients. Determine if it is a multiple-casualty incident and, if so, determine the approximate number of patients. Evaluate patients quickly to determine if they are high or low priority. Do you need to move patients immediately? Can it be done safely? Will you need more assistance? Let the dispatcher know what additional resources you are going to need as soon as possible.

Many EMS agencies are now using cellular phones as a backup to radio communications.

PHASE 5: TRANSFERRING PATIENTS

Emergency Medical Responders will help lift, carry, and load patients on appropriate devices and assist in preparing the patient for transport. While doing so, be sure to use appropriate lifting and moving procedures.

PHASE 6: AFTER THE EMERGENCY

The phases of emergency calls are cyclic. Once a call is finished, you will prepare for the next call, including cleaning and disinfecting equipment, restocking supplies, and refueling the unit. You will also complete paperwork and file reports, participate in debriefing, and, finally, notify the dispatcher that you are back in service.

Motor-Vehicle Collisions

Once you ensure your own safety, your main duty at the scene of an emergency is to provide patient care. At the scene of a motor-vehicle collision, however, you may have other duties to perform before you can reach the patients to provide this care. Your responsibilities at the scene may include:

7-1.3 Discuss the role of the Emergency Medical Responder in extrication.

- Making the scene safe, ensuring no one else is hurt as they approach.
- Evaluating the situation and calling the dispatcher for appropriate help.

- Gaining access to patients.
- Freeing trapped patients.
- Evaluating patients and providing emergency care.
- Moving patients who are in danger from fire, explosion, and other hazards.
- Determining which patients may be moved so that you can reach and provide care for another more critically injured patient.

Many Emergency Medical Responders are injured each year as they attempt to help at vehicle collisions. The Emergency Medical Responders are struck by another vehicle when they do not take initial steps to make the scene safe. Your first step is to secure an area around the scene so you can work safely.

Is It Safe ?

As you approach the scene of a vehicle collision, look carefully for signs of fluid spilling from any of the vehicles. Avoid driving through or parking over these spills or in the path of a fluid as it spreads. Consider all fluids as potentially flammable. Even if you think it might only be radiator coolant, it could still be mixed with fuel and ignite at any time. Be very aware of changing conditions. ■

FIRST ➤ Law enforcement officers and firefighters must follow their department's SOPs on vehicle collisions. However, if you are an Emergency Medical Responder without a special course in collision-scene procedures, use the items listed here as guidelines or follow your local protocols. Because each collision scene is unique, you will need to proceed with caution, carefully observe the scene, and decide what actions to take to control it.

1. Pull your vehicle completely off the road at least 50 feet from the scene. Turn on your vehicle's emergency flashers. You may want to use your headlights to light up the scene. If so, be sure to angle your vehicle so that it does not blind oncoming drivers.

2. Make certain that you have parked in a safe location. Look for fuel spills and fire. If you are downhill from the scene, fuel may run in your direction. Check the wind direction. Will the wind carry smoke or fire to where you have parked?

3. If your jurisdiction or agency has SOPs for positioning your unit and using warning lights, follow those guidelines. If you turn off the unit, you cannot leave your warning lights on.

4. Set out emergency warning devices, such as flashing lights or flares, to warn others (Figure 15.4). On high-speed roads, place one of these devices at least 250 feet from the scene. On low-speed roads, set one of these devices at least 100 feet from the scene. Add at least 25 feet to these measurements if the scene is on a curved road.

5. As you approach, check the scene again for safety. Is there fire, leaking fuel or gases, unstable vehicles, or downed electrical wires? If any of these conditions are present, make certain someone phones or radios for help. If a power line is down, get the nearest pole number so you may request that power be turned off. You may need fire services and a rescue squad at the scene. Some jurisdictions automatically dispatch these units for motor-vehicle collisions.

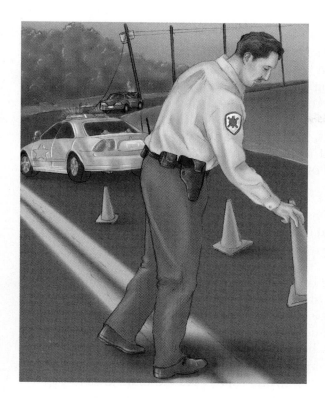

FIGURE 15.4 Warning devices.

FLARES

To ignite a flare, remove the small outer cap to expose the striker surface. Then remove the large plastic cap and hold it against the fuse on the end of the flare. Be sure to keep both caps because they will be used to keep the flare from rolling off the roadway once placed in position. Swipe the flare firmly against the striker in a downward motion to ignite it. This may take several attempts, much like striking a match. Once the flare has ignited, replace both plastic caps on the back end of the flare and place it on the road surface.

IMPORTANT: When carrying a lighted flare, always keep it pointing toward the ground and to one side to avoid being hit by burning sulfur. Watch out for spilled or leaking fuel, dry grass, and debris on the road surface. Remember that leaking fuel will flow downhill.

EMERGENCY FLASHERS

Use your vehicle's emergency flashers and set up emergency warning devices approved for highway use. For low visibility and night use, you must use flashing lights or flares.

CONES AND REFLECTORS

Set up cones or reflectors in a graduated line from the shoulder to the corner of your vehicle.

6. As you approach, observe the scene for clues. How many potential patients can you see? Could someone have been thrown from a vehicle? Could someone have walked away from the scene? Do you see signs indicating that children were in the vehicle (bottles, toys, school books, car seats)? Are there signs that a pedestrian or bike rider was involved? Have someone alert the dispatcher and report the number of possible patients.

7. If the scene is safe, stabilize the vehicle by chocking the wheels, gain access to the patients, perform your assessments, and begin care on those who appear to be most critical. ▪

Do not approach or attempt to gain access to patients if the scene is too dangerous. If you cannot control traffic, if electric lines are down, if there is fire at the scene, or if there are fuel or hazardous material spills, you are in danger. Call the dispatcher for additional resources for any of these conditions. If you are not trained to deal with fires, electricity, or hazardous materials, protect yourself and stay uphill and upwind from any spills.

FIRST ➤ An Emergency Medical Responder's first priority is personal safety. Your primary duty is to provide patient care at a safe scene. Do only what you have been trained to do. ▪

Is It Safe ?

Be very careful working in any vehicle with an undeployed airbag. These devices can deploy at any moment and could cause serious injury to rescue personnel. Make certain that all undeployed airbags have been identified and rendered safe by specially trained personnel. ▪

UPRIGHT VEHICLE

In most traffic collisions, the vehicles involved remain upright and are generally safer to approach than overturned vehicles. Even though the vehicles appear to be stable, with little chance of rolling or sliding away from the at-rest position, it is still necessary to take the safety precaution of stabilizing the vehicle.

Always evaluate vehicle stability when you assess the scene. As you look for traffic hazards, electrical hazards, spilled fuel, and fire, also see if there is any chance that the vehicle may roll away or flip over. Make sure vehicles are in "park" and the ignition is turned off, if you have immediate access. You may find the following situations:

- *Hills or slight inclines.* The vehicle may have come to rest on a surface that slants enough to allow forward or backward roll. To keep the vehicle from rolling, place wheel chocks, spare tires, logs, rocks, or similar objects under one or more wheels (Figure 15.5).
- *Slippery surfaces.* Ice, snow, or oil can produce a slippery road surface. If available, sprinkle dirt, sand, ashes, or kitty litter, or place newspapers around the wheels and chock the wheels to reduce the chances of slipping.
- *Tilted vehicle.* Even upright vehicles may be tilted to one side by their position or by the terrain. Do not work beneath a tilted vehicle or on the downhill side of one. Chocking the wheels may prevent the vehicle from tilting over, but tying the vehicle in place is safer. If strong rope is available, tie lines to the frame of the car (not the bumper) in front and back or to both sides. Then secure the lines to large trees or poles, guardrails, or heavier stable vehicles while waiting for fire services to arrive.
- *Stacked vehicles.* Part of one vehicle may be resting on top of another vehicle. There are several ways to stabilize them: chock the wheels of both vehicles; insert tires, lumber, blocks, or similar sturdy items between the road surface and the vehicles; use line or rope to tie and secure both vehicles.

FIRST ➤ Never try to enter or work around a vehicle until you are certain that it is stable.

FIGURE 15.5 A commercial chock device used to stabilize a vehicle prior to entry.

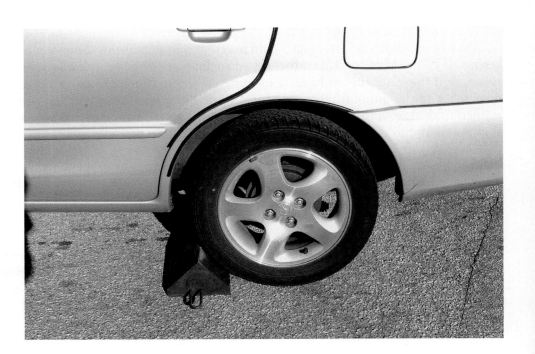

Once you stabilize the vehicle, there are two access methods to use for reaching a patient: **simple access** and **complex access**. Simple access does not require equipment; complex access requires tools and special equipment, which also calls for additional training. In most cases, you will approach an upright, stable vehicle and reach the patient by simple access. If the doors and windows are closed, there are four ways to gain access to the patients:

- *Open the doors.* Many people drive without locking the doors. However, many new models automatically lock once they reach a speed of five miles per hour. Some lock when the driver puts the transmission in "drive." Check all the doors, including side and rear doors on vans and hatchbacks, before trying another entry method. If all doors are locked, one of the occupants may be able to unlock a door. Try before you pry.

- *Enter through a window.* If doors are locked or jammed, the patient may be able to roll down a window. If not, you will have to break a window. When you begin using tools to access patients, the process becomes more complex.

- *Pry open the doors.* This method is very time consuming and not very practical given the technology available today. Access through windows is usually more practical.

- *Cut through the metal.* The only other access when entry through doors and windows is not possible is cutting through vehicle roofs, trunks, and doors. This entry method takes special tools that Emergency Medical Responders do not usually carry unless they are also members of fire services. If you cannot gain access through a door or window, it may be possible to cut around the lock of a door using a sharp tool (chisel or strong screwdriver) and a hammer. ■

Your instructor will teach you how to use these entry methods if they are Emergency Medical Responder skills in your jurisdiction.

Keep in mind that speed is sometimes crucial when you need to reach patients in a vehicle. Precious time is lost if you have to return to your vehicle to retrieve tools. Take all tools with you as you approach a vehicle. Many simple tools will help you gain access to a vehicle, including slotted and Phillips screwdrivers, chisels, hammers, pliers, wire, washers, and pry bars. Some Emergency Medical Responder tool kits include commercial "Slim Jims" for unlocking doors and spring-loaded center punches for breaking glass. Access with tools and special equipment is considered complex because it takes time, planning, and sometimes special training; and it requires taking additional safety precautions to protect the patient.

Unlocking Vehicle Doors

Special commercial tools for unlocking doors may be part of your Emergency Medical Responder kit. You might be able to unlock doors of older vehicles by slipping a commercial tool known as a "Slim Jim" between the window and the door. You also might be able to pry open the window with a wood wedge or pry bar and slip a wire coat hanger inside the window (Scan 15–1). Opening newer locks using these methods might be impossible, depending on the manufacturer. Some cars have a dead-bolt system that cannot be unlocked with special tools. These types of locks are designed to unlock on impact and allow rescuers to gain access. If you cannot unlock or open a door, gain access through a window.

Before you attempt to unlock a door, confirm that all doors are indeed locked and windows are up, preventing access any other way, or have an occupant on the inside unlock it. Check the doors for damage. A severely damaged door may not open easily even if you do unlock it. If all doors are damaged, be prepared to break glass and gain access through the window. Look in the windows to see if the car has buttons in the arm rest. It will not be easy to unlock doors with this type

7–1.4 List various methods of gaining access to the patient.

7–1.5 Distinguish between simple and complex access.

simple access ■ access gained to a vehicle or building without the use of equipment.

complex access ■ access gained to a vehicle or building with the use of specialized equipment.

REMEMBER

Try before you pry.

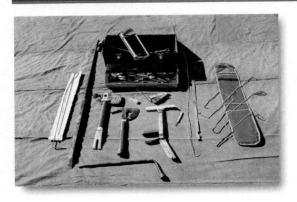

■ Various tools can be used to help unlock vehicle doors in older vehicles (check model years):

- ■ Wire hook.
- ■ Straight wire.
- ■ Slim Jim (or similar device).
- ■ Screwdriver.
- ■ Flat pry bar.

An oil dipstick or a keyhole saw may be used to help force up a locking button.

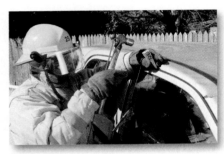

1 ■ a. **For framed windows,** pry the frame away from the vehicle body with a wood wedge and insert a wire hook.

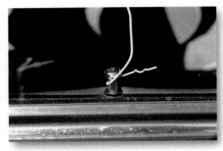

2 ■ **For flat-top locks,** use a hooked wire. Snag the locking button and pull upward.

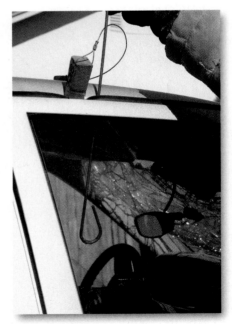

1 ■ b. Or use a wooden wedge to pry away the frame before inserting the wire hook.

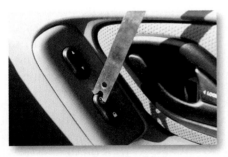

3 ■ **For rocker or push-button locks** on the door panel or on the arm rest, use a straight wire and press the lock open.

of locking device. Vehicles with electric locks and windows cannot be unlocked if the battery is disabled.

Gaining Access Through Vehicle Windows

To gain rapid access to patients who are unresponsive or unstable when the doors are locked, use a spring-loaded center punch on the rear or side windows. A heavy hammer may work, but it requires that you aim carefully and strike forcefully (possibly several times), which may shatter and spray glass. Always wear protective equipment, especially goggles and gloves, when breaking glass.

At the scene of a collision, most people consider breaking the windshield of a vehicle first if they cannot gain access through the doors. However, this is the wrong approach. Windshields are made of laminated safety glass, which has great strength. Even when shattered, the glass will still cling to an inner plastic layer. All cars have laminated safety glass windshields. Many foreign cars have this type of glass in all windows of a vehicle. If it is necessary to remove windshields, Emergency Medical Responders should leave that task to personnel trained in this rescue technique.

Rear and side windows are usually made of tempered glass. When this glass is broken, there is no plastic layer to hold the pieces. Tempered glass will not shatter into sharp pieces or shards. Instead, this glass will shatter into small rounded pieces and will often drop straight down into the vehicle, if you break it in a corner with a spring-loaded center punch. The small glass pieces can cut, but the cuts are usually minor.

If you must use a hammer, do not bash the center of the glass with it, or you will send pieces throughout the entire passenger compartment.

FIRST ➤ When gaining access through a vehicle window, you should (Figure 15.6 and Figure 15.7):

1. Make certain the vehicle is stable. If possible, have the driver turn off the ignition.
2. Confirm that all doors and windows are locked and secure.
3. Protect yourself by wearing gloves and eye protection.
4. If possible, select a window that is away from the patient. Place one gloved hand flat against the window, resting the heel of your hand on the corner of the door. Place the spring-loaded center punch between two fingers in one of the lower corners of the window, as close to the

REMEMBER

Wear gloves and protection for your eyes.

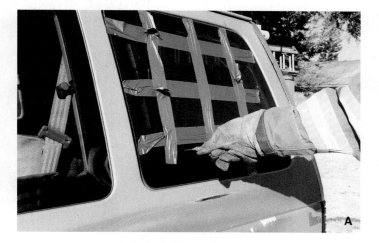

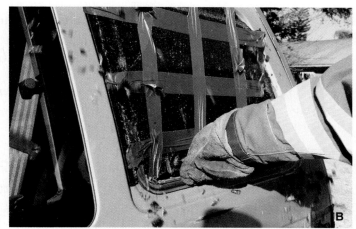

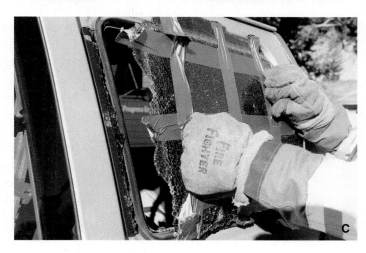

FIGURE 15.6 To break a window, **A.** place duct tape across the window to help keep the window intact after breaking with a center punch. **B.** Use a spring-loaded center punch in one of the corners to break the glass prior to removal. **C.** Once the glass has been broken, it can be pulled from the frame and removed.

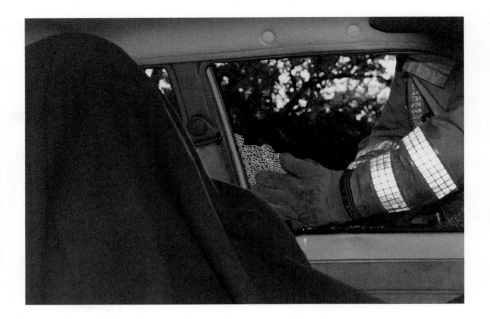

door as possible. Press the center punch with your other hand. When the window breaks, the hand pressing the center punch will not go through the window.

5. After breaking the window, reach in and try to open the door. You may only have to unlock the door to open it. Often, jammed doors that will not open from the outside will open from the inside.

6. Turn off the vehicle ignition, place the transmission in "park," and set the parking brake. ▪

OVERTURNED VEHICLE

Do not try to right an overturned vehicle. Even if you have enough help to turn the vehicle upright, moving it can cause further injury to the occupants. Stabilize the overturned vehicle while waiting for fire service units and before you try to reach the occupants. Always look for fuel spills, battery acid, and other chemical hazards around an overturned vehicle.

VEHICLE ON ITS SIDE

FIRST ➤ If you find a vehicle on its side and have some simple equipment, take the following precautions to stabilize it. You should (Figure 15.8):

1. Stabilize the vehicle with items such as tires, blocks, lumber, wheel chocks, cribbing, rocks, or similar available materials. Place these items between the road surface and the roofline. Also place stabilizing items between the road surface and the lower wheels if the wheels are not resting on the road surface.

2. If the vehicle is still unstable, use strong rope or line to tie the vehicle to secure objects.

3. Attempt to gain access to occupants of the vehicle. Entry through a door is dangerous because the door may be seven feet or more off the ground and your weight will move the vehicle as you climb on it. It will also be difficult to open the door with the vehicle on its side. Your first and more sensible entry point

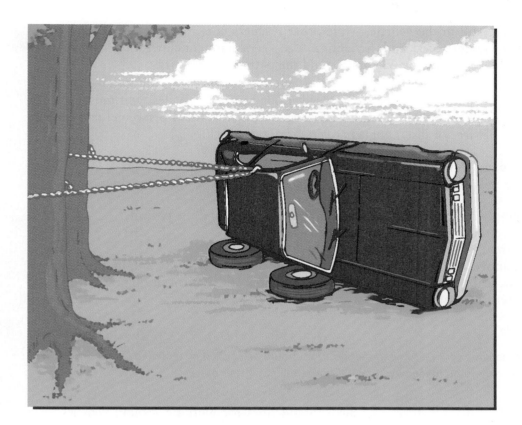

FIGURE 15.8 Stabilize the vehicle before trying to gain access to the patients. This requires special training. Do only what you have been trained to do.

will be through a window. The rear window is the best approach to take. Never attempt access to a damaged interior through broken glass without adequate protective clothing and equipment.

4. If you open a door, tie it securely open. Do not use a prop. Props can slip or be knocked away, causing the door to slam on you or the occupants. ∎

PATIENTS PINNED BENEATH VEHICLES

When a patient is pinned beneath a vehicle, call for a rescue squad immediately. Never place yourself in danger by reaching or crawling into the area where the patient is pinned. If it appears that the scene is too dangerous, Emergency Medical Responders can perform certain procedures to move the vehicle and free the patient, but this is often risky. Follow your department's SOPs in these situations.

A jack or pry bar and blocks can be used to raise a vehicle, which will enable rescuers to move the patient from beneath the vehicle. When lifting one side of the vehicle off the patient, be sure you are not causing the other side of the vehicle to press on another part of the patient, for example, his legs. With enough help, you may be able to lift the vehicle off the patient. In any attempt to raise a vehicle off a pinned patient, others must shore up the vehicle as you raise it so that it will not slip or fall back onto the rescuers or the patient. Use blocks, tires, lumber, or similar sturdy items at the scene. Do not attempt to enter the space to remove the victim until the entire vehicle is stable.

PATIENTS TRAPPED IN WRECKAGE

You may find patients with their arms, legs, or heads protruding through the window. Before trying to free them, you should use blankets to shield any patients who are still in the vehicle, while other rescuers continue to open the vehicle to provide better access and extrication. Use pliers, hammer claws, or a knife to carefully break or fold away glass around the patient's extremity.

FIRST ➤ When patients are trapped inside crushed vehicles, you must wait for special power tools and skilled rescue personnel. Trained personnel can quickly and easily free or disentangle patients from the wreck.

Emergency Medical Responders working on vehicles with occupants pinned inside will often be able to free some patients by way of the following:

- Simply remove wreckage from on top of and around the patient.
- Carefully move a seat forward or backward.
- Carefully lift out a back seat.
- Remove a patient's shoe to free a foot, or cut away clothing caught on wreckage.
- Cut seat belts, but be sure to properly support the patient during the cutting and after the tension has been released.

NOTE

In general, cervical spine immobilization should be applied by qualified personnel prior to performing maneuvers that will cause the patient to move.

- Follow manufacturer and agency guidelines for working around vehicles with deployed and undeployed airbags. Check the steering wheel beneath the deployed airbag for damage indicating that the patient might have struck it. Airbags may also activate in the front seat passenger area, and some more recent models have side air curtains. ◾

Is It Safe ?

Most late model cars and trucks have airbags in the steering column as well as several other locations within the passenger compartment. It is possible for these airbags to deploy after a collision has occurred. Many EMS and fire personnel have been injured when an airbag deployed while they were attempting to care for a patient. Consider this risk before deciding to enter a vehicle involved in a collision. ◾

In any attempt to free patients from vehicles, you must consider the immediate need for quick access. If immediate access and patient movement is necessary to save a life, make every attempt to reach the patient. If the patient's life is not at risk but immediate movement will cause further injury, then leave the patient in place until more highly trained personnel respond to the scene.

During the wait, talk to the patient to offer reassurance and explain why you are taking precautions. While you are talking to the patient, begin your initial patient assessment steps and provide oxygen while another Emergency Medical Responder stabilizes the head. If you must move the patient before more advanced care personnel arrive, make every attempt to maintain stabilization of the patient's spine during the move. Once EMTs and other EMS personnel arrive, report your patient assessment findings and provide them with any assistance they need, such as taking vital signs, controlling bleeding, gathering special equipment, or loading and lifting the patient.

Building Access

Gaining access to a patient in a locked building may require special skills and tools outside the range of Emergency Medical Responder duties. There are many types of gates, doors, windows, and locks that restrict access to buildings. In addition to access problems, older buildings may have many hidden and unsuspected dangers; security devices will present special barriers, and guard dogs will limit or halt your actions until they are contained.

Emergency Medical Responders are not expected to know how to open or destroy locks or have all the tools needed for the variety of windows, doors, and gates found in buildings. Unless you are trained in fire and rescue operations, you are not expected to know how to enter and make your way safely around an empty or abandoned building.

FIRST ➤ Follow the guidelines below for gaining access to patients inside any type of building (homes, offices, stores, schools). You will be expected to:

- Request additional resources, if necessary.
- Try opening and entering through open doors or windows first.
- Look for a key under mats or in mailboxes.
- Ask bystanders and neighbors if they have a key.
- Break glass to unlock doors or windows.

Follow your department's SOPs regarding notification of local law enforcement prior to and following any forcible entry. ◾

If you know or see that someone inside needs immediate care, do not try to gain access before calling for help. Your efforts to gain entry may fail, and you will need help as soon as possible. Call the dispatcher and request additional resources immediately.

While waiting for help, try different entry points. Try to open a door. If the door is locked, try opening a few low windows on your way to finding a second door. If the second door is locked, break the glass in a window or a door and enter as quickly but as safely as possible. Do not attempt to break through doors or windows made of large sheets of tempered glass. Some newer buildings and homes may have been constructed with Lexan resin (a type of plastic) or a special type of laminated glass that is designed to resist the forces of hurricanes and the debris carried by high winds. These materials are extremely difficult to break and can bounce a hammer back into your face. Do not try climbing up walls or posts to reach a high window. Do not try to gain access to a window by walking across roofs. Call and wait for special rescue personnel who will have the appropriate equipment.

FIRST ➤ When attempting to break a glass window, you should:

1. Make certain that the patient is not lying near the other side of the glass.

2. Use a hammer or similar blunt object to strike the glass near one of its edges (Figure 15.9). A nightstick or an aluminum flashlight will break most window glass. If you do not have tools, use a rock or a similar solid object to strike the glass.

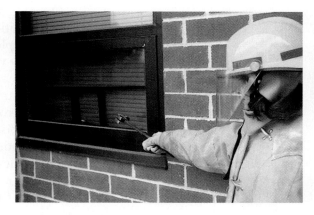

FIGURE 15.9 When doors and windows are locked, break glass to gain access to the locks.

3. Carefully clear all glass from the frame and reach in to unlock the door or window.

4. Make certain that you are stepping onto a safe floor. Be sure that you do not have an unusual drop when entering. Take a moment to visually inspect the floor for damage or poke the floor for signs of weakness. ▪

Hazards

FIRE

Television and movies have led people to believe that they should enter burning buildings or run up to burning vehicles in order to save victims. This is a dangerous tactic. Those in the fire service are highly trained to do their jobs. They are given special equipment and use special strategies to fight fires, which minimizes the risks to their safety. Firefighting requires special training, protective clothing, the right equipment, and usually more than one firefighter.

If you are a member of the fire service, follow SOPs for rescuing victims from vehicle and structure fires. If you are in law enforcement and have special training in rescuing victims from vehicle and structure fires, do only what you have been trained to do. If you are an Emergency Medical Responder without firefighting training, do not risk your life to approach a fire and provide care.

Motor-vehicle collisions do not usually produce fire, and most emergency calls to buildings do not involve fire. However, these events do occur, and you must be prepared to protect yourself. Your own safety is the first priority. Emergency Medical Responders with no training or little experience at fighting fires must follow the rules listed below to ensure their safety:

▪ Never approach a vehicle that is in flames. Using blankets, sand, or a fire extinguisher is appropriate if you know how to evaluate the fire and the danger of explosion and if you have protective clothing and know how to attack a fire. If you do not have the proper training to perform these tasks and do not have the necessary protection, stay clear. Make sure that the dispatcher knows there is a fire.

▪ Never attempt to enter a building that is obviously on fire or has smoke showing. Even a small fire can spread toxic fumes throughout the structure. If you enter, look and smell for signs of fire. Remember that fire could be hidden within the walls, floors, and ceilings.

▪ Never enter a smoky room or building or go through an area of dense smoke.

▪ Never attempt to enter a closed building or room giving off grayish-yellow smoke. Opening a door to this building or room will cause a back draft, which is a condition that immediately increases the intensity of the fire and can cause an explosion due to the sudden increase in oxygen supply.

▪ Do not work by yourself or enter a building unless others know that you are doing so. If you are injured or trapped, you are an unknown victim who may not be rescued until it is too late.

▪ Always feel the top of a door before opening it (Figure 15.10). If it is hot, do not open it. (Doorknobs and handles may also be hot.) If the door is cool, open it slowly and cautiously and avoid standing in its path as you open it.

▪ Never use the elevator if there is a possibility of a fire in a building. The elevator shaft can act as a flue and pull flames, hot toxic gases, and smoke into the shaft. Also, the fire can cause an electrical failure, which could trap you in the elevator. Some elevators have heat-activated call buttons. The elevator may take you to the fire floor, open, and expose you to lethal heat or toxic gases.

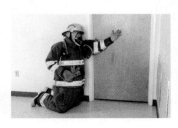

FIGURE 15.10 If a door is hot, do not open it.

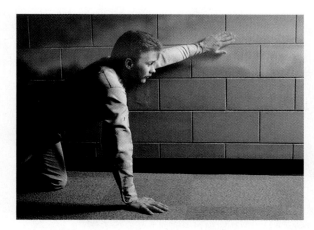

FIGURE 15.11 If trapped by fire or smoke, stay low and crawl to safety.

- If you find yourself in smoke, stay close to the floor and crawl to safety (Figure 15.11). If possible, cover your mouth and nose with a damp cloth.

NATURAL GAS

If you notice the odor of natural gas at any scene, move patients away from the area, keep bystanders away from the scene, and alert dispatch, so that other services can be activated, and request that gas in the area be shut off or diverted.

FIRST ➤ The smell of natural gas in a building is a signal for immediate action. Evacuate the building and call dispatch to report the odor of gas. If the gas is coming from a bottled source, do not try to turn off this source unless you have experience with this type of gas system. You can vent the area by opening windows and doors as you leave. Do not enter an area to rescue a patient. You must wear a self-contained breathing apparatus (SCBA) and be trained to handle such emergencies. Remember that there is always a danger of fire or explosion from simple acts such as turning on or off a light switch, or even from the spark of an appliance turning on. Play it safe and request the help you will need. ■

ELECTRICAL WIRES AND ABOVE-GROUND TRANSFORMERS

FIRST ➤ If electrical wires are down at a scene and block your pathway to a patient, or if they are lying across a car, do not attempt a rescue. As you approach a scene with downed wires, position your vehicle at least a pole away from the downed wires. If the power is restored, the wires can whip and arc in a circle as wide as their free length, which can be to the next pole (Figure 15.12).

Is It Safe?

When working in or around emergency scenes that involve utility poles and lines, be sure to evaluate the integrity of the power lines for several hundred yards in all directions. Damage to a single pole can affect the lines several poles away and create a hazard not immediately seen. ■

Never assume that power lines are dead or that a dead line will stay dead. Consider all downed lines as live. Do not be fooled by the fact that lights are out in the

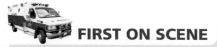

FIRST ON SCENE

As Robert was waiting for his cell phone call to be routed to the local dispatch center, he grabbed two of the fleeing technicians. "I need you guys to go down to the north entrance and make sure that nobody gets onto the studio property." The men immediately jogged off down the road toward the studio's only other gate.

"City fire dispatch, how can I help?" A man's voice came onto the line.

"Yes, my name is Robert, and I'm calling from Legend Studios over here on Cornell Boulevard. There's a fire on the exterior west side of our main sound stage building, and there are five or six large propane tanks in the danger zone."

After answering several questions from the dispatcher, Robert hung up and turned to the lead pyrotechnician who was staring back at the burning building expectantly. "Hey, Reed," Robert took a notepad and pen from his pocket. "Is there anything at all over in that area other than propane? Any chemicals or other flammable stuff? The fire department will need to know as soon as they get here."

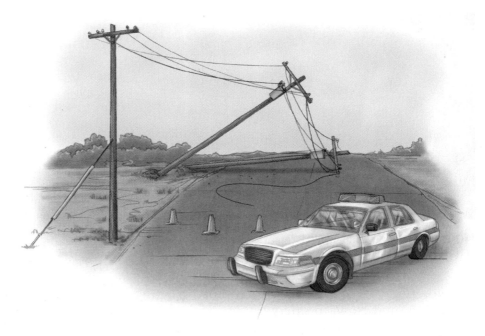

FIGURE 15.12 Place your vehicle at least a pole away from the pole with downed wires.

surrounding area. Even if lights are off all around you, the wire blocking your path may be live or could be re-energized as you pass by. Call or have someone alert dispatch to call the power company and request that the power be turned off. Even if you believe the power has been turned off, it is still best to wait for trained rescue personnel to arrive.

Many newer communities have underground electrical wires with access through an above-ground splice box or transformer. These above-ground transformer boxes are usually green, mounted on concrete pads, and often hidden by shrubbery (Figure 15.13). It may not be safe to approach a vehicle that has collided with an above-ground transformer box. Alert dispatch immediately and ask for special rescue assistance.

If patients are in a car that is touching a downed wire or is near one or has crashed into an above-ground transformer, tell them to stay in the vehicle and avoid touching any metal parts. If the patients have to leave the vehicle because of fire or other danger, you must tell them to jump clear of the car without touching

FIGURE 15.13 Pad-mounted transformer.

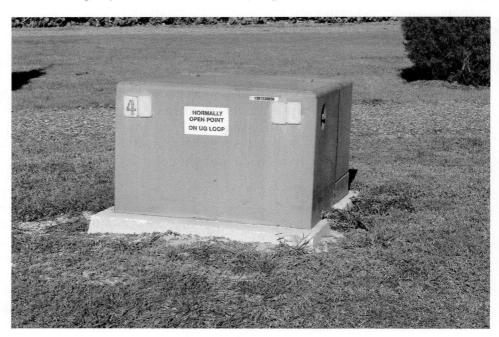

it and the ground at the same time. If they touch both simultaneously, they will complete a circuit and may be electrocuted. ∎

HAZARDOUS MATERIALS

There may be hazardous chemicals and other materials at the scene of an emergency. If so, do not attempt a rescue or perform patient care. No responders should enter a hazardous materials area unless they are trained to do so.

The possibility of hazardous materials incidents exists at every industrial site and every farm, truck, train, ship, barge, and airplane emergency incident. When responding to an emergency at these sites, assume that there are unsafe hazardous materials until their presence can be ruled out. When in doubt, stay clear and keep others clear of a hazardous material spill until trained rescuers arrive.

Emergency Medical Responder Responsibilities

Your role as an Emergency Medical Responder in a hazardous material situation is to first protect yourself and others around the scene. All emergency response vehicles should carry a current copy of the U.S. DOT's *Hazardous Materials: Emergency Response Guidebook*. At a hazardous material incident, refer to the guidebook for information on the chemical or substance and the perimeter of the safe area.

You may have to set up **safety zones**. Set up a hot (danger) zone, and keep all people out of this area. Set up a cold (safe) zone, which should be on the same level as and upwind from the hazardous material incident. Be aware that below-grade areas, such as ditches, trenches, and basements, will often have low-oxygen environments. Many gases are heavier than oxygen and will settle in low areas. The safe zone must not be downhill or downwind from the scene or on a high point that may be exposed to vapors if the wind shifts. Avoid low spots, streams, drainage fields, sewers, and sewer openings where spills may flow and fumes may collect.

Contact dispatch immediately with a description of the incident so you can get the appropriate help on the way. Advise the dispatcher of your position and stay on the line until you are told to disconnect. Ask and wait for information about the danger of the materials and for directions as to what you should do until the hazardous material (hazmat) teams arrive. Make certain you give your name and callback number.

If, for some reason, you cannot contact the dispatcher, call one of the following:

- CHEM-TEL on its 24-hour toll-free number at 800-255-3924 (for the United States and Canada).
- CHEMTREC on its 24-hour toll-free number at 800-262-8200 (for the United States and Canada).

When possible, provide the following information:

- Nature and location of the problem, an estimate of when the spill occurred, and if there are other possible hazardous materials near the scene.
- Type of material (gas, liquid, dry chemical, or a radioactive solid, liquid, or gas) and an estimate of how much material is at the scene.
- Name or identification number of the material. Look for labels or placards that are visible from your safe point. Use binoculars to help in reading this information.
- Name of the shipper or manufacturer. From a safe point or with binoculars, look for names on railroad cars, trucks, or containers. Ask bystanders, drivers, or railroad or factory personnel.
- Type of container. Is the material in a rail car or a truck? Is it in open storage, covered storage, or housed storage? Is the container still intact, or is liquid leaking, gas escaping, or a powder spilled? Report if the material is stable or if it is flaming, vaporizing, or blowing into the air.

7–1.7 State the role the Emergency Medical Responder should perform until appropriately trained personnel arrive at the scene of a hazardous materials situation.

REMEMBER

At hazardous material incidents, notify the dispatcher and stay a safe distance from the scene.

safety zone ∎ an area around the incident that is thought to be safe and free of hazards.

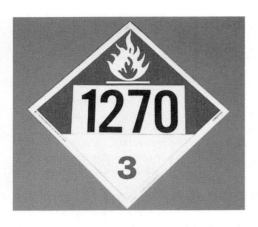

FIGURE 15.14 Hazardous materials placard.

- Weather conditions. Rain and wind are major concerns because they will carry hazardous materials to and contaminate other locations.
- Estimate of how many possible victims there are both in the hot zone (closest to the spill) and around the hot zone (in circles farther from the spill).
- Other significant problems at the scene such as fire, crowds, and traffic.

You may not be able to obtain and report most of this information, but any information you can provide is important to the responding units.

A major source of information at a hazardous material scene is the standard materials placard required by the U.S. DOT (Figure 15.14). This placard is on the vehicle, tank, or railroad car. The numbers, symbols, and colors provide information about the material in the container. Be aware that vehicles transporting hazardous materials insert placards into brackets. These placards may be made of metal or plastic and are hinged so they may be flipped to indicate a different cargo. During transportation or the incident, the placard may flip and show a different material. If possible, check with the driver, who must have a Material Safety Data Sheet (MSDS) on each hazardous material carried, to determine that the placard is correct. Some hazardous material transporters use placard stickers, which can be peeled off when the load is delivered. The driver applies another sticker for a different load of hazardous materials.

Refer to the U.S. DOT's *Hazardous Materials: Emergency Response Guidebook*. You may also want to become familiar with the National Fire Protection Association's (NFPA's) "Standard 473 Competencies for EMS Personnel Responding to Hazardous Materials Incidents."

Managing Patients

All contaminated victims must remain in the hot zone until the hazmat team decontaminates them and brings them to the cold zone for care by EMS personnel. If a victim of a hazardous material incident leaves the hot zone, you must first protect yourself from exposure. Victims may have chemicals on their bodies and clothing that could be harmful to you. *Do not* attempt to care for these patients unless you have the proper protection. Initial care includes flushing with water any contaminated areas, such as the skin, clothing, and eyes for at least 20 minutes, unless the material is dry lime. (Brush away excess dry lime first, then flush.) Remove contaminated clothing and jewelry as you flush the patient with water. Once the patient is flushed, use blankets to protect him from the environment and to maintain body temperature.

Victims may be able to wash themselves, or you may wash the victim. Use a small-diameter hose and make sure the victim stands in a large tub, small wading pool, or similar collection container so the contaminated rinse water does not run off into nearby sewers or streams. The hazmat team will manage all of the contaminated water by collecting it for transport and disposal. Perform wash operations uphill and upwind from the site, if possible. Do not place yourself at risk. If it is necessary to provide artificial ventilations, use an appropriate barrier device. Use resuscitation devices with one-way valves so contaminants do not blow back into your mouth or face.

The best thing for you to do at a hazardous material incident is to request the appropriate resources (Figure 15.15) and remain in the cold zone until the patient can be safely treated.

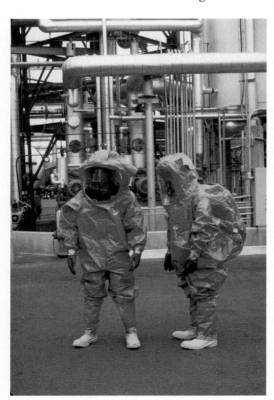

FIGURE 15.15 Special training and equipment, such as this fully encapsulated suit, are required at a hazardous materials incident.

Radiation Incidents

FIRST ➤ Stay clear of collisions involving radioactive materials. Your first duty is to protect yourself from exposure. Your next step should be to request the appropriate resources from a safe area away from the scene.

Look for radiation hazard labels (Figure 15.16). Stay upwind from any containers having these labels. Follow the same basic rules as you would when dealing with any hazardous material. The greater the distance you are from the source and the more objects that appropriately shield you from the source (concrete, thick steel, earth banks, heavy vehicles), the safer you will be.

When you are dispatched to hazardous material and radiation incidents, position your vehicle at a safe distance. Do not approach the scene unless you are specially trained to do so and are wearing the appropriate protective equipment (turnout coat, pants, boots, gloves, Nomex hood, helmet). Your protective equipment will provide some protection from most types of radiation, but be aware that it does not protect you enough to work close to a high-level radiation source for any period of time. ∎

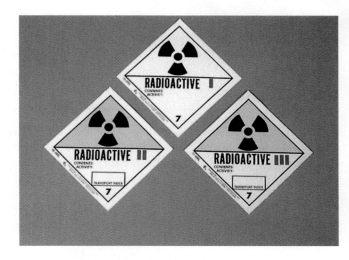

FIGURE 15.16 Radiation hazard labels.

Patients may be exposed to radiation, contaminated by it, or both. A patient who is exposed (not contaminated) was in the presence of radioactive material, but the material did not actually touch his clothing or body. Exposure to radiation may be harmful to the patient, but he is not radioactive and cannot pass on the exposure to you. However, the actual source of the radiation can be harmful to you. If the patient is still in the area of the radiation source, you must wait until the hazmat team brings him to the safe area.

Patients are contaminated when they come in contact with radiation sources, which may be gases, liquids, or particles. The radioactive materials may be on a patient's clothes, skin, or hair and will contaminate you when you touch the patient during assessment or care. The hazmat team will have to decontaminate the patient before you can provide care. Do not attempt to clean or care for radiation patients until they are in a safe area and are decontaminated.

FIRST ON SCENE WRAP-UP

Within minutes, the city streets leading to the studio had been closed by law enforcement, and fire services was cooling the propane tank battery with a jet of water from a distant truck. After about 15 minutes, the fabric of the blue screen had burned completely from the large, rectangular frame, and except for drifting grey ash and rapidly dissipating smoke, there was no sign of the once raging fire.

"Well, Robert," the Incident Commander put his hand on the safety officer's shoulder. "You couldn't have done anything better than you did: evacuating, blocking the two access points, and letting us know exactly what we were up against. You did a real fine job managing a pretty hazardous situation."

"Thank you," Robert smiled briefly. "Next time I'm only going to make one change."

"What's that?" the IC was pulling his orange vest off.

"Next time we do a shot like this," Robert said. "I'm going to have you guys already standing by.

Summary

As an Emergency Medical Responder, your first priority is your own safety, and your first duty is patient care. Before approaching a patient, make sure the scene is safe. Begin evaluating the scene as you approach. Evaluate for hazards, such as traffic, fire, downed electrical lines, hazardous materials, and unstable vehicles. Also size up the scene for ejected patients and for those who are standing or walking.

Always make certain that an upright vehicle will not roll. Stabilize vehicles that are on inclines or slippery surfaces. If one vehicle is stacked on another or on its side, stabilize both before trying to reach patients. Do not attempt to provide patient care in or around unstabilized vehicles or try to right overturned vehicles.

Gain access to patients in a stabilized vehicle by trying simple access first, such as doors and windows. If door access is not possible, attempt to gain access through a rear or side window. Break glass only after stabilizing the vehicle. Wear gloves and eye protection, or cover the glass and your face before breaking it. Break a window that is farthest from the patient. Wait for properly trained personnel if complex access is required.

Remove patients from vehicles only when there is danger or if life-saving care is required. Emergency Medical Responders may not have the skills or tools to remove patients trapped under a vehicle. If you must free a pinned patient, use a jack or pry bars to lift the vehicle and, while lifting, place blocks to stabilize and shore up the vehicle.

When caring for a patient with a body part protruding through a window, cover the body part first. Then break or fold the glass away before moving the patient.

Patients who are jammed or trapped in wreckage often can be freed by removing wreckage from around them, adjusting or removing seats, removing shoes, or cutting away clothing or seat belts.

The initial routes for gaining access to patients in buildings are doors and then windows. If you must break glass, protect yourself with gloves and goggles or cover the glass and your face. Be sure the patient is safe from flying glass and that you are stepping onto a safe floor.

At the scene of a fire, do not approach a burning vehicle or building unless you have the proper equipment and have been trained to assess the hazards and fight the fire. Do not enter a building that may be on fire. Do not try to go through smoke or potentially toxic gases. Do not attempt to enter a building or room that has any smoke coming from doors, windows, or vents. Do not open a door if it is hot. If caught in a burning building, stay low and crawl to safety.

Only trained personnel should shut off gas or electricity. If you smell natural gas, do not approach, but do alert dispatch. If there are electrical hazards, do not attempt a rescue. If electrical wires are touching a vehicle, have passengers stay in the vehicle and instruct them to avoid touching any metal objects inside the vehicle. If they must get out, warn them to jump clear without touching the vehicle and the ground at the same time.

If the scene contains hazardous or radioactive materials, stay in a safe area and request the appropriate resources. Provide the dispatcher with essential information.

Remember and Consider

➤ If you came upon a situation in which a person was trapped in a vehicle or a building, what would you do first? Remember that the first thing to consider is your own personal safety. Are you equipped to handle a rescue on your own? If not, what kind of help is available for different types of rescue situations?

Check with your department and find out what emergency support personnel and equipment are available to be sent to assist Emergency Medical Responders for emergencies where people are trapped.

➤ What tools do you carry in your vehicle or on your unit? Are they simple tools that typically do not need a special training class to show you how to use them? Or are the tools more mechanical with special attachments

that require training in order to use them properly? Regardless of the type of tool, will you know what to do with it when you need it to free a person from an entrapment situation?

Even simple tools are useless unless you know what to do with them or how to apply them effectively and safely in certain situations. If you have never actually removed a windshield with a putty knife, glazier's tool, or screwdriver, find out if your agency can get an old junked vehicle to practice on. Work under the guidance and instruction of someone who has had training or experience in auto extrication so that you can learn the appropriate techniques in a safe environment.

Investigate

Many response areas include a variety of building types in their residential, commercial, and industrial neighborhoods.

➤ Orient yourself and other department personnel to the different types of buildings in your response area by examining various neighborhoods and noting the type of construction, what the normal entry points are, and what other entry points there may be. Consider how you would enter different buildings if you could not gain access to trapped victims by the normal entry point.

Firefighters work with local businesses and industries to plan their fire attack and rescue operations in the event of a fire or other disaster. Emergency Medical Responders should do the same.

➤ Check with personnel at schools, stores, businesses, warehouses, and other commercial properties to find out the location of their first aid room; what medical personnel may be on duty and when; and what is the closest access point to work areas, first aid rooms, and offices or classrooms. Find out which areas will be difficult to access if there is an emergency and what hazards may hinder your care of any personnel or students.

Quick Quiz

1. The best way to approach a hazardous scene is to:
   a. do only what you feel comfortable doing.
   b. wear protective gear only if needed.
   c. do only what you have been trained to do.
   d. call dispatch if assistance is needed.

2. For Emergency Medical Responders, the phases of an emergency call in order are:
   a. preparation, dispatch, en route to scene, arrival at scene, transfer of patient, after the emergency.
   b. dispatch, en route to scene, arrival at scene, transfer of patient, after the emergency.
   c. preparation, dispatch, en route to scene, arrival at scene, transfer of patient, en route to hospital.
   d. dispatch, en route to scene, arrival at scene, preparation, transfer of patient, after the emergency.

3. When arriving at a motor-vehicle collision scene, the best place to park your vehicle is:
   a. off the road close to the scene in a safe location.
   b. as close to the scene as possible.
   c. off the road and far away from the scene.
   d. near other responding emergency vehicles.

4. When evaluating the stability of a vehicle before attempting to enter and care for patients, look for common hazards such as slippery surfaces, hills or slight inclines, and ___ vehicles.
   a. sturdy or stacked
   b. tilted or damaged
   c. parked or damaged
   d. tilted or missing

5. Which definition best defines both simple access and complex access?
   a. Simple access does not require equipment; complex access sometimes does.
   b. Simple and complex access both require special equipment.
   c. Simple access sometimes requires special equipment; complex access often does.
   d. Simple access does not require equipment; complex access requires specialized equipment.

6. There are four ways to access a patient in a vehicle with closed doors. They are enter through a window, pry open a door, cut through the metal, and:
   a. call an emergency locksmith.
   b. use the door handle to open a door.
   c. remove the engine and enter through the dash.
   d. wait until another responder opens a door.

7. The best way for the Emergency Medical Responder to manage a vehicle that is overturned is to:
   a. upright the vehicle, if enough help is available.
   b. upright the vehicle before gaining access to patients.
   c. never upright a vehicle because it can cause further injury to the patients inside.
   d. never upright a vehicle because it can cause further damage to the vehicle.

8. When a patient is pinned beneath a vehicle:
   a. attempt to upright the vehicle.
   b. call for a rescue squad immediately.
   c. stabilize the vehicle and then attempt to upright it.
   d. call for a rescue squad and then attempt to upright it.

9. When you must enter a locked building to gain access to a patient in need of immediate care:
   a. enter the building and then call for help.
   b. enter the building, stabilize the patient, and then call for help.
   c. attempt to enter the building, but if you fail, call for help.
   d. call for help before attempting entry into the building.

10. Specialized training is needed to manage fire, as well as:
   a. gas and bystanders.
   b. downed power lines and hazardous materials.
   c. smoke and blood.
   d. weather and hazardous materials.

CHAPTER 16

Multiple-Casualty Incidents, Triage, and the Incident Management System

This chapter discusses the role of the EMS system and that of the Emergency Medical Responder in emergencies involving multiple victims. Multiple-casualty incidents can be caused by anything, including vehicle collisions, hurricanes, and terrorist events such as those on September 11, 2001.

OBJECTIVES

This chapter is based on the objectives of the U.S. DOT's First Responder National Standard Curriculum. Note that cognitive objectives are listed below and beside corresponding text throughout the chapter. You will also notice as you read each objective that the term Emergency Medical Responder is used. This is simply a name change and reflects the new name for the First Responder.

By the end of this chapter, you should be able to (from cognitive or knowledge information):

7–1.8 Describe the criteria for a multiple-casualty situation. (pp. 554–555)

7–1.9 Discuss the role of the Emergency Medical Responder in the multiple-casualty situation. (p. 555)

7–1.10 Summarize the components of basic triage. (pp. 556–563)

By the end of this chapter, you should be able to show how to (through psychomotor skills):

7–1.12 Given a scenario of a mass-casualty incident, perform triage. (pp. 556–565)

ADDITIONAL LEARNING TASKS

Although relatively uncommon, multiple-casualty incidents, whether caused by nature or by humans, are a fact of life and will remain a part of our world. It is necessary for Emergency Medical Responders to understand their roles in such an incident and the overall structure of an incident management system. You should be able to:

➤ Define multiple-casualty incident (MCI).
➤ Describe the Emergency Medical Responders role at the scene of an MCI.
➤ Define incident management system (IMS).
➤ Describe the basic structure of an IMS.

When an emergency involves multiple patients and the available resources cannot care for all patients at one time, a method must be used to identify those patients most in need of immediate care. This process is called *triage*. After you learn about MCIs and how to triage patients, you should be able to:

➤ Define triage.
➤ Discuss the Emergency Medical Responder's role in the triage process.
➤ List the major steps of the triage process.
➤ Discuss how you might triage a simulated MCI.
➤ List the START triage criteria for assessing patients in an MCI.

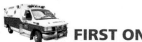

FIRST ON SCENE

Westside Mall security guard José Garza looked at his watch and then leaned on the polished wooden banister that borders the mezzanine level of the huge downtown shopping center. He watched as the crowds down on the main level bustled from store to store, swinging noisy plastic shopping bags and chatting on cell phones. It was like every other Saturday afternoon at Westside.

José stretched his back and walked toward the escalator that would take him down and out toward the mall's main entrance. If he didn't wander out and check the marble entry way to the mall every few hours, it would get too crowded with loitering kids and then he'd be dealing with everything from customer complaints to fights. It was definitely better to be proactive.

Just as he stepped off of the escalator, it happened. A thunderous explosion from the far end of the mall that sent screams and a boiling black cloud of smoke toward him. "Hey, Jerry!" José yelled into his shoulder mic. "We just had an explosion of some kind at the north end of the mall! Call 9-1-1 right away!"

"Already on it!" came the static-filled reply.

José tried to see through the wall of rancid smoke, which was rising slowly toward the high ceiling of the shopping center. The mall's automated evacuation message was echoing through the enormous building. He was surprised to see the smoke fade quickly, helped by the large vent fans located on the roof of the mall. As it did, José just stood and stared at the scene before him.

Shattered glass, colorful clothing, and people were scattered all over the tile floor at the end of the mall. Those who could move hurried past him to the clean and undamaged part of the mall. The rest, perhaps 15 or 20 people, just lay motionless on the floor, smoking, bleeding, and possibly dead.

José's stomach tightened as he realized that he was to be the first responder on this horrendous scene. He took a deep breath and moved toward the closest nonmoving person.

Multiple-Casualty Incidents

7–1.8 Describe the criteria for a multiple-casualty situation.

multiple-casualty incident (MCI)
■ any incident that results in enough patients to overwhelm immediately available resources. Also known as a *mass-casualty incident.*

If taken literally, the definition of a **multiple-casualty incident (MCI)** is any emergency with more than one victim (Figure 16.1). Although MCIs do indeed involve more than one victim, a more realistic definition is any emergency that involves multiple victims and overwhelms the first responding units. Most fire services, rescue squads, and ambulances are prepared and capable of managing a scene with more than one patient. However, can they manage a scene with three or four? How about five or six? What if the victims are all critical and need immediate transport?

In most cases, it is up to the first emergency personnel on the scene to make a judgment call and declare an MCI. If they feel that they can manage the number of patients with the resources immediately available, then an MCI may not be declared. If they cannot manage the number of patients, then an MCI is declared and an Incident Management System (IMS) is put into action.

The role of Emergency Medical Responders at an MCI will vary depending on several factors, such as when they arrive at the scene, the type of agency for whom they are working, and their specific level of training. Emergency Medical Responders who are first on scene may be dedicated to making the scene safe and keeping bystanders from becoming injured. Thus, they may not immediately become involved in patient care. For those who arrive after the scene has been made safe, their role will likely involve the triaging of patients. (Triage is discussed later in this chapter.) Other roles for the Emergency Medical Responder include treatment of patients and assisting with the transport of patients to appropriate receiving facilities. Other duties may include the setting up of landing zones if medical helicopters are used for patient evacuation.

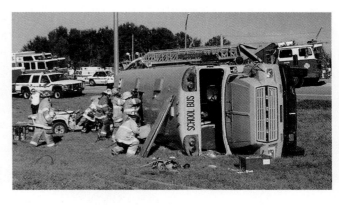

FIGURE 16.1 Plenty of resources have been called to the scene of this school bus wreck.

7–1.9 Discuss the role of the Emergency Medical Responder in the multiple-casualty situation.

Is It Safe?

Responding to any scene with multiple patients can be overwhelming for even the most experienced EMS provider. It is easy to let the sight of multiple patients distract you from your top priority, which is personal safety. Do your best to consciously set a deliberate pace as you enter and move through the scene. Every minute or so, look up and scan the scene for hazards. Be prepared to exit the scene as hazards appear. ∎

INCIDENT MANAGEMENT SYSTEM

The **incident management system (IMS)**, also called an incident command system (ICS), is a model tool for the command, control, and coordination of resources at the scene of a large-scale emergency involving multiple agencies. It consists of procedures for organizing personnel, facilities, equipment, and communications.

The first formal incident management systems were formed as a result of a mandate from Congress to analyze the aftermath of a devastating series of wildfires in southern California in the early 1970s. Since then, EMS, fire, and police agencies across the United States continue to develop and implement such plans.

Most incident management systems are based on well established management principles of planning, directing, organization, coordination, communication, delegation, and evaluation. They must be flexible enough to accommodate a single-agency or single-jurisdiction emergency, as well as multiagency or multi-jurisdictional events. Most incident management systems employ a top-down modular structure that can be scaled to any size event. Some of the modules that might be included in a typical incident management system are command, operations, planning, logistics, and finance.

incident management system (IMS) ∎ a model tool for the command, control, and coordination of resources at the scene of a large-scale emergency involving multiple agencies. Also known as *incident command system (ICS)*.

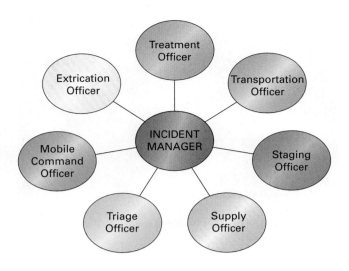

FIGURE 16.2 The incident manager delegates duties to the various sector officers.

National Incident Management System (NIMS) ■ a system that uses a unified approach to incident management and standard command and management structures, with an emphasis on preparedness, mutual aid, and resource management.

It is easy to imagine how chaos can occur when so many different agencies and departments respond to a single large-scale emergency. Designing and implementing an organized approach to such an event will ensure a more positive outcome for both the rescuers and the victims. See Figure 16.2 for an example of the EMS portion of a large incident management system.

NATIONAL INCIDENT MANAGEMENT SYSTEM

In response to the increased terrorist threat in the United States, the Federal Emergency Management Agency (FEMA) has developed its own incident management system known as the **National Incident Management System (NIMS)**. NIMS was developed so responders from different jurisdictions and disciplines can work together to respond to natural disasters and emergencies, including acts of terrorism. NIMS teaches a unified approach to incident management; standard command and management structures; and emphasis on preparedness, mutual aid, and resource management.

FEMA offers several free on-line instructional courses pertaining to both incident command systems and the new National Incident Management System (NIMS). You can find these courses and many others at the FEMA Web site (http://training.fema.gov/NIMS/).

7–1.10 Summarize the components of basic triage.

triage ■ a method of sorting patients for care and transport based on the severity of their injuries or illnesses.

Triage

When there are many victims at an emergency, it is nearly impossible to provide care to all those who need it when they need it. So a system called **triage** has been developed to help identify those victims who are most in need of immediate care. Triage is a process for sorting injured people into groups based on their need for or likely benefit from immediate medical care. Triage is used in hospital emergency departments, on battlefields, and at emergencies when there are multiple victims and limited medical resources (Figure 16.3).

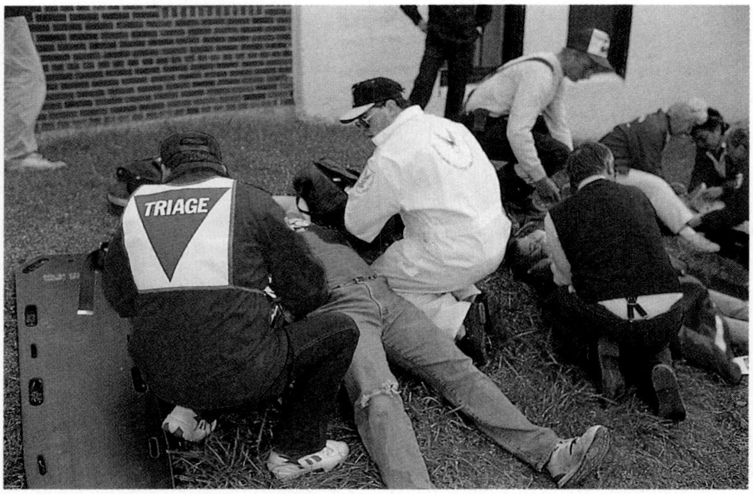

PRIORITIES

FIRST ➤ Triage is a process of sorting patients into categories and prioritizing their medical care and transport based on the severity of their injuries and medical conditions. This process is used at the scene of multiple-casualty incidents. When there are more victims than there are rescuers, the process of triaging helps ensure that the most critical but still salvageable patients are cared for first. ■

FIGURE 16.3 At the scene of a multiple-casualty incident, triage is the system used to identify victims who are most in need of immediate medical care.

For many MCIs, there may be a delay before additional help is on scene. If the emergency is large enough or in a remote area, an hour or more may pass before there are enough rescuers present to render care for all patients. So triage is also used to determine the order of transport for patients. Patients who appear to have serious medical- or trauma-related problems—such as heart attack, shock, major injuries, and heat stroke—must be transported quickly, while patients with minor injuries or illnesses are transported later.

Because Emergency Medical Responders are first on the scene, they must be able to triage patients and initiate care. When additional EMS personnel arrive, Emergency Medical Responders pass on information, continue to help complete the triage process, and help provide care to the worst patients first. You cannot begin to provide care to patients randomly. You must begin caring for those people who have the highest priority based on their condition. You will need to make brief notes on each patient while you are performing triage.

Is It Safe?

Triage is not an easy task. In an MCI, you will be expected to triage as many patients as possible without providing the care they need. It is not unusual for experienced providers to triage patients until they come to one that really needs life-saving care. At that point, they stop triaging and begin caring for the patient as they see fit. This is not always the best thing for all patients. Triaging is about saving as many patients as possible with the available resources. ■

Some jurisdictions have Emergency Medical Responders use triage tags for patient information (Figure 16.4). Even if you do not carry these tags, you should

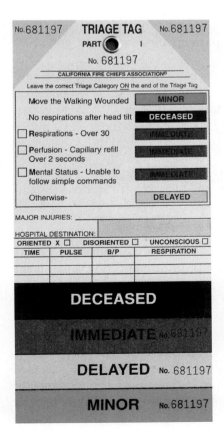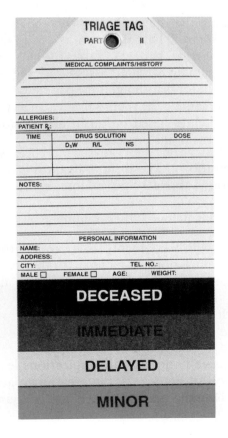

FIGURE 16.4 An example of a standard triage tag, front and back.

be familiar with them in case you are called to help when others are using triage tags. Use one triage tag per patient, and leave the tag attached to the patient so that others arriving at the scene can have immediate access to information. Do not delay the triage process in order to make elaborate notes.

TRIAGE PROCESS

FIRST ➤ There are several triage systems. Each uses slightly different criteria for classifying patients. Use the specific triage system and classifications that your jurisdiction has adopted. ■

START TRIAGE SYSTEM

START triage system ■ a system that uses respirations, perfusion, and mental status assessments to categorize patients into one of four treatment categories; letters stand for Simple Triage and Rapid Treatment.

One variation of a triage system that is common in fire departments and EMS is the **START triage system** developed by the Newport Beach, California, Fire and Marine Department and Hoag Hospital. The letters START stand for Simple Triage and Rapid Treatment. START is based on the rapid assessment of patients using the following three criteria: respirations, perfusion, and mental status (RPM). Patients are classified into one of four categories—immediate, delayed, minor, and deceased (Figure 16.5).

The first rescuers on the scene begin the triage process and quickly identify and separate those patients who are probably the least injured. They are initially classified as "minor." This is accomplished by directing all the walking wounded to a specific location away from the immediate emergency scene. By responding to the direction to move, patients who are able will move and therefore self-triage into the "minor" category, at least initially. It is important not to send these patients too far away because some of them may be able to assist with the care of more injured patients.

Once the walking wounded have exited the scene, the next step will be to begin triaging the remaining patients. START triage recommends you to "start where you stand." That is, begin assessing the patients closest to you and work your way out to all patients (Table 16–1).

Each remaining patient is assessed for the presence of respirations. Open the airway and check for breathing. If the patient takes a breath, he is tagged "immediate." If he is not breathing, he is not salvageable and is tagged "deceased." All respiratory rates are estimates based on quick observation. It is not necessary to take actual rates during the triage process.

- No respirations: dead or nonsalvageable (black or gray tag).
- Respirations above 30 per minute: immediate (red tag). No further assessment needed.
- Respirations below 30 per minute: assess perfusion.

Patients who were identified as ambulatory can assist in keeping the airway open for an unresponsive patient. If other patients cannot help, use items on the scene to position the head and maintain the airway.

FIRST ➤ It is important to understand that patients will constantly be reassessed as time and resources permit. ■

Responsive patients with respirations less than 30 per minute are assessed for perfusion status. Check the breathing patient's radial pulse. The presence of a radial pulse indicates a systolic blood pressure of at least 80 mmHg. Any patient

Simple Triage and Rapid Treatment

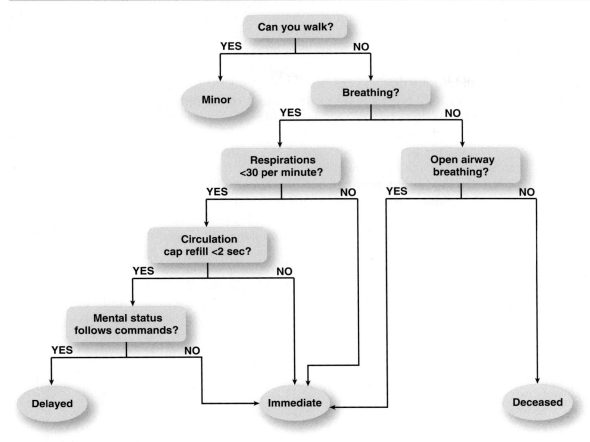

FIGURE 16.5 The START system.

TABLE 16–1	START Triage System			
	IMMEDIATE	**DELAYED**	**MINOR**	**DECEASED**
Respirations	>30 per minute	<30 per minute	<30 per minute	Absent
Perfusion	Capillary refill >2 seconds or radial pulse absent	Capillary refill <2 seconds or radial pulse present	Capillary refill <2 seconds or radial pulse present	Absent
Mental status	Unable to follow commands	Able to follow commands	Able to follow commands	Absent

with a radial pulse is assumed to have adequate perfusion. Therefore, assessment of mental status is the next step before categorizing the patient. Any patient without a radial pulse is assumed to have inadequate perfusion and is tagged "immediate."

Some triage systems use capillary refill to assess perfusion. However, it is often unreliable because of many variables, such as age, sex, and environment. If your protocols require that you check capillary refill, the following criteria will guide you: If capillary refill is greater than two seconds or the radial pulse is absent, categorize the patient as "immediate" and move on to the next patient. If capillary refill is less than two seconds and the patient has a radial pulse, continue to assess mental status.

During the perfusion assessment, if you find major bleeding, do what you can to attempt to control the bleeding. Have the patient or one of the walking wounded hold direct pressure over the wound. Elevate the legs of any patient with no radial pulse and keep him in this position.

The final step in the START triage process requires assessment of the patient's mental status. This is accomplished by determining if the patient can follow simple commands, such as "open or close your eyes" or "squeeze your fingers." If the patient is able to follow simple commands, he is categorized as "delayed" and you will move on to the next patient. If the patient is unable to follow simple commands, he is categorized as "immediate" and you will move on to the next patient.

NOTE

When working with the START triage process, it is good to know that all unresponsive breathing patients are automatically categorized as "immediate."

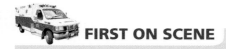

FIRST ON SCENE

The first person that José checked on was dead. That was bad, and he had to force himself to continue on. Luckily, the next five were alive. Some were hurt pretty seriously, but they were definitely alive. Of the last 10—those who had obviously been closest to the blast—he only found a pulse in three. He took the blue permanent marker from his shirt pocket and wrote either "RED," "YELLOW," or "D" on each person's forehead.

He was amazed at how quickly the triage training from his last Emergency Medical Responder class had come back to him. He was just returning to the first "RED" person to reassess him when a group of police officers moved systematically through the mall doors.

"I didn't have any tags, so I wrote on their foreheads," José shouted as the officers stood, unmoving, near the mall entrance. "What are you all waiting for? These people need help!"

"Step away from the area, son," a police officer ordered. "Go over by the escalator until we can clear the scene."

JumpSTART PEDIATRIC TRIAGE SYSTEM

The START triage system works well for rapidly assessing adults, but rescuers need to use different criteria to assess pediatric patients in multiple-casualty incidents. Using the START system, a respiratory rate of less than 30 breaths per minute in adults is a good sign, while a rate faster than 30 breaths a minute indicates a problem. Small children, especially crying infants, will normally have a respiratory rate greater than 30 breaths a minute. A child with a respiratory rate of 8 breaths a minute would be categorized "delayed" using the START system, when actually he is in respiratory failure and should be categorized "immediate."

There are similar assessment problems when checking circulation in children. Adults usually have circulatory failure followed by respiratory arrest. Children have respiratory failure followed by circulatory failure, meaning that a nonbreathing child could still have a pulse. But the START system would categorize the child with no respirations as "deceased." START also uses capillary refill as an assessment tool, and it can be a useful assessment for children in normal environments.

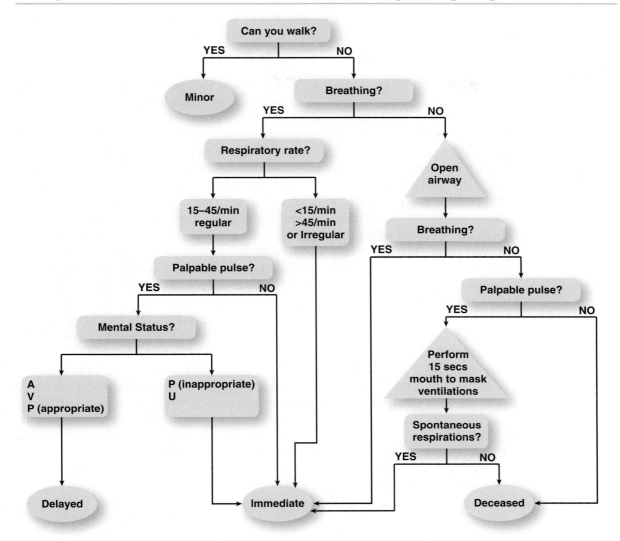

FIGURE 16.6 The JumpSTART Pediatric MCI Triage system.

However, the reliability of capillary refill as an assessment tool varies with age, sex, and the environment, and measuring it requires good lighting. The Jump-START system does not recommend using capillary refill for assessing perfusion.

When checking mental status in children, there is a broad range of responses possible, depending on the child's age. Infants will not be able to obey commands; small children do not have the developmental ability to respond appropriately to commands. However, rescuers can check for signs of mental status using the AVPU scale (alert, responsive to voice, responsive to pain, or unresponsive).

To meet the needs of children involved in MCIs, Dr. Lou Romig, medical director for the South Florida Regional Disaster Medical Assistance Team, developed a special triage system for pediatric patients, the **JumpSTART Pediatric MCI Triage system** (Figure 16.6). JumpSTART can be used on children from 12 months to eight years of age, although rescuers can use it on older children as well. The age ranges were determined by several criteria. Children from 12 to 18 months are beginning to walk and can be sorted as "walking wounded," or ambulatory patients. Children older than eight years of age have airway anatomy and physiology similar to that of an adult.

JumpSTART Pediatric MCI Triage system ■ a specialized pediatric triage system designed for patients from one to eight years of age.

Dr. Romig suggests that if the patient looks like a young adult, use START; if the patient looks like a child, use JumpSTART.

The assessment categories for the JumpSTART system are the same as for the START system: respirations, perfusion (peripheral pulses), and mental status (AVPU). The steps for JumpSTART are as follows:

1. Move all children who are able to walk to an area set aside for minor injuries. There, rescuers will perform a secondary triage, including respirations, pulse, and mental status. Infants who are not yet walking are assessed during initial triage, using the JumpSTART steps, or in the secondary triage area, if someone carries them there. Infants and children who are ambulatory (able to walk), have respirations, perfusion, and appropriate mental status, and have no significant external injury are categorized as "minor."

    In an MCI, it is possible to have a child with special health-care needs. These children may not be ambulatory and may also have chronic respiratory problems and elevated respiratory rates. Assess these special needs children the same as you would infants. It may also be difficult to assess mental status because of the child's special health-care or developmental status. Look for the child's parent or caregiver to get information if this person is present and uninjured.

2. a. Assess nonambulatory children for the presence or absence of spontaneous breathing. If there is breathing, assess the respiratory rate (see Step 3). Open the airway of any child who is not breathing or who is not breathing for more than 10 seconds. Clear a foreign body airway obstruction only if you see it. If the child begins to breathe spontaneously with an open airway, categorize the child as immediate, and move on to the next patient.

    b. If the child does not begin spontaneous breathing when you open the airway, palpate for a peripheral pulse (radial, brachial, or pedal). If there is no peripheral pulse, categorize the patient as deceased, and move on to the next patient.

    c. If the child does not begin spontaneous breathing when you open the airway, and the child has a pulse, ventilate the patient five times using an appropriate barrier device.

    Giving breaths is considered the "jumpstart" part of the pediatric triage system. Children may stop breathing or have a period of not breathing (apnea) but still maintain a pulse. The START system would categorize the nonbreathing child as "deceased," but the JumpSTART system modifies the process to include a pulse check for the nonbreathing child and five ventilations if there is a pulse. The ventilation is meant to jumpstart the child's breathing.

    However, if ventilations do not trigger spontaneous respirations, categorize the child as "deceased" and move on to the next patient. If the child begins to breathe spontaneously, categorize the child as "immediate" and move on without providing further ventilations. It is possible that the child may not be breathing when another rescuer arrives to begin secondary triage. This rescuer will determine the appropriate intervention based on the number of patients and the number of rescue personnel.

3. In this step, all patients have spontaneous respirations. If the respiratory rate is 15 to 45 breaths per minute, proceed to Step 4 and assess perfusion. If the respiratory rate is slower than 15 (slower than one breath every four seconds) or faster than 45 breaths a minute or very irregular, categorize the child as "immediate" and move on.

4. In this step, all patients have adequate respirations. Assess perfusion by palpating peripheral pulses on uninjured limbs. Check peripheral pulses rather than capillary refill because of the many variables that affect accuracy. If the child has palpable peripheral pulses, assess mental status (Step 5). If there are no peripheral pulses, categorize the patient as immediate, and move on.

5. In this step, all patients have adequate ABCs. Check the child's mental status by using a rapid AVPU assessment. Keep in mind that the developmental age of the child will affect results. If the child is alert, responds to your voice, or responds appropriately to pain (localizes the pain, or knows where you are pressing or grasping, and withdraws or pushes you away), categorize the patient as "delayed." If the child does not respond to your voice and responds inappropriately to pain (makes a noise, moves sporadically, or does not localize the pain), shows "posturing" (decorticate, with arms curled onto the chest toward the midline of the body; or decerebrate, with arms stiff at their sides and hands flexed away from the body), or is unresponsive, categorize as "immediate" and move on.

Patient Assessment

It is critical to consider the mechanism of injury and the findings from the initial and focused assessments when you determine order of care for multiple-casualty incidents. Vital signs and significant signs of injury will help you determine priority and care. Relate patient signs to possible injuries or illness (Figure 16.7).

NO APPARENT INJURY

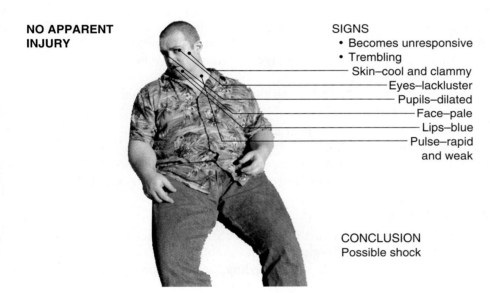

SIGNS
• Becomes unresponsive
• Trembling
Skin–cool and clammy
Eyes–lackluster
Pupils–dilated
Face–pale
Lips–blue
Pulse–rapid and weak

CONCLUSION
Possible shock

FIGURE 16.7 Emergency Medical Responders must be able to relate signs to specific illnesses and injuries.

NO APPARENT INJURY

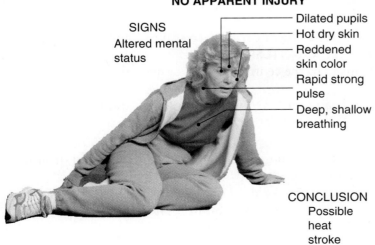

SIGNS
Altered mental status

Dilated pupils
Hot dry skin
Reddened skin color
Rapid strong pulse
Deep, shallow breathing

CONCLUSION
Possible heat stroke

FIRST ➤ As an Emergency Medical Responder, you must be able to apply the following information to the assessment and care of patients:

- Pulse (vital sign).

  — *Rapid, strong:* fear, overexertion, heat stroke and advanced heat exhaustion, high blood pressure, early stages of internal bleeding.
  — *Rapid, weak:* shock, blood loss, developing heat exhaustion, diabetic coma, falling blood pressure.
  — *Slow, strong:* stroke, possible skull fracture.
  — *No pulse:* carotid = cardiac arrest; distal = injury to the extremity (usually a possible fracture or dislocation) or shock with low blood pressure.

- Respiration (vital sign).

  — *Rapid, shallow:* shock, heart problems, heat exhaustion, insulin shock, congestive heart failure.
  — *Deep, grasping, labored:* airway obstruction, congestive heart failure, heart problems, lung disease, lung injury from excessive heat, chest injuries, diabetic coma.
  — *Snoring:* stroke, possible fractured skull, drug or alcohol abuse, airway obstruction.
  — *Stridor:* high-pitched sounds on inspiration.
  — *Crowing:* abnormal breathing sound indicating airway obstruction.
  — *Gurgling:* liquid in the airway, such as vomit, blood, or normal secretions, and inability to clear them, usually due to impaired mental status; airway obstruction; lung disease; lung damage due to excessive heat; fluids in lungs from pulmonary edema.
  — *Coughing blood:* chest wound, possible rib fracture, internal injuries.

- Skin temperature (vital sign).

  — *Cool, moist (clammy):* shock, heat exhaustion.
  — *Cool, dry:* exposure to cold.
  — *Hot, dry:* heat stroke, high fever, chemical (pesticide) exposure.
  — *Hot, moist:* heat exhaustion or heat stroke (but heat stroke may be either sweaty or dry), infectious disease.

- Skin color (vital sign).

  — *Red:* high blood pressure, heart attack, heat stroke, diabetic coma, minor burn, fever or infection, allergic reaction (anaphylaxis).
  — *Pale:* shock, heart attack, excessive bleeding, heat exhaustion, fright, insulin shock.
  — *Blue (cyanosis):* heart failure, airway obstruction, lung disease, certain poisonings, shock.

- Pupils (vital sign).

  — *Dilated, unresponsive to light:* cardiac arrest, unresponsiveness, shock, bleeding, heat stroke, drugs (LSD, uppers).
  — *Constricted:* damage to the central nervous system, drugs (heroin, morphine, codeine).
  — *Unequal:* stroke, head injury. Only useful in setting of profoundly altered mental status.

- Mental status.

  — *Confusion:* fright, anxiety, illness, minor head injury, alcohol or drug abuse, mental illness, shock, epilepsy, hypoxia.
  — *Stupor:* head injury, alcohol or drug abuse, stroke.
  — *Altered mental status:* head injury, fainting, epilepsy.

— *Unresponsiveness:* stroke, allergy shock, head injury, poisoning, drug or alcohol abuse, diabetic coma, heat stroke or advanced heat exhaustion, shock, heart attack.

■ Paralysis or loss of sensation.

— *One side of body:* stroke, head injury.
— *Arms only:* spine injury in neck.
— *Legs only:* spine injury along back.
— *Arms and legs:* spine injury in neck and possibly along back.
— *No pain, obvious injury:* spinal cord or brain damage, shock, anxiety, drug or alcohol abuse. ■

You have learned about the significance of the injuries and how to provide care for patients with these signs and symptoms throughout your Emergency Medical Responder course. When you are faced with multiple casualties at critical incidents, also be aware of your mental and physical stress levels. Critical incident stress debriefing (CISD) sessions or other qualified psychological support should be available after a disaster or unusual emergency to address the needs of rescuers who may have been influenced by the scene and the stress generated in providing emergency care.

 FIRST ON SCENE WRAP-UP

José sat on the frozen escalator for what seemed like an eternity as the mall slowly filled first with police officers and then with people in large, clumsy bomb suits. Finally, the firefighters and EMTs were allowed in to quickly carry out the wounded shoppers. The deceased ones, the ones on which José had written "D," were left sprawled on the beige tiles where they had fallen following the explosion.

José rubbed his eyes and noticed that his white uniform shirt was now covered in bloody smears and dark, pungent ash. He was taking it off when a police officer approached him. "Let's get you out to the treatment area, son."

"Oh, I'm not hurt," José rolled his shirt into a ball and put it under his arm.

"That's fine," the officer said, jabbing his thumb toward the main mall doors. "Let's just have you looked at, okay?"

José couldn't think of any good reason to stay in the mall or ever come back for that matter, so he walked to the door and, without looking back, walked out into the late afternoon sun. He was immediately overwhelmed by the number of emergency vehicles and rescuers hustling around on the marble entryway. He shaded his eyes from the sun and saw crowds of people, some with cameras, being held back by police barricades on the far side of the street.

"Are you the one who did the triaging in there?" A gruff voice startled José and he spun around.

"Uh yes, sir," he answered, seeing an older firefighter with a white helmet on.

"You did a real fine job," the man smiled, reached out, and shook José's hand. "I bet you saved some lives in there."

Summary

Although relatively rare multiple-casualty incidents (MCIs) can easily overwhelm the first responding units at the scene, it is up to those first units to quickly request additional resources and begin to establish command over the incident.

An incident management system (IMS), or incident command system (ICS), is a tool used to manage overall control of large scenes involving many resources and multiple agencies.

Triage is the sorting of patients based on the severity of their injuries and/or illnesses. The goal of triage is to save as many patients using the available resources. Triage systems vary by jurisdiction, but generally use a three- or four-category system. Typical categories include immediate for the most critical but salvageable patients, delayed for those less critical but still in need of care, minor for those who are generally ambulatory at the scene, and deceased for those who show no signs of life.

One variation of a triage system is the START system—a Simple Triage and Rapid Treatment program that uses respirations, perfusion, and mental status assessments to categorize patients into one of four treatment categories.

A variation of the START triage system designed specifically for pediatric patients is called the JumpSTART system, which takes into account the unique needs and presentation of pediatric patients.

Patient assessment is an important part of MCIs because patients will need continued care following the initial triage process. Taking multiple vital signs and other key signs will help determine the seriousness of the patient's injuries and whether they are getting worse or remaining stable. MCI patients must be continuously assessed by field personnel until they reach a destination hospital.

Remember and Consider

Any emergency that involves multiple victims and overwhelms the responders who arrive first on scene qualifies as an MCI. It is important to bring order to chaos; therefore, use the procedures within the incident management system to organize responding personnel and equipment. If you respond to an MCI, report to the Incident Commander or command post to receive instructions. Do not enter a declared MCI scene without being aware of and understanding potential life-threatening hazards or where you can have the greatest impact.

Victims at an MCI must be initially triaged to determine treatment priority. Care will be provided by other emergency personnel in an order that benefits the most critically injured first. Additional triage assessments will

follow and may result in documented changes in a patient's medical condition.

➤ It can be difficult to avoid providing immediate care to MCI victims. However, initial triage is necessary to determine how the greatest good can be provided for the greatest number of patients. By performing this task without distraction, more lives may potentially be saved.

Two popular triage systems—START and Jump-START—address the differences between acceptable pulse and respiratory values and mental status assessment. Understanding these variations will help your patient assessment skills in other areas of emergency medical care.

Investigate

Check your Emergency Medical Responder vehicle for triage tags. Take the time to understand the definition and values assigned to each tag. Ask an experienced rescuer to explain your agency's incident management system.

➤ Does your agency carry on-scene identifiers such as vests, tarps, or cones? Where are they located?

➤ Who in your department is best suited or appointed for leadership at an MCI?

Ask if you can participate in a table-top MCI exercise. This exercise will allow you to experience a multiple-casualty

response in a controlled setting, permit a global view of the incident, and perhaps give you an opportunity to sample various leadership roles.

➤ How often does the local EMS system perform a drill to test the system?

Many times the people coordinating such drills need volunteers to help serve as victims for the event. This would be a great opportunity to see how the system functions from the perspective of a patient. Contact your local EMS agency or fire service to inquire about helping with their next drill.

Quick Quiz

1. A multiple-casualty incident (MCI) involves ___ victims.
   a. more than one
   b. more than two
   c. fewer than 10
   d. fewer than 100

2. An incident management system (IMS) is a tool for the command, control, and ___ of resources at the scene of a large-scale emergency involving multiple agencies.
   a. constant monitoring
   b. care of victims
   c. coordination
   d. concerns of safety

3. The triage system was developed to assist in determining those victims needing:
   a. standard care.
   b. immediate transport.
   c. immediate care.
   d. long-term care.

4. Triage is a process of sorting patients into categories and prioritizing their medical care and transport based on:
   a. number of injuries and medical conditions.
   b. age, weight, and height of the patient.
   c. proximity to the mechanism of injury.
   d. severity of injuries and medical conditions.

5. During the triage process, patients will be placed into one of four categories—immediate, delayed:
   a. minor, or noninjury.
   b. minor, or deceased.
   c. noninjury, or deceased.
   d. minor, or walking wounded.

6. In the START triage system, patients are categorized based on the initial assessment of respirations and:
   a. perfusion and mental status.
   b. blood pressure and mental status.
   c. perfusion and signs of shock.
   d. signs of shock and mental status.

7. Patients may be classified as "walking wounded" if they are able to assist:
   a. in the triage of other patients.
   b. with hazard control.
   c. with the simple care of patients.
   d. in the extrication of victims.

8. The JumpSTART triage system was developed for:
   a. children age 12 months to the teenage years.
   b. children age 12 months to eight years of age.
   c. adult patients younger than 50 years of age.
   d. adult patients older than 50 years of age.

9. The JumpSTART triage assessment categories are:
   a. the same as for the START triage system.
   b. dependent on the age of the pediatric patient.
   c. very different from the START triage system.
   d. dependent on the injuries of the pediatric patient.

10. When determining the order of care for victims of multiple-casualty incidents, it is critical to consider the mechanism of injury and the findings from the:
    a. assessment of mental status.
    b. focused assessment only.
    c. initial assessment only.
    d. initial and focused assessments.

Determining Your Patient's Blood Pressure

In some localities, particularly those in which Emergency Medical Responders work in isolated areas, a special training program for learning to assess blood pressure may be included in the local Emergency Medical Responder course. If this is not part of your course, do not try to train yourself in the use of the blood pressure cuff. Do only what you have been trained to do in your program.

What Is Blood Pressure?

Blood pressure is one of five signs commonly referred to as vital signs. It is the measurement of the pressure of blood against the walls of the arteries. A single blood pressure reading that is significantly above or below the normal range for a patient can be a valuable tool in determining the current state or condition of the patient. Repeated blood pressure measurements are valuable for trending the patient's condition and can also help identify changes in the patient's condition over time.

Blood pressure is determined by measuring the pressure changes in the arteries. The left ventricle contracts forcing oxygen-rich blood into the aorta and other arteries to circulate throughout the body. The heart's contraction phase is called *systole*. The pressure generated in the arteries when the heart contracts is called the *systolic (sis-TOL-ik) blood pressure*. The systolic blood pressure is affected by many factors, such as the force of the heart's pumping action, the resistance and elasticity of the arteries, blood volume (blood loss means lower pressure), blood thickness or viscosity, and the amount of other fluids in the cells.

After the left ventricle of the heart contracts, it relaxes and refills. This relaxation phase is called *diastole*. During diastole, the pressure in the arteries falls. When measured, this pressure is called the *diastolic (di-as-TOL-ik) blood pressure*.

Blood pressure is measured in specific units called *millimeters of mercury (mmHg)*. These are the units on the blood pressure gauge. Because this system of measurement is standard and known to the people receiving patient information from Emergency Medical Responders, you will not have to say "millimeters of mercury" after each reading. Report the systolic pressure first and then the diastolic, as in 120 over 80 (120/80).

The reading of 120/80 is considered a normal blood pressure reading, which represents the average blood pressure obtained from a large sampling of healthy adults. There is a wide range of "normal" for adults and children. Blood pressures are not usually measured in the field for children younger than three years of age because very small equipment is required and accurate measurements are difficult to obtain.

You will not know the normal blood pressure for a patient unless the person is alert, knows the information, and can tell you what it is. Blood pressure varies greatly among individuals. However, there is a general rule for estimating what a patient's blood pressure should be. This rule works for adults up to the age of 40. To estimate the systolic blood pressure of an adult male at rest, add his age to 100. To estimate the systolic blood pressure of an adult female at rest, add her age to 90. To estimate children's systolic blood pressure, use the following formula: two times the age in years plus 80 (2 × age in years + 80). The diastolic estimate will be two-thirds of the systolic measurement. A normal diastolic pressure for adults is typically less than 90mmHg.

Because you will not know the normal reading for a particular patient, you will take several readings in order to identify a trend in the patient's condition. Only one blood pressure reading is of little use. The first reading may be high because of the effects of stress produced by the emergency. Taking several readings and comparing them is called *trending*.

An initial measurement may show that a patient has a blood pressure within normal range, but the condition may worsen. For example, a patient going into shock (hypoperfusion) may have a rapid pulse and a normal blood pressure reading when you first arrive at the scene. A few minutes later, the blood pressure may fall dramatically. Taking several readings while you are providing care is a way of identifying changes in the patient's status. Changes in blood pressure are significant and let you know that additional care is needed and transport is a priority.

A systolic blood pressure reading below 90 mmHg is considered lower than normal in most adults. However, some small adult females and small-build athletes may have a normal systolic blood pressure of 90 mmHg.

A systolic reading above 140 is typically considered high blood pressure, also referred to as *hypertension*. Many patients will show an initial rise in blood pressure at the emergency scene. This is usually due to anxiety, fear, or stress caused by the incident and will return to normal once the situation or condition is under control. You will need more than one reading to confirm high blood pressure. High blood pressure readings are typical in individuals who are obese or who have a history of high cholesterol. There are many other underlying medical conditions that cause high blood pressure that you will be unable to determine at the emergency scene. Several readings will help you determine patient status and guide your care and transport decisions.

In addition to the patient's overall appearance, use the following general guidelines at the emergency scene to help you make assessment decisions regarding the patient's current condition:

Adults
- Systolic above 140 is borderline high.
- Systolic below 100 is borderline low (depends on size and age of patient).
- Diastolic above 90 is borderline high.

Children: ages six to 14
- Systolic above 140 is borderline high.
- Systolic below 80 is borderline low.
- Diastolic above 70 is borderline high.

Children: ages three to five. (Blood pressure is not taken in a child under three years of age.)
- Systolic above 120 is borderline high.
- Systolic below 70 is borderline low.
- Diastolic above 70 is borderline high.

Measuring Blood Pressure

There are two common techniques used to measure blood pressure in emergency field situations. They are *auscultation (os-kul-TAY-shun)*, which is using a blood pressure cuff and a stethoscope (Figure A1.1) to listen for characteristic sounds; and *palpation*, which is using a blood pressure cuff and feeling the patient's radial pulse in the wrist or brachial pulse on the inner arm above the elbow. Palpating a blood pressure will only reveal the systolic pressure.

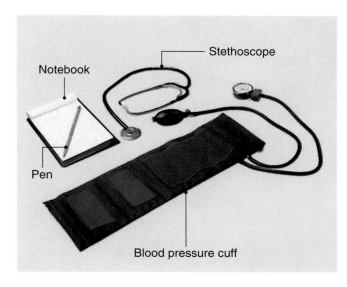

FIGURE A1.1 Blood pressure determination equipment.

DETERMINING BLOOD PRESSURE BY AUSCULTATION

To determine blood pressure using a blood pressure cuff and a stethoscope, you should:

1. Have the patient sit or lie down (Figure A1.2). Cut away or remove clothing over the arm. Support the arm at the level of the heart. Do not move the patient's arm if there is any possibility of spine injury. Check to be sure the arm to be used has not been injured.
2. Select the correct-size blood pressure cuff. Do not try to use an adult-size cuff on a child. The cuff should be two-thirds the width of the upper arm.
3. Wrap the cuff around the patient's upper arm. The lower border of the cuff should be about one inch above the crease in the patient's elbow. The center

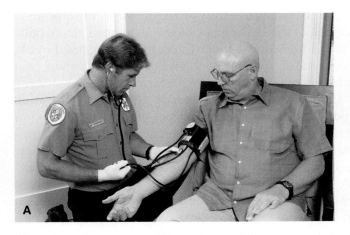
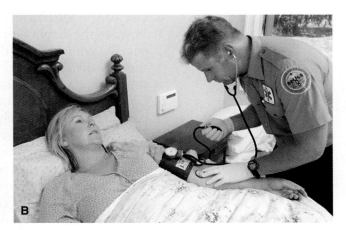

FIGURE A1.2 Positions for taking blood pressure: **A.** auscultation of a seated patient and **B.** of a supine patient.

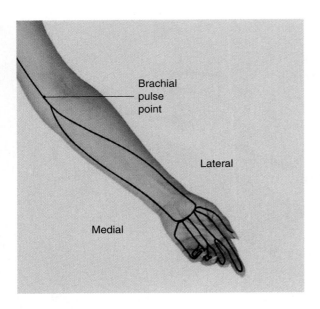

FIGURE A1.3 Brachial pulse point.

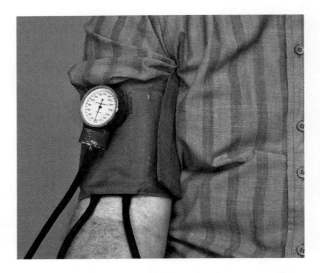

FIGURE A1.4 Positioning of the blood pressure cuff.

of the bladder inside the cuff must be placed over the brachial artery in the upper arm (Figure A1.3).

Some cuffs have a marker to tell you how to line up the cuff over the brachial artery. Know your equipment. Some cuffs have no markers, while others have inaccurate markers. The tubes entering the bladder in the cuff may not be in the correct location. The AHA recommends that you find the bladder center and line up the center of the bladder over the brachial artery.

4. Apply the cuff securely but not too tightly (Figure A1.4). You should be able to place one finger under the bottom edge of the cuff.

5. Place the ends of the stethoscope in your ears. Be sure to adjust the ear pieces so that they face forward into your ear canals. They are easily adjustable. If you are using a dual-head stethoscope, which has both a bell and a diaphragm, make certain to check that the appropriate side is activated before placing it on the patient.

6. Use your fingertips to locate the brachial artery at the crease in the elbow.

7. Position the diaphragm or bell of the stethoscope over the brachial artery pulse site. Do not let the head of the stethoscope touch the cuff. If it touches the cuff, the stethoscope will rub against it during inflation and deflation. You will hear the rubbing sounds, which may cause you to record a false reading.

8. Close the valve and inflate the cuff to approximately 180 mmHg for adult patients and 120 for children. The AHA preferred technique is to place your fingertips over the radial pulse as you inflate the cuff (explained below). When you can no longer feel the pulse, pump up the cuff pressure 30 more mmHg. Then slowly release the pressure as you listen for the pulse sounds.

9. Once the cuff is inflated, open the valve slowly to release pressure from the cuff. It should fall at a smooth rate of 2 to 3 mmHg per second or a little faster than the second hand on a watch.

10. Listen carefully as you watch the needle move. Note when you hear the sound of the pulse in the stethoscope. The first significant sound that you hear is the systolic pressure.

11. Let the cuff continue to deflate. Listen for and note when the sound of the pulse (clicking or tapping) fades (not when they stop). When the sound turns dull or soft, this is the diastolic pressure (Figure A1.5). (Some EMS systems have Emergency Medical Responders use the point where the sounds stop as the diastolic pressure.)

12. Let the rest of the air out of the cuff quickly. If practical, leave the cuff in place so you can take additional readings.

13. Record the time, the arm used, the position of the patient (lying down, sitting), and the patient's pressure. Round off the readings to the next highest number. For example, 145 mmHg should be recorded as 146 mmHg. (The markings on the gauge are in even numbers. You may "see" the first sound in between two markings and want to record it as an odd number, but all blood pressure readings are in even numbers.)

Some providers cannot find the brachial artery, or they cannot hear the pulse sounds when they inflate the cuff, but they can hear the sounds when they deflate the cuff. If you have this challenge, use your fingertips to find the radial pulse in the wrist of the arm to which you have applied the cuff. Inflate the cuff until you can no longer feel the radial pulse. Continue to inflate the cuff to a point 30 mmHg higher than where the pulse stopped. The rest of the procedure is the same.

If you are not certain of a reading, be sure the cuff is totally deflated and wait one or two minutes and try again, or use the patient's other arm. If you try the same arm again too soon, you may get a false high reading.

Sometimes patients with high systolic readings have sounds that disappear as you deflate the cuff, only to reappear again. This can lead to both false systolic and diastolic readings as you record the high systolic reading and record the first disappearance of sound as the diastolic reading. If you continued to listen, you might find that sounds start up again about 20 mmHg lower. Whenever you have a high diastolic reading, wait one or two minutes and take a second reading and be sure to listen for sounds until all air is deflated from the cuff. On a subsequent reading, feel for the disappearance of the radial pulse as you inflate the cuff (this will ensure that you did not measure a false systolic pressure), and listen as you deflate the cuff down into the normal range and until all air is released from the cuff. Use the last fade of sound as the diastolic pressure.

See Scan A1–1 for a summary of determining blood pressure by auscultation.

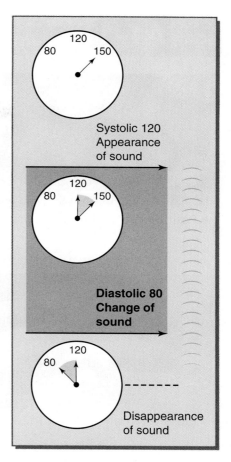

Systolic 120
Appearance of sound

Diastolic 80
Change of sound

Disappearance of sound

FIGURE A1.5 Example of blood pressure sounds.

DETERMINING BLOOD PRESSURE BY PALPATION

Using the palpation method (feeling the radial pulse) is not a very accurate method. It will provide you with one reading, an approximate systolic pressure. This method is used when there is too much ambient noise, making it difficult to hear with a stethoscope. To determine blood pressure by palpation, place the cuff in the same position on the arm as you would for auscultation and:

1. Find the radial pulse on the arm with the cuff.
2. Close the valve and inflate the cuff until you can no longer feel the pulse.
3. Continue to inflate the cuff to a point 30 mmHg above the point where the pulse disappeared.
4. Slowly deflate the cuff and note the reading when you feel the pulse return. This is the systolic blood pressure; you will not get a diastolic pressure reading by palpation.
5. Record the time, the arm used, the position of the patient, and the systolic pressure. Note that the reading was by palpation. If you give this information orally

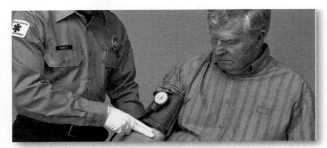

1 ■ Position cuff and find pulse site.

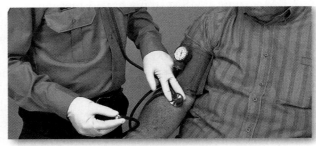

2 ■ Set diaphragm over pulse site.

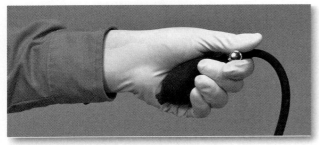

3 ■ Close valve and inflate cuff.

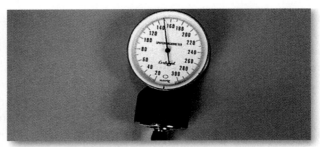

4 ■ Listen for sound to disappear. Inflate 30 mmHg beyond this point.

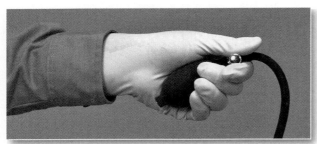

5 ■ Open valve to deflate 2 to 3 mmHg/sec.

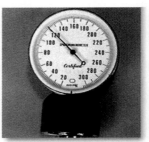

6 ■ (A) Listen for start of sound—systolic.
(B) Listen for sound to fade—diastolic.

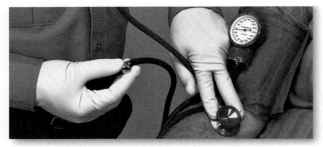

7 ■ Deflate cuff completely.

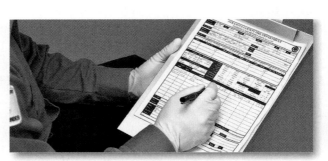

8 ■ Record results.

to someone, make sure they know the reading was by palpation, as in, "Blood pressure is 146 by palpation."

See Scan A1–2 for a summary of determining blood pressure by palpation.

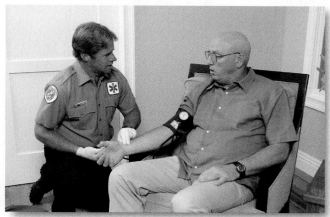

1 ■ Place the cuff and locate the radial pulse.

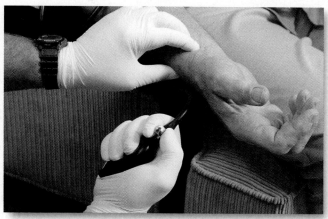

2 ■ Inflate the cuff until you feel the radial pulse go away.

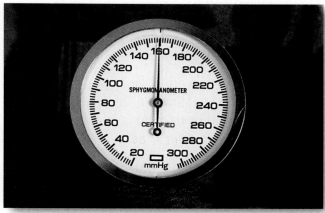

3 ■ Continue inflating cuff to approximately 30 mmHg beyond where the pulse went away.

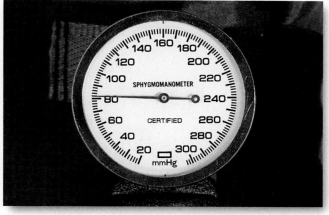

4 ■ Release the pressure in the cuff and note the pressure on the gauge when the radial pulse returns.

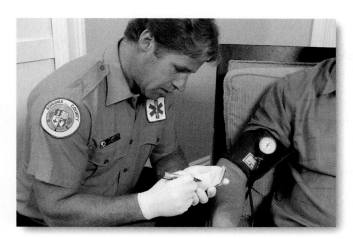

5 ■ Record your results along with the time.

Breathing Aids and Oxygen Therapy

The Emergency Medical Responder's Role

Some EMS systems do not train Emergency Medical Responders in the use of breathing aids and oxygen therapy. But in many jurisdictions, supplemental training programs are offered to meet community needs. Learning how to administer oxygen may be part of your course or may be offered as a special supplement or continuing education program. Your jurisdiction may require this training, especially if you are to perform your Emergency Medical Responder duties in an isolated area. You cannot train yourself to use oxygen administration equipment. Do only what you have been trained to do.

Basic life support (BLS) is possible without equipment and should never be delayed while you locate, retrieve, and set up airway adjuncts or supplemental oxygen. There is no doubt that the prompt and efficient use of certain pieces of equipment can assist you in maintaining an open airway, providing ventilations, and providing oxygen to the patient. But, the patient may suffer if you delay care, use faulty equipment, or use the wrong equipment.

New responsibilities come with the use of equipment in basic life support. You must:

- Be sure that the equipment is clean and operational before it will be needed at an emergency.
- Select the proper equipment for the patient.
- Monitor the patient more closely once you begin to use any device or delivery system.
- Make certain that the equipment is properly discarded, cleaned, refilled, replaced, or tested after each use.
- Practice and maintain the skills needed to use basic life support equipment in order to provide efficient emergency care.

The administration of oxygen may require orders from the medical director of your jurisdiction. This is because oxygen is a medication. As an Emergency Medical Responder, you may be given permission to initiate the use of oxygen by radio communications with a medical facility, or you may be able to begin oxygen administration without oral orders in very specific situations because you are operating under direction of local protocols. You may only be allowed to work with certain devices or administer oxygen while assisting EMTs. Your instructor will give you the guidelines for your jurisdiction.

Oxygen Therapy

IMPORTANCE OF OXYGEN

A patient may need oxygen for many reasons, including respiratory and cardiac arrest, shock, major blood loss, heart attack or heart failure, lung disease, injury to the lungs or the chest, airway obstruction, or stroke, just to name a few. The fact of the matter is that most victims of illness or injury will benefit from supplemental oxygen.

The 21% oxygen provided by room air is far more than the patient needs and is effective if the airway is open, the exchange surfaces of the lungs are working properly, there is enough oxygen available to be picked up by the blood, and the patient's heart and blood vessels are properly circulating blood to all the body tissues. When any one of these factors is missing or fails, a higher concentration of oxygen must be delivered to the patient so that the required amount reaches the body's tissues.

When performing CPR and using mouth-to-mask ventilations, your exhaled air delivers approximately 10% to 16% oxygen to the patient's lungs. This is enough to keep the patient alive for only a short time. CPR only provides approximately one-third the efficiency of a healthy, beating heart circulating blood and oxygen. Ventilating by mouth-to-mask provides the patient with only the minimum oxygen required for short-term survival. By providing oxygen from a supply source, nearly 100% oxygen can reach the lungs. With more oxygen in the patient's blood, CPR efficiency is improved and the patient has a better chance for survival.

NOTE

Oxygen is a medication. Providing oxygen is a special responsibility that can be given only to someone trained in its use.

HAZARDS OF OXYGEN

There are certain hazards associated with oxygen administration, including:

- Oxygen used in emergency care is stored under pressure (2,000 pounds per square inch [psi] or greater). If the tank is punctured or if a valve breaks off, the supply tank and the valve can become missiles.
- Oxygen supports combustion and causes fire to burn more rapidly. Oxygen can saturate linens and clothing and cause them to ignite quickly.
- Under pressure, oxygen and oil do not mix. When they come into contact with each other, there can be a severe reaction, which may cause an explosion. This can easily occur if you try to lubricate a delivery system or gauge with petroleum products.
- Long-term use of high oxygen concentrations can result in medical dangers. These dangers include lung tissue destruction (oxygen toxicity), seizure, lung collapse, eye damage in premature infants, and respiratory arrest in patients with chronic obstructive pulmonary disease (COPD), including emphysema, chronic bronchitis, and black lung disease.

Do not attempt to administer oxygen directly to newborn infants unless ordered to do so by a physician. When oxygen is required (difficult delivery, respiratory distress, very weak infant, premature birth, or other emergency), provide oxygen by blowing it into a foil tent formed over the infant's head, neck, and shoulders. If this is not practical, use a blow-by method by placing the mask near the side of the infant's mouth and nose (Figure A2.1).

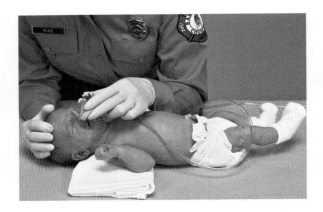

FIGURE A2.1 Blow-by oxygen technique.

Patients with a history of COPD have what is known as a "hypoxic" drive. That is, they have become used to the lower levels of oxygen in their lungs and blood. Prolonged use of high-flow oxygen can lower their drive to breathe, causing respiratory arrest in some patients. This is uncommon in the prehospital setting and is rarely a concern for the Emergency Medical Responder.

NOTE

Never withhold the concentration of oxygen that is appropriate for the patient. If you are in doubt as to how much oxygen to deliver, contact medical direction for advice.

EQUIPMENT AND SUPPLIES FOR OXYGEN THERAPY

An oxygen delivery system for the breathing patient includes a source (oxygen cylinder), pressure regulator, flow meter, and a delivery device (face mask or cannula) (Figure A2.2). When possible, a humidifier should be added to provide moisture to the oxygen if the patient will be on the system for more than 30 minutes. (Some EMS systems will not allow the use of humidifiers because of improper storage and potential contamination.)

The delivery system is the same for a nonbreathing patient, but a device must be added to allow the rescuer to force oxygen into the patient's lungs. This is known as a *demand valve* or as it is sometimes referred to, a *flow-restricted, oxygen-powered ventilation device (FROPVD)*. As an Emergency Medical Responder, you will probably use a pocket mask or bag-valve mask (BVM) connected to 100% oxygen when administering oxygen to the nonbreathing patient.

Oxygen Cylinders

When providing oxygen in the field, the standard source of oxygen is a seamless steel or aluminum cylinder filled with pressurized oxygen. The pressure is equal to 2,000 to 2,200 pounds per square inch (psi). Cylinders come in various sizes, identified by letters. The smaller sizes that are practical for the Emergency Medical Responder include (Figure A2.3):

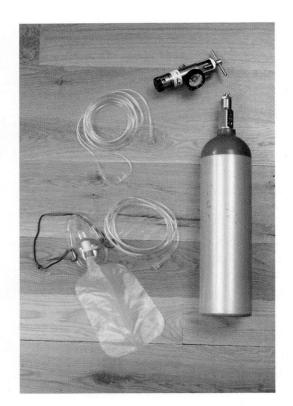

FIGURE A2.2 An oxygen delivery system.

- D cylinder, which contains about 425 liters of oxygen.
- Jumbo D cylinder, which contains about 640 liters of oxygen.
- E cylinder, which contains about 680 liters of oxygen.

Part of your duty as an Emergency Medical Responder is to make certain that the oxygen cylinders are full and ready for use before they are needed for patient care. In most cases, you will use a pressure gauge to determine the pressure remaining in the tank. The length of time that you can use an oxygen cylinder depends on the pressure in the cylinder and the flow rate. The method of calculating cylinder duration is shown in Table A2–1.

Oxygen cylinders should never be allowed to empty below the safe residual level. The safe residual level for an oxygen cylinder is determined when the pressure gauge reads 200 psi. (You cannot tell if an oxygen cylinder is full, partially full, or empty by lifting or moving the cylinder.) At this point, you must switch to a fresh cylinder; below this point, there is not enough oxygen for proper delivery to the patient.

Safety is of prime importance when working with oxygen cylinders. You should:

- Never allow a cylinder to drop or fall against any object. The cylinder must be well secured, preferably in a lying down position. Never let a cylinder stand by itself.
- Never allow smoking around oxygen equipment.
- Never use oxygen equipment around open flames or sparks.
- Never use grease or oil on devices that will be attached to an oxygen supply cylinder. Do not handle these devices when your hands are greasy.
- Never put tape on the cylinder outlet or use tape to mark or label any oxygen cylinder or oxygen delivery equipment. The oxygen can react with the adhesive left behind when it is torn from the cylinder and produce a fire.
- Never try to move an oxygen cylinder by rolling it on its side or bottom.
- Never store a cylinder near high heat or in a closed vehicle that is parked in the sun.
- Always use the pressure gauges and regulators that are intended for use with oxygen and the equipment you are using.
- Always ensure that the "O" ring is in good condition and free of cracks or divots. This will help prevent dangerous leaks.
- Always use medical-grade oxygen (USP). There are impurities in industrial-grade oxygen. The cylinder's label should state, "Oxygen USP."
- Always fully open the valve of an oxygen cylinder and then close it half a turn, when it is in use. This will serve as a safety measure in the event someone else thinks the valve is closed and tries to force it open.

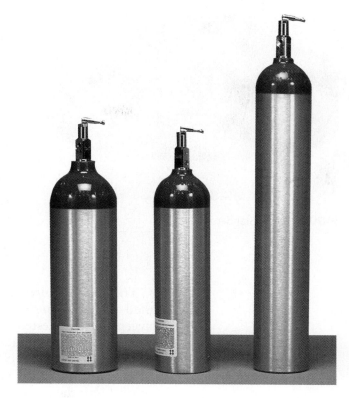

FIGURE A2.3 Various sized portable oxygen cylinders.

TABLE A2–1	Duration of Flow Formula

Simple Formula

$$\frac{\text{Gauge pressure in psi} - \text{residual pressure} \times \text{constant}}{\text{Flow rate in liters/minute}} = \text{Safe duration of flow in minutes}$$

Residual Pressure = 200 psi Cylinder Constant

D = 0.16	G = 2.41
E = 0.28	H = 3.14
M = 1.56	K = 3.14

Determine the life of a D cylinder that has a pressure of 2,000 psi and a flow rate of 10 LPM.

$$\frac{(2,000 - 200) \times 0.16}{10} = \frac{288}{10} = 28.8 \text{ minutes}$$

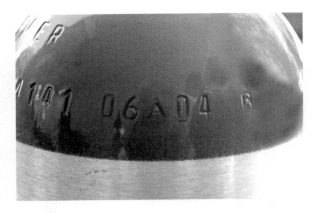

FIGURE A2.4 Standard test stamp.

- Always store reserve oxygen cylinders in a cool, ventilated room as approved by your EMS system.
- Always have oxygen cylinders hydrostatically tested. This should be done every five years for steel tanks (three years for aluminum cylinders). The date for retesting should be stamped on the top of the cylinder near the valve (Figure A2.4).

NOTE

Some oxygen cylinders have met more rigorous inspection and testing standards and are allowed to go up to 10 years between test dates. These cylinders have a five-pointed star immediately following the hydrostatic test date stamped into the crown.

The DOT requires that all compressed gas cylinders be inspected and pressure tested at specific intervals. The cylinders used in EMS that contain medical-grade oxygen must be tested every five years. This test is commonly referred to as a "hydrostatic" test because, following visual inspection, the tank is filled with water and pressurized to five-thirds the service pressure, or approximately 3,360 psi, to confirm that no leaks exist. The most recent hydrostatic test date must be stamped into the crown of the cylinder and easily readable.

Pressure Regulators

The pressure in an oxygen cylinder is too high to be used directly from the cylinder. A pressure regulator must be connected to the oxygen cylinder before it may be used to deliver oxygen to a patient (Figure A2.5). The safe working pressure for oxygen administration is 30 to 70 psi. The pressure regulator will reduce the pressure in the tank from 2,000 to a working pressure between 30 and 70 psi.

On cylinders of the "E" size or smaller, a yoke assembly is used to secure the pressure regulator to the cylinder valve assembly. The yoke has pins that must mate with the corresponding holes found in the valve assembly. This is called a *PIN-index safety system* (Figure A2.6). The position of the pins varies for

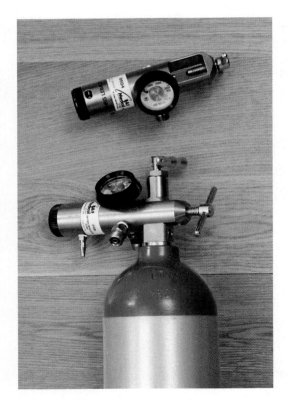

FIGURE A2.5 Pressure regulators, one on and one off the tank.

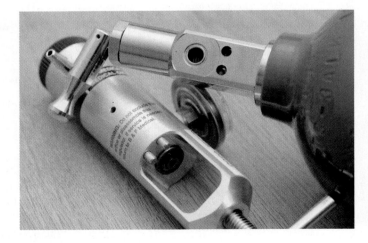

FIGURE A2.6 The PIN safety system.

different gases to prevent an oxygen delivery system from being connected to a cylinder containing another gas.

Before connecting the pressure regulator to an oxygen supply cylinder, open the cylinder valve slightly for just a second to clear dirt and dust out of the delivery port or threaded outlet. This is called "cracking" the cylinder valve. Part of the maintenance of the regulator includes cleaning the inlet filter. Checking the filter for damage and dirt will prevent damage to and contamination of the regulator.

Flowmeters

A flowmeter is connected to the pressure regulator to give the Emergency Medical Responder control over the flow of oxygen in liters per minute (LPM). The constant-flow selector valve is one of the most commonly used valves in the field today. However, many systems are still using the Bourdon-style flowmeter.

The constant-flow selector valve has no liter flow gauge. (For a photograph of this valve, refer to Figure A2.6). It allows for the adjustment of flow in liters per minute in stepped increments (2, 4, 6, 8, . . . 15 LPM). When using this type of flowmeter, make certain that it is properly adjusted for the desired flow. Monitor the dial to ensure that it stays properly adjusted. This type of meter should be tested for accuracy as recommended by the manufacturer.

The bourdon gauge flowmeter (Figure A2.7) is a pressure gauge calibrated to indicate flow of gas in liters per minute (LPM). It is inaccurate at low flow rates and has been criticized for being unstable. This device will not compensate for back pressure. A partial obstruction (as from a kinked hose) will produce a reading higher than the actual flow. The gauge may read 4 LPM and be delivering only 1 LPM. False high readings also can be produced when the filter in the gauge becomes clogged. The bourdon gauge is fairly sturdy and will operate in any position.

Humidifiers

A humidifier is an unbreakable container of sterile water that can be placed inline between the flowmeter and the oxygen delivery device. As the oxygen from the cylinder passes through the water, it is moisturized and becomes more comfortable for the patient to breathe. Unhumidified oxygen delivered to a patient over a long period of time (usually more than 20 minutes) will dry out the mucous membranes in the airway and lungs.

For the short period of time that the patient receives oxygen in the field, this is not usually a problem. A problem does arise, though, when humidifiers are not used appropriately. Too often, the task of changing them between patients is overlooked, or the device is opened but not used, which allows it to become contaminated over time. Because of this infection risk and the fact that they are not required for short transports, many EMS systems no longer use humidifiers.

Oxygen Delivery Devices for Breathing Patients

The nasal cannula and the nonrebreather mask are the main oxygen delivery devices used for the field administration of oxygen to breathing patients (Table A2–2).

The nasal cannula delivers oxygen into the patient's nostrils by way of two small plastic prongs (Figure A2.8). Its efficiency is greatly reduced by nasal injuries, colds, and other types of nasal airway obstruction. A flow rate of 1 to 6 LPM will provide the patient with 24% to 44% oxygen. The approximate relationship of oxygen concentration to liter per minute flow is:

1. LPM — 24% oxygen
2. LPM — 28% oxygen

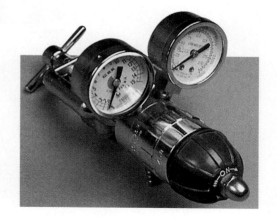

FIGURE A2.7 Bourdon gauge flowmeter (pressure gauge).

TABLE A2–2	Oxygen Delivery Devices		
Oxygen Delivery Device	**Flow Rate**	**% Oxygen Delivered**	**Special Use**
Nasal cannula	1 to 6 LPM	24% to 44%	Most medical and COPD patients at low concentrations
Nonrebreather mask	Start with 10 LPM, practical high is 15 LPM	80% to 95%	Good for patients with respiratory distress and shock; provides high-oxygen concentrations

3. LPM — 32% oxygen
4. LPM — 36% oxygen
5. LPM — 40% oxygen
6. LPM — 44% oxygen

For every 1 LPM increase in oxygen flow, you deliver a 4% increase in the concentration of oxygen. At 4 LPM and above, the patient's breathing patterns may prevent the delivery of the stated percentages. At 5 LPM, rapid drying of the nasal membranes is possible. After 6 LPM, the device does not deliver any higher concentration of oxygen and may be uncomfortable for most patients.

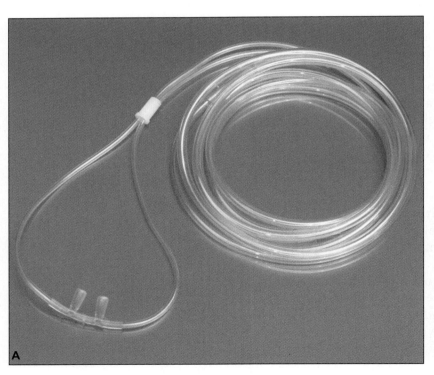
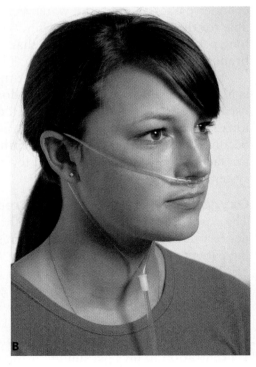

FIGURE A2.8 **A.** Example of a nasal cannula, and **B.** a nasal cannula properly placed on the face of the patient.

A nonrebreather mask is used to deliver high concentrations of oxygen. It is important that you inflate the reservoir bag before placing the mask on the patient's face (Figure A2.9). This is done by using your finger to cover the one-way valve inside the mask between the mask and the reservoir. Care must be taken to ensure a proper seal with the patient's face. The reservoir must not deflate by more than one-third when the patient takes his deepest inspiration. You can maintain the volume in the bag by adjusting the oxygen flow. The patient's exhaled air does not return to the reservoir; instead, it is vented through the one-way flaps or portholes on the mask. The minimum flow rate when using this mask is 8 LPM, but a higher flow (12 to 15 LPM) may be required.

ADMINISTERING OXYGEN

Scans A2–1 and A2–2 will take you step by step through the process of preparing the oxygen delivery system and administering oxygen.

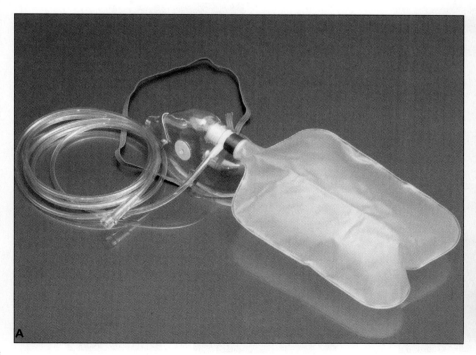
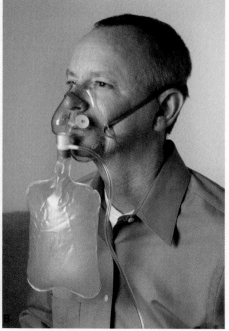

FIGURE A2.9 A. Example of a nonrebreather mask, and **B.** a nonrebreather properly placed on the face of a patient.

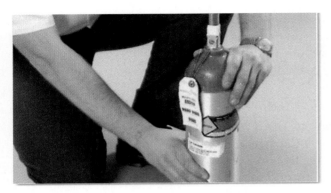

1 ■ Select desired cylinder and check label for "Oxygen USP."

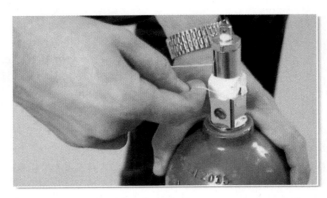

2 ■ Remove the plastic wrapper or cap protecting the cylinder outlet.

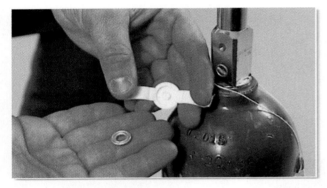

3 ■ Keep the plastic washer that is used in some setups.

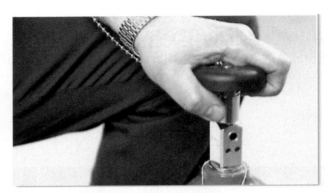

4 ■ "Crack" the main valve for one second.

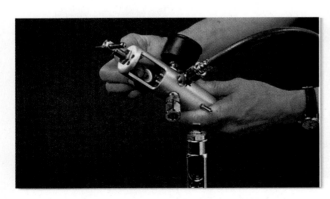

5 ■ Place cylinder valve gasket on regulator oxygen port.

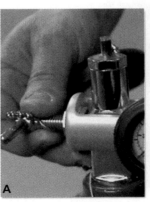
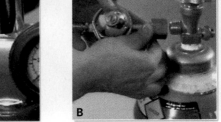

A

B

6 ■ (A) Align PINs or (B) thread by hand and . . .

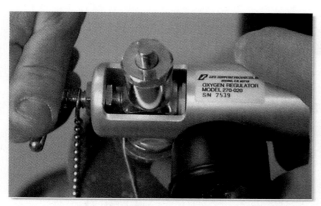

7 ■ Tighten T-screw hand-tight. Do not over-tighten because this can crush or crack the washer, thus causing a leak.

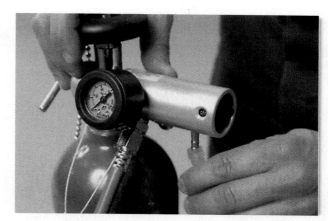

8 ■ Attach tubing and delivery device.

SCAN A2–2 Administering Oxygen

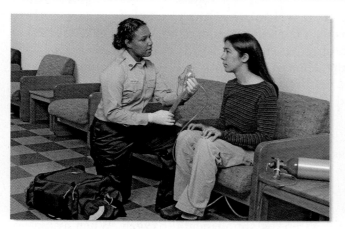

1 ■ Explain the need for oxygen therapy.

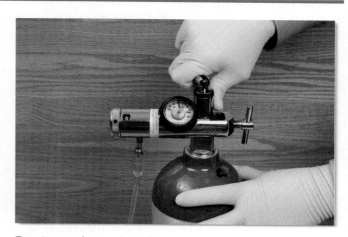

2 ■ Open the main valve.

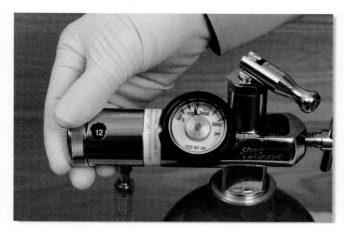

3 ■ Attach the delivery device and adjust flowmeter.

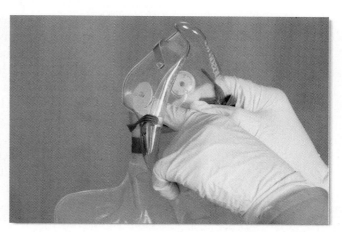

4 ■ Be sure to fill the reservoir bag prior to placing it on the patient by turning on the flow and placing your finger over the valve in the mask.

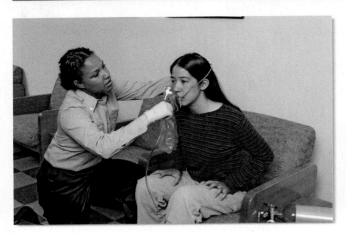

5 ■ Position the oxygen delivery device on the patient.

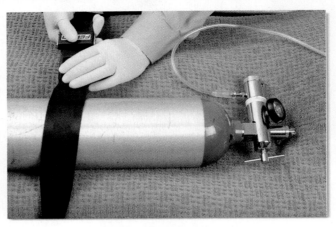

6 ■ Secure the cylinder during transfer.

Administration of Oxygen to a Nonbreathing Patient

The pocket face mask with oxygen inlet and your own breath can be combined to deliver oxygen to a nonbreathing patient. The BVM used alone or with 100% oxygen under pressure and the demand valve with 100% oxygen under pressure can be used in ventilating the nonbreathing patient. When using these devices, an oropharyngeal airway should be inserted.

> **NOTE**
>
> BVM and demand valve devices are not recommended when performing one-rescuer CPR. The preferred device for one-rescuer CPR is a pocket mask with supplemental oxygen.

Most BVMs are capable of accepting supplemental oxygen. When available, attach it to an oxygen source and adjust the flow to no less than 15 LPM. Many BVMs have an oxygen reservoir (long tube or bag) to increase the oxygen concentration delivered to the patient. Used without a reservoir, it will deliver approximately 50% oxygen. Used with a reservoir, it will deliver nearly 100% oxygen. Maintain an open airway, a tight mask-to-face seal, squeeze the bag to deliver oxygen, and release the bag to allow for a passive expiration. There is no need to remove the mask when the patient exhales. This device can also be used to assist the breathing efforts of a patient who has failing respirations (as in a drug overdose). This device works best when used by two rescuers. The first rescuer obtains a tight mask-to-face seal and keeps the airway open. The second rescuer squeezes the bag with both hands.

A demand valve device delivers oxygen through a regulator from a pressurized cylinder. By depressing a trigger on the device, the Emergency Medical Responder can deliver ventilations to the patient. Standard features of this device include a peak flow rate of 100% oxygen delivered at up to 40 LPM, inspiratory pressure relief valve that opens at approximately 60 cm of water pressure, a trigger that enables the rescuer to use both hands to maintain a mask seal while activating the device, and easy and effective operation during both usual and extreme environmental conditions.

To operate a demand valve, follow the same procedures for placing and sealing the mask as you would for the BVM. Then press the trigger to deliver oxygen until the chest rises and repeat as often as necessary for the specific patient. Release the trigger after the chest inflates and allow for passive exhalation. If the chest does not rise, reposition the head or reopen the airway, check for obstructions, reposition the mask, check for a seal, and try again. If the chest still does not rise, consider an alternative ventilation device or procedure.

Monitor your patient carefully whenever you are providing assisted ventilations. High pressure caused by forcing air or oxygen into a patient's airway can force air into the esophagus and fill the stomach. Air distends the stomach, which presses into the lung cavity and reduces expansion of the lungs. To avoid or correct this problem, carefully maintain and monitor airway, mask-to-face seal, and chest rise. Do not continue to provide ventilations after chest rise; allow passive exhalation and reventilate.

If you suspect neck injury, have an assistant stabilize the patient's head or use your knees to prevent head movement. Bring the jaw to the mask without tilting the head or neck and trigger the mask to ventilate the patient.

> **NOTE**
>
> The demand valve device should be used only on adults.

GENERAL GUIDELINES FOR OXYGEN DOSAGES

The following dosages of oxygen are recommended according to the nature of the patient's problem. The standing orders for oxygen vary slightly in different EMS systems. Follow your local protocols. In the following scenarios, when the nonrebreather mask is recommended and you only have a nasal cannula or the patient will not tolerate the mask, provide oxygen by cannula at a rate of 6 LPM.

Trauma

Provide oxygen by nonrebreather at 12 to 15 LPM to deliver 80% to 90% concentration (not necessary for minor scratches, scrapes and cuts, minor extremity injuries [finger or toe], strains, and sprains).

Childbirth

Provide oxygen by nonrebreather at 12 to 15 LPM to deliver 80% to 90% concentration for the mother with predelivery bleeding, excessive postdelivery bleeding, breech birth, or miscarriage or abortion with excessive bleeding.

For the newborn, provide oxygen into a tent placed over the infant's head and shoulders or by mask and blow-by method to premature infants, difficult breech births, infants with bleeding from the umbilical cord, weak infants, or those who have a lasting blue color (cyanosis) on other than hands and feet.

Environmental Emergencies

Provide oxygen by nonrebreather at 12 to 15 LPM to deliver 80% to 90% concentration for allergy (anaphylactic) shock, burns, drug overdose, near-drowning, poisoning, and scuba incidents.

If the patient is not breathing, provide oxygen through the pocket face mask with oxygen inlet while performing mouth-to-mask ventilations or by BVM attached to an oxygen cylinder. Use a reservoir with the BVM to provide nearly 100% oxygen concentration.

Medical Emergencies

Provide oxygen by nonrebreather at 12 to 15 LPM to deliver 80% to 90% concentration for chest pain, respiratory disorders and distress or trouble breathing,

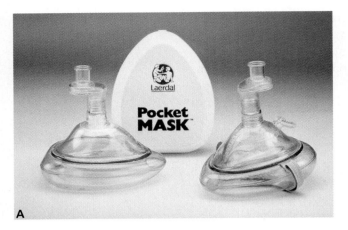

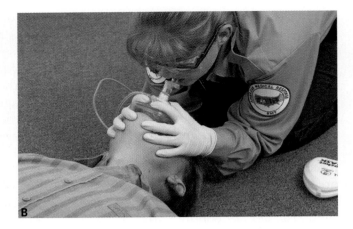

FIGURE A2.10 **A.** One mask without and one with an oxygen inlet. *(Photo courtesy of Laerdal Medical Corporation)* **B.** Rescuer delivering her own breath through the mask's chimney plus oxygen through the inlet.

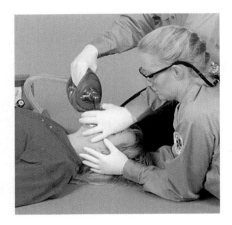

FIGURE A2.11 Bag-valve mask connected to an oxygen supply. *(Photo courtesy of Laerdal Medical Corporation)*

diabetic emergencies, patients recovering from seizure, and abdominal pain or distress.

If the patient is not breathing, provide oxygen through the pocket face mask with oxygen inlet (Figure A2.10) while performing mouth-to-mask ventilations or by BVM attached to an oxygen cylinder (Figure A2.11). Use a reservoir with the BVM to provide nearly 100% oxygen concentration.

Pharmacology

NOTE

This appendix is designed to aid Emergency Medical Responders who are being trained to assist patients in taking specific prescribed medications. This training is meant to be part of a formal training program that is under the guidance and supervision of a physician Medical Director. Any provider level in the EMS system that administers or assists patients in administering their own prescribed medications must follow either specific written protocols or oral medical direction. Emergency Medical Responders must not attempt to give any medication without specific medical direction.

Pharmacology is the study of drugs, their origins, nature, chemistry, effects, and use. Emergency Medical Responders will assess and care for many patients whose medical histories include the medications they take, and whose problems may be caused by the effects of taking or of not taking those medications properly. This appendix lists and describes the few medications that Emergency Medical Responders may be carrying and the few prescribed medications that you may assist a patient in administering. It also discusses how to give or assist the patient in administering the medications and the effects of these medications on the patients.

Remember that you may only give or assist in giving certain medications under the supervision of medical direction.

Medications

There are typically six medications that EMTs and Emergency Medical Responders may be trained to assist with or administer in the field. Three of the medications that are used commonly—and may be carried by Emergency Medical Responders—often are not even considered medications. They are *oxygen, activated charcoal*, and *oral glucose*. Many Emergency Medical Responders are allowed by their EMS Medical Director to administer these medications under specific conditions and circumstances. Activated charcoal and oral glucose are sold over the counter in most pharmacies and are found in many households.

The other medications described in this appendix must be prescribed by a physician and are usually carried by the patient. They are prescribed inhalers, nitroglycerin, epinephrine, and special transdermal patches sometimes called "transdermal infusion systems." Depending on the specific EMS system, Emergency Medical Responders may be able to assist a patient in taking any one of these medications with the approval of medical direction and under specific conditions and circumstances.

INDICATIONS, CONTRAINDICATIONS, ACTIONS, AND SIDE EFFECTS

For each medication, the Emergency Medical Responder must know and understand the specific indications, contraindications, and actions, as well as any expected side effects the medication may have on the patient. After a medication has been administered, it will be important to monitor the patient to see how the drug is affecting him. If taken properly, medications will usually ease the ill effects of the medical condition. But if the medications are expired or the patient's condition is beyond the help of the drug, the medication may be ineffective.

For each drug, there are *indications* for its use. Indications are specific signs or symptoms for which it is appropriate to use the drug. For example, nitroglycerin is indicated for patients experiencing cardiac chest pain, and an inhaler is indicated for someone having an asthma attack.

Also, there are *contraindications* for each drug's use. Contraindications are specific signs, symptoms, or conditions for which it is not appropriate to use the drug. For example, nitroglycerin is contraindicated in patients experiencing cardiac chest pain and who have a systolic blood pressure below 100. Because nitroglycerin reduces blood pressure, it is possible to cause the blood pressure to drop too low if it is not above 100 systolic before taking the dose. Administering oral glucose to an unresponsive patient may be contraindicated because it may cause an airway obstruction.

A medication's *action* is the specific effect it is designed to have on the patient. The action of nitroglycerin is to dilate the vessels. The action of activated charcoal is to bind with the poison, and the action of glucose is to raise the level of sugar in the blood.

Medications sometimes have *side effects*. A side effect is any unwanted action or reaction caused by the drug other than the desired effect. Some side effects are expected and predictable. Nitroglycerin will dilate vessels, not just in the heart, but also throughout the body. This may cause a large enough drop in blood pressure to make the patient dizzy or light headed. Another common side effect of nitroglycerin is a headache. You must anticipate side effects and document them when they occur, especially before administering a second dose. It is good practice to advise or remind the patient about the possible side effects before administering any medication. This could minimize the chances of any surprises that could further add to the patient's anxiety. If the patient has taken any of these medications before, they probably will know what side effects to expect.

MEDICATIONS CARRIED ON THE EMERGENCY MEDICAL RESPONDER UNIT

Activated Charcoal

Activated charcoal (Scan A3–1) is not the kind of charcoal you find in the barbecue grill. It is most often found in a slurry form, which is a powder premixed with water for use in the prehospital emergency situation. (Some brands require you to add the water.) Activated charcoal is administered to patients who have ingested a poison or who took an overdose of oral drugs or medications. When the patient drinks the activated charcoal slurry, it binds with the poisonous substance and also helps prevent the poison or drug from being absorbed by the body. Follow local protocols for administration.

Oral Glucose

Glucose is a simple sugar, which is found in many common foods such as fruit, bread, and vegetables, and is the body's main source of energy. The brain, in

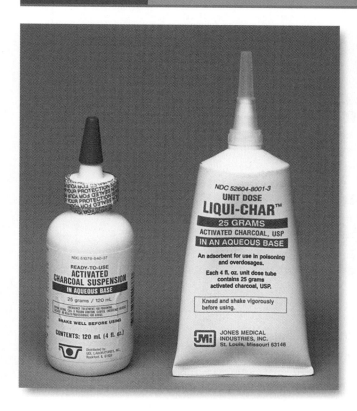

Medication Name

1 ■ Generic: activated charcoal.
2 ■ Trade: SuperChar, InstaChar, Actidose, Liqui-Char, and others.

Indications

Poisoning by mouth (ingestion).

Contraindications

1 ■ Altered mental status.
2 ■ Ingestion of acids or alkalis.
3 ■ Unable to swallow.

Form

1 ■ Premixed in water, frequently available in plastic bottle containing 12.5 grams of activated charcoal.
2 ■ Powder, which should be avoided in field.

Dosage

1 ■ Adults and children: 1 gram activated charcoal/kg of body weight.
2 ■ Usual adult dose: 25–50 grams.
3 ■ Usual pediatric dose: 12.5–25 grams.

Steps for Administration

1 ■ Consult medical direction.
2 ■ Shake container vigorously.
3 ■ Because medication looks like mud, patient may need to be persuaded to drink it. Providing a covered container and a straw will prevent the patient from seeing the medication and so may improve patient compliance.
4 ■ If patient does not drink the medication right away, the charcoal will settle. Shake or stir it again before administering.
5 ■ Record the name, dose, route, and time of administration of the medication.

Actions

1 ■ Activated charcoal binds to certain poisons and prevents them from being absorbed into the body.

Side Effects

1 ■ Causes black stools.
2 ■ Some patients, particularly those who have ingested poisons that cause nausea, may vomit. If patient vomits, repeat the dose once.

Reassessment Strategies

Be prepared for the patient to vomit or further deteriorate. If the patient worsens, provide oxygen as you have been trained to do.

particular, is very sensitive to abnormal levels of glucose and functions poorly without it. A patient with abnormal glucose levels will commonly have an altered mental status.

Glucose levels can be raised by giving oral glucose (Scan A3–2), a form of glucose that comes in a gel or chewable tablet. It is indicated for patients with an altered mental status and a history of diabetes. It is taken orally.

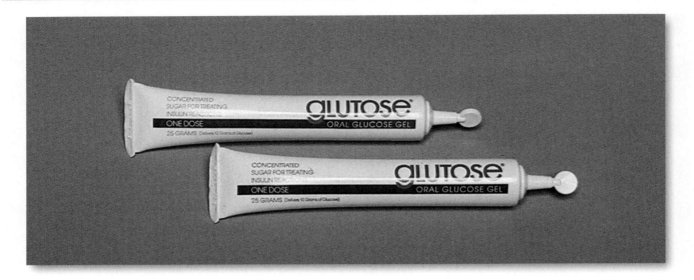

Medication Name

1 ■ Generic: glucose, oral.
2 ■ Trade: Glutose, Insta-glucose, BD Glucose Tablets.

Indications

1 ■ Patients with altered mental status with a known history of diabetes.
2 ■ Patient has taken insulin but no food recently and may have been very physically active.

Contraindications

1 ■ Unresponsiveness or unable to swallow or otherwise manage own airway.
2 ■ Known diabetic who has not taken insulin for days.

Medication Form

Gel, in toothpaste-type tubes; chewable tablets.

Dosage

One tube; three 5.0 gram chewable tablets. This dose can be used for both adults and children. Tubes can come in 15 mg, 30 mg, and 45 mg dosages.

Steps for Administration

1 ■ Ensure signs and symptoms of altered mental status with a known history of diabetes.
2 ■ Ensure patient is alert enough to swallow.
3 ■ Administer glucose.
   a. Self-administered into mouth and swallowed.
   b. Place on tongue depressor between cheek and gum.
   OR
   c. Have patient chew one to three tablets.
4 ■ Perform ongoing assessment.

Actions

Increases blood sugar levels.

Side Effects

None when given properly.

Reassessment Strategies

Continue to monitor the patient's mental status and signs and symptoms. If patient becomes less responsive, discontinue administration. Continue to provide oxygen as you have been trained to do.

NOTE

Glucose tablets may be colored. If the patient reports having asthma or an allergy to aspirin, note if the tablet is made with FD&C Yellow Dye No. 5. This dye causes the same reaction as aspirin in patients who have allergies to aspirin. It also is believed to set off bronchospasms in some asthma patients.

To assist in the administration of oral glucose, have the patient hold the tube and instruct him to squeeze small amounts into his mouth and swallow. You want him to ingest the entire tube as quickly as possible, but without choking. An alternative method for administration is to apply some of the gel to a tongue depressor and spread it between the patient's cheek and gum. Continue to apply small doses until the tube is empty. The mucous membrane inside the mouth is rich in blood vessels, which quickly absorb the glucose and carry it through the bloodstream. Once the level of glucose is elevated, the patient's condition usually begins to improve.

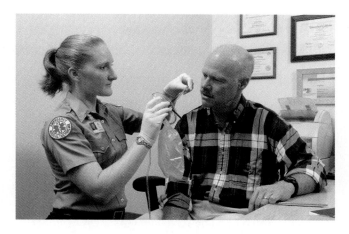

FIGURE A3.1 Oxygen is a powerful drug.

For tablets, the typical strength is 5.0 grams of D-glucose (dextrose). This form of glucose passes through the mucosa (lining) of the mouth, esophagus, and stomach so that no special digestion is needed. It does not have to enter the small intestine to be absorbed. The manufacturer's recommended dosage is three tablets or 15.0 grams of D-glucose. *Do not* try to administer glucose tablets to anyone who is unresponsive and unable to manage his own airway.

The patient should respond quickly to the tablets. Fatigue may remain for various periods of time, depending on the patient and how rapidly the blood glucose level fell during the hypoglycemic (low blood sugar) episode. Some patients have feelings of uneasiness that remain for up to one-half hour. Most are able to eat additional foods that help with their symptoms. However, do not allow someone to ingest foods if he has been given glucose and reports nausea. The nausea should subside shortly, and, if the patient requests food and remains alert, most protocols for hypoglycemic events allow it.

Oxygen

One hundred percent oxygen (Figure A3.1) is used as a drug to treat patients who have low oxygen levels in their blood because of medical or traumatic conditions. Oxygen and oxygen therapy are briefly described in Appendix 2. If your Emergency Medical Responder unit carries oxygen and oxygen delivery devices, you must participate in a training program to learn how and when to use them properly. Be sure to follow your jurisdiction's guidelines, protocols, and medical direction.

PRESCRIPTION MEDICATIONS

Metered-Dose Inhalers

Many patients have chronic respiratory diseases—such as asthma, emphysema, or bronchitis—that cause the airway passages in the lungs to narrow or become constricted. Such patients usually carry a device called a *metered-dose inhaler* (Scan A3–3). It typically contains medication called a *bronchodilator*. This medication enlarges, or dilates, the airway passages so the patient can breathe easier. The inhaler device holds the medication in an aerosol form, which can be sprayed into the mouth and inhaled.

You must have medical direction to help a patient self-administer this medication. You must also make sure that this medication belongs to the patient and was not lent to him by a well-meaning family member or friend with a similar problem. Also, checking for an expiration date is important because expired medication is less effective.

It is essential that you not let bystanders or family members volunteer their own medications for your patients and that you do not let couples share a single

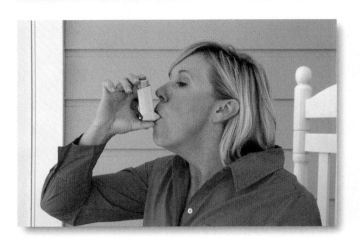 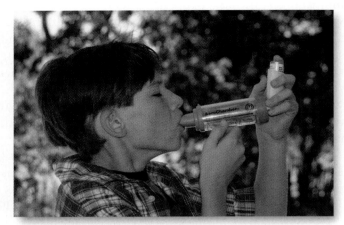

Medication Name

1 ■ Generic: albuterol, ipratropium, metaproterenol.
2 ■ Trade: Proventil, Ventolin, Atrovent, Alupent, Metaprel.

Indications

Meets all of the following criteria:
1 ■ Patient exhibits signs and symptoms of respiratory difficulty.
2 ■ Patient has physician-prescribed inhaler.
3 ■ Medical direction gives Emergency Medical Responder specific authorization to use.

Contraindications

1 ■ Altered mental status (such that the patient is unable to use the device properly).
2 ■ No permission has been given by medical direction.
3 ■ Patient has already taken maximum prescribed dose prior to rescuer's arrival.

Medication Form

Handheld metered-dose inhaler.

Dosage

Number of inhalations based on medical direction's order or physician's order.

Steps for Administration

1 ■ Obtain order from medical direction.
2 ■ Confirm patient is alert enough to use inhaler.
3 ■ Ensure it is the patient's own prescription.
4 ■ Check expiration date of inhaler.
5 ■ Check if patient has already taken any doses.

6 ■ Shake inhaler vigorously several times.
7 ■ Have patient exhale deeply.
8 ■ Have patient put lips around the opening of the inhaler.
9 ■ Have patient depress the handheld inhaler when beginning to inhale deeply.
10 ■ Instruct patient to hold breath for as long as is comfortable so that medication can be absorbed.
11 ■ Allow patient to breathe a few times and repeat second dose if so ordered by medical direction.
12 ■ If patient has a spacer device for use with the inhaler (device for attachment between inhaler and patient to allow for more effective use of medication), it should be used.
13 ■ Provide oxygen as appropriate.

Actions

Dilates bronchioles, reducing airway resistance.

Side Effects

1 ■ Increased pulse rate.
2 ■ Anxiety.
3 ■ Nervousness.

Reassessment Strategies

1 ■ Monitor vital signs.
2 ■ Adjust oxygen as appropriate.
3 ■ Reassess level of respiratory distress.
4 ■ Observe for deterioration of patient. If breathing becomes inadequate, provide artificial ventilations.

prescription. Patients should only take their own medications as directed by their physicians.

Nitroglycerin

Nitroglycerin is a chemical that is well known as an explosive, but it also has medical uses. It dilates blood vessels and relieves certain types of pain, particularly the type caused by a heart condition called *angina pectoris*. Patients who have heart conditions that cause recurring chest pain or who have a history of heart attack may have a prescription for nitroglycerin (Scan A3-4). Nitroglycerin dilates, or enlarges, the constricted vessels in the heart muscle to increase the available supply of blood and oxygen, which help ease the pain.

SCAN A3-4 Nitroglycerin

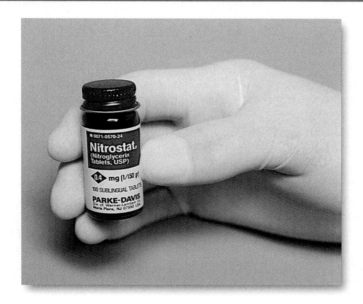

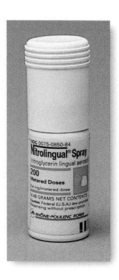

Medication Name

1 ■ Generic: nitroglycerin.
2 ■ Trade: Nitrostat, NitroTab, Nitrolingual.

Indications

All of the following conditions must be met:

1 ■ Patient complains of chest pain.
2 ■ Patient has a history of cardiac problems.
3 ■ Patient's physician has prescribed nitroglycerin.
4 ■ Systolic blood pressure is greater than 100 systolic. (Local protocols may vary.)
5 ■ Medical direction authorizes administration of the medication.

Contraindications

1 ■ Patient has a systolic blood pressure below 100 mmHg. (Local protocols may vary.)
2 ■ Patient has a head injury.
3 ■ Patient has already taken the maximum prescribed dose.

Medication Form

Tablet or sublingual spray.

Dosage

One dose is equal to 0.4 mg, repeat in three to five minutes. If no relief, systolic blood pressure remains above 100 (local protocols may vary), and if authorized by medical direction, up to a maximum of three doses. Spray is typically prescribed for one metered spray followed by a second in 15 minutes.

Steps for Assisting Patient

1 ■ Perform focused assessment for cardiac patient.
2 ■ Take blood pressure. (Systolic pressure must be above 100; local protocols may vary.)
3 ■ Contact medical direction if no standing orders.
4 ■ Ensure right medication, right patient, right dose, and right route. Check expiration date.
5 ■ Ensure patient is alert.

(Continued on next page)

6 ■ Question patient on last dose taken and effects. Ensure understanding of route of administration.

7 ■ Ask patient to lift tongue and place tablet or spray dose on or under tongue (while you are wearing gloves) or have patient place tablet or spray under tongue.

8 ■ Have patient keep mouth closed with tablet under tongue (without swallowing) until dissolved and absorbed.

9 ■ Recheck blood pressure within two minutes.

10 ■ Record administration, route, and time.

11 ■ Perform reassessment.

Actions

1 ■ Dilates blood vessels.

2 ■ Decreases workload of heart.

Side Effects

1 ■ Hypotension (lowers blood pressure).

2 ■ Headache.

3 ■ Pulse rate changes.

4 ■ Dizziness, lightheadedness.

Reassessment Strategies

1 ■ Monitor blood pressure.

2 ■ Ask patient about affect on pain relief.

3 ■ Seek medical direction before readministering.

4 ■ Record assessments.

5 ■ Provide oxygen as appropriate.

Often, Emergency Medical Responders will arrive at the scene to find out during the assessment that the patient with chest pain has taken a dose of nitroglycerin. Just as often, the patient with chest pain is carrying the medication and has not thought to take it. Patients are typically instructed by their physician to take up to three tablets—one every five minutes—over a 15-minute period.

You will need to consult medical direction to help administer nitroglycerin or to get permission to give more after the patient has taken three doses. As with the inhaler, be sure to check that the nitroglycerin is actually the patient's medication and that it has not reached the expiration date.

The patient may have a bottle of nitroglycerin sublingual spray (e.g., Nitrolingual Pumpspray). At the onset of suspected cardiac chest pain, one to two metered sprays may be administered onto or under the tongue within 15 minutes.

The patient may have nitroglycerin transdermal patches (transdermal infusion system). These are for daily application and help prevent angina attacks, but they are not meant to relieve and correct an acute event (Figure A3.2).

Sometimes the medication may not be effective because the patient has not stored it properly or it has expired. Even if the patient's pain diminishes, you

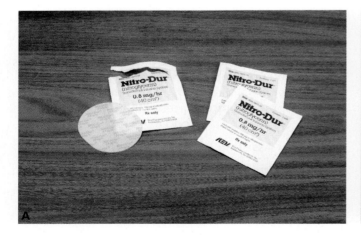
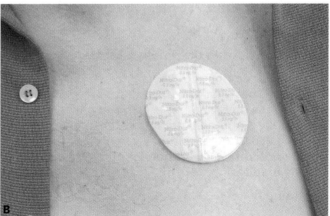

FIGURE A3.2 Transdermal nitroglycerin patches may be found applied to the patient's chest, upper arm (usually medially), or upper back.

should request an EMT response. In fact, you should arrange for patient transport every time. Anytime a patient complains of chest pain—regardless of whether it persists or whether the patient has a history of chest pain—arrange for immediate transport to a medical facility.

In recent years, the use of aspirin for the treatment of suspected heart attack has become commonplace in most hospitals and EMS systems. In fact, several pharmaceutical companies have created television and radio commercials encouraging the use of aspirin for this purpose. As an Emergency Medical Responder, you may encounter patients who have recently taken aspirin or who may want to take some while in your care. You must follow your local protocols when assisting any patient with the administration of medication.

Epinephrine Autoinjectors

Many people have allergies and will react severely to certain foods, medicines, or the poisons of insect stings or snakebites. Those reactions may be life threatening when they cause the airway to become swollen and blood vessels to dilate. Epinephrine (Scan A3–5) is a medication that can reverse those reactions. It dilates the air passages so breathing becomes easier, and it constricts the blood vessels.

Reactions to allergens can have a very sudden onset, and any reaction that causes breathing and circulation problems must be recognized and treated quickly. As a result, the patient must take his prescribed epinephrine immediately.

Those patients who are aware of their allergies and expect severe reactions generally carry a prescription with them in a device called an *autoinjector*. This is a syringe with a spring-loaded needle that will release and inject epinephrine into a muscle when the patient presses it against his skin (usually in the thigh). If you need to assist the patient in taking epinephrine, first check to see if the injector is prescribed for that patient and get permission from medical direction. Also, check the expiration date.

> **NOTE**
>
> An expired medication will be ineffective, but an allergic reaction may not be the reason for the patient's problem. Even when a patient reports that he feels better, he must be transported to a hospital as soon as possible by EMTs.

Rules to Follow When Administering Medications

Before you give any of the three medications you may carry (activated charcoal, oral glucose, or oxygen), or before you assist a patient in taking any of the three prescribed medications (metered-dose inhaler, nitroglycerin, or epinephrine), there are a few more things you need to know.

You will check the five "rights" that are rules for giving any medication. Often, you will have to rely on the patient's word. Ask the following questions:

- *Right patient?* Is this the right patient for this medication? Read aloud the name written on the medication bottle: "Is your name Henry Smith?" If the patient does not have a labeled box or bottle, simply ask if this is his own medication. If he says "yes," you may believe him.
- *Right medication?* Is this the right medication for this patient? The patient is having chest pain but hands you a bottle of penicillin, or the patient has strep throat but hands you a bottle of nitroglycerin.

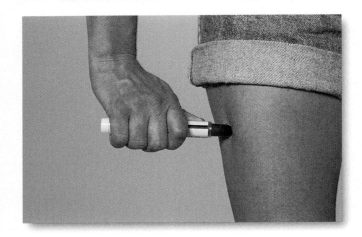

Medication Name

1 ■ Generic: epinephrine.
2 ■ Trade: Adrenalin, Epi-Pen.

Indications

Must meet the following three criteria:
1 ■ Patient exhibits signs of a severe allergic reaction, including either respiratory distress or shock.
2 ■ Medication is prescribed for this patient by a physician.
3 ■ Medical direction authorizes use for this patient.

Contraindications

No contraindications when used in a life-threatening situation.

Medication Form

Liquid administered by an autoinjector, which is an automatically injectable needle-and-syringe system.

Dosage

Adults: one adult autoinjector (0.3 mg).
Infant and child: one infant/child autoinjector (0.15 mg).

Steps for Assisting Patient

1 ■ Obtain patient's prescribed autoinjector. Ensure:
   a. Prescription is written for the patient who is experiencing the severe allergic reaction.
   b. Medication is not expired or discolored (if visible).
2 ■ Obtain order from medical direction.
3 ■ Remove cap from autoinjector.
4 ■ Place tip of autoinjector against patient's lateral thigh, midway between hip and knee.
5 ■ Push the injector firmly against the thigh until the injector activates.
6 ■ Hold the injector in place until the medication is injected (at least 10 seconds).
7 ■ Record activity and time.
8 ■ Dispose of injector in biohazard container.

Actions

1 ■ Dilates the bronchioles.
2 ■ Constricts blood vessels.

Side Effects

1 ■ Increased heart rate.
2 ■ Dizziness.
3 ■ Chest pain.
4 ■ Headache.
5 ■ Nausea.
6 ■ Vomiting.
7 ■ Excitability, anxiety.
8 ■ Pale skin.

Reassessment Strategies

1 ■ Arrange for transport.
2 ■ Continue focused assessment of airway, breathing, and circulatory status. If patient's condition continues to worsen (decreasing mental status, increasing breathing difficulty, decreasing blood pressure):
   a. Obtain medical direction for an additional dose of epinephrine.
   b. Provide care for shock, including administration of oxygen per local protocols.
   c. Prepare to initiate basic life support (CPR, AED).
3 ■ If patient's condition improves, provide supportive care:
   a. Continue oxygen.
   b. Provide care for shock.

- *Right dose?* Is this the right dose for this patient? The dosage is usually written on the label, but the patient does not always carry the original box or bottle the medication came in.
- *Right route?* Is this the right route for taking the medication? Different types of medications, such as tablets, powders, sprays, gels, slurries, and pastes, are given by different routes—swallowed by mouth, inhaled by mouth, dissolved under the tongue, and injected into or absorbed through the skin.
- *Right time?* Is this the right time to be giving the medication? In the case of nitroglycerin, has enough time elapsed since the last dose was given?

Routes for Administering Medications

The way a patient takes a medication has an effect on how quickly the medication enters the bloodstream and begins to relieve the medical condition. Medications are administered by the following routes:

- *Oral or swallowed,* usually in some solid form (a tablet or pill), or in some liquid form (powder dissolved in or mixed with a liquid such as the activated charcoal slurry).
- *Intramuscular,* or injected into a muscle, like the epinephrine autoinjector.
- *Sublingual,* or dissolved under the tongue, like the nitroglycerin tablets.
- *Inhaled,* or breathed into the lungs, from an inhaler or oxygen delivery device, such as the medication given for chronic respiratory problems or the oxygen gas given for respiratory distress and for most medical and trauma patients.
- *Endotracheal,* or sprayed into a tube inserted into the trachea (windpipe), so it can more directly reach the lungs and be absorbed quickly. (Emergency Medical Responders will not administer medication in this form.)
- *Transdermal patches or transdermal infusion systems,* affixed to the skin by an adhesive backing on one side of the patch. Another chemical is mixed in with the medication, usually a form of alcohol that will carry the medication or drug through the patient's skin into the bloodstream. These patches are slow to react and are not meant for acute attacks such as the onset of chest pain. They are meant to stay in place for one to three days or longer, depending on the type of medication. Be careful not to remove a patch, and do not leave a patch at the scene. Some can stop children from breathing. Some patches contain high enough doses to be poisonous if ingested by children and animals.
- *Intranasal,* or sprayed directly into the nasal cavity through the nostril. Studies have shown that certain medications can be rapidly and effectively absorbed through the nasal mucous membranes and into the bloodstream.

You can see there is a lot to know and understand about medications. Once you do, you will become more confident in giving the ones that you carry and the prescribed ones you can assist patients in taking. Remember, you may only administer or assist with specific medications and then only with medical direction.

Air Medical Operations

Many EMS systems across the United States use air medical resources such as helicopters (rotor-wing) and airplanes (fixed-wing) to transport critically ill and injured patients (Figure A4.1). It is estimated that there are approximately 500,000 patients transported by helicopter and another 150,000 transported by airplane in the United States each year.

Although it is unlikely for an Emergency Medical Responder to be hired to work on an EMS aircraft, your training can be the first step in becoming qualified to work there. However, as an Emergency Medical Responder, you may be in a position to request a helicopter or at the very least assist in the landing of a helicopter at the scene of an emergency.

Crew Configurations

The majority of EMS aircraft being flown in the United States are staffed with a nurse and a paramedic. The following is a list of other common medical crew configurations:

- Nurse and nurse.
- Doctor and nurse.
- Nurse and respiratory therapist.
- Paramedic and paramedic.

The specific crew configuration is often determined by local regulations and/or the type of patient being cared for. These configurations are common for both helicopters and planes.

Air Medical Resources

ROTOR-WING RESOURCES (HELICOPTER)

Most EMS helicopters fly two types of missions, the scene call and the inter-facility transport (IFT). The scene call is made when a helicopter is requested to respond to the scene of an emergency, such as a vehicle collision on the freeway or a near-drowning incident at a lake or the beach. In these cases, the helicopter is requested to respond to the scene just as a ground ambulance might. If all goes well, the helicopter will land near the patient, allowing the medical crew to exit the aircraft, begin caring for the patient, and prepare him for transport (Figure A4.2).

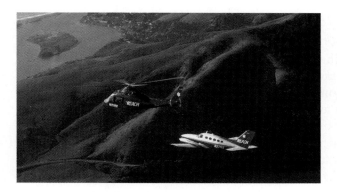

FIGURE A4.1 Both helicopters and airplanes are used in EMS today.
(© REACH, Inc./Tony Irvin)

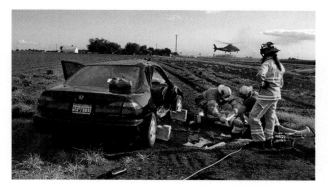

FIGURE A4.2 In many cases, a helicopter can land right at the emergency scene.
(© REACH, Inc./Rick Roach)

The *interfacility transport (IFT)* occurs when a patient is already at a hospital but needs to be transported to another hospital. In most cases, the patient is in need of a higher level of care than the sending hospital is capable of providing. For example, a patient with significant trauma transported by ground ambulance to a hospital five minutes away may need to be transported to the regional trauma center 60 miles away. An interfacility transport by aircraft would be required.

There are many different types of EMS helicopters in use today. They differ in many ways, including size, shape, number of engines, and how high or fast they can fly (Figure A4.3). Regardless of size or performance capabilities, EMS helicopters all share one very important characteristic—they are designed to carry critically ill or injured patients. The vast majority of them are configured to carry just one patient lying on a stretcher. Although some can carry two patients, the ability to provide care while in flight is greatly minimized due to the limited space. Because a helicopter can fly from hospital pad to hospital pad, it is ideal for short transports (under 200 miles).

FIXED-WING RESOURCES (AIRPLANES)

Like helicopters, fixed-wing resources vary in size and performance capabilities as well and include jets, turboprops, and piston-driven aircraft (Figure A4.4). The reason to choose an airplane over a helicopter is most often distance. Airplanes can fly much faster and farther than the typical helicopter, due largely to their ability to carry much more fuel. The airplane is ideal when there is no helipad at either hospital and the hospitals are more than 200 miles apart. Unlike the helicopter, the airplane is only capable of performing interfacility transports. This is due to the fact that it is not feasible for an airplane to land at the scene of an emergency. It can, however, land at an airport and meet a waiting ambulance.

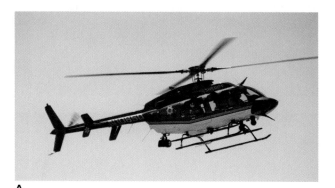

A.

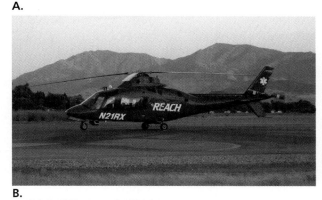

B.

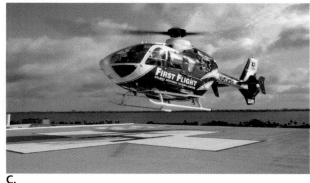

C.

FIGURE A4.3 EMS helicopters come in many shapes and sizes: **A.** Bell 407, **B.** Agusta 109, and **C.** Eurocopter EC 135
(© REACH, Inc.).

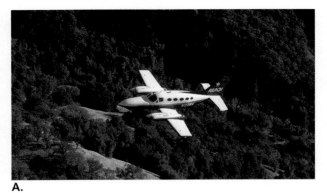

A.

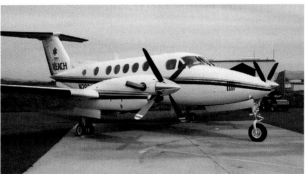

B.

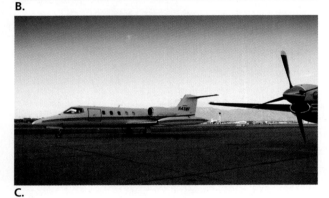

C.

FIGURE A4.4 Fixed-wing aircraft (airplanes) are used for longer transports: **A.** Cessna 421 *(© REACH, Inc./Tony Irvin)*; **B.** KingAir B200 *(© REACH, Inc.)*; and **C.** Lear Jet *(© Med Flight Air Ambulance)*.

REQUESTING AIR MEDICAL RESOURCES

In most cases, it is the first responding units that determine the need for a helicopter response. This is why it is important for you as an Emergency Medical Responder to become familiar with the air medical resources in your region and understand their capabilities and limitations.

In most cases, a helicopter is appropriate whenever expedient transport is necessary or advanced providers are required. Most helicopter medical personnel receive specialized training over and above their counterparts on an ambulance or in a hospital. This training gives them an advanced scope of practice and allows them to deliver medications and perform procedures beyond the typical nurse or paramedic.

Most EMS systems that have air medical resources will have specific protocols and/or guidelines for deciding when it is appropriate to activate an air resource. These protocols often define specific patient types such as severe trauma and critical medical, or they may also define areas of the region that are remote and thus may take hours for a typical ground ambulance transport. It is important that you familiarize yourself with your local protocols for the use of air medical resources.

Just because you request a helicopter does not mean that one will respond. EMS helicopters are a limited resource, and many things can prevent them from responding to your request. They could be committed to another emergency and therefore may be unable to respond to your request, or there could be weather in the area of the scene or at the receiving hospital that would prevent the pilot from completing the transport safely and legally.

Visual Flight Rules

All pilots must operate aircraft based on specific and clearly defined rules established by the Federal Aviation Administration (FAA). The ability to fly any particular mission will depend on at least two factors: the training and capabilities of the pilot, and the design and configuration of the aircraft. It is safe to say that most EMS aircraft operate under what are known as *visual flight rules*, or *VFR*. This means that conditions along the intended route must be clear and free of weather such as fog or clouds. A VFR mission can be flown day or night so long as there is no significant weather anywhere along the intended route of flight.

Instrument Flight Rules

Many EMS air medical programs have specially trained pilots and specially configured aircraft so they can accept a request for transport even when the weather is bad. The rules that must be followed are called *instrument flight rules*, or more simply *IFR*. Being IFR capable allows the pilot to fly into and through known weather along the route of flight. There are limitations as to the type and extent of weather an IFR pilot can fly in. For instance, there must be at least some visibility on the ground for the pilot to take off and land safely. In conditions where the fog is so thick that the pilot cannot see more than a few hundred yards, he or she may decline the request due to extreme weather conditions.

What Happens After a Request Is Made?

EMS flight programs use specially trained dispatchers called the *Flight Communication Specialist*. It is the Communication Specialist who receives the request for transport, provides an ETA to the caller, and relays the request on the flight crew in the form of a dispatch. Once the flight crew receives a dispatch, several events must take place prior to the launch of the aircraft. The pilot will perform a weather check and confirm that weather conditions along the intended route of flight are within acceptable minimums. The medical crew will gather any needed equipment and head to the aircraft. In many programs, a specific risk assessment is performed prior to each flight to ensure the highest level of safety (Figure A4.5).

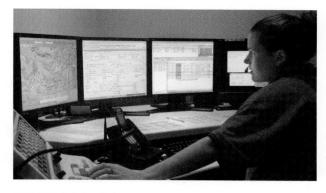

FIGURE A4.5 Flight Communication Specialists are responsible for dispatching and tracking EMS aircraft on each mission.

If the weather is acceptable and the medical crew has everything they need, all crew members approach the aircraft and perform a series of specific preflight safety checks prior to engine start and launch. If all goes well, they will be in the air and headed to their destination within minutes.

Occasionally, there will be factors that require the team to decline a request. Some of the most common reasons a crew might decline a request are poor weather conditions, mechanical failure, or patient size and weight.

Selecting an Appropriate Landing Zone

One of the characteristics that make helicopters so versatile is their ability to land nearly anywhere. The term "nearly" is used because helicopters do need a clear, flat space to set down. An appropriate space for a helicopter to land has several important characteristics and is referred to as a *landing zone, or LZ*. The following characteristics are simply general guidelines and may differ slightly from program to program. It is best to learn the specific requirements of the programs operating in your area (Figure A4.6). Characteristics of a good landing zone include:

- As close to the incident as possible.
- 100 feet × 100 feet for daytime use, or 125 feet × 125 feet for nighttime use.
- Little or no slope.
- Free of dry sand or dirt and loose debris.
- Free of utility wires near or around the site.
- Free of tall trees or poles around the site.
- Free of roaming animals.

One of the most important things you can do as an Emergency Medical Responder at the scene where a helicopter has been requested is to provide the dispatch

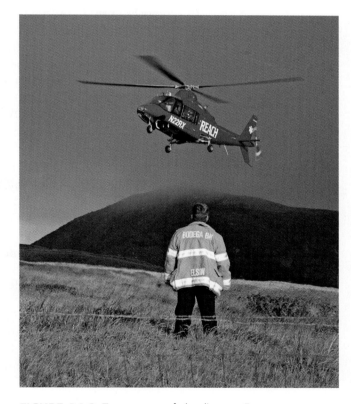

FIGURE A4.6 To ensure a safe landing, an Emergency Medical Responder should assist in the landing process. *(© REACH, Inc.)*

center with accurate GPS coordinates (latitude and longitude). If the flight crew can simply find the scene from the air based on your coordinates, they may be able to see other areas near the scene that could serve as ideal landing zones.

Once an LZ has been selected, it is important to perform a quick checklist and report the findings to the flight crew. The acronym HOTSAW is a common tool used to remember this LZ checklist:

H — Hazards. Be sure the area is free of obvious hazards such as loose debris and traffic.
O — Obstacles. Confirm that there are no obstacles such as tall trees, poles, or wires.
T — Terrain. Ensure that the area selected is firm and even.
S — Slope. Ensure that the area is as flat as possible.
A — Animals. Check to see that there are no roaming animals in the area.
W — Wind. Estimate wind speed and direction and relay that information to the flight crew.

If the area chosen for the LZ is a dirt surface, try to wet the area down prior to landing. This will avoid a big dust storm caused by the downwash from the rotor blades. An excessive amount of dirt or snow can cause the pilot to lose site of the ground, which can be very dangerous.

In most instances, a single person will be designated as the landing officer for the aircraft. This person should maintain radio contact with the flight crew during the entire landing phase whenever possible. He should stand at one side of the LZ and wave his arms to signal to the flight crew that he is the landing officer. It is important for the landing officer and others to wear proper eye and ear protection whenever working around a helicopter. Remove any hats or other loose clothing that could be blown off during the landing or departure.

If the helicopter is to land at night, *never* shine any kind of light, such as a flashlight, at the aircraft. This could temporarily blind the pilot, which could have catastrophic consequences. In most cases, the lights of your emergency vehicle will be all the pilot needs to locate the scene.

Once the aircraft is safely on the ground, maintain direct eye contact with the pilot or other flight crew members. Do not approach the aircraft until someone from the flight crew has specifically directed you to do so.

Safety Around the Aircraft

Depending on several factors, the pilot may decide to shut down at the scene or remain "hot" with the rotors spinning. Regardless of the circumstances, follow these important guidelines when working around an aircraft at an LZ:

- Never approach an aircraft unless specifically directed to do so by the flight crew.
- Never shine any light at the aircraft.
- Never walk behind an aircraft, regardless of whether or not it is shut down.
- If on a slight slope, never approach the aircraft from the uphill side.
- Always remove your hat before approaching the aircraft.

Response to Terrorism and Weapons of Mass Destruction

Terrorism

The U.S. government defines *terrorism* as "the use of force or violence against persons or property to intimidate or coerce a government, the civilian population, or any segment thereof to further political or social objectives." For years, the people of the United States remained somewhat insulated from the effects of terrorists and terrorism because they only viewed such events on the nightly news. However, terrorism is no longer something that only happens in distant countries.

In recent years, the effects of terrorism have hit home with incidents such as the bombing of the Federal Building in Oklahoma City, the spread of anthrax through the U.S. Postal Service, and the events of September 11, 2001, in New York City (Figure A5.1), Washington, DC, and Pennsylvania.

INCIDENTS INVOLVING NUCLEAR/ RADIOLOGICAL AGENTS

Until recently, the potential for a terrorist organization to obtain or develop nuclear devices was thought to be minimal. With the growing supply of nuclear waste on a worldwide scale and the developing technology of Third World countries, the likelihood of a nuclear threat by a terrorist organization is ever increasing.

There are two types of potential nuclear incidents. One is the possible detonation of a nuclear device, and the other is the detonation of a conventional explosive incorporating nuclear material. A plausible scenario involves the detonation of a *radiological dispersal device (RDD)*, which would spread radioactive material across a wide area surrounding the blast site. Another scenario involves the detonation of a large *explosive device* (such as a truck bomb) near a nuclear power plant or radiological cargo transport.

Nuclear incidents emit three main types of radioactive particles: alpha, beta, and gamma.

- *Alpha particles* are the heaviest and most highly charged of the nuclear particles. They are easily stopped by human skin but can become a serious hazard if ingested or inhaled.
- *Beta particles* are smaller and travel much faster and farther than alpha particles. Beta particles can penetrate through the skin but rarely reach the vital organs. Although they can cause burns to the skin if exposure lasts long enough, the biggest threat occurs when they are ingested or inhaled into the body. Beta particles also can enter the body through unprotected open wounds.
- *Gamma rays* are a type of radiation that travels through the air in the form of waves. The rays can travel great distances and penetrate most materials,

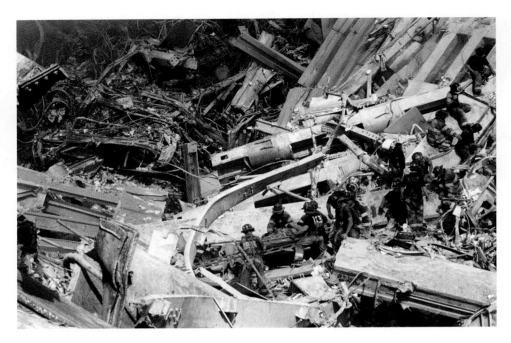

FIGURE A5.1 World Trade Center, September 2001
(© David Turnley/Corbis)

including the human body. Acute radiation sickness occurs when someone is exposed to large doses of gamma radiation over a short period of time and can cause symptoms such as skin irritation, burns, nausea, vomiting, high fever, and hair loss.

INCIDENTS INVOLVING BIOLOGICAL AGENTS

Biological agents pose one of the most serious threats due to their accessibility and ability to spread rapidly. The potential is also very high for widespread casualties. Biological agents are most dangerous when either inhaled (spread through the air) or ingested (through contaminated food or water supplies).

There are four common types of biological agents: bacteria, rickettsia, viruses, and toxins:

- *Bacteria* are single-celled organisms that can quickly cause disease in humans. Some of the more common bacteria used for terrorist activities are anthrax, cholera, the plague, and tularemia.
- *Rickettsia* are smaller than bacteria cells and live inside individual host cells. An example of rickettsia is *Coxiella burnetii*, which is the organism that causes Q fever.
- *Viruses* are the simplest of microorganisms and cannot survive without a living host. The most common viruses that have served as biological agents include smallpox, Venezuelan equine encephalitis, and Ebola, among others.
- *Toxins* are substances that occur naturally in the environment and can be produced by an animal, plant, or microbe. They differ from biological agents in that they are not manufactured. The four common toxins with a history of use as terrorist weapons are botulism, SEB (staphylococcal enterotoxin), ricin, and mycotoxins. Ricin has been used in several well-publicized incidents in the United States and Japan. It is a toxin made from the castor bean plant, which is grown around the world.

INCIDENTS INVOLVING CHEMICAL AGENTS

The primary routes of exposure for chemical agents are inhalation, ingestion, and absorption or contact with the skin, with inhalation being the most common. The five classifications of chemical agents are nerve agents, vesicant (blister) agents, cyanogens agents, pulmonary agents, and riot-control agents.

Nerve Agents

Nerve agents disrupt the nerve impulse transmissions throughout the body and are extremely toxic in very small quantities. In some cases, a single small drop can be fatal to an average human. Nerve agents include sarin (GB), which has been used against Japanese and Iraqi civilians; soman (GD); tabun (GA); and V agent (VX). These are liquid agents that are typically spread in the form of an aerosol spray.

In the case of GA, GB, and GD, the first letter "G" stands for the country (Germany) that developed the agent. The second letter indicates the order in which the agent was developed. In the case of VX, the "V" stands for venom and the "X" represents one of the chemicals that make up the compound. These agents resemble water or clear oil in their purest form and possess no odor. Sometimes small explosives are used to spread them, which can cause widespread death. Many dead animals at the scene of an incident may be an outward warning sign or detection clue. Early signs of nerve agent exposure are:

- Uncontrolled salivation.
- Urination.
- Defecation.
- Tearing.

Other later signs and symptoms include:

- Blurred vision.
- Excessive sweating.
- Muscle tremors.
- Difficulty breathing.
- Nausea, vomiting.
- Abdominal pain.

Vesicant Agents

Vesicant agents are more commonly referred to as blister or mustard agents due to their unique smell. They can easily penetrate several layers of clothing and are quickly absorbed into the skin. Mustard (H, HD, HN) and Lewisite (L, HL) are common vesicants. Although less toxic than nerve agents, it takes only a few drops on the skin to cause severe injury. The signs and symptoms of vesicant exposure include:

- Reddening, swelling, and tearing of the eyes.
- Tenderness and burning of the skin followed by the development of fluid-filled blisters.
- Nausea, vomiting.
- Severe abdominal pain.
- After about two hours, victims will experience runny nose, burning in the throat, and shortness of breath.

Cyanogens

Cyanogens are agents that interfere with the ability of the blood to carry oxygen and can cause asphyxiation in victims of exposure. Common cyanogens are hydrogen cyanide (AC) and cyanogens chloride (CK). All cyanogens are very toxic in high concentrations and can lead to rapid death. Under pressure, these agents are in liquid form. In their pure form, they are a gas. Cyanogens are common industrial chemicals used in a variety of processes, and all have an aroma similar to bitter almonds or peach blossoms. Signs and symptoms of cyanogens exposure include:

- Severe respiratory distress.
- Vomiting.
- Diarrhea.
- Dizziness, headache.
- Seizures, coma.

It is essential that victims of exposure be quickly moved to fresh air and treated for respiratory distress.

Pulmonary Agents

Pulmonary agents are sometimes called *choking agents*. They directly affect the respiratory system, causing fluid buildup (edema) in the lungs, which in turn causes asphyxiation similar to that seen in drowning victims. Chlorine and phosgene are two of the most common of these agents and are commonly found in industrial settings. Chlorine is a familiar smell to most people. Phosgene has an aroma of freshly cut hay. Both chemicals are in a gaseous state in their pure form and are stored in bottles or cylinders. Signs and symptoms include:

- Severe eye irritation.
- Coughing.
- Choking.
- Severe respiratory distress.

Riot Control Agents

Riot-control agents include both irritating and psychedelic agents, both of which are designed to incapacitate the victim. For the most part, they are not lethal. However, under certain circumstances, irritating agents have been known to cause asphyxiation. In some individuals, psychedelic agents have been known to cause behavior that can lead to death.

Common irritating agents include mace, tear gas, and pepper spray. These agents will typically cause severe pain when they come in contact with the skin, especially moist areas such as the nose, mouth, and eyes.

Signs and symptoms of exposure to irritating agents include:

- Burning and irritation in the eyes and throat.
- Coughing, choking.
- Respiratory distress.
- Nausea.
- Vomiting.

Psychedelic agents include lysergic acid diethylamide (LSD), 3-quinuclidinyl benzilate (BZ), and benctyzine. These agents alter the nervous system, causing visual and aural hallucinations and severe changes in thought processes and behavior. The effects of these agents can be unpredictable, ranging from overwhelming fear to extreme belligerence.

Role of the Emergency Medical Responder

Terrorist attacks are meant to cause fear, and they are likely to occur when they are least expected. Having a high index of suspicion and recognizing the outward warning signs of a possible terrorist attack is of utmost importance for the first units on scene. Donning the appropriate personal protective equipment (PPE) early will minimize the chances of all emergency responders becoming victims themselves.

Firefighters are probably the best prepared of all Emergency Medical Responders because of the wide range of duties they are trained and expected to perform. Ambulance personnel are probably the least equipped to respond to a terrorist attack because their personal protective equipment is primarily designed to minimize exposure to body fluids and aerosolized droplets from coughing patients.

Without the proper training and equipment, Emergency Medical Responders are likely to become victims if they enter the scene too quickly. In most cases, the best action will be to recognize the danger as soon as possible and retreat to a safe distance from the scene. Requesting appropriate resources such as specialized hazardous materials teams will be important.

NOTE

Many terrorists will set a secondary device that is meant to incapacitate or kill responders. These devices may be set to go off 10 to 15 minutes after the first one. By doing this, terrorists will be sure that the device will go off while rescuers are caring for patients who were injured by the first one. Make sure that the scene is truly safe before entering.

Decontamination

Decontamination is the process by which chemical, biological, and/or radiological agents are removed from exposed victims, equipment, and the environment. Regardless of whether the incident is a hazardous materials release or an intentional terrorist act, prompt decontamination can be the single most important aspect of the operation to minimize exposure and limit casualties.

Depending on the size and scope of the incident, Emergency Medical Responders may be asked to assist with the decontamination process. If not part of the decontamination process, they will certainly play an important role in the emergency care given to patients after coming out of decontamination. It will be important for Emergency Medical Responders assisting at such an event to continue to wear the appropriate personal protective equipment, even after a victim has been decontaminated. This will minimize any contamination from residual agents remaining on the victim or equipment.

Swimming and Diving Incidents

The amount of time spent on this subject in your Emergency Medical Responder course will depend on the area in which you live and the length of your course. There are few new procedures to learn about caring for patients who have had swimming or diving emergencies. Of key importance to you will be learning the types of injuries associated with water incidents and knowing the care skills used when the patient is a near-drowning victim.

Do not attempt a water rescue unless you have been trained to do so, you are a good swimmer, and others are on hand to help. Never attempt a water rescue by yourself. A personal flotation device (PFD) should be worn by all those involved in a water rescue. Except for shallow pools and open, shallow waters with uniform bottoms, the problems faced in water rescue are too great and too dangerous for the poor swimmer or untrained person to attempt. If not being able to help bothers you, take a course in water safety and rescue. Otherwise, you will probably become a victim yourself, rather than the person who rescues and provides care.

Mouth-to-mask techniques and CPR are not practical while the patient is in the water. Follow your EMS system guidelines.

Water-Related Incidents

Most people, when they think of water-related incidents, tend to think only of drowning. There is no doubt that drowning must be the number one consideration, even when the first problem faced by a person in the water is an injury or a medical emergency.

Injuries occur on, in, and near the water. Boating, water skiing, and diving incidents produce airway obstructions, fractures, bleeding, and soft-tissue injuries. Other types of incidents, such as falls from bridges and motor-vehicle collisions, also may involve the water. In these cases, the victims suffer injuries normally associated with the underlying mechanism of injury plus the effects of the water hazard (drowning, hypothermia, delayed care because of complicated rescue, and so on).

Sometimes, the mishap or drowning may have been caused by a medical emergency that took place while the patient was in the water or on a boat. Knowing how the incident occurred may give you clues to detecting the medical emergency. As with all aspects of Emergency Medical Responder care, consider the mechanism of injury or nature of illness and perform a thorough patient assessment. They may be critical in deciding the procedures to be followed when caring for a patient.

Learn to associate the problems of drowning with scenes other than swimming pools and beaches. Remember, bathtub drownings do occur. Only a few inches of water are needed for an adult to drown. Even less is required for an infant.

As an Emergency Medical Responder, take particular care to look for the following when your patient is the victim of a water-related mishap:

- Airway obstruction may be from water, foreign matter in the airway, or a swollen airway (often seen if the neck is injured in a dive). Spasms along the airway are common in cases of near-drowning.
- Cardiac arrest is usually related to respiratory arrest.
- Through overexertion, the patient may have greater problems than the obvious near-drowning. Often, inexperienced rescuers are fooled into thinking that chest pains reported by the patient are due to muscle cramps produced during swimming or the panic of a near-drowning situation.
- Injuries to the head and neck are to be expected in boating, water skiing, and diving incidents, but they also occur in cases of near-drowning.
- While performing a patient assessment, be on the alert for suspected fractures or dislocations, soft-tissue injuries, and internal bleeding. The fact that the patient is suffering from internal bleeding is often missed during the first stages of care because of the concern for other problems associated with near-drowning. Constantly monitor patients for the signs and symptoms of shock.
- The water does not have to be overly cold and the length of stay in the water does not have to be very long for hypothermia to occur.

REACHING THE VICTIM

The U.S. Coast Guard, the American Red Cross, and the YMCA offer water safety and rescue courses. Unless you are a good swimmer and have been trained in water rescue, do not go into the water to save someone.

Reach, Throw, Then Go

If the patient is close to shore or poolside, attempt to reach and pull the patient from the water. If unable to reach the victim with your hand, attempt to use a branch, a fishing pole, an oar, a stick, or other such object. A towel, a shirt, or an article of your own clothing may work as well. In cases where there is no object near at hand or conditions are such that you may only have one opportunity to grab the person (for example, strong currents), lie down flat on your stomach and extend your arm or leg (not recommended for the nonswimmer). In all cases, make sure that your position is secure and that you will not be pulled into the water. This is critical if you are extending an arm or leg to the person. If the victim is some distance away from the shore or edge, attempt to throw something to him. In this case, it is best to use a rope (line).

If the person is alert but too far away to be pulled from the water, then you must carefully throw an object that will float. A personal flotation device (PFD), life jacket, or ring buoy (life preserver) is ideal, but these objects may not be at the scene. If that is the case, then the best course of action is to throw anything that will float and to do this as soon as possible (Figure A6.1). Objects you might use include inflated automobile tubes, foam cushions, plastic jugs, logs, boards, plastic picnic containers,

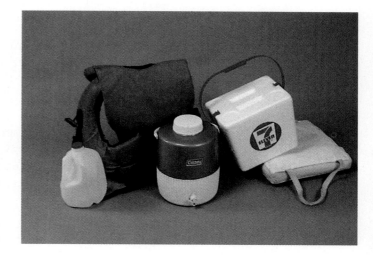

FIGURE A6.1 Throw the patient anything that will float.

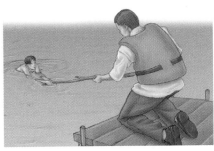
Reach

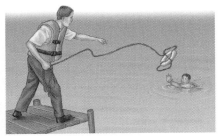
Throw

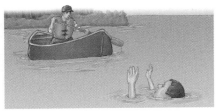
Then go

FIGURE A6.2 Pull the patient from the water, throw an object that will float, and try to tow, or, if necessary and you are properly equipped and trained, go to the patient.

surfboards, pieces of wood, large balls, and plastic toys. Two empty, capped plastic milk jugs can keep an adult afloat for hours. It is best to tie rope to the objects so that they can be retrieved if they do not land near the patient. You may have to add some water to lightweight plastic jugs so that you can throw them the required distance.

Once you are sure that the person has a flotation device or floating object to hold on to, try to find a way to tow the patient to shore. Throw the patient a line or another flotation device attached to a line. Make sure that your own position is a safe one. If conditions are safe and you are a strong swimmer, wade no deeper than your waist if you must reduce the distance for throwing the line.

You may find that the near-drowning victim is too far from shore to allow for throwing and towing, or the victim may be unresponsive and unable to react to your efforts. In such cases, if there is a boat at the scene, you may be able to take the boat to the patient. Do not go to the patient if you cannot swim. Even if you are a swimmer, you must wear a personal flotation device while you are in the boat. In cases where the patient is alert, try to have the patient grab an oar or the rear of the boat. Take great care in helping the person into the boat. This is a tricky process in a canoe. If the canoe or boat tips over, stay with the vessel, holding on to its bottom or side. It will almost certainly stay afloat. If you take a boat out and find that the patient is unresponsive, assume that the patient has a neck or spine injury.

Again, in water rescue situations (Figure A6.2), begin by trying to pull the patient from the water. If this cannot be done, throw objects that will float and try to tow the patient from the water. Do not try to take a boat to the victim if you cannot swim. Wear a personal flotation device while in the boat. Unless you are a good swimmer and trained in water rescue and life-saving, do not swim to the patient. Even so, wear a personal flotation device.

CARE FOR THE PATIENT

Patient with No Neck or Spine Injuries

In all cases of shallow-water incidents, assume that the unresponsive patient has neck and spine injuries. If the patient can be removed quickly from the water using a cervical collar and spine board or if the patient is out of the water when you arrive, you should:

1. Start your initial assessment of the patient.
2. If needed, provide mouth-to-mask resuscitation as quickly as possible. Check for airway obstruction.

> **NOTE**
>
> Mouth-to-mask techniques are usually not practical when the patient is in the water because much of your effort will be in keeping the patient's face above the surface. It is most practical to use the mouth-to-mouth procedure, but know that this might expose you to potentially infectious body fluids. *Follow your local EMS guidelines.*

3. Once the patient is out of the water, provide CPR, if needed. As in all such cases, make certain that someone has activated the EMS system.
4. If the patient is breathing and has a pulse, check for bleeding and attempt to control any serious bleeding that you find.

5. If there is breathing and a pulse, perform a patient assessment. But first cover the patient to conserve body heat. Also be sure to put something under the patient to prevent heat loss. Uncover only those areas of the patient's body involved in assessment. Care for any problems you may find. Remove wet clothing if there are no injuries that must first be stabilized.

6. If the patient can be moved, take him to a warm place. Do not allow the near-drowning patient to walk. Handle the patient gently at all times.

7. Provide care for shock and check again to make certain that the EMS system has been activated.

You may find more resistance than expected to your efforts to provide breaths to someone with water in the airway. Apply more force, if necessary, once you are certain that no foreign objects are obstructing the airway. Watch the patient's chest rise and fall. Adjust your ventilations as needed to help prevent gastric distention. Remember, you must not delay ventilating the patient.

Many times, a patient with water in the airway will also have water in the stomach. This may provide resistance to your efforts to resuscitate the patient. When this happens, you may find that some of the air from your breaths will go into the patient's stomach, even when you adjust your ventilations. Current American Heart Association and American Red Cross guidelines indicate that you should not attempt to relieve water or air from the patient's stomach (unless immediate suctioning is available) due to the risk of forcing material from the stomach to enter the patient's airway, even to the point of entering the lungs. When gastric distention occurs, reposition the airway and continue with resuscitation, making sure the breaths are slow and full.

NOTE

Drowning victims who are resuscitated are likely to vomit. Rescuers should have suction ready and be prepared to clear the airway when this occurs.

Humans have a reaction in cold water that is similar to other mammals. This reaction is called the *mammalian diving reflex*. When the face of a person or other mammal is submerged in cold water, the mammalian diving reflex slows down the body's metabolism, which results in a decrease in oxygen consumption. At the same time, the reflex causes a redistribution of blood to more vital organs—the brain, heart, and lungs. The diving reflex is more pronounced in infants and children, and they may fare better in cold-water drowning than adults. Start CPR on all drowning victims as soon as they are pulled from the water. CPR should continue while en route to the hospital. Cases have been reported in which cold-water drowning victims, especially children, were revived and fully recovered after being in the water for longer than 30 minutes. Never believe that a person has drowned; rather, consider the victim to be a near-drowning patient.

As an Emergency Medical Responder, you must be realistic when dealing with drownings. Many patients cannot be successfully resuscitated. The effects of water in the airway and the lack of oxygen to the brain may be too harsh for the body to endure. You may resuscitate some patients only to find out that they died within 48 hours due to pneumonia, lung damage, or brain damage. Even when you provide the best of care, some patients will die. However, you must give patients every opportunity for survival. You will not be able to tell which patient will survive. Provide resuscitation for all drowning victims.

Patient with Neck or Spine Injuries

Injuries to the neck (cervical spine) and the rest of the spinal column occur during many water-related incidents. For Emergency Medical Responder care, you will not be expected to know how to use long spine boards and other floating, rigid devices for rescue situations. But you will be able to take certain actions to protect a patient's neck and spine during both rescue and care.

If a patient is unresponsive, neck and spine injuries may not be easily detected. In such a situation, assume that the patient has them and provide care accordingly. Also assume neck and spine injuries whenever you assess a water emergency patient and find head injuries. Learn to quickly evaluate the patient for possible neck and spine injuries. Remember that you will not have time to do a complete test for such injuries in patients who are in the water. Likewise, a complete assessment will not be possible for any patient you find in respiratory or cardiac arrest.

When a patient with possible neck and spine injuries is responsive and you are in shallow warm water, stabilize the patient until the EMS system responds with personnel trained to remove the patient from the water. Simply keep the patient floating in a face-up position while you support the back and stabilize the head and neck (Scan A6–1). However, seldom will this be the case. Too often, the water will be too cold or too deep, or there will be dangerous tides or currents. Often, in those conditions, the patient will need resuscitation and will have to be removed from the water as quickly as possible. Even so, it is better to wait for trained, equipped rescue personnel to help remove a breathing patient from the water rather than risk injuring the patient's spine by doing it yourself.

If you arrive at the scene and find the unresponsive patient has already been removed from the water, have someone activate the EMS system and begin your initial assessment. Provide life support care as needed, using the jaw-thrust maneuver rather than the head-tilt, chin-lift maneuver. After breathing and circulation are ensured, and bleeding is cared for, perform a patient assessment, providing care as needed. Keep the patient warm and provide care for shock. Unless absolutely necessary, do not move the patient if there is any chance of neck or spine injuries.

If the patient is still in the water, do not attempt a rescue unless you are a good swimmer, are trained to do so, and have others on hand who can help you. Make certain that someone activates the EMS system. This should be done immediately. Do not wait until after the rescue is attempted. Valuable time will be lost if the rescue fails. Providing care for a possible spine injury patient still in the water requires you to:

1. Turn the patient face up in the water. This should be done while you are in the water and wearing a personal flotation device. To turn the patient, you should:
   a. Position yourself at the patient's side, as shown in Scan A6–1. Grasp the patient's arms midway between the elbow and shoulder and gently float them above the patient's head.
   b. Clasp the patient's arms firmly against his head to brace the neck and keep the head in line. Move forward in the water to bring the patient's body to the surface and in line.
   c. Rotate the patient by pushing down on the near arm and pulling the far arm toward you, making sure you brace the patient's head firmly with his arms. Do not lift the patient.
   d. Once the patient is face up, maintain pressure on the patient's arms to brace the head.
   e. In shallow water, you can hold the patient's arms with one hand and support the hips with the other.

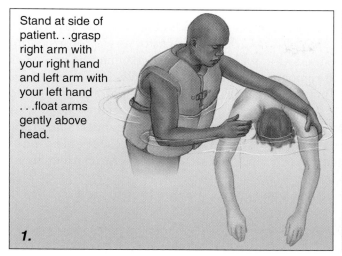

1. Stand at side of patient. . .grasp right arm with your right hand and left arm with your left hand . . .float arms gently above head.

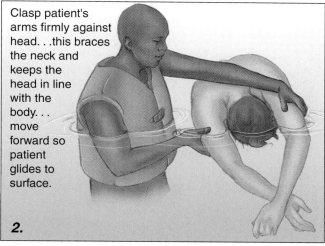

2. Clasp patient's arms firmly against head. . .this braces the neck and keeps the head in line with the body. . . move forward so patient glides to surface.

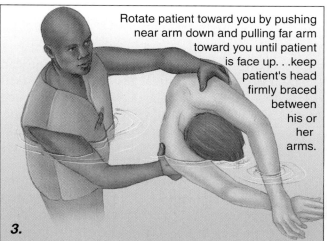

3. Rotate patient toward you by pushing near arm down and pulling far arm toward you until patient is face up. . .keep patient's head firmly braced between his or her arms.

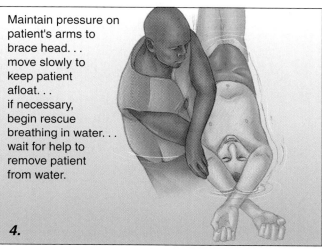

4. Maintain pressure on patient's arms to brace head. . . move slowly to keep patient afloat. . . if necessary, begin rescue breathing in water. . . wait for help to remove patient from water.

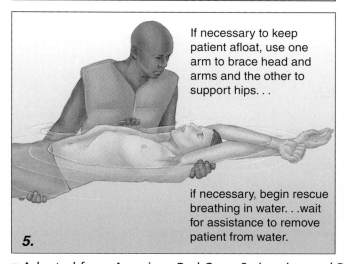

5. If necessary to keep patient afloat, use one arm to brace head and arms and the other to support hips. . .

   if necessary, begin rescue breathing in water. . .wait for assistance to remove patient from water.

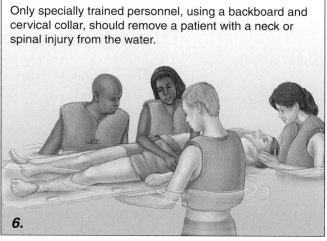

6. Only specially trained personnel, using a backboard and cervical collar, should remove a patient with a neck or spinal injury from the water.

■ Adapted from American Red Cross *Swimming and Diving*.

f. In deeper water, continue to move toward shallow water where you can stand or can be supported by someone else.

2. If necessary, begin your initial assessment while the patient is still in the water. Do not delay the detection of respiratory arrest.

3. If needed, provide rescue breathing as soon as possible. Use the jaw-thrust maneuver to protect the patient's neck and spine. Check for airway obstruction. CPR and mouth-to-mask resuscitation will not be effective while the patient is in the water. Give priority to removing the patient from the water.

4. If someone is there to help you, have him support the patient along the midline of the back while you provide support to the patient's head and neck. Float the patient to shore and continue to provide back and neck support as shown in Scan A6–1. Wait for trained rescue personnel equipped with a backboard and cervical collar to remove the patient from the water.

> **NOTE**
>
> Attempt to remove the patient from the water yourself *only* if trained rescue personnel will not arrive soon and the patient has no heartbeat. You must make every effort to maintain in-line stabilization of the patient's body. Support the patient's head and neck while those helping you lift the patient from the water.

5. Once the patient is out of the water, attempts at respiratory resuscitation can begin. Check for a pulse to see if CPR should be started. If you are by yourself and must row a cardiac arrest patient to shore, delay CPR until you reach shore. You cannot row a boat and perform CPR. Also, CPR will be more effective on shore. In some cases, depending on the boat's stability and water conditions, you may be able to provide effective CPR in the boat until other rescuers arrive.

6. If the patient is breathing, check for and control all serious bleeding. Cover the patient to conserve body heat and perform a patient assessment, caring for any injuries you may find. Do not move the patient if there are any signs of possible neck or spine injuries.

7. Give care for shock and make sure the EMS system has been activated.

Diving Incidents

DIVING BOARD INCIDENTS

Each year, many people are injured as they attempt dives or enter the water from diving boards. These same injuries are seen in dives from poolsides, docks, boats, and the shore. A large number of such cases involve teenagers.

Most diving board incidents involve the head and neck. As an Emergency Medical Responder, you will also see injuries to the spine, hands, feet, and ribs occurring with great frequency. Any part of the body can be injured in these types of emergencies, requiring complete assessment of all patients unless you are providing life support measures. Remember, a medical emergency may have led to the diving incident.

Once the patient is out of the water, care will be the same as for any victim of trauma. Care in the water and while removing the patient from the water is the same as for any patient who may have skull, neck, or spine injuries. Be sure to look for delayed reactions, particularly weakness, tingling sensations, or numbness in the limbs.

SCUBA DIVING INCIDENTS

The word *scuba* is short for self-contained underwater breathing apparatus. Scuba diving emergencies have increased with the popularity of the sport and with inexperienced divers going into the water without the benefit of proper training. Scuba diving emergencies can produce body injuries or near-drownings. Medical problems can lead to a scuba diving emergency. However, two special problems are seen in scuba diving incidents. They are gas bubbles in the diver's blood and the "bends."

An air embolism, or gas bubbles in the blood, occurs when gases leave a diver's injured lung and enter the bloodstream. This happens for many reasons, although it is most often associated with divers who hold their breath because of inadequate training, equipment failure, underwater emergency, or when trying to conserve air during a long dive. An air embolism can develop in the automobile collision victim who is trapped below water, as he takes gulps of air from air bubbles held inside the vehicle.

Air embolism can develop in both shallow and deep waters. The onset is rapid, with signs of personality changes and distorted senses sometimes giving the impression of drunkenness. The patient may have convulsions and rapidly become unresponsive. There may be signs of air outside the lungs being trapped in the chest cavity.

You should suspect possible air embolism when the patient has any of the following signs or symptoms:

- Personality changes.
- Distorted senses. Blurred vision is most common.
- Chest pains.
- Numbness and tingling sensations in the arms and/or legs.
- Total body weakness, or weakness of one or more limbs.
- Frothy blood in the mouth or nose.
- Convulsions.

The bends are really part of what is called *decompression sickness*. Patients with decompression sickness usually are those individuals who have come up too quickly from a deep, prolonged dive. When they do this, nitrogen gas is trapped in their tissues and may find its way into the bloodstream. The onset of the bends is usually slow for scuba divers, taking from one to 48 hours to appear. Because of this delay, the patient interview and reports from the patient's family and friends may be your only clue to relate the patient's problems to a dive.

NOTE

Scuba divers increase the risk of decompression sickness if they fly within 12 hours following a dive.

The signs and symptoms of decompression sickness include:

- Fatigue.
- Pain to the muscles and joints (the bends).
- Numbness or paralysis.
- Choking, coughing, and/or labored breathing.
- Chest pains.
- Collapse and unresponsiveness.
- Blotches on the skin (mottling). Sometimes, these rashes keep changing appearance.

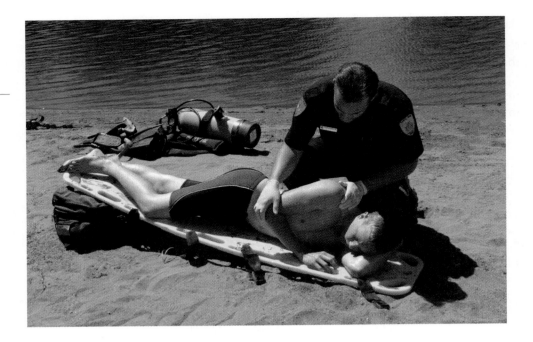

If you think a patient has gas bubbles in the blood or decompression sickness due to a dive, be certain that the dispatcher is aware of the problem. The patient will need EMT transport to a medical facility as soon as possible. Dispatch may want to direct the EMTs to take the patient to a special facility (hyperbaric trauma center) where a patient is exposed to oxygen under greatly increased pressure conditions. This procedure is done in a sealed hyperbaric chamber.

While waiting for the EMTs to arrive, provide care for shock and constantly monitor the patient. Respiratory and cardiac arrest are possible. Positioning of the patient is critical in order to avoid gas bubbles in the blood damaging the brain. Place the patient on the left side. The patient may be placed in a slight head-down position, but for no more than 10 minutes and only if it can be maintained without impairing breathing or other resuscitative measures (Figure A6.3). Provide oxygen as per local protocols.

Ice-Related Incidents

Ice rescues require special training. Unless you are trained specifically to work on ice, do not attempt a rescue. If you cannot swim, you have no business going onto the ice. You may walk on an undetected thin spot, fall through the ice, and quickly drown. All rescuers who are on or at the edge of the ice must wear personal flotation devices.

The major problem faced in ice rescue is reaching the victim. Never walk out to the person or attempt to enter the water through a hole in the ice in order to find the victim. Never attempt an ice rescue by yourself unless you have some basic equipment, such as a personal flotation device and a ladder, and you are specifically trained in one-rescuer techniques. Never go onto ice that is rapidly breaking up. Your best course of action will be to work with others from a safe ice surface or the shore (Figure A6.4).

As the first choice of action, throw a line to the victim or reach out with a stick or a pole. If the victim is not holding on to the ice, but trying to keep afloat in open water, throw anything that will float. Do not try to go onto the ice to rescue the victim. Call for help immediately. Ice rescues require special training, protective clothing, and rescue equipment.

If you have had specialized training and the necessary equipment and personnel and you have to go onto the ice to get the patient, it is strongly recommended that you work with other trained help. Pushing a long ladder out onto the ice and then crawling along the ladder is a very effective method of safe rescue, providing someone is holding the ladder from a safe position. If enough people are on hand, a human chain can be formed to reach the patient; however, these people should be trained and wearing PFDs.

One of the few methods of ice rescue that can be tried by the single rescuer is the use of a light boat. This craft can be moved along the ice by riding inside of the boat and pushing the ice with your hands or with a stick or an oar. This is often a slow and awkward method, but if the ice cracks, at least you are safe in a boat.

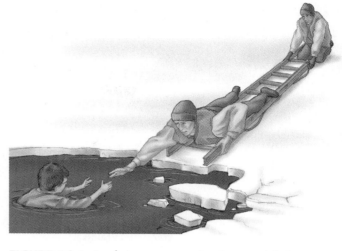

FIGURE A6.4 A safe ice rescue requires teamwork between specially trained Emergency Medical Responders.

Expect to find injuries with any patient who has fallen through the ice. Broken leg bones are common. Hypothermia is often a problem and should always be considered. Do not attempt to rewarm the severely hypothermic patient.

Activate the EMS system for all patients who have had incidents on ice or have been in cold water. There may be injuries that are difficult to detect and problems because of the cold that may be delayed.

ASSISTING THE EMTs

You may be the first on the scene of a water or an ice rescue and have the EMTs arrive during rescue or care. At other times, you may arrive at the scene after the EMTs. Some of the things you can do to help, if directed to do so, might be to:

- Interview bystanders. The information gained could indicate the number of victims, a hidden medical emergency, or the cause of the incident.
- Both the curiosity seeker and those wanting to help may come to the scene. Unless controlled, they may hinder rescue, fall into the water, or place too much weight on the ice surface.
- Additional help is usually required in emergencies involving ice.
- You may have to look for a ladder or a boat.
- Two-rescuer CPR, positioning the patient, and splinting the patient may require your aid.
- If you are a good swimmer and have been trained in water rescue, the EMTs may need you in the water. Remember that a spine board will float and will pop up easily from below the surface of the water. If you are called on to help place a spine board under a patient who is still in the water, make sure of your position so as not to slip, and keep a firm grip on the board. If you have any doubts as to what the EMTs want you to do, ask questions.

Student Learning Skill Sheets

Bleeding Control/Shock Management

STEPS TO BE PERFORMED	ACTION/VERBAL RESPONSE	POINTS
*Takes or verbalizes appropriate BSI precautions.	I am taking appropriate BSI precautions.	(1)
Applies direct pressure to wound.	Using an appropriate dressing, I am applying direct pressure to the wound.	(1)
Elevates the extremity.	I am now elevating the extremity to help slow the bleeding.	(1)
The examiner states: The wound continues to bleed.		
Applies additional dressing to the wound.	I will now apply an additional dressing to the wound without removing the original dressing.	(1)
The examiner states: The wound continues to bleed. The second dressing does not control the bleeding.		
Applies appropriate pressure point.	I am locating and applying pressure to the appropriate arterial pressure point.	(1)
The examiner states: The bleeding is now controlled.		
Applies clean dressing.	I am replacing the outer blood-soaked dressings with fresh ones.	(1)
Applies appropriate pressure bandage.	I am applying a clean bandage to secure the dressing to the wound.	(1)
The examiner states: The patient is showing signs and symptoms of shock.		
Properly positions the patient.	I will now lay the patient down with feet elevated.	(1)
Initiates appropriate oxygen therapy.	I will now place the patient on supplemental oxygen.	(1)
Initiates steps to prevent heat loss from the patient.	I will now cover the patient with a blanket to preserve heat.	(1)
Indicates need for immediate transportation.	I will categorize this patient as high priority for transport.	(1)

Bleeding Control/Shock Management *(continued)*

* = CRITICAL CRITERIA *(Must Perform to Pass)*	TOTAL POINTS (11 pts) PASSING: 80% = (8 pts)	

Start Time: _____ Date: _____

Stop Time: _____

Student's Name: _____

Evaluator's Name: _____

_____ **Did not take or verbalize BSI precautions**

_____ **Applies tourniquet before attempting other methods of bleeding control**

_____ **Did not control hemorrhage in a timely manner**

_____ **Did not indicate a need for immediate transportation**

Bag-Valve Mask—Nonbreathing Patient

STEPS TO BE PERFORMED	ACTION/VERBAL RESPONSE	POINTS
*Takes or verbalizes appropriate BSI precautions.	I am taking appropriate BSI precautions.	(1)
Opens airway (manually or with adjunct).	I will ensure an open airway either manually or by inserting an appropriate adjunct device.	(1)
Selects appropriate mask.	I will select an appropriate mask and connect it to the BVM device.	(1)
Connects to oxygen supply.	I will now connect the BVM to the liter flow valve on the regulator and adjust to 15 LPM.	(1)
Establishes and maintains a proper mask-to-face seal.	I will now place the mask over the patient's face and ensure a tight seal around the mask.	(1)
Instructs assistant to ventilate patient.	I will now instruct my assistant to ventilate the patient once every five seconds or approximately 12 times per minute. I will watch for chest rise and fall to determine proper volume.	(1)

NOTE: Examiner must observe proper ventilations for at least 30 seconds.

* = CRITICAL CRITERIA (Must Perform to Pass)	TOTAL POINTS (6 pts) PASSING: 80% = (5 pts)	

Start Time: _____ Date: _____

Stop Time: _____

Student's Name: _____

Evaluator's Name: _____

_____ Did not take or verbalize BSI precautions

_____ Did not immediately ventilate the patient

_____ Interrupted ventilations for more than 20 seconds

_____ Did not provide high-concentration oxygen

_____ Did not provide adequate tidal volume during ventilations

_____ Did not allow for adequate exhalation

Immobilization—Long Bone Injury

STEPS TO BE PERFORMED	ACTION/VERBAL RESPONSE	POINTS
*Takes or verbalizes appropriate BSI precautions.	I am taking appropriate BSI precautions.	(1)
Directs application of manual stabilization of injury.	I will either direct the patient to continue holding the injury still or ask my partner to take over for the patient.	(1)
Assesses circulation, sensation, and motor function.	I will now assess circulation, sensation, and motor function of the extremity.	(1)

Examiner states: Circulation, sensation, and motor function are present and normal.

Measures immobilization device.	I will now select an appropriate device and size it to ensure that it will fit the extremity.	(1)
Applies device.	I will now apply the device to the extremity, ensuring that it is well padded.	(1)
Immobilizes joint above the injury site.	I will now immobilize the joint above the injury site.	(1)
Immobilizes the joint below the injury site.	I will now immobilize the joint below the injury site.	(1)
Secures entire extremity.	I will now secure the entire extremity to minimize movement.	(1)
Ensures hand/foot in position of function.	I will now ensure that the hand/foot is in the position of function.	(1)
Reassess circulation, sensation, and motor function.	I will now reassess circulation, sensation, and motor function.	(1)

Examiner states: Circulation, sensation, and motor function are present and normal.

* = CRITICAL CRITERIA (Must Perform to Pass)	TOTAL POINTS (10 pts) PASSING: 80% = (8 pts)	

Start Time: _____ Date: _____

Stop Time: _____

Student's Name: _____

Evaluator's Name: _____

_____ **Grossly moves the injured extremity**

_____ **Did not immobilize the joint above and below the injury site**

_____ **Did not reassess circulation, sensation, and motor function before and after immobilization**

Mouth-to-Mask Ventilation

STEPS TO BE PERFORMED	ACTION/VERBAL RESPONSE	POINTS
*Takes or verbalizes appropriate BSI precautions.	I am taking appropriate BSI precautions.	(1)
Connects one-way valve to mask.	I am placing an appropriate one-way valve to the mask.	(1)
Opens airway (manually or with adjunct).	I will now ensure an open airway either manually or by inserting an appropriate airway.	(1)
Establishes and maintains a proper mask-to-face seal.	I will now place the mask over the patient's face and ensure a tight seal around the mask.	(1)
Ventilates the patient at the proper volume and rate (10–20 breaths per minute)	I will now ventilate the patient once every five seconds or approximately 12 times per minute. I will watch for chest rise and fall to determine proper tidal volume.	(1)

NOTE: The examiner must witness ventilations for at least 30 seconds.

* = CRITICAL CRITERIA (Must Perform to Pass)	TOTAL POINTS (5 pts) PASSING: 80% = (4 pts)	

Start Time: _____ Date: _____

Stop Time: _____

Student's Name: _____

Evaluator's Name: _____

_____ Did not take or verbalize BSI precautions

_____ Did not provide proper volume per breath

_____ Did not ventilate the patient at 10–20 breaths per minute

_____ Did not allow for complete exhalation

Oxygen Administration

STEPS TO BE PERFORMED	ACTION/VERBAL RESPONSE	POINTS
*Takes or verbalizes appropriate BSI precautions.	I am taking appropriate BSI precautions.	(1)
Assembly of Regulator to Tank		
Assembles regulator onto tank.	I will now assemble the regulator onto the tank, ensuring the presence of an "O" ring and proper alignment of pins.	(1)
Opens tank.	I will now open the tank valve by turning one full turn counter-clockwise. I will make certain that the gauge is facing away.	(1)
Checks for leaks.	I am confirming there are no leaks around the regulator.	(1)
Checks tank pressure.	I will now state the pressure in the tank as determined from the reading on the pressure gauge.	(1)
Nonrebreather Mask		
Attaches device to regulator.	I will now attach the device to the liter flow valve on the regulator.	(1)
Adjusts flow.	I will now adjust the flow to between 10 and 15 LPM.	(1)
Fills reservoir.	I will now place my finger over the valve inside the mask to allow the reservoir to fill.	(1)
Applies device to patient's face.	I will now place the mask over the patient's face and place the strap around his head.	(1)
NOTE: Examiner advises that the patient is not tolerating the mask and to place a cannula on the patient.		
Removes mask and connects cannula to regulator.	I will now remove the nonre-breather mask and connect the cannula to the liter flow valve on the regulator.	(1)
Adjusts flow.	I will now adjust the flow to between 1 and 6 LPM.	(1)
Applies cannula to patient.	I will now place the prongs into the patient's nose, wrap the tubing around his ears, and cinch the tube under the neck.	(1)

Oxygen Administration *(continued)*

| ** = CRITICAL CRITERIA*
(Must Perform to Pass) | *TOTAL POINTS (12 pts)*
PASSING: 80% = (10 pts) | |

Start Time: _____ Date: _____

Stop Time: _____

Student's Name: _____

Evaluator's Name: _____

_____ **Did not take or verbalize BSI precautions**

_____ **Did not assemble regulator without leaks**

_____ **Did not fill reservoir**

_____ **Did not adjust liter flow to appropriate rates**

Suctioning

STEPS TO BE PERFORMED	ACTION/VERBAL RESPONSE	POINTS
*Takes or verbalizes appropriate BSI precautions.	I am taking appropriate BSI precautions.	(1)
Oral Suction		
Selects appropriate suction device.	I am selecting the appropriate suction device.	(1)
Ensures that suction is working.	I am now testing to make certain that the device is working.	(1)
Inserts device into mouth.	I will now insert the device into the patient's mouth, ensuring not to stimulate a gag reflex.	(1)
Activates suction.	I will activate suction only after insertion in the mouth.	(1)
Maintains sight of tip throughout suctioning.	I will not insert the device any further than I can see.	(1)
Nasal Suction		
Selects appropriate suction device.	I am selecting the appropriate suction device.	(1)
Ensures that suction is working.	I am now testing to make certain that the device is working.	(1)
Measures device prior to insertion.	I will now measure the device from the patient's nose to the earlobe.	(1)
Inserts device.	I will now insert the device. If I meet resistance, I will try the other side.	(1)
Activates suction.	I will activate suction while rotating and pulling the device out.	(1)
*** = CRITICAL CRITERIA (Must Perform to Pass)**	**TOTAL POINTS (11 pts) PASSING: 80% = (9 pts)**	

Start Time: _____ Date: _____

Stop Time: _____

Student's Name: _____

Evaluator's Name: _____

_____ **Did not demonstrate an acceptable suction technique**

_____ **Did not select an appropriate suction device**

Patient Assessment—Trauma

DETERMINES PROPER BSI	ACTION/VERBAL RESPONSE	POINTS
*Takes or verbalizes appropriate BSI precautions. (CRITICAL CRITERIA)	I am taking appropriate BSI precautions.	(1)
SCENE SIZE-UP	*ACTION/VERBAL RESPONSE*	
*Assesses scene safety. (CRITICAL CRITERIA)	I am determining if the scene is safe.	(1)
Determines mechanism of injury.	I am determining the mechanism of injury.	(1)
Determines number of patients.	I am determining the number of patients.	(1)
Assesses need for additional help.	I am determining the need for additional help.	(1)
Takes cervical spine precautions as necessary.	I am taking/directing appropriate c-spine precautions.	(1)
INITIAL ASSESSMENT	*ACTION/VERBAL RESPONSE*	
Verbalizes general impression of patient.	I observe an approximately ___ -year-old male/female patient who appears to be in *mild/moderate/severe* distress **(determine one and state it).**	(1)
Determines responsiveness/ level of consciousness.	EYES OPEN/AWAKE: "Hello, my name is _____, and I am an EMR. May I take care of you? What is your name? How old are you?" I have determined the patient is awake and alert. (If eyes are open but patient seems confused, state it.)	(1)
	EYES CLOSED: Determine responsiveness using: Alert—Verbal— Painful—Unresponsive	(1)
Determines chief complaint.	"What seems to be the problem?"	(1)
Identifies apparent life threats.	I am identifying and managing apparent life threats.	(1)
Assesses airway/initiates appropriate airway management. (CRITICAL CRITERIA)	IF PATIENT SPEAKS TO YOU: I have determined the airway is patent. IF PATIENT DOES NOT SPEAK OR IS UNCONSCIOUS: I am assessing the airway for patency.	(1)

***Assesses breathing/initiates appropriate oxygen therapy.* (CRITICAL CRITERIA)**	I am assessing breathing for adequate rate and tidal volume, labored or easy.	(1)
	At this time, I would initiate oxygen therapy if appropriate. (Specify the device and appropriate flow rate.)	(1)
***Assesses circulation.* (CRITICAL CRITERIA)**	I am assessing for presence of a pulse at the carotid artery (unconscious patient) or radial artery (conscious patient), assessing approximate rate, strength, and regularity.	(1)
***Assesses and controls severe bleeding.* (CRITICAL CRITERIA)**	I am assessing for and controlling severe bleeding.	(1)
Assesses skin signs.	I am assessing the skin for color, temperature, and moisture.	(1)
States priority of patient for transport.	At this time, I have determined the patient is *low or high* priority *(select one).*	(1)
OBTAINS BASELINE VITAL SIGNS.	I will obtain a baseline blood pressure, pulse, and respirations. Skin signs have already been noted. Pupils will be noted in detailed physical exam.	(1)
DETERMINES APPROPRIATE ASSESSMENT PATH.	***FOCUSED HISTORY and PHYSICAL EXAM or RAPID TRAUMA ASSESSMENT***	
Performs focused history and physical exam or, if indicated, completes a rapid trauma assessment.	I am focusing my history and examination on the body part or body system relating to the chief complaint. In the case of a significant MOI, I will perform a rapid trauma assessment.	(1)
Obtains SAMPLE history if patient is conscious. *(Otherwise, moves to rapid trauma assessment.)*		
*S—Signs and symptoms (Assesses history of present injury.)	I am observing for obvious trauma and questioning the patient about his complaints.	(1)
*A—Allergies	Is the patient allergic to foods or medications?	(1)
*M—Medications	Does the patient take any medications (prescribed/ nonprescribed, vitamins, herbal remedies, birth control pills, illegal drugs)?	(1)

*P—Past pertinent medical history	Does he have history of other medical conditions, such as diabetes, high blood pressure, cardiac or breathing problems, seizures?	(1)
*L—Last oral intake	When and what did the patient last eat or drink?	(1)
*E—Event(s) leading to present complaint	What was he doing right before this happened?	(1)
*OPQRST *(as pertinent)*		(1)
DETAILED PHYSICAL EXAMINATION	**BOLD** items make up the Rapid Trauma Assessment *Italicized* items make up the Physical Examination	
Place an "X" in the box if the student performs an appropriate physical exam while stating the appropriate findings.	**D**eformities, **C**ontusions, **A**brasions, **P**unctures/ penetrations, **B**urns, **T**enderness, **L**acerations, **S**welling	
Head	**I am examining the head for DCAP-BTLS** + *scars*	(1)
Face	**I am examining the face for DCAP-BTLS** + *equality of facial muscles*	(1)
Eyes	**I am examining the eyes for size, equality, reactivity to light** + *color, pink-moist conjunctiva.*	(1)
Ears	**I am examining the ears for DCAP-BTLS, drainage.**	(1)
Nose	**I am examining the nose for DCAP-BTLS, drainage, singed nostrils, flaring.**	(1)
Mouth	**I am examining the mouth for DCAP-BTLS, loose/broken teeth, blood** + *mucus, foreign body, pink, moist soft tissue.*	(1)
Neck	**I am examining the neck for DCAP-BTLS, jugular vein distention, tracheal deviation, accessory muscle use** + *medical identification device, stoma.*	(1)
Chest	**I am examining the chest for DCAP-BTLS, chest rise, paradoxical movement.**	(1)

Patient Assessment—Trauma *(continued)*

Abdomen	**I am examining the abdomen for DCAP-BTLS, distention, rigidity, guarding.**	(1)
Pelvis	**I am examining the pelvis for DCAP-BTLS** + *incontinence of urine.*	(1)
Legs	**I am examining the legs for DCAP-BTLS; distal circulation, sensation, motor function; equal pulses bilaterally** + *capillary refill, track marks, medical identification jewelry.*	(1)
Arms	**I am examining the arms for distal DCAP-BTLS; distal circulation, sensation, motor function; equal pulses bilaterally** + *capillary refill, scars, track marks, medical identification jewelry.*	(1)
Back	**I am examining the back for DCAP-BTLS, paradoxical chest movement.**	(1)
Manages injuries and wounds appropriately (*verbalizes*).	I would perform or delegate the following interventions.	(1)
ONGOING ASSESSMENT (verbalized)		
Obtains second set of vital signs and compares to baseline.	I would record second set of vital signs and compare with the first set.	(1)
**** = CRITICAL CRITERIA (Must Perform to Pass)***	***TOTAL POINTS (42 pts) PASSING: 80% = (34 pts)***	

Point deductions for times greater than 10 minutes.

11 minutes: −1 point; 12 minutes: −3 points; 13 minutes: −6 points; 14 minutes: −10 points; 15 minutes: −15 points.

Start Time: ________ Date: ________

Stop Time: ________

Student's Name:

____

Evaluator's Name:

____

Abdominal Distention (abdomen)	Swelling of the abdomen. Can be caused by bleeding or trapped air.
Accessory Muscle Use (neck and chest)	Contraction of the muscles of the neck, chest, and abdomen. Indicative of moderate to severe respiratory distress.
Pink Moist Conjunctiva (eyes)	The area around the eye that is visible when the lower eyelid is pulled down.
Guarding (abdomen)	When a patient tightens the abdominal muscles during palpation.
Incontinence of Urine (pelvis)	Loss of bladder control.
Jugular Vein Distention (neck)	Abnormally bulging neck veins. May be indicative of heart failure.
Nasal flaring (nose)	Indicative of moderate to severe respiratory distress.
Paradoxical Movement (chest and back)	When a section of ribs in the chest or back moves opposite from the normal movement of breathing.
Patent Airway (mouth)	Open and clear airway.
Abdominal Rigidity (abdomen)	A stiff or tight abdomen when the patient is at rest. May be indicative of abdominal trauma/bleeding.
Singed Nares (nose)	Burning and/or soot around the nostrils. May be indicative of inhalation of hot air and smoke.
Stoma (neck)	Hole in anterior neck from which patient breathes.
Subcutaneous Emphysema (chest and back)	Air that has become trapped beneath the skin. Typically secondary to severe chest trauma.
Tracheal Deviation (neck)	Movement of the trachea away from the midline of the neck. Indicative of severe chest trauma.

Upper Airway Adjuncts

STEPS TO BE PERFORMED	ACTION/VERBAL RESPONSE	POINTS
*Takes or verbalizes appropriate BSI precautions.	I am taking appropriate BSI precautions.	(1)

Oropharyngeal Airway (OPA)

STEPS TO BE PERFORMED	ACTION/VERBAL RESPONSE	POINTS
Selects appropriate airway.	I am selecting the appropriate airway and the approximate size.	(1)
Measures airway.	I am now measuring the airway from the corner of the mouth to the earlobe.	(1)
Inserts airway.	I will now insert the airway in a manner that will not push the tongue back into the patient's airway.	(1)

The examiner states: The patient is gagging and becoming conscious.

STEPS TO BE PERFORMED	ACTION/VERBAL RESPONSE	POINTS
Properly removes airway.	I will now pull the airway straight out.	(1)

Nasopharyngeal Airway (NPA)

STEPS TO BE PERFORMED	ACTION/VERBAL RESPONSE	POINTS
Selects appropriate airway.	I am selecting the appropriate airway and the approximate size.	(1)
Measures airway.	I am now measuring the airway from the tip of the nose to the earlobe.	(1)
Lubricates airway.	I will now lubricate the airway prior to insertion.	(1)
Inserts airway.	I will now fully insert the airway with the bevel facing toward the septum.	(1)

The examiner states: What if you meet resistance while attempting to insert the airway?

STEPS TO BE PERFORMED	ACTION/VERBAL RESPONSE	POINTS
Attempts to insert on other side.	I will attempt to insert the airway in the other nostril.	(1)
* = CRITICAL CRITERIA (Must Perform to Pass)	TOTAL POINTS (10 pts) PASSING: 80% = (8 pts)	

Start Time: _____ Date: _____

Stop Time: _____

Student's Name:

_____

Evaluator's Name:

_____

_____ **Did not take or verbalize BSI precautions**

_____ **Did not obtain a patent airway with either airway**

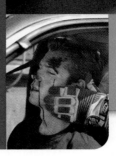

Answers to Quick Quiz Questions

CHAPTER 1

1. c	2. a	3. b	4. d	5. d
6. b	7. c	8. a	9. a	10. b

CHAPTER 2

1. b	2. c	3. d	4. b	5. d
6. d	7. b	8. c	9. a	10. b

CHAPTER 3

1. c	2. a	3. a	4. d	5. c
6. c	7. b	8. a	9. b	10. d

CHAPTER 4

1. c	2. b	3. a	4. d	5. a	6. c	7. b	8. c
9. a	10. d	11. c	12. a	13. d	14. b	15. c	16. d
17. a	18. d	19. c	20. a				

CHAPTER 5

1. a	2. c	3. b	4. b	5. a
6. b	7. d	8. a	9. b	10. d

CHAPTER 6

1. b	2. a	3. a	4. d	5. c	6. d	7. b	8. c
9. a	10. b	11. c	12. d	13. a	14. d	15. a	16. c
17. d	18. a						

CHAPTER 7

1. b	2. d	3. c	4. a	5. c	6. c	7. d	8. b
9. c	10. b						

11. Step 1—c, Step 2—u, Step 3—f, Step 4—p, Step 5—k, Step 6—g, Step 7—r, Step 8—t, Step 9—a, Step 10—v, Step 11—I, Step 12—m, Step 13—n, Step 14—o, Step 15—j, Step 16—b, Step 17—h, Step 18—s, Step 19—o, Step 20—L, Step 21—d, Step 22—e

CHAPTER 8

1. c	2. c	3. b	4. a	5. a	6. d	7. a	8. a
9. c	10. b	11. b	12. a	13. a	14. d	15. c	

CHAPTER 9

1. b   2. d   3. d   4. b   5. a   6. c   7. a   8. c
9. a   10. d   11. c   12. c   13. b   14. d   15. a   16. a
17. b   18. c   19. b   20. d

CHAPTER 10

1. b   2. c   3. b   4. a   5. d   6. c   7. d   8. a
9. a   10. d   11. b   12. a   13. c   14. c   15. a

CHAPTER 11

1. a 2. a 3. b 4. d 5. d 6. c 7. b 8. a 9. d 10. b 11. c 12. d
13. a 14. d 15. c 16. b 17. a 18. c 19. b 20. d

CHAPTER 12

1. a   2. c   3. b   4. c   5. d
6. b   7. a   8. c   9. d   10. b

CHAPTER 13

1. a   2. c   3. b   4. b   5. c   6. a   7. d   8. c
9. a   10. b   11. b   12. d   13. b   14. d   15. c

CHAPTER 14

1. b   2. a   3. b   4. d   5. b   6. c   7. a   8. d
9. d   10. d   11. c   12. b   13. b   14. c   15. a

CHAPTER 15

1. c   2. a   3. a   4. b   5. d
6. b   7. c   8. b   9. d   10. b

CHAPTER 16

1. a   2. c   3. c   4. d   5. b
6. a   7. c   8. b   9. a   10. d

Glossary

A

abandonment to leave a sick or injured patient before equal or more highly trained personnel can assume responsibility for care.

ABCs the patient's airway, breathing, and circulation as they relate to the initial assessment.

abdominal cavity the anterior body cavity that extends from the diaphragm to the pelvic cavity.

abdominal quadrants four divisions of the abdomen used to pinpoint the location of pain or injury: right upper quadrant (RUQ), left upper quadrant (LUQ), right lower quadrant (RLQ), and left lower quadrant (LLQ).

abdominal thrusts manual thrusts delivered to create pressure that can help expel an airway obstruction in an adult or child.

abortion a spontaneous miscarriage or induced loss of the embryo or fetus.

abrasion (ab-RAY-zhun) the simplest form of open wound that damages the skin surface but does not break all layers of skin; scratches and scrapes.

absorption taking into the body through the skin and body tissues.

accessory muscles muscles of the neck, chest, and abdomen that can assist during respiratory difficulty.

ACLS advanced cardiac life support.

acute rapid onset; severe.

acute abdomen the sudden onset of severe abdominal pain; abdominal pain related to one of many medical conditions or a specific injury to the abdomen. Also called *acute abdominal distress*.

adequate breathing breathing that is sufficient to support life, characterized by a normal respiratory rate, depth, and effort.

advanced life support (ALS) prehospital emergency care that involves the use of intravenous fluids, drug infusions, cardiac monitoring, defibrillation, intubation, and other advanced procedures.

AED automated external defibrillation.

afterbirth the tissues that deliver after the birth of the baby; consists of placenta, umbilical cord, tissues from the amniotic sac, and some tissues from the lining of the uterus.

AIDS acquired immune deficiency syndrome.

altered mental status (AMS) a medical condition characterized by a decrease in the patient's alertness and responsiveness to his surroundings. Also called *altered level of responsiveness*.

ALS advanced life support.

amniotic (am-ne-OT-ik) sac the fluid-filled sac that surrounds the developing embryo and fetus.

amputation injury that involves the cutting or tearing off of a limb or one of its parts.

anaphylactic (AN-ah-fi-LAK-tik) shock a severe allergic reaction in which a person goes into shock. Also called *allergy shock*.

anatomical (AN-ah-TOM-i-kal) position the standard reference position for the body in the study of anatomy. The body is standing erect, facing the observer. The arms are down at the sides, and the palms of the hands are forward.

anatomy the study of body structure.

angina pectoris (an-JI-nah PEK-to-ris) chest pain caused by an insufficient blood supply to the heart muscle.

anterior the front of the body or body part.

apnea (ap-ne-ah) temporary cessation of breathing.

appendicular (ap-en-DIK-u-ler) skeleton bones and joints that form the upper and lower extremities.

artery any blood vessel that carries blood away from the heart.

artificial ventilation process of forcing air or oxygen into the lungs. Also called *pulmonary resuscitation* or *rescue breathing*.

asystole (ah-SIS-to-le) no electrical activity in the heart; cardiac arrest. Also called *flatline*.

auscultation (os-kul-TAY-shun) listening to sounds that occur within the body.

automated external defibrillator (AED) an electrical device that can detect certain abnormal heart rhythms and deliver a shock through the patient's chest. This shock may allow the heart to resume a normal pattern of beating. See *defibrillation*.

AVPU scale a memory aid for the classifications of mental status, or levels of responsiveness. The letters stand for alert, verbal, painful, and unresponsive.

avulsion (ah-VUL-shun) a soft-tissue injury in which flaps of skin are torn loose or torn off.

axial (AK-si-al) skeleton bones and joints that form the center or upright axis of the body. It includes the skull, spine, breastbone, and ribs.

B

bag-valve mask (BVM) an aid for pulmonary resuscitation; made up of a face mask, self-refilling bag, and valves that control the one-way flow of air.

bandage any material that is used to hold a dressing in place.

baseline vital signs the first determination of vital signs; used to compare with all further readings of vital signs in order to identify trends.

behavioral emergency a situation in which an individual exhibits abnormal behavior that is unacceptable or intolerable to the patient, family, or community.

biological death occurs approximately four to six minutes after onset of clinical death and results where there is an excessive amount of brain cell death.

BLS basic life support.

blunt trauma an injury caused by an object that was not sharp enough to penetrate the skin.

body mechanics the proper use of the body to facilitate lifting and moving and to prevent injury.

body substance isolation (BSI) precautions practice that minimizes contact with a patient's blood and body fluids.

BP-DOC a memory aid used to recall what to look for in a physical exam. The letters stand for bleeding, pain, deformities, open wounds, and crepitus.

brachial (BRAY-ke-al) pressure point a location in the upper arm, where the brachial artery is close to the skin surface and lies over a bone. It can be used to help control serious external bleeding from the upper limb.

brachial pulse (BRAY-ke-al) the pulse that can be felt in the medial side of the upper arm between the elbow and shoulder.

breech birth a birth in which the buttocks or both feet deliver first.

bronchitis (bronk-I-tus) inflammation of the bronchi; a form of chronic obstructive pulmonary disease (COPD).

bruise a simple closed wound in which blood leaks between soft tissues, causing a discoloration. Also called *contusion*.

BSI body substance isolation.

bulky dressing a thick dressing or a buildup of thin dressings used to help control profuse bleeding, stabilize impaled objects, or cover large open wounds.

burnout an extreme emotional state characterized by emotional exhaustion, a diminished sense of personal accomplishment, and cynicism.

C

capillaries the microscopic blood vessels that connect arteries to veins; where exchange takes place between the bloodstream and the body tissues.

capillary refill the return (refill) of blood into the capillaries after it has been forced out by fingertip pressure. Normal refill time is two seconds or less.

cardiac arrest when the heart stops beating. Also, the ineffective circulation caused by erratic muscle activity in the lower chambers of the heart (ventricular fibrillation).

cardiac compromise a term used to describe specific signs and symptoms that indicate some type of emergency relating to the heart.

cardiopulmonary resuscitation (KAR-de-o-PUL-mo-ner-e re-SUS-ci-TA-shun) (CPR) combined compression and breathing techniques that maintain circulation and breathing.

carotid (kah-ROT-id) pulse the pulse that can be felt on either side of the neck.

central nervous system (CNS) the brain and spinal cord.

cephalic (sef-FAL-ik) position at the top of the supine patient's head.

cerebrospinal (ser-e-bro-SPI-nal) fluid (CSF) the clear fluid that surrounds the brain and spinal cord.

cervical (SER-vi-kal) spine the neck bones.

chain of survival the idea that the survival of the patient in cardiac arrest depends on the linkage of early access, early CPR, early defibrillation, and early advanced life support.

chest compressions putting pressure on the chest to artificially circulate blood to the brain, lungs, and the rest of the patient's body.

chest thrusts manual thrusts delivered to create pressure that can help expel an airway obstruction in an infant or in pregnant or obese patients.

CHF congestive heart failure.

chronic long and drawn out; recurring.

chief complaint the reason EMS was called in the patient's own words.

chronic obstructive pulmonary disease (COPD) a variety of lung problems related to diseases of the airway passages or exchange levels, including emphysema complicated by chronic bronchitis.

clinical death the moment when breathing and heart actions stop.

closed injury an injury with no associated opening of the skin.

CNS central nervous system.

competence the state of being competent, or properly or sufficiently qualified or capable of making appropriate decisions about one's own health or condition.

complex access access gained to a vehicle or building with the use of specialized equipment.

concussion (kon-KUSH-un) injury to the brain that results from a blow or impact from an object but does not cause permanent neurological damage.

confidentiality refers to the treatment of information that an individual has disclosed in a relationship of trust and with the expectation that it will not be divulged to others.

consent See *expressed consent* and *implied consent*.

contraction time the period of time that a contraction of the womb lasts during labor. It is measured from the start of the uterus contracting until it relaxes.

contusion (kon-TU-zhun) bruising; in the case of the brain, bruising caused by a force of a blow great enough to rupture blood vessels on the surface or deep within the brain.

convulsions uncontrolled muscular contractions.

COPD chronic obstructive pulmonary disease.

CPR cardiopulmonary resuscitation.

cranium (KRAY-ne-um) the bones that form the forehead and the floor, back, top, and upper sides of the skull.

cravat a triangular bandage that is folded to a width of three or four inches and used to tie soft or rigid splints in place.

crepitus (KREP-i-tus) a grating noise or the sensation felt when broken bone ends rub together.

critical incident any situation that causes a rescuer to experience unusually strong emotions that interfere with the ability to function either during the incident or after; a highly stressful incident.

critical incident stress debriefing (CISD) a process in which teams of professional and peer counselors provide emotional and psychological support to EMS personnel who are or have been involved in a critical (highly stressful) incident.

critical incident stress management (CISM) an in-depth, broad plan designed to help rescue personnel cope with the stress resulting from a highly stressful incident.

croup (KROOP) acute respiratory condition found in infants and children, which is characterized by a barking type of cough or stridor.

crowning the bulging out of the vagina caused by exposure of the baby's head or other presenting part during contractions.

crush injury a soft-tissue injury produced by crushing forces. Soft tissues and internal organs are crushed, and hard tissues are usually damaged.

CSF cerebrospinal fluid.

CVA cerebrovascular accident. Also called *brain attack* or *stroke*.

cyanotic (sy-ah-OT-ik) bluish discoloration of the skin and mucous membranes; a sign that body tissues are not receiving enough oxygen. The condition is called *cyanosis (sy-ah-NO-sis)*.

D

DCAP-BTLS a memory aid used to recall what to look for in a physical exam. The letters stand for deformities, contusions, abrasions, punctures and penetrations, burns, tenderness, lacerations, and swelling.

defibrillation the application of an electric shock to a patient's heart in an attempt to convert a lethal rhythm into a normal one.

deformed injury an injury that causes a bone or joint to take on an unnatural shape or bend. Also called *angulated injury*.

dehydration excessive loss of body water (fluids).

delirium tremens (DTs) temporary state of mental confusion characterized by sweating, anxiety, trembling, and hallucinations.

detailed physical exam a complete head-to-toe exam.

diabetes usually refers to diabetes mellitus, a disease that prevents individuals from producing enough insulin or from using insulin effectively.

diaphoresis perspiration, especially when it is heavy and caused by a medical condition.

diaphragm (DI-uh-fram) the muscular structure that divides the chest cavity from the abdominal cavity.

dilate enlarge; expand in diameter.

direct force a force that causes injury at the site of impact.

direct pressure the quickest, most effective way to control most forms of external bleeding. Pressure is applied directly over the wound site.

dislocation the pulling or pushing of a bone end partially or completely free of a joint.

distal farther away from the torso.

dorsalis pedis (dor-SAL-is PEED-is) pulse the pulse located lateral to the large tendon of the big toe.

downers depressants that affect the central nervous system to relax the user.

dressing any material used to cover a wound; helps control bleeding and reduce contamination.

DTs delirium tremens.

duty to act a legal requirement that Emergency Medical Responders while on duty must provide care according to their department's standard operating procedures.

dyspnea difficulty breathing.

dysrhythmias (dis-RITH-mee-uhs) a disturbance in heart rate or rhythm.

E

elderly a person age 65 or older.

emergency care the prehospital assessment and basic care for the sick or injured patient. The physical and emotional needs of the patient are considered and attended to during care.

Emergency Medical Dispatcher (EMD) a member of the EMS system who provide pre-arrival instructions to callers, thereby helping to initiate life-saving care before EMS personnel arrive.

Emergency Medical Responder a member of the EMS system who has been trained to render first aid care for a patient and help EMTs at the emergency scene.

emergency medical services (EMS) system the chain of human resources and services linked together to provide continuous emergency care from the onset of care at the prehospital scene, during transport, and on arrival at the medical facility.

Emergency Medical Technician (EMT) a member of the EMS system whose training emphasizes assessment, care, and transportation of the ill or injured patient. Depending on the level of training, emergency care may include starting IV (intravenous) lines, inserting advanced airways, and administering some medications.

emergency move a patient move that is carried out quickly when the scene is hazardous, care of the patient requires immediate repositioning, or you must reach another patient who needs life-saving care.

emphysema (emf-a-ZEE-muh) disease that causes a loss of elasticity in the lungs; a form of chronic obstructive pulmonary disease (COPD).

epiglottis (EP-i-GLOT-is) a flap of cartilage and other tissues located above the larynx. It helps close off the airway when a person swallows.

epiglottitis (ep-i-glot-I-tis) swelling of the epiglottis that may be caused by a bacterial infection, which can obstruct the airway; potentially life threatening.

evisceration (e-VIS-er-a-shun) protrusion of the intestines through the abdominal wall.

expiration refers to the passive process of breathing out, or exhaling.

expressed consent consent to emergency care that is given to an Emergency Medical Responder by a competent adult who has made an informed decision. Also referred to as *informed consent*.

F

femoral (FEM-o-ral) pressure point a location at the anterior pelvis in the thigh, which can be used to help control serious external bleeding from the lower limb.

fetus (FE-tus) the developing unborn baby. The fertilized egg is an embryo until the eighth week after fertilization, when it becomes a fetus.

fibrillation a disorganized electrical activity within the heart that renders the heart incapable of pumping blood.

flail chest the condition that results when there are two or more ribs fractured in two or more places, or the breastbone separates from the chest and produces a loose segment of the chest wall. This segment will move in the opposite direction of the chest during breathing.

focused history and physical exam part of patient assessment that includes the patient history, a physical examination, and vital signs.

focused trauma assessment an examination of the area the patient tells you is injured.

fontanel an area on the infant's skull where the bones have not yet fused. Also called *soft spot*.

fracture any break, crack, chip, split, or splintering of a bone.

frostbite localized cold injury in which the skin is frozen.

full-thickness burn a burn involving all layers of skin. Muscle layers below the skin and bones may also be damaged. Also called *third-degree burn*.

G

gag reflex a retching action, hacking, or vomiting that is induced when something touches a certain level of the patient's throat.

gastric distention inflation of the stomach.

generalized seizure a seizure characterized by unresponsiveness and full body convulsions.

genitalia (jen-i-TA-le-ah) the external reproductive organs.

glucose (GLU-kohs) a simple sugar that is the primary source of energy for the body's tissues.

Good Samaritan laws state laws designed to protect care providers who deliver care in good faith, to the level of their training, and without compensation.

guarding the protection of an area of injury or pain by the patient; the spasming of muscles to minimize movement that might cause pain.

H

hallucinogens mind-altering drugs that act on the central nervous system to excite the user or to distort perception of surroundings.

hazardous materials incident the release of a harmful substance into the environment. Also called a *hazmat incident.*

HBV hepatitis B virus.

head-tilt, chin-lift maneuver technique used to open the airway of a patient with no suspected neck or spine injury.

heat cramps common term for muscle cramps in the lower limbs and abdomen associated with the loss of fluids and salts while active in a hot environment.

heat exhaustion prolonged exposure to heat, which creates moist, pale skin that may feel normal or cool to the touch.

heat stroke prolonged exposure to heat, which creates dry or moist skin that may feel warm or hot to the touch.

HEPA respirator high-efficiency particulate air respirator.

hyperglycemia a condition in which the sugar (glucose) level increases in the blood and decreases in the tissue cells. The problem can be serious enough to produce a coma.

hyperthermia an increase in body core temperature above its normal temperature.

hyperventilation uncontrolled, rapid, deep breathing that is usually self-correcting; may occur by itself or as a sign of a more serious problem.

hypoglycemia too little sugar in the blood.

hypoperfusion the lack of adequate perfusion; shock.

hypothermia (HI-po-THURM-e-ah) a general cooling of the body. Also called *generalized cold emergency.*

hypoxic (hi-POX-ik) refers to an insufficient level of oxygen in the blood and tissues. The condition is called *hypoxia.*

I

implied consent a legal position that assumes an unresponsive or incompetent adult patient would consent to receiving emergency care if he could. This form of consent may apply to other types of patients (for example, the mentally ill).

inadequate breathing breathing that is not sufficient to support life.

incident management system (IMS) a model tool for the command, control, and coordination of resources at the scene of a large-scale emergency involving multiple agencies. Also known as *incident command system (ICS).*

incision a laceration with smooth edges, usually caused by very sharp objects such as a razor blade, knife, or broken glass.

incontinence (in-CON-ti-nents) loss of bladder and/or bowel control.

indirect force a force that is transmitted along bones, causing injury away from the point of impact.

inferior away from the head (for example, the lips are inferior to the nose).

informed consent *See expressed consent.*

ingestion taking into the body by swallowing.

inhalation taking into the body by breathing in.

injection taking into the body by puncturing the skin.

inspiration refers to the process of breathing in, or inhaling.

insulin (IN-su-lin) a hormone produced in the pancreas that is needed to move sugar (glucose) from the blood into the cells.

insulin shock severe hypoglycemia. A form of shock usually caused by too high a level of insulin in the blood, producing a sudden drop in blood sugar.

interval time the period of time from the start of one contraction until the beginning of the next.

interventions actions taken to correct or stabilize a patient's illness or injury.

IV intravenous.

J

jaw-thrust maneuver technique used to open the airway of a trauma patient with possible neck or spine injury.

jugular vein distention (JVD) an abnormal bulging of the veins of the neck indicating possible injury to the chest or heart.

JumpSTART Pediatric MCI Triage system a specialized pediatric triage system designed for patients from one to eight years of age.

L

L liter.

laceration a soft-tissue injury in which all layers of skin are opened and the tissues immediately below the skin are damaged.

laryngectomy (lar-in-JEK-to-me) the total or partial removal of the larynx.

larynx (LAR-inks) the section of the airway between the throat and the trachea. Also called *voice box*.

lateral to the side, away from the midline of the body.

lateral position at the supine patient's side.

lateral recumbent position the patient is lying on his side.

LPM liters per minute.

lucid (LOO-sid) clear perception or understanding.

M

mandible (MAN-di-bl) the lower jaw bone.

manual stabilization restricting the movement of an injured person or body part with your hands.

manual traction process of drawing or pulling; a stabilizing procedure that precedes the application of a splint.

MCI multiple-casualty incident. Also called *mass-casualty incident*.

mechanism of injury (MOI) the force or forces that may have caused injury.

meconium staining amniotic fluid that is green or brownish-yellow from fetal fecal contamination, which occurs when the fetus is stressed.

medial toward the midline of the body.

Medical Director a physician who assumes the ultimate responsibility for medical oversight of the patient care aspects of the EMS system.

medical patient one who has or describes symptoms of an illness; a patient with no injuries.

MI myocardial infarction. Also called *heart attack*.

midline an imaginary vertical line used to divide the body into right and left halves.

miscarriage the natural loss of the embryo or fetus before the twenty-eighth week of pregnancy. Also called a *spontaneous abortion*.

mobility (mo-BIL-i-tee) ability to move.

MOI mechanism of injury.

motor function the ability to move without pain or restriction.

multiple-casualty incident (MCI) any incident that results in enough patients to overwhelm immediately available resources. Also known as a *mass-casualty incident*.

musculoskeletal system all the muscles, bones, joints, and related structures such as tendons and ligaments that enable the body and its parts to move and function.

myocardial infarction (MI) a condition in which the heart has suffered tissue damage due to a lack of adequate circulation to the heart muscle.

N

narcotics a class of drugs for the relief of pain. Illicit use is to provide an intense state of relaxation.

nasopharyngeal (na-zo-fah-RIN-je-al) airway (NPA) a flexible tube that is lubricated and then inserted into a patient's nose to the level of the nasopharynx (back of the throat) to provide an open airway. Also called *nasal* airway.

National Incident Management System (NIMS) a system that uses a unified approach to incident management and standard command and management structures, with an emphasis on preparedness, mutual aid, and resource management.

nature of illness (NOI) what is medically wrong with the patient; a complaint not related to an injury.

neglect failure of the parents or caregivers to provide for the child's basic physical, social, emotional, medical, and/or medical needs.

negligence a failure to provide the expected standard of care.

NOI nature of illness.

nonemergency move the preferred choice when the situation is not urgent, the patient is stable, and you have adequate time and personnel for a move.

NPA nasopharngeal airway. Also called *nasal airway*.

O

occlusive dressing a dressing used to create an airtight seal or to close an open wound of a body cavity.

off-line (indirect) medical direction standing orders and protocols developed by an EMS system that authorize rescuers to perform particular skills in certain situations without actually speaking to the Medical Director.

on-line (direct) medical direction orders to perform a skill or administer care from the on-duty physician, given to the rescuer in person, by radio, or by phone.

ongoing assessment the last step in patient assessment, which is used to detect changes in a patient's condition; includes repeating initial assessment, reassessing and recording vital signs, and checking interventions.

OPA oropharyngeal airway. Also called *oral airway*.

open injury an injury with an associated opening of the skin.

OPQRST a memory device used for assessing the responsive medical patient. It stands for *onset, provocation, quality, region/radiate, severity, and time.*

oropharyngeal (or-o-fah-RIN-je-al) airway (OPA) a curved breathing tube inserted into the patient's mouth. It will hold the base of the tongue forward. Also called *oral airway.*

P

palpation feeling or sensing by touch.

Paramedic a member of the EMS system whose training includes advanced life support care, such as inserting endotracheal (ET) tubes and starting IV lines. Paramedics also administer medications, interpret electrocardiograms, monitor cardiac rhythms, and perform cardiac defibrillation.

partial complex seizure a seizure characterized by a temporary loss of concentration with no dramatic body movements.

partial-thickness burn a burn in which the outer layer of skin is burned through and the second layer (dermis) is damaged. Also called *second-degree burn.*

PASG pneumatic antishock garment.

pathogens organisms such as viruses and bacteria that cause infection and disease.

patient assessment the gathering of information to determine a possible illness or injury. It includes interviews and physical examinations.

patient history information relating to a patient's current complaint or condition, as well as information about past medical problems that could be related.

pediatric patients refers to infants and children. For the purposes of CPR, patients from birth to one year of age are considered infants. Patients from one year old to the onset of puberty are considered children.

pelvic cavity the anterior body cavity surrounded by the bones of the pelvis.

perfusion the adequate supply of well oxygenated blood to body tissues.

personal protective equipment (PPE) equipment such as gloves, mask, eyewear, gown, turnout gear, and helmet, which protect rescuers from infection and/or from exposure to hazardous materials and the dangers of rescue operations.

pharynx (FAR-inks) the throat.

physical abuse inflicting any type of physical injury or performing any physical act that harms or disfigures the child.

placenta (plah-SEN-tah) an organ of pregnancy that is composed of maternal and fetal tissues by which exchange between the circulatory systems of the mother and fetus can take place without the mixing of their blood.

plasma (PLAZ-mah) the fluid portion of the blood.

pocket face mask a device used to help provide ventilations. It has a chimney with a one-way valve and HEPA filter. Some have an inlet for supplemental oxygen.

poison any substance that can be harmful to the body.

position of function the natural position of the body part, specifically the hand or foot.

posterior the back of the body or body part.

posterior tibial (TIB-e-al) pulse the pulse felt behind the medial ankle.

PPE personal protective equipment.

premature baby any baby that is born with a birth weight of less than 5.5 pounds or before the thirth-seventh week (prior to the ninth month) of pregnancy.

prolapsed cord a potential birth complication in which the umbilical cord presents through the vaginal opening before the baby's head.

prone the patient is lying face down.

protocols written guidelines that direct the care that EMS personnel provide for patients.

proximal closer to the torso.

psychological abuse persistent emotional or verbal abuse that affects a child's emotional development, self-esteem, and emotional well-being.

pulmonary resuscitation (PUL-mo-ner-e re-SUS-si-TAY-shun) a technique by which breaths are provided to a patient in an attempt to artificially maintain normal lung function. Also called *rescue breathing* or *artificial ventilation.*

puncture an open wound that tears through the skin and damages tissues in a straight line.

R

radial pulse the pulse that can be felt on the thumb side of the wrist.

rapid physical exam a quick head-to-toe assessment of the most critical patients.

rapid trauma assessment a quick, safe head-to-toe exam of the trauma patient.

recovery position the position in which a patient with no suspected spine injuries may be placed, usually on the left side.

referred pain pain spread out over one or more areas.

respiration the act of breathing; the exchange of oxygen and carbon dioxide that takes place in the lungs.

rigid splint a stiff device made of a material with little flexibility (such as metal, plastic, or wood) that is long enough to immobilize an extremity and the joints above and below the injury site.

roller bandage a long strip of soft, self-adherent gauze, a few inches wide and some yards long; used to secure dressings in place.

rule of nines a system used for estimating the amount of skin surface that is burned. The body is divided into 12 regions. For adults, each of 11 regions equals 9% of the body surface, and the genital section is classified as 1%.

S

safety zone an area around the incident that is thought to be safe and free of hazards.

SAMPLE history a system of information gathering that allows the rescuer to ask questions about past or present medical or injury problems. Letters stand for signs/symptoms, allergies, medications, pertinent past medical history, last oral intake, and event leading to the illness of injury.

scene size-up an overview of the scene to identify any obvious or potential hazards; consists of taking BSI precautions, determining the safety of the scene, identifying the mechanism of injury or nature of illness, determining the number of patients, and identifying additional resources.

scope of practice the care that an Emergency Medical Responder, an EMT, or Paramedic is allowed and supposed to provide according to local, state, or regional regulations or statutes. Also called *scope of care*.

seizure irregular electrical activity in the brain that can cause a sudden change in behavior or movement.

sensation the ability of the skin to have feeling.

sexual abuse physical sexual contact with or exposure to children and sexual exploitation of children by exposing, displaying, or photographing them for sexual purposes or with sexual intent.

shock the reaction of the body to the failure of the circulatory system to provide enough blood to the vital organs. Also referred to as *hypoperfusion*.

SIDS sudden infant death syndrome.

signs objective indications of illness or injury that can be seen, heard, felt, and smelled by another person.

simple access access gained to a vehicle or building without the use of equipment.

skeletal system all the bones and joints of the body.

sling a large triangular bandage or other cloth device that is applied as a soft splint to immobilize possible injuries to the shoulder girdle and upper extremity.

soft splint a device, such as a sling and swathe or a pillow secured with cravats, that can be applied to immobilize a painful extremity.

soft tissues the tissues of the body that make up the skin, muscles, nerves, blood vessels, fat, and the cells that line and cover organs and glands.

SOPs standard operating procedures.

splinting applying a device that will immobilize an injured extremity.

sprain a partial or complete tearing of a ligament.

standard of care the care that should be provided for any level of training based on local laws, administrative orders, and guidelines and protocols established by the local EMS system.

standard operating procedures (SOPs) written directions that define how one should act given specific situations.

standing orders specific instructions developed by the Medical Director, which authorize the Emergency Medical Responder, EMT, or Paramedic to provide care for specific medical conditions or injuries.

START triage system a system that uses respirations, perfusion, and mental status assessments to categorize patients into one of four treatment categories; letters stand for Simple Triage and Rapid Treatment.

stoma (STO-mah) any permanent opening that has been surgically made; the opening in the neck of a neck breather.

strain the overstretching or tearing of a muscle.

stress an emotionally disruptive or upsetting condition that occurs in response to adverse external influences.

stressor the part of a situation or the situation that causes stress.

stroke the blocking or bursting of a vessel that supplies blood to the brain. A portion of the brain is damaged or destroyed by this event. Also known as *cerebrovascular accident (CVA)* or "brain attack."

sucking chest would an open chest wound in which air is sucked through the wound opening and into the chest cavity each time the patient breathes.

superficial burn a burn involving only the outer layer of skin (epidermis). Also called *first-degree burn*.

superior toward the head (for example, the chest is superior to the abdomen).

supine the patient is lying face up.

swathe a large cravat, usually made of cloth, used to secure a sling or rigid splint and sling to the body.

symptoms subjective indications of illness or injury that cannot be observed by another person but are felt and reported by the patient.

syncope (SIN-ko-pe) collapse or fainting.

T

TB tuberculosis.

thoracic (tho-RAS-ik) cavity the anterior body cavity that is above (superior to) the diaphragm. Also called *chest cavity*.

tidal volume the amount of air being moved in and out of the lungs with each breath.

tourniquet a wide, flat band or belt used to constrict blood vessels to help stop the flow of blood.

toxic (TOK-sik) poisonous.

trachea (TRAY-ke-ah) the windpipe.

tracheal deviation a shifting of the trachea to either side of the midline of the neck caused by the buildup of pressure inside the chest.

trauma patient one who has a physical injury caused by an external force.

trending monitoring the patient's signs and symptoms and documenting any changes, both good and bad.

triage a method of sorting patients for care and transport based on the severity of their injuries or illnesses.

triangular bandage a piece of triangular cloth material about 50 to 60 inches long at its base and 36 to 40 inches long on each side. It can be folded and used as a sling, a swathe, or a cravat.

tripod position sitting forward, leaning on hands or elbows.

twisting force a force that occurs when one part of an extremity remains in place while the rest moves or twists.

U

umbilical (um-BIL-i-kal) cord the structure that connects the fetus to the placenta. It contains fetal blood vessels.

unresponsive no reaction to verbal or painful stimuli.

uppers stimulants that affect the central nervous system to excite the user.

uterus (U-ter-us) the womb. The muscular structure in which the fetus develops.

V

vagina (vah-JI-nah) the birth canal.

vein any blood vessel that returns blood to the heart.

ventilation the supplying of air to the lungs. See *pulmonary resuscitation*.

ventricular fibrillation (ven-TRIK-u-ler fib-ri-LAY-shun) (VF) uncoordinated electrical activity, causing rapid ineffective contractions of the lower heart chambers and the absence of a pulse. See *defibrillation*.

ventricular tachycardia (ven-TRIK-u-ler tak-e-KAR-de-ah) the abnormally rapid contraction of the heart's lower chambers, resulting in very poor circulation. Also called *V-tach*.

vital signs objective signs that include assessment of the patient's pulse, respirations, skin, blood pressure, and pupils.

Index

A

Abandonment, 29–32, 35
Abdominal cavity, 65
Abdominal injuries, 353–354, 363
Abdominal pain, 272–274
Abdominal quadrants, 65
Abdominal thrusts, 131–133
Abnormal delivery, 471–474. *See also* Childbirth
  breech birth, 471–472
  limb presentation, 472
  meconium staining, 471
  multiple births, 473
  premature births, 473–474
  prolapsed cord, 473
  stillborn deliveries, 474
Abortion, 469, 470
Abrasions, 332–333
Absorbed poisons, 274, 279–280. *See also* Poisons
Abuse
  alcohol, 293–294, 299
  drug, 294–297, 299
  physical, 519, 521–522
  sexual, 520–521
  stress and, 42
Acquired immune deficiency syndrome (AIDS), 47, 49, 50
Activated charcoal, 589–591. *See also* Medications
Acute abdomen, 272–273, 298
Acute CHF, 254
Adequate breathing, 119, 259. *See also* Breathing
Advanced directives, 27
Advanced Emergency Medical Technicians (AEMTs), 7
Advanced life support (ALS)
  defined, 207
  early, 241
  in priority dispatching, 176
Afterbirth, 452
Aged. *See* Geriatric patients
Age-related physical changes
  cardiovascular system, 437
  integumentary system (skin), 440
  musculoskeletal system, 439
  nervous system, 438–439
  respiratory system, 437
Air embolism, 617
Air medical operations, 600–604
  crew configurations, 600

fixed-wing resources (airplanes), 601, 602
  Flight Communication Specialist and, 603
  instrument flight rules (IFR), 602
  interfacility transport (IFT), 600, 601
  landing zone selection, 603–604
  requesting resources, 602
  resources, 600–602
  rotor-wing resources (helicopters), 600–601
  safety around aircraft, 604
  visual flight rules (VFR), 602
Air splints. *See* Inflatable splints
Airborne pathogens, 49–52
Airway assessment, 172–173
Airway, breathing, and circulation (ABCs), 84, 168, 241
Airway management, 112–152
  breathing, 115–119
  obstructions, 130–137
  opening, 120–121, 223–224
  pediatric patients, 496
  pulmonary resuscitation, 119–130
  resuscitation aids, 138–146
  suction systems, 146–148
Airway obstructions, 130–137
  allergic reaction, 131
  causes, 130–131
  complete, 131
  epiglottis, 130
  finger sweeps, 137
  foreign objects, 130
  infection, 131
  obese patients, 135–137
  partial, 131
  pediatric patients, 501
  pregnant patients, 135–137
  tissue damage, 130–131
  tongue, 130
Airways, artificial
  nasopharyngeal (NPA), 138, 141–142
  oropharyngeal (OPA), 138–141
Alcohol abuse, 293–294, 299
Allergic reactions, in airway obstructions, 131
Altered mental status (AMS), 263–274, 298
  defined, 263
  diabetes, 268–271
  elderly patients, 436–437
  pediatric patients, 504
  seizures, 267–268
  stroke, 264–267

Alzheimer's disease, 442
Ambulance Volante, 5
Amniotic sac, 452
Amputations, 334, 338–339
Anaphylactic shock, 282, 298, 326
Anatomical position, 60
Anatomy, 59
Aneurysm, 441
Angina pectoris, 252–254, 595–597
Angulated injuries. *See* Deformed injuries
Ankle injuries, 404, 405
Anterior, 61
Anterior hip dislocation, 400
Apical pulse, 465
Apnea, 501
Appendicular skeleton, 371–381
Arteries, 306, 307. *See also* Blood vessels
Aspirin, 597
Assessment. *See also* Initial assessment; Ongoing assessment; Patient assessment
  airway, 172–173
  behavioral emergency, 290, 291–292
  breathing, 119, 172–174, 188, 224, 328
  cardiac compromise and, 257
  chest pain and, 257
  child and, 175–176, 486–488, 495–499
  childbirth and, 454–455, 469
  circulation, 174–175, 210
  documentation and, 163
  extremity injury and, 391
  focused, 177, 178, 196
  heat emergency and, 283
  internal bleeding and, 321–324
  medical patient and, 157–158
  mental status, 169, 170–172, 210
  newborn and, 462
  poison and, 276–281
  pupils, 191
Asthma signs and symptoms, 502
Asystole, 233
Auscultation method, 571–574. *See also* Blood pressure
Autoinjectors, 597, 598
Automated external defibrillators (AEDs), 232–240
  assessment and, 240
  attaching to patient, 236–237
  basic warnings, 235–236
  defined, 207, 232
  fully automated, 232, 237–238